50% OFF
Online FNP Prep Course!

By Mometrix

Dear Customer,

We consider it an honor and a privilege that you chose our FNP Study Guide. As a way of showing our appreciation and to help us better serve you, we are offering **50% off our online FNP Prep Course**. Many FNP courses cost hundreds of dollars and don't deliver enough value. With our course, you get access to the best FNP prep material, and **you only pay half price**.

We have structured our online course to perfectly complement your printed study guide. The FNP Prep Course contains **in-depth lessons** that cover all the most important topics, **90+ video reviews** that explain difficult concepts, over **600 practice questions** to ensure you feel prepared, and more than **750 digital flashcards**, so you can study while you're on the go.

Online FNP Prep Course

Topics Covered:
- Assessment
    - Pediatric Illness and Injury Prevention
    - Functional Status and Rehabilitation
- Diagnosis
    - Cardiovascular Pathophysiology
    - Fever and Fibromyalgia
- Planning
    - Pediatric Response to Illness
    - Principles of Pharmacology
- Implementation
    - Infection Control
    - Therapeutic Relationships
- Evaluation
    - Ethical Behavior
    - Evidence-Based Practice

Course Features:
- FNP Study Guide
    - Get content that complements our best-selling study guide.
- Full-Length Practice Tests
    - With over 600 practice questions, you can test yourself again and again.
- Mobile Friendly
    - If you need to study on the go, the course is easily accessible from your mobile device.
- FNP Flashcards
    - Our course includes a flashcard mode consisting of over 750 content cards to help you study.

To receive this discount, visit our website at mometrix.com/university/fnp or simply scan this QR code with your smartphone. At the checkout page, enter the discount code: **fnp50off**

If you have any questions or concerns, please contact us at support@mometrix.com

Mometrix
TEST PREPARATION

ACCESS YOUR ONLINE RESOURCES

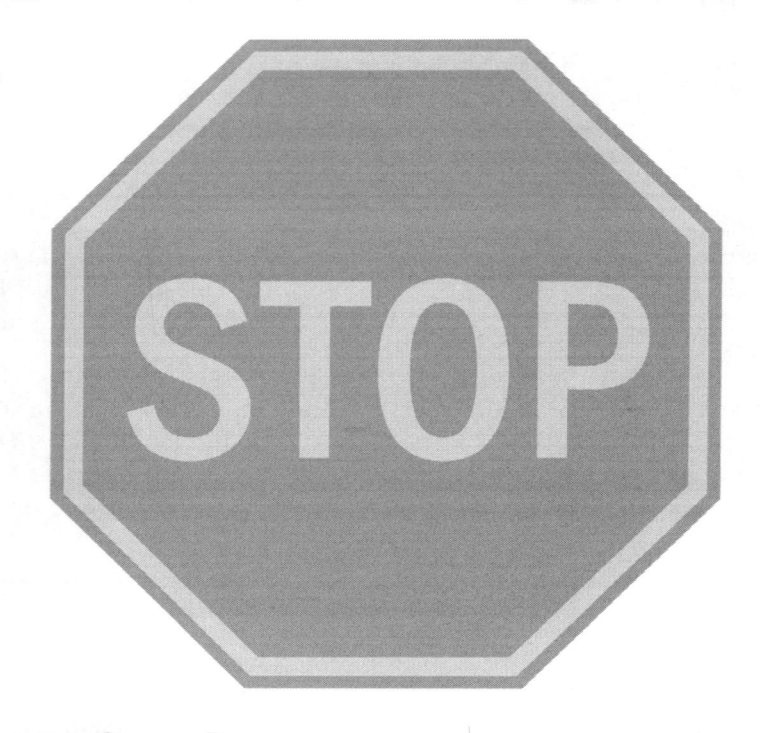

DON'T MISS OUT ON THE ONLINE RESOURCES INCLUDED WITH YOUR PURCHASE!

Your purchase of this product unlocks access to our Online Resources page. Elevate your study experience with our **interactive practice test interface**, along with all of the additional resources that we couldn't include in this book.

Flip to the Online Resources section at the end of this book to find the link and a QR code to get started!

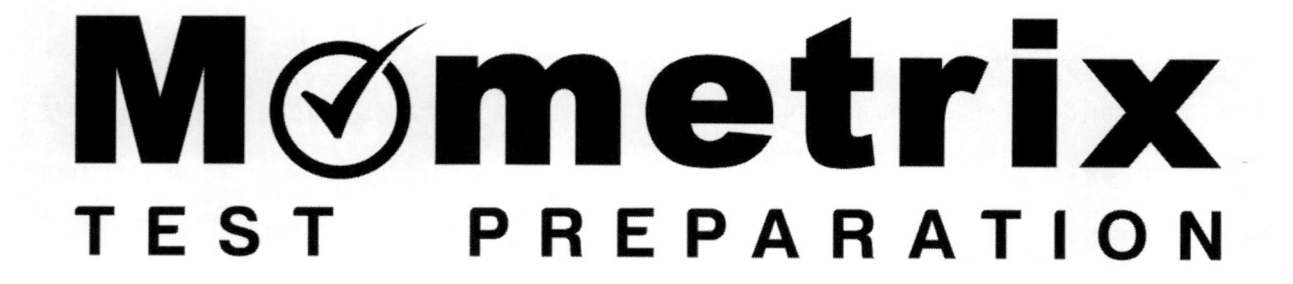

Mometrix
TEST PREPARATION

Mometrix
TEST PREPARATION

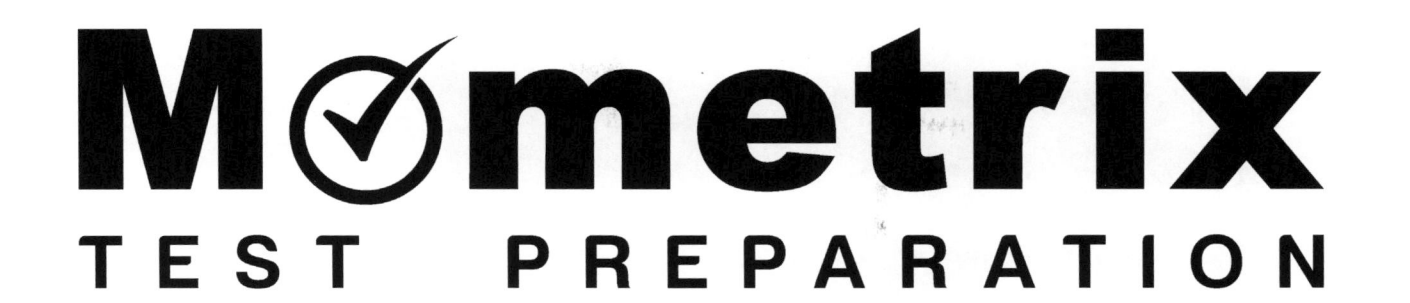

FNP
Certification Review 2025-2026

Family Nurse Practitioner Secrets Study Guide

3 Full-Length Practice Test

75+ Online Video Tutorials

7th Edition

Copyright © 2025 by Mometrix Media LLC

All rights reserved. This product, or parts thereof, may not be reproduced, stored in a retrieval system, or transmitted in any form or by any means—electronic, mechanical, photocopy, recording, scanning, or other—except for brief quotations in critical reviews or articles, without the prior written permission of the publisher.

Written and edited by Matthew Bowling

Printed in the United States of America

This paper meets the requirements of ANSI/NISO Z39.48-1992 (Permanence of Paper).

Mometrix offers volume discount pricing to institutions. For more information or a price quote, please contact our sales department at sales@mometrix.com or 888-248-1219.

Mometrix Media LLC is not affiliated with or endorsed by any official testing organization. All organizational and test names are trademarks of their respective owners.

Paperback
ISBN 13: 978-1-5167-2864-0
ISBN 10: 1-5167-2864-5

Dear Future Exam Success Story

First of all, **THANK YOU** for purchasing Mometrix study materials!

Second, congratulations! You are one of the few determined test-takers who are committed to doing whatever it takes to excel on your exam. **You have come to the right place.** We developed these study materials with one goal in mind: to deliver you the information you need in a format that's concise and easy to use.

In addition to optimizing your guide for the content of the test, we've outlined our recommended steps for breaking down the preparation process into small, attainable goals so you can make sure you stay on track.

We've also analyzed the entire test-taking process, identifying the most common pitfalls and showing how you can overcome them and be ready for any curveball the test throws you.

Standardized testing is one of the biggest obstacles on your road to success, which only increases the importance of doing well in the high-pressure, high-stakes environment of test day. Your results on this test could have a significant impact on your future, and this guide provides the information and practical advice to help you achieve your full potential on test day.

Your success is our success

We would love to hear from you! If you would like to share the story of your exam success or if you have any questions or comments in regard to our products, please contact us at **800-673-8175** or **support@mometrix.com**.

Thanks again for your business and we wish you continued success!

Sincerely,
The Mometrix Test Preparation Team

Need more help? Check out our flashcards at:
http://mometrixflashcards.com/NP

Table of Contents

Introduction 1
Secret Key #1 – Plan Big, Study Small 2
Secret Key #2 – Make Your Studying Count 3
Secret Key #3 – Practice the Right Way 4
Secret Key #4 – Pace Yourself 6
Secret Key #5 – Have a Plan for Guessing 7
Test-Taking Strategies 10
Assessment 15
    Evidence-Based Health Promotion and Screening 15
    Pediatric Illness and Injury Prevention 19
    Comprehensive History and Physical Assessment 36
    Pediatric History and Physical Assessment 40
    Geriatric History and Physical Assessment 51
    Cardiovascular Assessment 55
    Endocrine Assessment 63
    Gastrointestinal Assessment 65
    Hematologic Assessment 70
    Genitourinary Assessment 72
    Integumentary Assessment 76
    Musculoskeletal Assessment 81
    Neurological Assessment 83
    EENT Assessment 88
    Respiratory Assessment 90
    Psychological Assessment 95
    Pain Assessment 99
    Functional Status and Rehabilitation 108
    Pediatric Growth and Development 111
    Family Dynamics 117
    Abuse and Neglect 123
Diagnosis 127
    Cardiovascular Pathophysiology 127
    Ear, Nose, and Throat Pathophysiology 159
    Pediatric EENT Pathophysiology 167
    Endocrine Pathophysiology 172
    Fever and Fibromyalgia 182
    Gastrointestinal Pathophysiology 183
    Genitourinary Pathophysiology 199
    Hematologic Pathophysiology 215
    Immunologic Pathophysiology 219
    Integumentary Pathophysiology 222
    Musculoskeletal Pathophysiology 226

iii

Neurological Pathophysiology	233
Respiratory Pathophysiology	251
Multisystem Pathophysiology	267
Acid Base Imbalances	280
Fluid and Electrolyte Imbalances	283
Infectious Diseases	287
Geriatric Pathophysiology	300
Psychosocial Pathophysiology	304
Diagnostic Testing	317
Cardiovascular Diagnostics	320
Endocrine Diagnostics	321
Gastrointestinal Diagnostics	323
Genitourinary Diagnostics	325
Hematologic Diagnostics	327
Neurological Diagnostics	330

Planning — 332

Nursing Care Planning	332
Adult Age/Disease-Related Factors that Influence Findings	335
Pediatric Response to Illness	337
Impact of Pediatric Chronic Illness on the Family	339
Pediatric Evidence-Based Practices	341
Grief and Loss	343
Principles of Pharmacology	347
Principles of Adult Medication Administration	351
Principles of Pediatric Medication Administration	354
Cultural Sensitivity Practice	357
Nursing Research	360

Implementation — 363

Legal and Ethical Implications for Healthcare	363
Cardiovascular Procedures and Interventions	367
Gastrointestinal Procedures and Interventions	370
Genitourinary Procedures and Interventions	377
Integumentary Procedures and Interventions	382
Musculoskeletal Procedures and Interventions	385
Psychosocial Interventions	389
Respiratory Procedures and Interventions	392
Cardiovascular Pharmacology	399
Endocrine Pharmacology	401
Gastrointestinal Pharmacology	402
Integumentary Pharmacology	405
Respiratory Pharmacology	406
Infectious Disease Pharmacology	409
Pharmacologic Pain Management	413
Psychosocial Pharmacology	421
Immunizations	426
Infection Control	433
Alternative, Complementary, and Non-Pharmacologic Interventions	435
APRN Scope and Standards	440

PATIENT EDUCATION	445
TELEHEALTH	449
THERAPEUTIC RELATIONSHIPS	452

EVALUATION — 457
- ETHICAL BEHAVIOR — 457
- EVIDENCE-BASED PRACTICE — 460

FNP PRACTICE TEST #1 — 463

ANSWER KEY AND EXPLANATIONS FOR TEST #1 — 494

FNP PRACTICE TESTS #2 AND #3 — 514

ONLINE RESOURCES — 515

Introduction

Thank you for purchasing this resource! You have made the choice to prepare yourself for a test that could have a huge impact on your future, and this guide is designed to help you be fully ready for test day. Obviously, it's important to have a solid understanding of the test material, but you also need to be prepared for the unique environment and stressors of the test, so that you can perform to the best of your abilities.

For this purpose, the first section that appears in this guide is the **Secret Keys**. We've devoted countless hours to meticulously researching what works and what doesn't, and we've boiled down our findings to the five most impactful steps you can take to improve your performance on the test. We start at the beginning with study planning and move through the preparation process, all the way to the testing strategies that will help you get the most out of what you know when you're finally sitting in front of the test.

We recommend that you start preparing for your test as far in advance as possible. However, if you've bought this guide as a last-minute study resource and only have a few days before your test, we recommend that you skip over the first two Secret Keys since they address a long-term study plan.

If you struggle with **test anxiety**, we strongly encourage you to check out our recommendations for how you can overcome it. Test anxiety is a formidable foe, but it can be beaten, and we want to make sure you have the tools you need to defeat it.

Secret Key #1 – Plan Big, Study Small

There's a lot riding on your performance. If you want to ace this test, you're going to need to keep your skills sharp and the material fresh in your mind. You need a plan that lets you review everything you need to know while still fitting in your schedule. We'll break this strategy down into three categories.

Information Organization

Start with the information you already have: the official test outline. From this, you can make a complete list of all the concepts you need to cover before the test. Organize these concepts into groups that can be studied together, and create a list of any related vocabulary you need to learn so you can brush up on any difficult terms. You'll want to keep this vocabulary list handy once you actually start studying since you may need to add to it along the way.

Time Management

Once you have your set of study concepts, decide how to spread them out over the time you have left before the test. Break your study plan into small, clear goals so you have a manageable task for each day and know exactly what you're doing. Then just focus on one small step at a time. When you manage your time this way, you don't need to spend hours at a time studying. Studying a small block of content for a short period each day helps you retain information better and avoid stressing over how much you have left to do. You can relax knowing that you have a plan to cover everything in time. In order for this strategy to be effective though, you have to start studying early and stick to your schedule. Avoid the exhaustion and futility that comes from last-minute cramming!

Study Environment

The environment you study in has a big impact on your learning. Studying in a coffee shop, while probably more enjoyable, is not likely to be as fruitful as studying in a quiet room. It's important to keep distractions to a minimum. You're only planning to study for a short block of time, so make the most of it. Don't pause to check your phone or get up to find a snack. It's also important to **avoid multitasking**. Research has consistently shown that multitasking will make your studying dramatically less effective. Your study area should also be comfortable and well-lit so you don't have the distraction of straining your eyes or sitting on an uncomfortable chair.

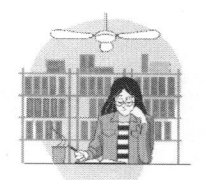

The time of day you study is also important. You want to be rested and alert. Don't wait until just before bedtime. Study when you'll be most likely to comprehend and remember. Even better, if you know what time of day your test will be, set that time aside for study. That way your brain will be used to working on that subject at that specific time and you'll have a better chance of recalling information.

Finally, it can be helpful to team up with others who are studying for the same test. Your actual studying should be done in as isolated an environment as possible, but the work of organizing the information and setting up the study plan can be divided up. In between study sessions, you can discuss with your teammates the concepts that you're all studying and quiz each other on the details. Just be sure that your teammates are as serious about the test as you are. If you find that your study time is being replaced with social time, you might need to find a new team.

Secret Key #2 – Make Your Studying Count

You're devoting a lot of time and effort to preparing for this test, so you want to be absolutely certain it will pay off. This means doing more than just reading the content and hoping you can remember it on test day. It's important to make every minute of study count. There are two main areas you can focus on to make your studying count.

Retention

It doesn't matter how much time you study if you can't remember the material. You need to make sure you are retaining the concepts. To check your retention of the information you're learning, try recalling it at later times with minimal prompting. Try carrying around flashcards and glance at one or two from time to time or ask a friend who's also studying for the test to quiz you.

To enhance your retention, look for ways to put the information into practice so that you can apply it rather than simply recalling it. If you're using the information in practical ways, it will be much easier to remember. Similarly, it helps to solidify a concept in your mind if you're not only reading it to yourself but also explaining it to someone else. Ask a friend to let you teach them about a concept you're a little shaky on (or speak aloud to an imaginary audience if necessary). As you try to summarize, define, give examples, and answer your friend's questions, you'll understand the concepts better and they will stay with you longer. Finally, step back for a big picture view and ask yourself how each piece of information fits with the whole subject. When you link the different concepts together and see them working together as a whole, it's easier to remember the individual components.

Finally, practice showing your work on any multi-step problems, even if you're just studying. Writing out each step you take to solve a problem will help solidify the process in your mind, and you'll be more likely to remember it during the test.

Modality

Modality simply refers to the means or method by which you study. Choosing a study modality that fits your own individual learning style is crucial. No two people learn best in exactly the same way, so it's important to know your strengths and use them to your advantage.

For example, if you learn best by visualization, focus on visualizing a concept in your mind and draw an image or a diagram. Try color-coding your notes, illustrating them, or creating symbols that will trigger your mind to recall a learned concept. If you learn best by hearing or discussing information, find a study partner who learns the same way or read aloud to yourself. Think about how to put the information in your own words. Imagine that you are giving a lecture on the topic and record yourself so you can listen to it later.

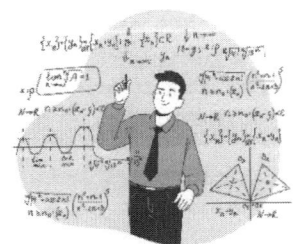

For any learning style, flashcards can be helpful. Organize the information so you can take advantage of spare moments to review. Underline key words or phrases. Use different colors for different categories. Mnemonic devices (such as creating a short list in which every item starts with the same letter) can also help with retention. Find what works best for you and use it to store the information in your mind most effectively and easily.

Secret Key #3 – Practice the Right Way

Your success on test day depends not only on how many hours you put into preparing, but also on whether you prepared the right way. It's good to check along the way to see if your studying is paying off. One of the most effective ways to do this is by taking practice tests to evaluate your progress. Practice tests are useful because they show exactly where you need to improve. Every time you take a practice test, pay special attention to these three groups of questions:

- The questions you got wrong
- The questions you had to guess on, even if you guessed right
- The questions you found difficult or slow to work through

This will show you exactly what your weak areas are, and where you need to devote more study time. Ask yourself why each of these questions gave you trouble. Was it because you didn't understand the material? Was it because you didn't remember the vocabulary? Do you need more repetitions on this type of question to build speed and confidence? Dig into those questions and figure out how you can strengthen your weak areas as you go back to review the material.

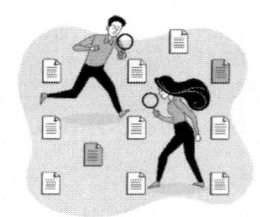

Additionally, many practice tests have a section explaining the answer choices. It can be tempting to read the explanation and think that you now have a good understanding of the concept. However, an explanation likely only covers part of the question's broader context. Even if the explanation makes perfect sense, **go back and investigate** every concept related to the question until you're positive you have a thorough understanding.

As you go along, keep in mind that the practice test is just that: practice. Memorizing these questions and answers will not be very helpful on the actual test because it is unlikely to have any of the same exact questions. If you only know the right answers to the sample questions, you won't be prepared for the real thing. **Study the concepts** until you understand them fully, and then you'll be able to answer any question that shows up on the test.

It's important to wait on the practice tests until you're ready. If you take a test on your first day of study, you may be overwhelmed by the amount of material covered and how much you need to learn. Work up to it gradually.

On test day, you'll need to be prepared for answering questions, managing your time, and using the test-taking strategies you've learned. It's a lot to balance, like a mental marathon that will have a big impact on your future. Like training for a marathon, you'll need to start slowly and work your way up. When test day arrives, you'll be ready.

Start with the strategies you've read in the first two Secret Keys—plan your course and study in the way that works best for you. If you have time, consider using multiple study resources to get different approaches to the same concepts. It can be helpful to see difficult concepts from more than one angle. Then find a good source for practice tests. Many times, the test website will suggest potential study resources or provide sample tests.

Practice Test Strategy

If you're able to find at least three practice tests, we recommend this strategy:

Untimed and Open-Book Practice

Take the first test with no time constraints and with your notes and study guide handy. Take your time and focus on applying the strategies you've learned.

Timed and Open-Book Practice

Take the second practice test open-book as well, but set a timer and practice pacing yourself to finish in time.

Timed and Closed-Book Practice

Take any other practice tests as if it were test day. Set a timer and put away your study materials. Sit at a table or desk in a quiet room, imagine yourself at the testing center, and answer questions as quickly and accurately as possible.

Keep repeating timed and closed-book tests on a regular basis until you run out of practice tests or it's time for the actual test. Your mind will be ready for the schedule and stress of test day, and you'll be able to focus on recalling the material you've learned.

Secret Key #4 – Pace Yourself

Once you're fully prepared for the material on the test, your biggest challenge on test day will be managing your time. Just knowing that the clock is ticking can make you panic even if you have plenty of time left. Work on pacing yourself so you can build confidence against the time constraints of the exam. Pacing is a difficult skill to master, especially in a high-pressure environment, so **practice is vital**.

Set time expectations for your pace based on how much time is available. For example, if a section has 60 questions and the time limit is 30 minutes, you know you have to average 30 seconds or less per question in order to answer them all. Although 30 seconds is the hard limit, set 25 seconds per question as your goal, so you reserve extra time to spend on harder questions. When you budget extra time for the harder questions, you no longer have any reason to stress when those questions take longer to answer.

Don't let this time expectation distract you from working through the test at a calm, steady pace, but keep it in mind so you don't spend too much time on any one question. Recognize that taking extra time on one question you don't understand may keep you from answering two that you do understand later in the test. If your time limit for a question is up and you're still not sure of the answer, mark it and move on, and come back to it later if the time and the test format allow. If the testing format doesn't allow you to return to earlier questions, just make an educated guess; then put it out of your mind and move on.

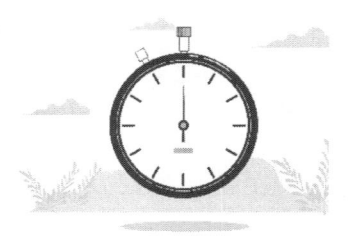

On the easier questions, be careful not to rush. It may seem wise to hurry through them so you have more time for the challenging ones, but it's not worth missing one if you know the concept and just didn't take the time to read the question fully. Work efficiently but make sure you understand the question and have looked at all of the answer choices, since more than one may seem right at first.

Even if you're paying attention to the time, you may find yourself a little behind at some point. You should speed up to get back on track, but do so wisely. Don't panic; just take a few seconds less on each question until you're caught up. Don't guess without thinking, but do look through the answer choices and eliminate any you know are wrong. If you can get down to two choices, it is often worthwhile to guess from those. Once you've chosen an answer, move on and don't dwell on any that you skipped or had to hurry through. If a question was taking too long, chances are it was one of the harder ones, so you weren't as likely to get it right anyway.

On the other hand, if you find yourself getting ahead of schedule, it may be beneficial to slow down a little. The more quickly you work, the more likely you are to make a careless mistake that will affect your score. You've budgeted time for each question, so don't be afraid to spend that time. Practice an efficient but careful pace to get the most out of the time you have.

Secret Key #5 – Have a Plan for Guessing

When you're taking the test, you may find yourself stuck on a question. Some of the answer choices seem better than others, but you don't see the one answer choice that is obviously correct. What do you do?

The scenario described above is very common, yet most test takers have not effectively prepared for it. Developing and practicing a plan for guessing may be one of the single most effective uses of your time as you get ready for the exam.

In developing your plan for guessing, there are three questions to address:

- When should you start the guessing process?
- How should you narrow down the choices?
- Which answer should you choose?

When to Start the Guessing Process

Unless your plan for guessing is to select C every time (which, despite its merits, is not what we recommend), you need to leave yourself enough time to apply your answer elimination strategies. Since you have a limited amount of time for each question, that means that if you're going to give yourself the best shot at guessing correctly, you have to decide quickly whether or not you will guess.

Of course, the best-case scenario is that you don't have to guess at all, so first, see if you can answer the question based on your knowledge of the subject and basic reasoning skills. Focus on the key words in the question and try to jog your memory of related topics. Give yourself a chance to bring the knowledge to mind, but once you realize that you don't have (or you can't access) the knowledge you need to answer the question, it's time to start the guessing process.

It's almost always better to start the guessing process too early than too late. It only takes a few seconds to remember something and answer the question from knowledge. Carefully eliminating wrong answer choices takes longer. Plus, going through the process of eliminating answer choices can actually help jog your memory.

Summary: Start the guessing process as soon as you decide that you can't answer the question based on your knowledge.

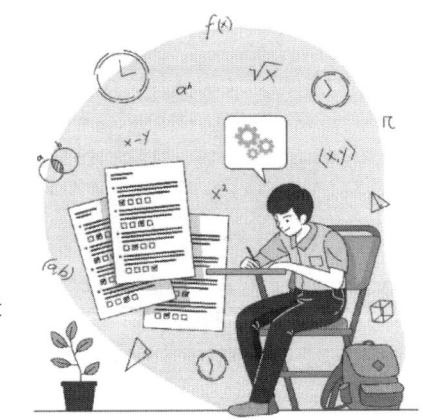

How to Narrow Down the Choices

The next chapter in this book (**Test-Taking Strategies**) includes a wide range of strategies for how to approach questions and how to look for answer choices to eliminate. You will definitely want to read those carefully, practice them, and figure out which ones work best for you. Here though, we're going to address a mindset rather than a particular strategy.

Your odds of guessing an answer correctly depend on how many options you are choosing from.

Number of options left	5	4	3	2	1
Odds of guessing correctly	20%	25%	33%	50%	100%

You can see from this chart just how valuable it is to be able to eliminate incorrect answers and make an educated guess, but there are two things that many test takers do that cause them to miss out on the benefits of guessing:

- Accidentally eliminating the correct answer
- Selecting an answer based on an impression

We'll look at the first one here, and the second one in the next section.

To avoid accidentally eliminating the correct answer, we recommend a thought exercise called **the $5 challenge**. In this challenge, you only eliminate an answer choice from contention if you are willing to bet $5 on it being wrong. Why $5? Five dollars is a small but not insignificant amount of money. It's an amount you could afford to lose but wouldn't want to throw away. And while losing $5 once might not hurt too much, doing it twenty times will set you back $100. In the same way, each small decision you make—eliminating a choice here, guessing on a question there—won't by itself impact your score very much, but when you put them all together, they can make a big difference. By holding each answer choice elimination decision to a higher standard, you can reduce the risk of accidentally eliminating the correct answer.

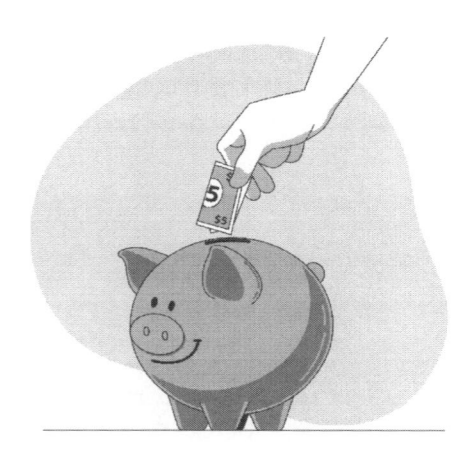

The $5 challenge can also be applied in a positive sense: If you are willing to bet $5 that an answer choice *is* correct, go ahead and mark it as correct.

Summary: Only eliminate an answer choice if you are willing to bet $5 that it is wrong.

Which Answer to Choose

You're taking the test. You've run into a hard question and decided you'll have to guess. You've eliminated all the answer choices you're willing to bet $5 on. Now you have to pick an answer. Why do we even need to talk about this? Why can't you just pick whichever one you feel like when the time comes?

The answer to these questions is that if you don't come into the test with a plan, you'll rely on your impression to select an answer choice, and if you do that, you risk falling into a trap. The test writers know that everyone who takes their test will be guessing on some of the questions, so they intentionally write wrong answer choices to seem plausible. You still have to pick an answer though, and if the wrong answer choices are designed to look right, how can you ever be sure that you're not falling for their trap? The best solution we've found to this dilemma is to take the decision out of your hands entirely. Here is the process we recommend:

Once you've eliminated any choices that you are confident (willing to bet $5) are wrong, select the first remaining choice as your answer.

Whether you choose to select the first remaining choice, the second, or the last, the important thing is that you use some preselected standard. Using this approach guarantees that you will not be enticed into selecting an answer choice that looks right, because you are not basing your decision on how the answer choices look.

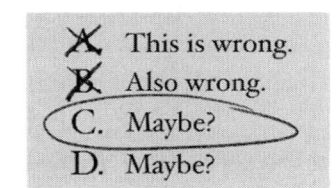

This is not meant to make you question your knowledge. Instead, it is to help you recognize the difference between your knowledge and your impressions. There's a huge difference between thinking an answer is right because of what you know, and thinking an answer is right because it looks or sounds like it should be right.

Summary: To ensure that your selection is appropriately random, make a predetermined selection from among all answer choices you have not eliminated.

Test-Taking Strategies

This section contains a list of test-taking strategies that you may find helpful as you work through the test. By taking what you know and applying logical thought, you can maximize your chances of answering any question correctly!

It is very important to realize that every question is different and every person is different: no single strategy will work on every question, and no single strategy will work for every person. That's why we've included all of them here, so you can try them out and determine which ones work best for different types of questions and which ones work best for you.

Question Strategies

⊘ READ CAREFULLY

Read the question and the answer choices carefully. Don't miss the question because you misread the terms. You have plenty of time to read each question thoroughly and make sure you understand what is being asked. Yet a happy medium must be attained, so don't waste too much time. You must read carefully and efficiently.

⊘ CONTEXTUAL CLUES

Look for contextual clues. If the question includes a word you are not familiar with, look at the immediate context for some indication of what the word might mean. Contextual clues can often give you all the information you need to decipher the meaning of an unfamiliar word. Even if you can't determine the meaning, you may be able to narrow down the possibilities enough to make a solid guess at the answer to the question.

⊘ PREFIXES

If you're having trouble with a word in the question or answer choices, try dissecting it. Take advantage of every clue that the word might include. Prefixes can be a huge help. Usually, they allow you to determine a basic meaning. *Pre-* means before, *post-* means after, *pro-* is positive, *de-* is negative. From prefixes, you can get an idea of the general meaning of the word and try to put it into context.

⊘ HEDGE WORDS

Watch out for critical hedge words, such as *likely, may, can, sometimes, often, almost, mostly, usually, generally, rarely,* and *sometimes*. Question writers insert these hedge phrases to cover every possibility. Often an answer choice will be wrong simply because it leaves no room for exception. Be on guard for answer choices that have definitive words such as *exactly* and *always*.

⊘ SWITCHBACK WORDS

Stay alert for *switchbacks*. These are the words and phrases frequently used to alert you to shifts in thought. The most common switchback words are *but, although,* and *however*. Others include *nevertheless, on the other hand, even though, while, in spite of, despite,* and *regardless of*. Switchback words are important to catch because they can change the direction of the question or an answer choice.

⊘ FACE VALUE

When in doubt, use common sense. Accept the situation in the problem at face value. Don't read too much into it. These problems will not require you to make wild assumptions. If you have to go beyond creativity and warp time or space in order to have an answer choice fit the question, then you should move on and consider the other answer choices. These are normal problems rooted in reality. The applicable relationship or explanation may not be readily apparent, but it is there for you to figure out. Use your common sense to interpret anything that isn't clear.

Answer Choice Strategies

⊘ Answer Selection

The most thorough way to pick an answer choice is to identify and eliminate wrong answers until only one is left, then confirm it is the correct answer. Sometimes an answer choice may immediately seem right, but be careful. The test writers will usually put more than one reasonable answer choice on each question, so take a second to read all of them and make sure that the other choices are not equally obvious. As long as you have time left, it is better to read every answer choice than to pick the first one that looks right without checking the others.

⊘ Answer Choice Families

An answer choice family consists of two (in rare cases, three) answer choices that are very similar in construction and cannot all be true at the same time. If you see two answer choices that are direct opposites or parallels, one of them is usually the correct answer. For instance, if one answer choice says that quantity x increases and another either says that quantity x decreases (opposite) or says that quantity y increases (parallel), then those answer choices would fall into the same family. An answer choice that doesn't match the construction of the answer choice family is more likely to be incorrect. Most questions will not have answer choice families, but when they do appear, you should be prepared to recognize them.

⊘ Eliminate Answers

Eliminate answer choices as soon as you realize they are wrong, but make sure you consider all possibilities. If you are eliminating answer choices and realize that the last one you are left with is also wrong, don't panic. Start over and consider each choice again. There may be something you missed the first time that you will realize on the second pass.

⊘ Avoid Fact Traps

Don't be distracted by an answer choice that is factually true but doesn't answer the question. You are looking for the choice that answers the question. Stay focused on what the question is asking for so you don't accidentally pick an answer that is true but incorrect. Always go back to the question and make sure the answer choice you've selected actually answers the question and is not merely a true statement.

⊘ Extreme Statements

In general, you should avoid answers that put forth extreme actions as standard practice or proclaim controversial ideas as established fact. An answer choice that states the "process should be used in certain situations, if..." is much more likely to be correct than one that states the "process should be discontinued completely." The first is a calm rational statement and doesn't even make a definitive, uncompromising stance, using a hedge word *if* to provide wiggle room, whereas the second choice is far more extreme.

⊘ Benchmark

As you read through the answer choices and you come across one that seems to answer the question well, mentally select that answer choice. This is not your final answer, but it's the one that will help you evaluate the other answer choices. The one that you selected is your benchmark or standard for judging each of the other answer choices. Every other answer choice must be compared to your benchmark. That choice is correct until proven otherwise by another answer choice beating it. If you find a better answer, then that one becomes your new benchmark. Once you've decided that no other choice answers the question as well as your benchmark, you have your final answer.

⊘ Predict the Answer

Before you even start looking at the answer choices, it is often best to try to predict the answer. When you come up with the answer on your own, it is easier to avoid distractions and traps because you will know exactly what to look for. The right answer choice is unlikely to be word-for-word what you came up with, but it should be a close match. Even if you are confident that you have the right answer, you should still take the time to read each option before moving on.

General Strategies

⊘ Tough Questions

If you are stumped on a problem or it appears too hard or too difficult, don't waste time. Move on! Remember though, if you can quickly check for obviously incorrect answer choices, your chances of guessing correctly are greatly improved. Before you completely give up, at least try to knock out a couple of possible answers. Eliminate what you can and then guess at the remaining answer choices before moving on.

⊘ Check Your Work

Since you will probably not know every term listed and the answer to every question, it is important that you get credit for the ones that you do know. Don't miss any questions through careless mistakes. If at all possible, try to take a second to look back over your answer selection and make sure you've selected the correct answer choice and haven't made a costly careless mistake (such as marking an answer choice that you didn't mean to mark). This quick double check should more than pay for itself in caught mistakes for the time it costs.

⊘ Pace Yourself

It's easy to be overwhelmed when you're looking at a page full of questions; your mind is confused and full of random thoughts, and the clock is ticking down faster than you would like. Calm down and maintain the pace that you have set for yourself. Especially as you get down to the last few minutes of the test, don't let the small numbers on the clock make you panic. As long as you are on track by monitoring your pace, you are guaranteed to have time for each question.

⊘ Don't Rush

It is very easy to make errors when you are in a hurry. Maintaining a fast pace in answering questions is pointless if it makes you miss questions that you would have gotten right otherwise. Test writers like to include distracting information and wrong answers that seem right. Taking a little extra time to avoid careless mistakes can make all the difference in your test score. Find a pace that allows you to be confident in the answers that you select.

⊘ Keep Moving

Panicking will not help you pass the test, so do your best to stay calm and keep moving. Taking deep breaths and going through the answer elimination steps you practiced can help to break through a stress barrier and keep your pace.

Final Notes

The combination of a solid foundation of content knowledge and the confidence that comes from practicing your plan for applying that knowledge is the key to maximizing your performance on test day. As your foundation of content knowledge is built up and strengthened, you'll find that the strategies included in this chapter become more and more effective in helping you quickly sift through the distractions and traps of the test to isolate the correct answer.

Now that you're preparing to move forward into the test content chapters of this book, be sure to keep your goal in mind. As you read, think about how you will be able to apply this information on the test. If you've already seen sample questions for the test and you have an idea of the question format and style, try to come up with questions of your own that you can answer based on what you're reading. This will give you valuable practice applying your knowledge in the same ways you can expect to on test day.

Good luck and good studying!

Assessment

Evidence-Based Health Promotion and Screening

HEALTH PROMOTION

Nurses promote health when they assist individuals to change behavior in ways that help them to attain and maintain the highest level of wellbeing possible. Health promotion is a very popular way to control healthcare costs and reduce illness and early death. Health is increasingly the topic of newscasts and literature. The public is demanding more information pertinent to the maintenance of health and to the ways in which the average person can act independently to do so. Health promotion is centered on ideal personal habits, lifestyles, and environmental control that decrease the risk for disease. The US Public Health Service periodically identifies national health goals and most recently published a program called **Healthy People 2030**, with measurable goals to increase the general quality and years of life for all and to increase the health status of all groups to an equal level of wellness. Health promotion programs in the community are now offered by workplaces, clinics, schools, and churches, not just by hospitals as in the past.

HEALTHY PEOPLE 2030

The 5 **main goals** of *Healthy People 2030* are

- Attaining healthy, thriving lives free of preventable disease, disability, injury, and premature death
- Eliminating health disparities, achieving health equality, and increasing health literacy
- Creating environments conducive to health-promotion
- Improving health in all life stages
- Collaborating with leadership and key stakeholders in policy design that improves the health and well-being of all

Healthy People 2030 has 62 topic areas with 355 total objectives divided across five sections:

- Health Conditions
- Health Behaviors
- Populations
- Settings and Systems
- Social Determinants of Health

MAIN COMPONENTS OF HEALTH PROMOTION

Health promotion efforts are concentrated in four areas:

- Individuals must be educated to realize that their **lifestyle and choices** have a large impact on their health. They must then be motivated to choose to modify their personal risk factors and take the responsibility to do so.
- The emphasis on **good nutrition** as the biggest factor that impacts health and the length of life must be brought into general awareness. This is occurring via the media through numerous books and articles educating people about the essential nutrients needed to maintain health.
- **Stress** is a constant in a production-driven society. Individuals must learn ways to manage and decrease stress to achieve and maintain health and to decrease the effects of stress upon chronic illness, risk of infections, and trauma.
- **Physical fitness** helps cardiovascular status, relieves stress, controls weight, delays aging, promotes strength and endurance, and improves appearance and performance. Individuals must have programs that increase activity gradually to prevent injury and are designed to meet individual needs.

HEALTH SELF-MANAGEMENT

Health self-management includes health maintenance, disease prevention, and health promotion. Health maintenance is defined as strategies that help maintain and/or improve health over time. Health maintenance is dependent on three factors, which include health perception, motivation for behavioral change, and compliance to set goals. Disease prevention is an effort to limit the development or progression of lifestyle-related illness. **Disease prevention** can be categorized into primary, secondary, and tertiary prevention.

- **Primary prevention** measures are employed prior to disease onset and are used in health populations.
- **Secondary prevention** measures are used to screen, detect, and treat disease in earlier stages to prevent further progression or development of other complications.
- **Tertiary prevention** measures are used to prevent the worsening of a disease and the onset of other complications or comorbid conditions secondary to that disease.

Health promotion strategies include risk reduction strategies applied to the general population.

INFLUENCES ON DECISION TO MODIFY BEHAVIOR TO ACHIEVE AND MAINTAIN HEALTH

Many factors have an influence on people's efforts to change behavior in a way that improves and maintains their health status. These factors include age, ethnicity, gender, lifestyle, level of education, self-esteem, motivation, and self-image. The patient's support network and the availability of health promotion programs and healthcare systems also have an influence on healthcare behaviors. Some people may be prevented from accessing health promotion programs because of lack of medical insurance. Financial status and employment are important as well. The presence of addictions and diseases, the length of illness, and the severity of disabilities are all factors to be considered. The value placed on health, the threat of potential losses, and the perceived benefits of behavior modification are important motivating factors.

STRATEGIES TO ENCOURAGE SMOKING CESSATION

The **health impact associated with smoking** varies among smokers and can be affected by the number of cigarettes used daily, exposure to smoking-associated stimuli, and educational level. The presence of stress and depression, psychosocial problems, lack of coping mechanisms, low income, and long-term habitual behavior are problematic for the quitter. Nurses can promote smoking cessation by taking every opportunity to bring up the subject, educating about the dangers of smoking and benefits of quitting, and providing **resources** to help patients quit. Strategies include:

- Educating about the personal effects of smoking upon that individual
- Encouraging patients to set a quit date
- Referring to programs and smoking cessation information
- Educating about the use of nicotine replacements including nicotine gum, lozenges, inhalers, transdermal patches, and nasal sprays
- Educating about the use of medications such as Zyban, Catapres, and Chantix
- Providing support via phone calls or office visits
- Discovering the reason for relapses
- Praising and rewarding any success in the quitting process

HEALTHY NUTRITION PRINCIPLES

Healthy nutrition principles include the following:

- Eating a range of different kinds of foods, and eating increased amounts fruits, vegetables, whole grains, poultry, and fish.
- Diets should consist of 55–60% **carbohydrates**, less than 30% **fat**, and the rest should be **protein** (0.8–1.0 g/kg).
- Restrict **saturated fat** to <10%. Restrict **cholesterol** to 300 mg/day.
- Utilize moderate amounts of sugar, salt, and sodium.
- Take a **multivitamin** including folic acid if the patient is female and able to have children. Get 200–800 IU/day of vitamin D in order to absorb calcium.
- **Calcium** intake should be: 1,300 mg/day for women age 13–18 or those who are pregnant/nursing; 1,000 mg/day for women age 19–50 years; 1,500 mg/day for age 51 years and older.
- **Weight loss** may improve diabetes, joint pain, inflammation, cardiovascular disease, hypothyroidism, or renal disease.

YOUNG ADULT HEALTH SCREENINGS

Health screening is encouraged for conditions that are very likely to occur and diseases that are likely to kill if they are not identified early. The assessment should be supported by evidence using standardized techniques and proper follow-up.

Young adult (ages 20-39 years) screenings, according to the US Preventive Services Task Force (USPSTF), should include:

- A full head-to-toe physical (every 5-6 years)
- Routine blood pressure screening
- Cholesterol screening (every 5 years; more frequently when total cholesterol is higher than 200 mg/dL)
- PPD test for tuberculosis when patient has had known contact with TB or is at increased risk (health care workers, prisoners, homeless, or immunocompromised)
- Dental check-up (annually)
- Thyroid palpation (every 3 years)
- Depression screening (at every visit)
- Men perform self-testicular exam every month
- Women conduct a self-breast exam every month; should receive a clinical breast exam every 3 years
- Pap smear and pelvic assessments every 3 years (or up to 5 years in conjunction with HPV testing)
- Screening for gonorrhea and chlamydia for all sexually active individuals
- Health education and promotion (every time patient is seen)
- Influenza vaccination (annually)
- Td immunization every 10 years

ADULT SCREENINGS

Adults (age 40 and older) screenings, according to the USPSTF, should maintain the same schedule as young adults (unless indicated below) in addition to the following:

- A full head-to-toe physical (annually)
- Blood pressure screening (annually)
- ECG (over 40, annually; only when there are cardiac risks)
- Clinical breast exam (annually in women over 40)
- Mammogram (biennially in women over 40)
- General colorectal cancer screening for risks (annually), and colorectal cancer screening via colonoscopy (every 10 years starting at age 45 until age 75)
- Prostate-specific antigen screening (men over 50 with average risk, or younger if higher risk; upon the patient's informed request only)

DISEASE PREVENTION FOR THE ELDERLY

Although life spans are longer, **ongoing (chronic) diseases** are still the primary reason patients die. Elderly patients have more of an absolute chance of getting a disease, but they also react well to prevention. Keep good records of the elderly patient's history, including updating every year and following advice for patients over the age of 65 years. Evaluate nutrition, functional ability, alcoholic beverage intake (more than 2 alcoholic beverages a day constitutes abuse), smoking, illegal drugs, misuse of prescriptions, and exercise level.

- **Preventative measures** include a physical, screening assessments, and immunizations.
- Some **routine screenings** include: fasting glucose, papanicolaou smear, dipstick urinalysis, mammography, PPD, fecal occult blood/sigmoidoscopy, electrocardiogram, thyroid function, glaucoma and sight, hearing, and cholesterol.
- **Immunizations** include yearly flu shot, pneumococcal vaccine, and tetanus; respiratory syncytial virus (RSV) vaccination at age 75.

The following screens are controversial: depression for someone with no symptoms, dementia for someone with no symptoms, osteoporosis including bone densitometry for postmenopausal females (counsel females regarding hormone prophylaxis), colon and prostate cancer, and cholesterol for someone with no symptoms.

Pediatric Illness and Injury Prevention

WELLNESS EVALUATION

A wellness evaluation is a complete assessment and report of the general health profile of the child, compiling all available pertinent information. A **health profile** should include the following:

- Basic measurements, such as height, weight, and head circumference, and the percentile ranking for age.
- Vital signs, including pulse, respiration, and blood pressure. Body temperature should be included as well.
- Nutrition profile that outlines the child's normal diet and any dietary modifications or adverse reactions, such as allergies or intolerances.
- Mobility/activity level that explains the infant's mobility in accordance to expected development for age. For older children, the type of activities and physical exercise the child engages in and their frequency should be noted.
- Results of any screening tests and, if elective rather than standard, the reason for the test.
- Health promotion/disease prevention activities, including duration, results, and compliance with prescribed interventions.

INFANTS

WELL BABY CHECKUPS DURING THE FIRST YEAR OF LIFE

Most pediatricians will want to check the breastfed baby's weight at one week of age, and the bottle-fed baby's weight at 2 weeks. If the PKU, thyroid, hematocrit and hemoglobin tests were not done after birth, they should be completed at the first visit. Well baby checkups are usually scheduled at 2, 4, 6, 9, and 12 months. A home health assessment and physical exam will be done, along with weight, height, and head circumference. Development, expectations, and concerns are discussed and immunizations will be given according the latest recommendations. If lead testing is warranted, it will be done at 9 or 12 months.

DENTAL HEALTH OF INFANTS

As teeth erupt, the parents can clean them by gently rubbing with a clean wet cloth. Supplemental fluoride is prescribed beginning at 6 months if the parent's water does not contain fluoride or if the baby is breastfed only. Parents should be warned of the dental problems (bottle-mouth caries) that may occur when babies are given a bottle to sleep with or breast feedings are prolonged to pacify the baby. Discuss with parents the symptoms of teething (slight fever, fussiness, drooling) and ways to make the baby more comfortable and facilitate teething (allow baby to chew on a rubber teething ring, rub a clean finger on the baby's gums, and give acetaminophen). Dental visits, by recommendation of the American Academy of Pediatrics, should begin at 6 months.

VISION AND HEARING HEALTH OF INFANTS

Vision will be assessed by having the baby track an object or familiar face. Lack of the following would indicate visual problems: blink reflex, doll's eye reflex (the head is moved to one side and the eyes will not follow right away—disappears as infant grows), tracking by one month, following own hands and feet by 4 months, reaching for toys at 5 months, or good hand-eye coordination at 7 months. Lack of the following would indicate hearing problems: startle or blink reflex at loud noise, responding in some way to loud noises when asleep, turning head toward sound at 6 months, making babbling sounds at 7 months, or general response to human voice or sound.

TODDLERS AND PRESCHOOLERS

WELL CHILD CHECK UP FOR TODDLERS

Well child visits are scheduled at 15, 18, 24, and 36 months, encompassing a physical exam, home health assessment and immunizations, as appropriate. DTP (DTaP), Hib, polio, and hepatitis B boosters are given by

18 months of age. Other vaccines are given if not begun earlier. The MMR and varicella vaccines are started. Blood pressure, height, weight, head circumference (until anterior fontanel closes), vision, and hearing are checked. Hemoglobin will be tested to detect iron-deficiency anemia and lead levels may be tested in those who live in a high-risk area or show signs of lead poisoning (poor growth or neurological irritability).

COMMON ISSUES FACED BY PARENTS OF TODDLERS AND DISCIPLINE TECHNIQUES TO USE

Toddlers have learned the word "no" and will use it often. Asking open-ended questions, giving choices and ignoring the behavior are ways to handle this frustrating negativism. Toddlers also enjoy rituals (same bedtime routine, same cup, spoon, or bowl) and this helps them to maintain some control over their environment. When routines are altered, the toddler may show signs of regression. Allowing for routines within reason and ignoring regression while giving praise for accomplishments will help the child get through this stage. Sibling rivalry can occur with the birth of a new baby. Setting limits, introducing the concept of a new baby gradually, spending time with both children together, and encouraging the toddler to help with small tasks (get a diaper for mommy) will help with the transition. Temper tantrums begin around 2 years of age and are best ignored, making sure the child does not harm himself. Time-outs can be used before behavior escalates; this may prevent the temper tantrum.

DENTAL HEALTH OF TODDLERS AND PRESCHOOLERS

Toddlers should have regular dental visits. The parents should be brushing their teeth with a small, soft toothbrush, using either water or a very small amount of toothpaste (fluoridated toothpaste, if swallowed, can be harmful). Flossing should be done by the parent to remove food below the gum line and to establish good dental hygiene habits early.

Preschoolers can begin to help with brushing and flossing, although the parents need to supervise and assist them to make sure that all teeth are clean. A pea-sized squeeze of toothpaste should be used to prevent harmful effects of swallowed fluoride. Dental visits every 6 months should be established. Cavities can be prevented with good brushing and flossing habits, limiting foods with lots of sugar, chewing sugar-free gum, and brushing after eating foods with lots of sugar. Teeth-grinding at night is fairly common during these years. If it seems to last longer than it takes the child to fall asleep, a dentist should be consulted. A mouthpiece worn during the night may be needed.

WELL CHILD VISIT AND ANTICIPATORY GUIDANCE FOR PRESCHOOLERS

Checkups are scheduled every year from **age 3 to 6** and include a physical exam, height, weight, vision, hearing, and blood pressure checks. If all immunizations are up-to-date, boosters for DTaP (diphtheria, tetanus, and pertussis), polio, and MMR (measles, mumps, rubella) vaccines will be given. Before entering school, a tuberculin test is required. Lead testing is indicated if the child is at risk (older homes may have lead paint or lead water pipes), as well as hyperlipidemia testing if indicated.

Toilet training is usually completed by age 5. Discipline can be achieved by time-outs, consistency, firm limits, and short explanations of why certain behaviors are wrong. Continue with consistent routines, allowing imaginative play, and limiting TV watching. Read to the child daily. Teach proper hand washing and allow children to do simple chores around the house. Talk to the parents about what to expect when the child begins school.

SCHOOL AGE CHILDREN

WELL CHILD VISITS AND ANTICIPATORY GUIDANCE FOR SCHOOL AGE CHILDREN

Checkups should be scheduled at least every 2 years starting at **age 6 until age 10** and every year thereafter. Included in these visits should be a physical exam, dietary intake, height, weight, hearing, vision, blood pressure, and heart and respiratory rates. The child and family should be questioned about any alcohol, drug, or tobacco use. Assess the home and family dynamics, any extracurricular activities, changes in thought processes (depression), academics, and sexuality problems. High risk children are screened for TB (tuberculosis), and all are screened for scoliosis. The tetanus booster is given at age 11 or 12, along with any missed boosters from the preschool years. The parents should be preparing the child for puberty changes, discussing sex education, as well as talking about drugs, alcohol, and tobacco. TV viewing and computer usage should be limited and monitored for content. Encourage exercise at least one hour a day.

DENTAL HEALTH OF SCHOOL AGE CHILDREN

It is during these years that the baby teeth are lost and replaced by the permanent teeth. Continue with proper brushing (twice a day with fluoride toothpaste) and flossing, assisting as needed until the child is proficient, along with regular dental visits. Make sure the child's toothbrush is small, soft and replaced every 2-3 months. Braces may be needed when the teeth are too crowded or out of alignment. Any permanent tooth that is knocked out should be rinsed in water, placed back into the socket and held in place so that it can be saved. As an alternative, the tooth can be placed in a cup of milk or held in the child's mouth, under the tongue. A dentist should be consulted immediately.

DISCIPLINE AND STRESSORS OF SCHOOL AGE CHILDREN

Set clear limits; taking away privileges is often a successful discipline method for school age children. Use lots of praise for good behaviors. The parent should role model appropriate behaviors and social skills. Show the child that she is a unique person, with much to contribute to the family, and take her thoughts seriously. Explain the whys of rules and consequences. A common misbehavior of this age is dishonesty, which, while distressing to the parents, is a common phase for children to go through.

School age children are exposed to more stress today than ever before. The nurse needs to assess for stressors and whether the child is able to cope or if there is a need for assistance in coping.

SEXUALITY OF SCHOOL AGE CHILDREN

Children of this age are exposed to a great deal of sexual material on TV, in music, in newspapers, and elsewhere. It is common for them to experiment with their own bodies. If parents do not dwell on these behaviors, answer questions honestly, and make themselves available for discussions, the school age child will develop a healthy attitude toward his own sexuality. If the parents do not talk openly with their children, the children will seek answers from their peers, who are not always reliable sources.

ADOLESCENTS

HEALTH CHECKUP AND DENTAL HEALTH FOR ADOLESCENTS

Providing privacy for the adolescent during doctor visits is helpful in gaining a full assessment. A physical exam, including assessing puberty changes, height, weight, vital signs, and growth trajectory, should be done yearly. Consider meningococcal, pneumococcal, influenza, and varicella vaccines for this age. A booster dose of tetanus and diphtheria vaccine is needed 10 years after the pre-kindergarten dose. Hepatitis B vaccines should be started if not given earlier, and hepatitis A vaccines are considered for those at high-risk. The teen should be screened for scoliosis and goiter.

Dental visits should occur every 6 months. Proper brushing and flossing are important, especially when orthodontic devices are in place. Gingivitis is common, usually due to improper cleaning of braces, sugary foods, and hormones. The teen should be encouraged to take special care with their dental hygiene. Trauma to the mouth and teeth is common in sports activities. If the tooth is knocked out, it should be rinsed and placed back in the socket and the teen should be seen by a dentist immediately.

ADOLESCENT ISSUES TO DISCUSS DURING ROUTINE CHECKUPS

Discuss the nutrition requirements of the adolescent and how they are being met. Athletes, teens with eating disorders, and females with heavy menstrual cycles will need additional counseling and possibly supplements to meet their nutritional needs. Ask how much sleep the teen is getting, explain that teens need more sleep than children who are school aged, encourage them to get plenty of rest, and address any sleep problems they might be having. Ask about any risk-taking behaviors (alcohol, drugs, cigarette smoking) and educate as to the consequences of these. Talk about accident prevention, automobile safety, appropriate equipment for sports, and gun safety. Discuss issues of violence and how to prevent date rape. Discuss sexuality and address any issues or concerns such as birth control and STIs. Assess for abnormalities in menstruation. Talk about masturbation and, in males, nocturnal emissions. Assist the teen in addressing any acne concerns.

RISK ANALYSIS AS PART OF DISEASE PREVENTION

Risk analysis is an important part of health promotion and disease prevention because it can help to identify those factors (normed for age and sex) that put a child at risk for current or future disease. Typically, risk analysis uses observations, interviews, and questionnaires to gain information about a child and their family so that interventions and diagnostic testing can be targeted to areas of increased risk. Risk factors may be controllable (diet and exercise) or non-controllable (genetic), but once identified, a plan of care can be formulated. Risk analysis is an important component of cost-containment because early identification and treatment or intervention can reduce future costs of care. **Areas for risk analysis** may include:

- Nutrition
- Exercise
- Cardiovascular
- Diabetes
- Hypertension
- Cancer
- Osteoporosis
- Vision
- Behavior and lifestyle

Results of risk analysis are not diagnostic, but they indicate if the child is at a low, medium, or high risk of developing a disease or health problem.

COMPONENTS OF RISK ANALYSIS

Risk analysis can be used to assess individual risks or to assess the risk and effectiveness of different treatments and programs in a broader sense. Risk analysis should be carried out for all new treatments and procedures to determine if the benefits outweigh the risks and if they are cost-effective. Risk analysis should be an ongoing part of the nurse's role. There are three primary **components** to risk analysis:

- **Assessing** requires gaining information by questioning, observing, or analyzing data, which may be derived from active study or review of the research.
- **Intervening** involves taking information from the assessment and making changes in management, treatments, or procedures to reflect the risk analysis with the aim of providing the most beneficial and cost-effective care.
- **Communicating** requires publishing the results or sharing those with the organization, family, child, or the general public, depending on the scope of the risk analysis.

RISK FACTORS FOR NEONATES ASSOCIATED WITH MATERNAL DISEASE

There are a number of **maternal factors** that put the infant at increased risk:

- **Diabetes mellitus**: Both gestational and pre-existing diabetes put the infant at risk of stillbirth, hypoglycemia, and macrosomia (larger size than normal) as well as birth injury. Maternal pre-existing diabetes is also associated with birth defects, including abnormal development of the cardiovascular and gastrointestinal systems, neurological and spinal cord disorders, and urinary tract abnormalities.
- **HIV/Hepatitis B**: Infectious diseases may be transmitted during pregnancy or delivery.

IMPLICATIONS OF FETAL DRUG EXPOSURE

There are many drugs that can profoundly affect the growing fetus. Some are prescribed drugs, such as Accutane, but the greatest numbers are illicit drugs, such as crack, heroin, or cocaine. Increasing numbers of children are born to addicted mothers. While each drug has specific effects, there are many effects that are common with any type of fetal drug exposure:

- Premature weight and low birth weight with infants who are small for gestational age (SGA)
- Failure to thrive often related to poor sucking and dysphagia
- Increased risk of congenital infectious disease (HIV, hepatitis, CMV)
- Increased risk of SIDS
- Withdrawal symptoms typically manifest within 72 hours of birth:
    - Tremors, excitability, seizures
    - Vomiting, diarrhea, diaphoresis
    - Dry, red, irritated skin
- Developmental and cognitive problems that vary with age. Initial problems often subside within the first couple of years, but in a small number of children learning disabilities and behavioral problems persist.

IMPLICATIONS OF FETAL ALCOHOL SYNDROME

Fetal alcohol syndrome (FAS) is a syndrome of birth defects that develop as the result of maternal ingestion of alcohol. Despite campaigns to inform the public, women continue to drink during pregnancy, but no safe amount of alcohol ingestion has been determined. FAS results in:

- **Facial abnormalities**: Hypoplastic (underdeveloped) maxilla, micrognathia (undersized jaw), hypoplastic philtrum (groove beneath the nose), and short palpebral fissures (eye slits between upper and lower lids).
- **Neurological deficits**: May include microcephaly, intellectual disability, motor delay, and hearing deficits. Learning disorders may include problems with visual-spatial and verbal learning, attention disorders, and delayed reaction times.
- **Growth retardation**: Prenatal growth deficit persists with slow growth after birth.
- **Behavioral problems**: Irritability and hyperactivity. Poor judgment in behavior may relate to deficit in executive functions.

Indication of brain damage without the associated physical abnormalities is referred to as alcohol-related neurodevelopmental disorder (ARND).

INFANT WITHDRAWAL FROM FETAL EXPOSURE TO DRUGS

Fetal exposure to drugs, such as opioids, methadone, cocaine, crack, and other recreational drugs causes **withdrawal symptoms** in about 60% of infants. There are many variables, which include the type of drug, the extent of drug use, and the duration of maternal drug use. For example, children may have withdrawal symptoms within 48 hours for cocaine, heroin, and methamphetamine exposure, but there may be delays of up to 2-3 weeks for methadone. Short hospital stays after birth make it imperative that children who are at risk are identified so that they can receive supportive treatment, particularly since they often feed poorly and can quickly become dehydrated and undernourished. Polydrug use makes it difficult to describe a typical profile of **symptoms**, but they usually include:

- Tremors
- Irritability
- Hypertonicity
- High-pitched crying
- Diarrhea
- Dry skin
- Seizures (in severe cases)

Treatment is supportive, but children with opiate exposure may be given decreasing doses of opiates, such as morphine elixir, with close monitoring until the child is weaned off of the medication.

FETAL NICOTINE/CARBON MONOXIDE EXPOSURE

About 25% of women who smoke regularly before becoming pregnant continue to smoke throughout pregnancy, and others are exposed to second-hand smoke, putting the fetus at risk for a number of abnormalities from **exposure to nicotine and carbon monoxide**:

- Fetal growth retardation with damage to neurotransmitters accompanied by nervous system cell death with concomitant damage to peripheral autonomic nervous system
- Vasoconstriction from nicotine and interference with oxygen transport caused by carbon monoxide can lead to fetal hypoxia
- Vasoconstriction leading to increased risk of spontaneous abortion, prematurity, and low birth weight
- Increased risk for perinatal death and SIDS
- Cognitive deficiency and learning disorders, such as auditory processing defects (Children of mothers who smoke have a 50% increase in idiopathic intellectual disability.)
- Increased cancer risk, especially for acute lymphocytic leukemia and lymphoma

CARDIOVASCULAR RISK REDUCTION

Some children, specifically those with diabetes mellitus, Kawasaki disease, and familial hypercholesterolemia, are at increased risk of developing **cardiovascular disease**, which can lead to severe coronary artery disease in less than ten years from onset. Screening children who are at risk should begin at age 2 and include cholesterol levels to assess for an elevation of low-density lipoprotein (LDL):

- Total cholesterol <170 and LDL <110: Normal level
- Total cholesterol 170-199 and LDL 110-120: Borderline elevation
- Total cholesterol >200 with LDL >130: Elevated

Early dietary intervention to reduce cholesterol and prevent further increase in LDLs can significantly reduce morbidity and mortality. Dietary recommendations to reduce LDLs include guidelines provided in the *Therapeutic Lifestyle Changes* diet created by the National Institutes of Health for those at risk or with elevated cholesterol.

- 25–30% of diet should be from fat and <7% from saturated fat
- 10–25 g of soluble fiber per day
- <200 mg dietary cholesterol per day
- ≥2 g of plant sterols or stanols per day (found in vegetables, fruits, and nuts)
- 30 minutes of moderate to vigorous exercise per day

ENVIRONMENTAL ASSESSMENT
ENVIRONMENTAL HEALTH HISTORY

The environmental health history is important to determine potential hazards in the child's surroundings that may contribute to poor health or injuries. Examples of potential exposures that should be considered when taking a pediatric environmental health history include air pollution, including industrial exposure, cigarette smoke, carbon monoxide from furnaces or machinery; lead exposure through paint or plumbing in older homes; allergen exposure, such as pet dander, pollen, or mold; exposure to ultraviolet radiation during outdoor activities; water quality; and nutrition.

ENVIRONMENTAL INFLUENCES ON THE PEDIATRIC PATIENT'S HEALTH

Safety in the home environment is a big influence on the health of the child. Accidental injuries in and around the home can include burns from scalding liquids or cooking appliances, drownings in pools or bathtubs, falls from climbing or from bicycles, and motor vehicle accidents or pedestrian-car accidents. Children who spend a great deal of time watching TV or playing video games are at risk for obesity and health issues that accompany obesity. Some children may try to be like characters they see on TV shows or other media, which can lead to aggressive behavior and risk-taking.

CONSIDERATION OF ENVIRONMENTAL FACTORS PRIOR TO A CHILD'S RETURN HOME

Environmental factors should be assessed within the **actual environment** if at all possible. If not, careful questioning and drawing of diagrams and approximate floor plans with the patient (or the patient's parent)—or asking for a drawing—can be useful, especially when showing the patient needed modifications. Family members may also assist with the assessment, providing useful information. Some patients or their parents, may be reluctant to admit that the home is cluttered or that they are unable to maintain the home environment in a sanitary condition. Brochures and handouts about home safety and assistive devices should be provided to the patient and caretaker as well as contact names and numbers for equipment needed in the home. A checklist should be compiled of all necessary changes or additions, with specific details, such as "Install 18-inch grab bar across from toilet." In some cases, a social worker or occupational therapist should visit the home.

GENERAL ELEMENTS OF ENVIRONMENTAL SAFETY

Some elements of an environmental assessment are not specific to rooms in the house but are **general needs** that must be met in order for individuals, especially the disabled child and their caregivers, to remain safe:

- **Environmental hazards** such as piles of papers or junk on the floors, loose carpet or rugs, and cluttered pathways can cause falls and must be cleared, organized, or repaired.
- **Lighting** should be adequate enough for reading in all rooms and stairways.
- **Heat and air conditioning** must be adequate. The young and the elderly are especially susceptible to heat and cold injury.
- **Sanitation** should ensure that health hazards do not exist, such as from rotting food or infestations of cockroaches or rodents.

- **Animals** should be cared for adequately with access to food, water, toileting, and routine veterinary care.
- **Smoke/chemicals** in the environment may pose a hazard, such as exposure to cigarette smoke or cleaning materials.

DANGEROUS WEAPONS AND TOYS

Parents should be advised that any guns kept in the home must be secured, with the guns unloaded and with the ammunition separately secured in a different location. All children, from an early age, should be taught to never pick up a gun or point it at anyone, even in play, and to immediately tell a trusted adult if they see anyone with a gun or know of anyone, such as a peer, who is carrying a gun or intends to harm someone with a gun.

Children should be protected from **dangerous toys**, which can include toys with small parts that may cause choking, especially for infants and toddlers. Toys that shoot projectiles, have cords or strings attached, or have sharp edges may pose a risk as well. Some products, such as some types of slime, have been found to contain toxins, so parents should regularly check with the US Consumer Product Safety Commission for alerts and should always read and adhere to warning labels. Smart toys and electronic devices that connect to the internet may provide identifying information about the child to unauthorized individuals.

RECOMMENDATIONS FOR PARENTS AND CHILDREN REGARDING SOCIAL SITUATIONS

Recommendations for social situations include:

- **Strangers**: Parents should stress the importance of going places and playing outside with a friend or an adult and not being alone. Children should know to run and yell if a stranger asks them to carry something, help get something out of a car, or to help look for or see a puppy or kitten. Parents should stress that children should never get into a car with a stranger or an acquaintance who says that the child's parent has sent the person unless this person uses a password. Children should know to yell what is happening ("This woman is taking me!") and should know their full name, address, and phone number as soon as they are old enough to learn them.
- **Violence**: Parents should limit children's exposure to violent media content (TV, movies, video games) and use blocking tools when appropriate. Parents should encourage children to talk about their feeling if they've experienced or observed violence and to reassure them. If violence is common, children should play only in safe areas and learn safety rules, such as dropping to the ground if they hear gunshots.
- **Bullying**: Parents should recognize the signs that a child is being bullied (depression, withdrawal, dislike of school, change in affect, lack of friends, change of sleep patterns, bruises) and teach children the impact that bullying has on others. Advise parents to teach children to tell an adult if they are being bullied and to respond assertively, act unimpressed, make a joke out of mean comments, and get involved in activities, such as clubs, where they feel safe. If children are cyberbullied, they should block the senders, change passwords, and report it to an adult.
- **Automobile safety/distracted driving**: Children should be seated and secured properly for their age and size and should be taught to avoid yelling, throwing things, and scuffling while in the car as this may distract the driver. Teenage drivers should be taught safe driving (including never driving while drinking), should have clear consequences for unsafe driving (such as a loss of driving privileges), and should have an app on their phones that prevents texting while driving and provides their location to their parents.

Recommendations for Sports and Recreation

Recommendations regarding sports and recreation include:

- **Concussion risks**: Greatest risks are from sports activities (football, hockey, soccer, lacrosse) and accidents (fall, car/bicycle). Parents should ensure that any sports team a child participates in has adequate safety rules (limits to tackling, for example) and that coaches carefully monitor the children. Children should always wear appropriate safety gear, such as helmets, when engaged in sports activities and should never continue playing if exhibiting any signs of head injury (headache, dizziness, confusion).
- **Helmet use**: Helmets (the appropriate type) should be worn for sports activities that may involve falls or blows to the head (hockey, football, skateboarding, baseball, bicycling). Helmets should fit snuggly so that they don't move if they are rotated, turned, or tilted, and the helmet should be pressed down at the crown to check for fitting of the jaw pads and chin straps. Football helmets may be air/fluid filled or padded.

Vehicle Safety

Boat Safety

According to the US Coast Guard's recommendations for **boat safety**, infants who are not of the appropriate weight and size to wear approved personal flotation devices (PFDs) should not be taken on recreational boats (rowboats, motorboats, kayaks, sailboats). All other children should wear life jackets that are properly fitted and secured. PFDs do not include swimming aids intended for play, such as water wings or pool noodles. If an infant is on a boat, a caregiver wearing a life jacket should hold the infant at all times and should not place the child in a car seat (which will not float). Infants and young children are more likely to develop hypothermia, so they should be wrapped with a dry blanket or towel if cold and shivering. Children by about age 3 should be taught safety rules, such as keeping hands and feet inside the boat and walking instead of running. All children should take swimming lessons. Older children should take a boat safety course if possible. Adolescents should be cautioned to never engage in drinking or recreational drug use while boating.

Car Seats

All infants, regardless of age, must be placed properly in an **infant car seat** during transit. Holding an infant while the car is in motion is not safe. Car seats should be new or in very good condition and fastened according to manufacturer's guidelines to ensure safety:

- Place the car seat in the back seat and away from any side airbags.
- Always securely buckle the child into the seat.
- Face the infant seat toward the rear of the car.
- Recline the seat so that the infant's head does not fall forward.
- Place padding around (not under) the infant if the infant slouches to one side.
- Place blankets OVER the straps and buckles, not under.

The infant/toddler should be placed in the rear-facing seat to the maximum weight and height allowed by the seat (some accommodate up to 65 pounds). Once transitioned to front-facing seats, children should be placed in belt-positioning booster seats until the vehicle's seat/shoulder belts fit properly (usually until 4' 9" and 8-12 years old). Until age 13, children should sit secured in the back seat and not the front.

Leading Causes of Death By Age Group

Birth to 10-Year Age Group

For the **birth to 10-year** age group, the US Preventive Services Task Force has assembled a list of the **five leading causes of death**. The number one cause of death in this age group is actually a group of conditions that arise in the time period surrounding birth (the "**perinatal period**"). There are a number of conditions that arise surrounding birth that are fatal, including placental problems (premature separation, abruption), umbilical cord problems (cord prolapse, nuchal cord, single umbilical artery), infections (chorioamnionitis, congenital pneumonia), trauma during the birthing process (nerve damage, intracranial hemorrhage), and hemolytic disease of the newborn. The second leading cause of death is attributed to **congenital defects**, including tetralogy of Fallot, transposition of the great arteries, spina bifida, and anencephaly. Other leading causes of death include **sudden infant death syndrome (SIDS), motor vehicle injuries**, and **other unintentional injuries**.

INJURY PREVENTION COUNSELING

Injury prevention counseling is a strong recommendation for the **birth to 10-year** age group, owing to the fact that motor vehicle accidents and other unintentional accidents are leading causes of death for this population. Children and their parents should be advised to use car safety seats until the age of 5 (this is subject to state law, however, as some states require the use of booster seats until a certain height or age is reached). After the age of 5, standard safety belts should always be used. When biking, skating, or skateboarding, a helmet should always be worn; these activities should not take place in the street. Parents should be advised to become CPR certified. They should also be advised to keep drugs, poisons, guns, other weapons, and matches out of the reach of children; to install smoke detectors and plan an escape route in the event of fire; and to make sure that stairs, windows, and pools are safe for children.

11- TO 24-YEAR AGE GROUP

The list of the top five leading causes of death in the **11-24** age population differs significantly from the leading causes of death in the birth to 10-year age population. Leading the list for ages 11-24 are deaths caused by either **motor vehicle accidents or other unintentional accidents**. Second on the list is **homicide**, followed by **suicide**. The fourth leading cause of death in the 11-24 age population is **cancer**. The most common fatal cancers in this age group include leukemia (acute lymphocytic leukemia and acute myeloid leukemia), brain tumors (medulloblastoma, astrocytoma, and brainstem glioma), rhabdomyosarcoma, neuroblastoma, Wilms tumor, Ewing sarcoma, and Hodgkin's lymphoma. The fifth leading cause of death in this age population is due to **general heart diseases**, which may include cardiomyopathies and faulty valves.

YOUTH RISK BEHAVIOR SURVEILLANCE SYSTEM

The **Youth Risk Behavior Surveillance System** (YRBSS) is a program conducted through the CDC that monitors eight different categories of health-risk behaviors of adolescents:

- Unintentional injuries and violence
- Tobacco use
- Alcohol and other drug use
- Sexual behaviors
- Dietary behaviors
- Physical activity
- Obesity, overweight, and weight control
- Other health topics

The YRBSS gathers data from participating states and local surveys (such as large cities) from grades 9-12 and then compiles the information, assessing for trends. Current results reflect data collected in 2021 and released in 2023. Responses are either weighted (≥60% participation) or unweighted (relates only to those completing survey). Weighted results can be generalized to the teenage population at large in the area of the survey. The data obtained in the YRBSS is used to determine progress in national health objectives for health promotion.

YRBSS 2021 RESULTS
TOBACCO USE

The CDC conducts the Youth Risk Behavior Surveillance System to determine health-risk behaviors that contribute to significant morbidity in adolescents. **Tobacco,** often thought of as an adult issue, is a cause of concern for children and teenagers. Tobacco use is one of the leading preventable causes of death in the United

States, but 2021 results showed that about 6.3% of children (down from 9.5% in 2019) have tried smoking before high school, often beginning by age 12, putting themselves at risk for heart and lung disease as adults. Almost 18% of children have tried smoking in total according to 2021 results, which is a downward trend. A newer trend is the use of electronic vapor products, with 36% of children reporting having tried this product at some point, and 18% reporting current use. Those most at risk are males in low-income families with parents who smoke. Male adolescents may smoke to be rebellious, but females often smoke to lose weight. Other factors include the desire to be part of a group, lack of supervision, and accessibility of tobacco. Intervention includes identifying those smoking, providing information about the dangers of smoking, beginning with children at about 9 years old, and providing programs to help teenagers quit smoking.

DRUG USE

Drug use continues to be a serious problem for children and teenagers, with some starting as young as 9 or 10, using a wide variety of drugs, including marijuana, crack, prescription drugs, cocaine, inhalants (such as glue and lighter fluid), hallucinogens, and steroids. Marijuana is the most reported drug in the high school data, with about 28% of children reporting having used marijuana in their lifetime. Approximately 13% of children reported having used illicit drugs (e.g., cocaine, heroin, inhalants, methamphetamines, ecstasy, or hallucinogens) at least once in their lifetime. Risk factors for drug use include aggressive behavior, poor social skills, and poor academic progress coupled with lack of parental supervision, poverty, and availability of drugs. Small children who use drugs are often reacting to circumstances within the family, while teenagers are more likely to use drugs in response to peer pressure from outside the family. Studies have shown that early intervention to teach children better self-control and coping skills is often more effective than trying to change behavior patterns that are established, so family-based programs often show positive results. Teenagers may need help with basic academic skills and social skills to improve communication. Methods of resisting drugs must be provided and reinforced. Drug recovery programs can be helpful but are often too expensive or not available for those who need them.

ALCOHOL USE

Alcohol use is a significant problem in adolescence and even in younger children. It is the most-commonly abused substance. Of high schoolers who responded to the survey question in 2021, about 23% reported having had at least one drink within the past 30 days (down from 30% in 2019). While alcohol can impair development of almost all body systems in a growing child, it is of particular concern for the effects on the neurological system and liver. Additionally, because it interferes with impulse control, adolescents who drink are often involved in violence, abuse, and at-risk sexual behavior. Drinking should be suspected if a child has memory problems, changes in behavior, poor academic progress, emotional lability, and physical changes, such as slurring of speech, general lethargy, or lack of coordination. Intervention includes teaching children from around age 9 about the dangers of drinking, identifying those who are drinking, identifying underlying problems, and providing programs to help teenagers stop drinking, such as counseling or Alcoholics Anonymous.

HIGH-RISK SEXUAL BEHAVIOR

High-risk sexual behavior in teenagers is often coupled with other health-risk behaviors, such as drinking and drug use. In 2021, about 30% of high school students reported having previously had sex (a significant decline from the 38.4% reported in 2019), with around 3% becoming sexually active before the age of 13. Risk factors include poverty, single-family homes, lack of supervision, and siblings or peers who are sexually active. Those who have sex before age 15 are especially vulnerable, often having multiple partners and unprotected sex, leading to sexually transmitted infections (STIs) and pregnancy. They are often emotionally vulnerable and unable to deal effectively with relationships. Intervention should begin early with age-appropriate honest sex education. Abstinence education, while the ideal, has not been successful in changing the sexual behavior of teenagers, with studies showing that many of those signing pledges to remain virgins are already sexually active. Teenagers who are sexually active should be advised regarding the use of condoms, birth control, and protection from STIs in a non-judgmental manner.

PREVENTION OF STIs

The **CDC** has developed five strategies to prevent and control the spread of STIs:

- **Educate** those at risk about how to make changes in sexual practices to prevent infection.
- **Identify** symptomatic and asymptomatic infected persons who might not seek diagnosis or treatment.
- **Diagnose** and treat those who are infected.
- **Prevent infection** of sex partners through evaluation, treatment, and counseling.
- Provide pre-exposure **vaccination** for those at risk.

Practitioners are advised to inquire of patients' **sexual histories** and to assess risk. The 5-P approach to questioning is advocated. Practitioners should ask about:

- **Partners**: Gender and number
- **Pregnancy prevention**: Birth control
- **Protection**: Methods used
- **Practices**: Type of sexual practices (oral, anal, vaginal) and use of condoms
- **Past history of STIs**: High-risk behavior (promiscuity, prostitution) and disease risk (human immunodeficiency virus [HIV]/ hepatitis)

The CDC recommends a number of specific preventive methods as part of the clinical guidelines for prevention of sexually transmitted infections:

- **Abstinence or reduction** in number of sex partners.
- Pre-exposure **vaccination**: All those evaluated for STIs should receive hepatitis B vaccination, and men who have sex with men (MSM) and illicit drug users should receive hepatitis A vaccination.
- **Male latex (or polyurethane) condoms** should be used for all sexual encounters with only water-based lubricants used with latex.
- **Female condoms** may be used if a male condom cannot be used properly.
- Condoms and diaphragms should not be used with spermicides containing **nonoxynol-9 (N-9)**, and N-9 should not be used as a lubricant for anal sex.
- **Non-barrier contraceptive measures** provide no protection from STIs and must not be relied on to prevent disease.

MEASURES TO PREVENT INJURY/ILLNESS OF TODDLERS
HOME AND AUTO SAFETY

Toddlers are curious and very mobile, so accidents can occur easily in and outside the home. **Auto safety** includes using the appropriate size child-safety seat in the back seat, and buckling the child up every time they are in a moving vehicle. Toddlers need to be supervised closely when playing outside, to prevent them from running into the street in front of moving vehicles. Parents can begin to teach them how to stop, look, and listen before crossing a street.

The home environment needs to be child-proofed, moving all poisonous substances well away from the toddler's reach (keeping in mind that toddlers will learn to climb). Poisons should be stored in a locked or inaccessible location to the child. Medication should be stored up high and children should not be told that medication is candy when they are taking it.

Water, Toy, and Gun Safety, and Burns

The following are some measures the parents can take to prevent injury and illness of their toddler, focusing on burns and water, toy, and gun safety:

- Never leave a toddler alone in or near water, as they can drown in as little as one inch of water. Toddlers are still unstable and prone to falling, possibly into a puddle or bucket.
- When appropriate, life jackets should be worn by toddlers (in a boat or near a lake, pond, or pool).
- Toddlers should wear helmets when riding tricycles.
- Make sure any toys given to toddlers are appropriate for their age and safe. Balloons, small toys, and plastic bags are potential choking hazards.
- A big concern today is guns kept in the home. Toddlers don't know the difference between a toy gun and a real gun, so all guns kept in the home must be properly secured.
- Teach the toddler the meaning of "hot," while using safety plugs on appliances, keep matches and lighters up high, turn pot handles toward the back of the stove, and don't use tablecloths in the home (toddlers can pull on these and topple hot food/liquids on themselves).

Measures to Prevent Injury/Illness of Preschoolers
Home and Auto Safety

Preschoolers are aware of potential dangers and can be taught safety rules. Poisonous substances, including medicines, need to have safety caps and be locked up. Watch for unsafe areas at playgrounds. Enforce the wearing of safety equipment when playing sports. Use the appropriate safety seat (booster) in the back seat until the child weighs 80 lb. After 80 lb, use a seat belt in the back seat. Do not leave a child alone in a car or home. Use close supervision when playing outside and near streets. Have the child wear a bike helmet when riding and teach him the rules for safe riding. Parents should have the poison control number saved to their phones or written down somewhere it can be quickly accessed.

Auto, Sports, and Water Safety

School age children are especially prone to accidents, due to their mobility and participation in sports and other physical activities. The following rules should be taught to children and enforced by the parents/caregivers:

- Children should always wear a seatbelt, and sit in the backseat, in a moving vehicle.
- When riding anything with wheels, the child should always wear a helmet and elbow and knee pads.
- The child must obey traffic signals when walking on or across streets.
- The school-aged child should participate in swim lessons and be taught to swim with a buddy, wear a life jacket when in a boat, and not dive into shallow water.

Measures to Prevent Injury/Illness of School Age Children

The following are some measures parents can take to prevent injury/illness of their school age child, focusing on drug, fire, stranger, and gun safety:

- Keep medicine locked and teach children the dangers of taking any medicine without adult supervision.
- Begin teaching the child about illegal drug use and smoking.
- Use sunscreen when playing outside.
- Establish an escape route for each member of the family in case of fire and practice the route monthly.
- Don't allow the child to use the stove without adult supervision.
- Teach the child to stay away from guns. Parents should keep guns unloaded and in a locked location with ammunition stored in a separate location.
- Teach the child to not talk to strangers or approach strange vehicles.
- Make sure the child knows their phone number, their address, and how to call 911.
- Find a neighbor's house that can serve as a safe place for the child if needed.

Measures to Prevent Injury/Illness of Adolescents

Adolescents think they are invincible, which can contribute to risk-taking behaviors.

- Motor vehicle accidents claim many teenagers' lives every year. Teens should take driver's education courses, wear seat belts at all times, obey traffic laws, and refrain from drinking and driving.
- If an adolescent legally uses firearms, they need to be taught safety rules and how to use and store firearms.
- Adolescents should be taught the risks of using drugs, alcohol, and nicotine.
- Sports teams should focus on safety, proper equipment, and appropriate conditioning.
- Adolescents should know proper swimming and water safety and use sunscreen when outside.
- Sexual activity is a high-risk behavior that should be addressed on a family level. If appropriate, the adolescent should be taught sexual responsibility.

Appropriate Sunscreen Use

While children need some exposure to the sun, sunscreen protects against harmful ultraviolet rays that can cause burns, sun damage, premature aging, and skin cancer. Sunscreen should be generously applied before children go out in the sun, covering the parts of the body that are exposed, including the face, lips, tops of the ears, and back of the neck. It should be reapplied at least every 2 hours, and if children are going to be around water, the sunscreen should be waterproof. The sun protection factor (SPF) should be a minimum of 30 for children older than 6 months, as recommended by the American Academy of Dermatology. The American Academy of Pediatrics recommends that children under the age of 6 months be kept out of direct sunlight. If they must be in direct sunlight, children should be covered by clothing and hats. A small amount of SPF 15 sunscreen is allowed on children under the age of 6 months, but only to small areas such as their face and the backs of their hands.

Guidelines for Using Insect Repellant

Insect repellant may be used on children to prevent insect bites, but it should be used with caution. Many insect repellants contain N,N-diethyl-meta-toluamide (DEET), which has been shown to be safe for limited use with children over 2 months of age. Repellants used on children should have less than a 30% concentration of DEET and should only be applied once a day. It should be sprayed on a caregiver's hand and then put on the child, rather than spraying the child directly. This decreases the likelihood of the child ingesting the repellant. Insect repellant can also be applied to clothing to provide some protection without applying it directly to the skin.

Screening Procedures for Children Throughout Childhood

Many screening procedures are available, including extensive laboratory testing that may be indicated if there is cause for concern that a child may have a disorder. However, some basic screening should be done for all children:

- **Genetic disorders:** Screening is usually done at birth according to state guidelines, and further testing may be indicated if there is concern that a child has a disorder that requires treatment.
- **Hearing:** Testing is usually done with newborns, between ages 3 and 8, and then every 2-3 years until age 18.
- **Height and weight:** These are monitored monthly during the first year and then at least yearly until age 18 to determine if the child's development is within the normal range.
- **Vision:** This is screened at birth, at 3-4 years, and periodically between 5-18. Vision problems may become obvious when the child enters school and can't see the board or has trouble reading.
- **Fasting blood sugar:** Done every 2 years for those at risk.
- **Head circumference:** Measurement is done at birth, 1 year, and 2 years.
- **Blood pressure:** This is usually checked during infancy (6-12 months) and then periodically throughout childhood.
- **Dental screening:** Bottle fed babies may require earlier screening as they often fall asleep with the bottle in their mouths, leading to infant caries. Dental screening is done periodically throughout childhood, especially after the new teeth come in, to evaluate for malocclusion or other problems.
- **Alcohol/drug use:** Screening may be done periodically for children between 11-18 years, especially if they are at risk.
- **Developmental screening:** There are a number of screening tests that are available and can be used if a child appears to have a developmental delay or abnormality. Screening tests must be age-appropriate. The tests are not diagnostic, but can help to confirm developmental abnormalities. Tests may assess motor skills, language, and cognitive ability.

Screening Children for Celiac Disease

Celiac disease is gluten-sensitive enteropathy with a chronic malabsorption syndrome caused by damage to the villi from toxic reactions to gluten in wheat, barley, rye, and oats. Symptoms normally don't appear until the child begins a diet of solid foods and exhibits chronic diarrhea, vomiting, and failure to thrive. A careful family history may indicate a genetic disposition, but these warning symptoms should trigger screening even without such history. Additionally, 4-13% of children with trisomy 21 (Down syndrome) have celiac disease, so screening is recommended for all infants with trisomy 21. Identifying children with celiac disease early and providing dietary counseling for the parents can prevent the damage to the intestines that will otherwise occur. Parents and eventually the child should be taught dietary substitutions and referred to national organizations, such as the American Celiac Society and the Celiac-Sprue Association, which can provide information and support.

Screening of Teenagers for Scoliosis

Scoliosis is the lateral curvature ≥11° of the spine, usually occurring (in 2-3% of adolescents) during the period between 10-15 when the child goes through a growth spurt, so screening should be done at least twice during this period. Scoliosis is more common in girls than boys. Screening includes:

- Child stands upright and shoulders, waist, and hips are assessed.
- Adams forward bending test, in which the child bends over at the waist (as in toe touching) and the screener observes the hips to determine if there is a difference in height.
- Scoliometer measures the curvature of the spine in the thoracic and lumbar area when the child bends over.
- Moire topography uses a grating positioned near the child so it casts shadows that show contour lines.
- X-rays are used to confirm positive screenings.

Positive findings may include one shoulder lower than another, uneven waistline, prominence of shoulder blade(s), one hip higher than another, or lateral leaning when upright.

COLLECTION OF BLOOD SPECIMENS
COLLECTION OF CAPILLARY BLOOD SAMPLES

The **heel stick** is used in infants up to 6 months of age. The heel is warmed for 5 to 10 minutes, followed by cleaning with an alcohol wipe. Special lancets should be used that ensure the puncture goes no deeper than 2 mm. The outside or inside edge of the heel should be used to prevent osteochondritis. After the specimen is collected, apply pressure until bleeding has stopped and apply a bandage. A colorful bandage will help reassure school age children and keep dirt out of the wound. Pain control should be provided to reduce the pain and stress associated with blood draws.

COLLECTION OF VENOUS AND ARTERIAL BLOOD SPECIMENS

The nurse is responsible for overseeing that the **blood specimens** are collected according to protocol, including the timing of collections, the equipment used, and the transportation and storage of the specimens. Venous samples are obtained from an access line (the type of fluid being infused may affect the blood values) or by venipuncture. Pressure is applied after venipuncture to prevent bruising, followed by a bandage. Central lines are the preferred access lines, as peripheral lines are prone to being replaced more often when used to collect blood. Arterial samples are useful for measuring blood gases, using an arterial catheter inserted into the femoral, brachial, or radial arteries or using deep heel stick. Always assess for circulatory problems before attempting an arterial draw. Make sure the child is calm, as crying can affect the values. Heparinized tubes are used to prevent clotting of the blood, and care is taken to ensure that no air bubbles enter the tube. Provide explanations to children according developmental level. Provide pain control as needed.

POSITIONING TECHNIQUES FOR VENIPUNCTURES IN PEDIATRIC PATIENTS

Painful procedures require adequate pain relief. Older children can cooperate and need little restraint. Babies and younger children need good positioning to comfort them and decrease movement. A jugular venipuncture requires that the infant be placed in a mummy restraint (wrapped in a blanket in such a way that restrains the arms and legs) or that the older child's arms and legs are restrained. A small pillow is placed under the neck, the neck is extended, and the head positioned and held still. After the procedure, pressure is applied to the site for 3-5 minutes without compromising breathing or circulation. A femoral venipuncture requires the infant to be supine with the legs turned out. The legs are restrained. For a venipuncture in an extremity, stabilize the arm or leg while another person hugs the child to prevent movement and helps to hold the extremity.

DIAGNOSTIC PURPOSE OF IMAGING TESTS
X-Ray

X-rays are used for diagnosis and evaluation of treatment and to determine correct placement of medical devices. **X-rays** pass more readily through soft tissue than dense tissue, so dense tissue, which has less radiation exposure, appears as white against the darker background of soft tissue. Therefore, x-rays are most commonly used for evaluation of bones, such as for fractures or dislocations. They may also be used for soft tissue when a disease or disorder alters density of tissue, such as with pneumonia in the lungs or gallstones, kidney stones, or tumors although small tumors may go undetected. Different types of tissue have different color gradations. For example, organs with high fluid content (stomach, liver) appear gray while muscles (which have more fat) appear slightly darker. Spaces filled with air (such as the lungs) appear very dark. X-rays may also be used with contrast medium to take images of the cardiovascular or GI systems.

CT Scan

Computerized tomography (CT) involves scanning tissue in successive layers through a narrow-beam x-ray, providing a cross-sectional view. CTs can demonstrate differences in soft-tissue density. CT scans may be done with fluoroscopy or contrast material, such as iodine dye, to evaluate for infections, tumors, or other abnormalities. CT scans can differentiate between cellulitis and formation of abscesses better than a routine x-ray.

MRI

Magnetic resonance imaging (MRI) uses magnetic fields and radiofrequency signals to create a cross-sectional view, and the images are more detailed than with CT. MRI may be done with or without contrast material. MRI uses radio waves and magnetic fields to create images of internal structures, providing information about infections, tumors, or other abnormalities that may not be obvious with x-rays, CT scans, or ultrasounds. MRIs are more expensive than x-rays, CTs, or ultrasounds, so they are often done after other testing has been inconclusive.

Ultrasound

Ultrasound uses ultrasonic sound waves transmitted by a transducer, which picks up reflected sound waves that a computer converts to electronic images. **Ultrasound** can show fluid accumulation, the movement of blood through the organs, masses, malformations (congenital abnormalities), change in size of the organs or other structures, and obstructions.

Overnight Polysomnogram

An overnight polysomnogram (PSG) is a sleep study, which is often used when a child presents with some type of sleep disorder, such as night terrors or sleepwalking. A PSG requires an overnight stay in a sleep lab. Sensors are connected to the child's head to measure brain activity and eye movement during the study. Pulse oximetry may also be used to assess oxygen levels during sleep. The child is connected to the sensors and then goes to sleep in the room. Typically, a parent is allowed to sleep in the same room during the study to reduce the child's fears.

Differential Diagnosis

Process

The differential diagnosis is an important tool that allows the clinician to become familiar with the patient's condition, understand the condition, create an effective treatment plan, and follow the progress of the patient. To start, thoroughly examine the patient's chart, making a list of all of the abnormal test results and laboratory values. Add to this list all of the patient's complaints. Once this list is complete, organize the test results, labs, and complaints by anatomic location or organ system. After breaking the list down by organ site, look for any relationships between symptoms and/or results. Create another list of those data that seem to be related, and list all of the diseases or conditions that explain the findings, eliminating any that do not fit.

Influences on the Clinical Decision-Making Process

Although one would like to think that there isn't much variation in the **clinical decision-making process**, this simply is not true. The process, of course, will differ depending on the patient, the differential diagnosis, and the clinician. Let's start with the clinician. The way the clinician conducts the clinical decision-making process is influenced by the knowledge base of the clinician, as well as the level of his experience, the ability he possesses to think both critically and creatively, and the confidence that he has in his ability to make educated decisions. The acuity level of the patient is also a factor in the clinical decision-making process, as is the length of the differential. A time stressor is placed on the clinician when the condition of the patient is critical, and when there are more diseases that must be eliminated from the differential. An element of stress may also exist if the clinician has a high number of patients, especially if there are multiple high-acuity patients.

Comprehensive History and Physical Assessment

COMPONENTS OF HEALTH HISTORY

There are several different components that must be included in a nursing **health history**:

- The **biographic element** of the nursing health history includes the patient's name, age, physical address, sex, marital status, occupational status, religious preference, healthcare financing, and regular physician.
- The **chief complaint** is the next aspect of the history and involves the reason the patient is seeking care.
- Following this, the **history of the present illness** details the current health problem, including date of onset, description of symptoms, and any aggravating factors.
- **Past medical history** entails asking about the patient's usual health status, past medical or surgical problems, immunization status, current medications, allergies (including medication allergies), and family history.
- A detailed **family history** is important as it may reveal risk factors for certain medical conditions such as heart disease, diabetes, arthritis, hypertension, or mental disorders.
- The **review of systems** is used to obtain a full, systematic report by the patient on subjective symptoms. For example, in inquiring about the cardiovascular system, the nurse notes positive or negative answers regarding chest pain and other symptoms or problems that are pertinent to heart function and circulation.

SOCIAL DETERMINANTS OF HEALTH

Social determinants of health refer to the non-medical elements of a person's social environment that have a direct impact on his or her physical health and tendencies. The heavy influence of this component of health is reflected in its being listed as one of the five main sections of *Healthy People 2030*, an initiative of the US Department of Health and Human Services (HHS) that aims to allow people to have longer and healthier lives, to reduce health disparities, to create environments that promote health, and to improve the quality of life and health across all age groups. According to HHS, social determinants of health are "the conditions in the environments where people are born, live, learn, work, play, worship, and age that affect a wide range of health, functioning, and quality-of-life outcomes and risks." For these reasons, a health history should inquire into the patient's social determinants of health also:

- The patient's **lifestyle** is an important component of the nursing health history and includes habits, diet, sleep, hobbies, and the patient's ability to perform the activities of daily living.
- A **social history** is the component of the nursing health history that details family relationships, ethnicity, educational level, economic status, and the condition of the patient's home and environment.
- The nursing health history also includes the patient's **psychological status** and the patient's **usual means of obtaining healthcare**.

Obtaining a Health History

The health history assessment and review of systems help to identify nursing care needs:

- First, check the patient's chart for information gathered by other health professionals and note any areas that need clarification prior to the patient interview.
- Use the written or electronic template provided by the facility to record the history, customizing it to the patient.
- Record any changes in this information during the patient's hospital stay.
- Plan the time of the interview with the patient when there are not critical care needs that must be met first.
- Take time to alleviate patient's anxiety and establish rapport and trust.
- Approach the patient with an attitude of respect and sincere caring.
- Listen to the patient and use effective therapeutic communication skills during the interview.
- Review all areas of the health history with the patient and then ask for any other information that may be important. The family may be able to fill in missing information if the patient is unable to do so.

Organs That Maintain Homeostasis in the Body

The organs of homeostatic function include the following:

- **Lungs**: The lungs help maintain acid-base balance by releasing CO_2. They also remove water via expired air.
- **Kidneys**: The kidneys maintain fluid balance in the body by filtering the blood and releasing fluid as needed. Electrolyte levels are maintained in the same way. Wastes and toxins are removed from the blood and body in the urine. The pH of the blood is maintained via the retention of hydrogen ions.
- **Heart**: The heart must pump blood with sufficient force to properly perfuse all organs and to push enough blood through the kidneys for filtering.
- **Adrenal glands**: Aldosterone and cortisol are produced by the adrenals to cause the kidneys to retain sodium and fluids.
- **Pituitary gland**: The pituitary stores and releases antidiuretic hormone (ADH) from the hypothalamus to direct the kidneys to retain fluids to maintain cellular osmotic pressure.
- **Parathyroid glands**: Parathyroid hormone maintains calcium and phosphate levels by causing calcium absorption by the intestines and renal tubules and from the bones as needed.

Daily Gain and Loss of Fluids

The body's fluid gains and losses should be about equal on a daily basis to maintain fluid and electrolyte balance. This can be monitored by measuring **intake** and **output** (I&O), but a number of other factors must be considered as well:

Fluid gains are as follows:

- Food people eat each day contains about 1000 mL of fluid.
- Fluids they drink average 1300 mL per day.
- Metabolic processes produce about 300 mL of fluid per day.

Fluid losses are as follows:

- Fluid is lost via the kidneys by production of 1–2 L of urine daily.
- The skin sweats and this evaporates an average of 600 mL daily, but this can increase up to 1000 mL/hr in hot and dry climates, during fever, during exercise or as a result of burns. Fluid loss can decrease in hot humid conditions.
- Exhaled air accounts for 300–400 mL of fluid loss daily.
- Fluids lost in stools total about 100–200 mL daily.

PHYSICAL EXAMINATION TECHNIQUES

The **physical exam** is an important element of nursing assessment. The physical assessment needs to be organized and systematic and should be age- and developmentally-appropriate. The physical exam may be a complete physical exam, a system-specific exam, or an exam of a specific body part. The basic **techniques** of a physical exam are inspection, palpation, auscultation, and percussion. The nurse makes a visual, aural, and olfactory assessment of the patient. This includes paying attention to the patient's skin tone, breathing sounds, and breath odor. Palpation includes techniques for touching the patient's body in order to get physical information such as temperature, skin tone and condition, or swelling in the glands. Auscultation is the examination of sounds within the body, such as heart tones, wheezing or crackling in the lungs, or bowel sounds. Auscultation is usually performed with a stethoscope. Percussion involves making quick taps to parts of the body with the fingers to ascertain the shape and condition of organs, identify areas of tenderness, or assess reflexes.

PALPATION

Use of palpation can provide valuable details during physical assessment of the patient:

- Be sure to wash and warm the hands prior to touching the patient.
- Do not use gloves unless you anticipate contact with bodily fluids.
- Explain the process and how it will feel and instruct the patient to relax the muscles if appropriate. Provide warmth and privacy during palpation.
- Use light palpation to feel the cervical lymph nodes and thyroid glands and to feel the superficial blood vessels for thrills.
- Place your hands on the chest to detect heart vibrations and to feel tactile fremitus during speech.
- Palpate the relaxed abdomen to identify structures and their borders and any masses or nodules on otherwise smooth organ surfaces. Of note, the abdomen should be auscultated prior to palpation since palpation may cause bowel sounds that would not otherwise exist and may be misunderstood.
- Utilize both hands to palpate the female reproductive organs by pushing organs into the reach of the other hand.

Palpation to identify organs and structures takes practice. Each patient is different but after you palpate many patients, the similarities in organ borders and consistency can be determined.

PALPATING FOR TACTILE FREMITUS

The act of speaking causes the chest wall to vibrate. This vibration can be felt by placing your hands lightly on the chest wall over a section of the lungs bilaterally while the patient repeats the letter "e" or the numbers "99." The amount of vibration felt depends on the weight of the patient, the muscle mass of the chest and back, gender, deepness of the voice, and condition of the lungs. **Tactile fremitus** is greater over major airways and normal lung tissue. It is less over lungs full of air or with emphysema or a pneumothorax. Lung consolidation will produce increased fremitus. The nurse should not feel for fremitus over the sternum or scapula. The areas above and below the breasts and above, medial to, and below the scapulae should be tested.

PERCUSSION

Percussion is striking part of the body to set the chest or abdominal wall into motion, producing sound that helps to locate underlying organs and reveal whether they are dense or filled with air or fluid. The sounds produced include:

- **Tympany**: Hollow drum sound produced when the organ contains air (stomach, intestines)
- **Resonance**: Hollow, low-pitched sound of normal lungs
- **Hyperresonance**: Low-pitched sound of lungs with emphysema or pneumothorax (louder than resonance)
- **Dullness**: "thud" heard over dense structures such as the liver
- **Flatness**: sound heard over muscles or bones such as in the thigh

Percussion is performed by placing the middle finger of one hand over the area and striking it with the middle finger of the opposite hand. It can be used to find the margins of an organ or area of pathology by repeatedly striking areas near to each other and listening for changes in sound representing the edge of the organ. The extent of lung consolidation can be determined in this manner.

AUSCULTATION

Auscultation is listening to sounds within the body through either the bell or the diaphragm of the stethoscope. These sounds differ in the following ways:

- **Intensity**: The level of sound in terms of loudness
- **Frequency**: Low or high pitch of the sound
- **Quality**: Helps to distinguish between rumbling and musical-type sounds

The **bell** of the stethoscope is best when listening for the lower frequency sounds of heart murmurs or bruit, with the bell placed lightly on the skin. The **diaphragm** is best for high-pitched sounds, such as heart or lung sounds or bowel sounds, with the diaphragm placed firmly on the skin. The nurse should not touch the tubing or place the end of the stethoscope in contact with cloth or hair, or extra sounds will be heard that may obscure the sounds transmitted.

Pediatric History and Physical Assessment

MEDICAL AND SURGICAL HISTORY

The pediatric nurse is expected to demonstrate competency in assessment, including **medical and surgical history**, as part of identifying and managing health concerns in infants and children. Complete and accurate documentation of findings is an essential element of the plan of care. **History** may be collected in the classic manner that begins with a complaint and includes health history, surgical history, review of systems, nutrition, developmental status, family history, and socioeconomic factors that may affect the health issue. This should include detailed information about medical conditions, treatments, and surgery.

A **problem-oriented history** builds upon the classic history by focusing on developmental health problems, functional problems, and diseases, moving from subjective information (history) to objective (physical/laboratory data):

- Developmental assessment includes motor, speech, cognitive, social, and adaptive behaviors.
- Functional assessment includes issues related to basic health behavior patterns, such as diet, sleeping, coping, sexuality, and elimination.
- Diseases are those diagnoses according to the *International Classification of Diseases,* Clinical Modification (ICD-10-CM, used to classify morbidity data), and interventions are planned based on diagnosis.

MEDICAL AND SURGICAL HISTORY OF THE ADOLESCENT

While the essential elements of assessment and medical and surgical history for **adolescents** are similar to those for infants and children, there are some differences because often the adolescent is providing, or in some cases withholding, information. Additionally, the risk factors associated with adolescence vary from those of infancy or earlier childhood. Assessment should include lifestyle information, such as whether the teenager has been homeless, engaged in high-risk sexual behavior, violence, tobacco use, or drug use. Documenting nutrition, weight concerns, peer relationships, and coping mechanisms can help to identify health concerns. A complete history should include information about medical conditions, treatment, and surgery. Successful assessment includes:

- Listen and show respect for the adolescent
- Question adolescent/parent cause for concern
- Interview both the adolescent and the parent(s) alone
- Observe nonverbal behavior and interactions among children and parents

DIFFERENCE FROM ADULT HISTORY

Pediatric histories differ from adult histories in both their content and the method of obtaining the history. The content differs because of the patient's age, and parents are the most likely source of information for a pediatric history. Differences between a pediatric history and an adult history include the following: the prenatal history, including significant events during pregnancy and the history of the child's development, including the ages of developmental milestones.

TYPES OF HEALTH HISTORIES

Depending on the status of the child at the exam, the nurse may need to take one or more of three different **types of health histories**.

- The **initial history** is the child's health history from gestation until the present time; it includes the birth history, developmental milestones, and any illnesses. The initial history is often taken at a preliminary visit to a pediatric practitioner when no other history is available.
- The **well interim history** is taken when an initial history is on file. The well interim history outlines any significant health events that have occurred since the last visit.

- The **episodic history** is taken to confirm events that have led up to the current visit. For example, an episodic history for a child with an arm fracture would involve a description of the activities that resulted in the injury.

ENVIRONMENTAL CONSIDERATIONS WHEN COLLECTING HISTORY

Obtaining a pediatric history may be challenging because of the time it takes to gather data while managing the behavior of a child. If siblings are also present, there may be more distractions. An **environment** that is most suitable for taking a pediatric history is one that is conducive to gaining information in the quickest and most accurate way possible, with minimal distractions. Depending on the age of the child, the nurse may take the history in a quiet room that is separate from others, which protects the privacy of the family as well. While minimal distractions may help with collecting information, some locations may offer toys or activities to keep the child busy so the nurse has adequate time to talk with the caregiver without interruption.

METHODS OF GATHERING INFORMATION FOR PEDIATRIC HISTORY

The information from a pediatric history may be **gathered** through several means, depending on the location. Some offices have preprinted forms that allow parents to fill out the information about their child, whether it is before the office visit or on admission. With these forms, parents must "fill in the blanks," but there is also space to describe illnesses and conditions that may be affecting the child. A face-to-face interview is another method of gathering information when no forms are available; this is suitable when the child is seen emergently or when the present illness or injury must be addressed quickly.

TYPES OF INFORMANTS

The **most common person to give information** about the pediatric patient is the parent. Foster parents, adoptive parents, and legal guardians may also be informants; however, depending on the length of time the adult has known the child, the information may not be as comprehensive as that from a parent who has cared for the child since birth. Older children and teens may provide information about themselves if they are capable of answering questions. In emergent situations or if a parent is not available, the person who has brought the child for care may be the informant. This may be emergency personnel, teachers, neighbors, or friends. In the absence of parents, a child's medical record may also be a source of valuable information.

IN LOCO PARENTIS

In loco parentis is a Latin term used to describe a person standing in place of the parent. Legally, the term means the responsibility of a caregiver for a child whose parent may be unavailable during assessment or treatment. Examples of *in loco parentis* include cases where a child is taken for medical treatment by someone in authority at school, daycare, or another organization, when the parent is unavailable or in cases of guardianship or foster placement. In these situations, the caregiver would provide as much information about the patient's history as possible.

EFFECTS OF FAMILY MEMBERS ON PATIENT HISTORY AND ABILITY TO GAIN INFORMATION

Family members can be great sources of information when taking a patient history, but they may also be distracting or disruptive, prohibiting attempts at gathering information. The nurse should assess the situation before attempting the patient history to minimize distractions as much as possible. Ideas include providing toys and activities that may keep the patient's siblings busy during the interview; offering reading materials, television, or other pursuits during the interview to prevent interruptions; or asking another nurse or professional to monitor or talk with family members while assessing the patient.

Identifying Caregivers' Perception of Child's Baseline

During times of emergency, a child's caregivers may be stressed, but the nurse must have information regarding the caregivers' perception of the **child's baseline status**, especially with infants and younger children or those who are developmentally delayed. The nurse should ask specific questions rather than very general questions, such as "What behavior or activity is normal for your child?" Questions relate to the child's age, but those for infants and young children should include:

- **Height (length) and weight:** Considered in conjunction with one another to establish appropriate nutritional status and growth/development. These are compared against standardized curves.
- **Diet:** Whether the child is nursing or bottle-fed, including the frequency and duration of nursing or ounces of milk per feeding. Question the number of meals daily and typical diet and eating habits.
- **Mobility:** Varies by age, but includes the ability to grasp, roll, turn, sit up, walk, run, and manipulate items.
- **Elimination:** Includes bowel and urinary output, problems, habits, routine, and continence. If the patient is an infant, include the number of wet diapers daily.
- **Sensory:** Includes age-appropriate indications of hearing and vision.
- **Communication:** Includes age-appropriate communication, such as vocalizing, babbling, saying words, saying sentences, comprehension.

Using Developmentally Appropriate Communication

Children, even toddlers, should always receive an explanation of treatment or other aspects of care, but the explanations should be given with **developmentally appropriate communication**, avoiding technical terms the child may not understand. Short explanations are better for small children as they may become very anxious. If more detailed explanations are needed for the parents, these explanations should be given away from the child.

Avoid	Use
Shot, injection, bee sting, needle stick	Medication under the skin
Incision, cut	Special opening
Pain	Hurt, "owie," or other term used by the child
Take temperature	See how warm you are
Monitor	TV/Computer screen
Stool, feces	Use child's term (poop, doo-doo)
Urine	Use child's term (pee-pee)
Gurney	Rolling bed
X-ray	Special pictures
Catheter	Tube
Anesthetize, deaden	Make sleepy, numb
Treat	Fix, make better

Potential Barriers When Taking a Pediatric History

When taking a pediatric health history, several **barriers** can inhibit the nurse's ability to gather information:

- The **environment** may not be conducive to conducting an examination or talking to the family because of noise or an inadequate space.
- **Parents** often are a great source of background information for the pediatric patient, but cultural differences, ethnic practices, and language barriers may all inhibit gathering information. Parents who are under the influence of medication or alcohol, those with psychiatric histories, those who are very young, and those who face financial pressures, illness, or time constraints may have difficulty supplying accurate information.
- **Siblings** or other **family members** who are present in the room may also be a distraction when trying to obtain a history.

Chief Complaint Taken During Medical History

The **chief complaint** is a description of symptoms that brought the patient in for treatment, such as shortness of breath, nausea, vomiting, abdominal pain, rash, or headache. Determining the chief complaint is part of taking the patient history, as this explains the reasons for seeking medical care. Other parts of the history related to the chief complaint include circumstances that may have led to the current symptoms, factors that make the symptoms better or worse, and a history of illnesses that may exacerbate the current chief complaint.

History of Present Illness

The history of the present illness follows a description of the chief complaint. The history of the present illness explains circumstances that drove the patient and family to seek care. Determining the history of the present illness is important for diagnostic purposes and for guiding treatment plans. The nurse can ask questions such as the following:

- How long have you experienced these symptoms?
- What makes the symptoms worse or better?
- Are symptoms worsening?
- What does the family believe to be the cause of the symptoms?

Pregnancy and Birth History

The **history of health during pregnancy and delivery** is an important component of the pediatric history. If the information is available, the nurse should record all significant events that occurred during pregnancy, labor, and delivery. Components of this type of history include the following:

- The health of the mother, such as any illnesses associated with pregnancy, bed rest, medication use, or complications
- The infant's gestational age at birth and whether the child was considered pre-term or full-term
- The type of delivery and any complications that occurred during delivery, such as fetal distress, cord compression, or emergent cesarean section
- The infant's health after birth, including Apgar scores, health complications, or time spent in the neonatal intensive care unit

Neonatal History

The parents of young infants and children should give an account of any significant events that occurred during the neonatal period, which may impact the child's health and behavior at the visit. The **neonatal history** should include the following:

- Complications associated with delivery, such as cord compression or excessive bleeding
- Assistance needed in delivery, such as vacuum extraction or forceps
- Apgar scores
- The need for oxygen or resuscitation at birth
- Complications in the prenatal period, such as hypoglycemia, transient tachypnea, infection, or jaundice
- Medications
- Periods of apnea
- Time spent in the neonatal intensive care unit, if applicable

Pediatric Feeding History

The pediatric feeding history indicates the type of feedings the child has taken from birth until the present visit. The feeding history is important because it determines whether the child has met developmental milestones for feeding, if the child is gaining weight appropriately, and if there are any health issues that may interfere with feedings, such as gastrointestinal issues or allergies. The pediatric nutrition portion of the history includes whether the child was breastfed or bottle-fed. If the child was fed by bottle, the type and amount of formula are noted. Any feeding issues, such as reflux or breast milk jaundice, are also noted. Older infants and toddlers have complete health histories concerning the introduction of solid foods, the timing of these foods, and the variety of foods eaten. Older child histories describe the number of meals and snacks each day, food preferences and dislikes, and any health problems associated with certain foods, such as gluten intolerance or food allergies.

Pediatric Behavioral History

The pediatric behavioral history describes social or environmental situations that may affect children's health, both physically and emotionally. Behavioral issues at home may lead to increased risks of injury or may be the result of physical illnesses that affect the children's ability to cope. Components of a behavioral history for the pediatric patient include assessing the children's environment at home, such as the number of siblings; family dynamics (e.g., parents together, divorced, separated); behavioral concerns, such as excessive temper tantrums, breath holding, controlling or manipulative behavior, responses to strangers, relationships with peers, and rapport with teachers and persons of authority. Sleep issues should be assessed to determine how much sleep the children are getting each night, if they still take naps, their bed times and waking times, and the state of their sleeping quarters. Older children and adolescents should be assessed for tobacco, alcohol, or drug use, peer relationships, and sexual development.

Medication Reconciliation During Collection of Patient History

Maintaining an **accurate list of current and previous medications** is an essential component of medication reconciliation. A patient (or parent) who maintains a list of personal medications becomes more involved in the care received and serves alongside the health care team as part of managing this care. The patient may have better health or improved outcomes when medication use is tracked and communicated to the health care team. In addition, maintaining a knowledge base of medications will benefit the patient/family and allow the opportunity for education about side effects and complications associated with certain medications. This also supports long-term compliance with the prescribed medication regimen.

Assessing for Drug and Food Allergies When Collecting Patient History

Assessing for **drug allergies** is especially important when collecting patient history in order to identify drugs that may cause reactions and to predict what other drugs may also trigger allergic reactions. For example, a patient who is allergic to penicillin may have cross reactivity to other antibiotics as well. The list of drug allergies should be reviewed with every new prescription. Food allergies should also be assessed, as they may provide indications of possible drug allergies. For example:

- Allergic reaction to bananas, kiwi, melons, papaya, raw potatoes, tomato and/or avocado increases the risk of allergy to latex.
- Allergic reaction to eggs or chicken is a contraindication for use of hyaluronic acid intra-articular injections because the substance is derived from chicken.
- The culture media for some vaccines can include eggs and horse serum.
- Allergic reaction to seafood may be associated with allergic reaction to IV iodine contrast.

Interaction Between Some Food/Food Elements and Medications

Grapefruit may interact with many drugs (statins, SSRIs, CCBs, sildenafil, sirolimus, tacrolimus, buspirone, midazolam, cyclosporine), and the interaction may occur up to 3 days after ingestion of grapefruit. Grapefruit inhibits CYP3A4, an isoenzyme of cytochrome P450, which is found in the wall of the intestines and the liver, but the inhibitory action takes place primarily in the intestines, decreasing the intestinal metabolism of various drugs and increasing absorption so that blood levels rise. This may intensify therapeutic effects or result in toxicity.

Vitamin K (phytonadione) may also interact with drugs. It is used to reverse excessive doses of warfarin but may decrease the effects of other drugs as well (anisindione, dicumarol). Some drug interactions decrease the effects of the vitamin K (cholestyramine, colesevelam colestipol, and sevelamer).

Tyramine-containing foods can cause a severe reaction when taken with MAOIs. Neuronal MAO is inhibited, resulting in increased levels of norepinephrine in sympathetic nerve terminals. Because MAO is inhibited in the intestinal walls and liver, dietary tyramine enters the circulatory system intact and promotes release of the epinephrine that has built up, resulting in severe vasoconstriction and stimulation of the heart.

ASSESSING HISTORY FOR GENETIC OR FAMILIAL RISKS

Assessing family history for **genetic or familial risks** is an important part of disease prevention because, in some cases, early identification and intervention may reduce future health risks. Creating a genogram with the family is helpful. A thorough history should be broad and include assessment of the following:

- Early onset disorders, such as cardiovascular disease, hypertension, or Alzheimer's disease
- Progressive neurological or neuromuscular diseases
- Diabetes mellitus
- Mental illness, such as depression, bipolar disorder, and schizophrenia
- Intellectual disability, including Trisomy 21 (Down syndrome)
- Any unusual disabilities or abnormalities, such as birth defects

Once risk factors are determined, then the question of screening tests arises. If there is a possibility that the child is a carrier, then screening is usually deferred until the child can give informed consent. Screening is done with parental permission when it is in the best interests of the child, allowing for appropriate care and intervention.

RELATIONSHIP BETWEEN ETHNICITY AND RISK OF GENETIC DISORDERS

Some ethnic groups have increased risk for **genetic disorders** with high carrier rates, ranging from 1:6 to 1:40. The nurse should be aware of these risks and observant for symptoms in the child. A careful maternal and paternal family history may provide information about occurrence of the disease in other family members. Some disorders are covered in routine neonatal screening, but others are not. In some cases, it may be appropriate to recommend testing to ensure that early diagnosis is made so that treatment can be initiated. The following groups are at increased risk for specific genetic disorders:

- Ashkenazi Jews: Canavan disease, Tay-Sachs disease, cystic fibrosis, and familial dysautonomia
- African Americans: Sickle cell disease (carrier rate 1:6 to 1:12), other hemoglobinopathy
- European Caucasians: Cystic fibrosis
- Mediterranean: Beta thalassemia
- South Asian: Beta thalassemia
- Southeast Asian: Alpha and beta thalassemia

USE OF INFORMATION FROM PEDIATRIC HISTORY IN CURRENT PRACTICE

Information from the pediatric history can be a valuable resource for the nurse and offers a **framework for providing treatment**. The pediatric history not only gives clues to the current complaint and offers direction for treatment, but it may also be used to educate parents about better health practices at home. Thus, the history serves as a teaching tool for better parenting. Additionally, a pediatric history may identify patterns of illness that can be genetic, which may indicate further testing for other family members who may be at risk. Finally, the pediatric history supports public health measures for identifying and treating children who are at risk for chronic disease, such as diabetes, asthma, or obesity.

Primary Survey

Elements of the primary survey, which can be remembered using the **ABCDE mnemonic**, include the following:

- **Airway**: Check airway for obstruction. Open airway with head tilt chin maneuver (lift chin with one hand and apply pressure to forehead with the other) or if trauma is present, the jaw thrust (stabilize cervical spine and pull mandible forward).
- **Breathing**: Look, listen, and feel for breathing for no more than 10 seconds. If not breathing, institute bag-valve-mask (BVM) ventilation followed by nasotracheal or orotracheal intubation if there is no response to BVM.
- **Circulation**: Provide basic life support (BLS). Check the carotid pulse in children >1 year of age, the brachial pulse in infants, and the umbilical pulse in neonates. Begin CPR: 120 compressions per minute in neonates and 100-120 per minute for infants and children. Defibrillate. If no response, institute Pediatric Advanced Life Support (PALS).
- **Disability**: Evaluate neurological status by checking pupillary response, level of alertness, Glasgow Coma Scale, CT for suspected stroke, blood glucose level and naloxone for suspected narcotic overdose.
- **Exposure/environmental control**: Remove clothes, check body for lesions, rashes, and trauma and maintain thermoregulation.

Secondary Survey

Elements of the secondary survey include the following:

- **History**: Question medical problems, current medications, onset of illness or injury, allergies, time of last meal, and pregnancy status when applicable.
- **Head**: Examine eyes, ears, nose, throat, skull, and skin for lacerations and bruises.
- **Neck**: Note carotid pulses, stiffness, bruit, jugular venous distention and trauma.
- **Chest**: Complete inspection, palpation, percussion, and auscultation. Note hyperresonance, dullness, adventitious sounds, or absent breath sounds.
- **Heart**: Note rhythm, heart sounds, and murmurs.
- **Abdomen**: Complete careful examination with supporting laboratory (blood counts) and imaging assessment (ultrasound, radiograph, CT, MRI) as needed.
- **Rectal, genital, perineal**: Perform examination if indicated.
- **Musculoskeletal**: Inspect and palpate all extremities for fractures, lacerations, dislocations, motor function, sensation, and pulses with supporting imaging as indicated. Multiple trauma patients should have pelvis x-ray.
- **Neurological**: Assess level of consciousness and complete evaluation of pupils and cranial nerves, reflexes, motor function, and sensory level with supporting imaging, such as CT scans. Note evidence of spinal cord injury.

Height, Weight, Head Circumference, and Chest Circumference

Height and weight are plotted on a standard growth chart. If the child is below the 5th percentile or above the 95th percentile, or falls two standard deviations below his normal curve, further investigation is required.

Normal head growth is 1.0-1.5 cm per month during the first year. A smaller than normal head circumference could be due to prematurity or microcephaly, a congenital abnormality resulting in mental deficits due to a small brain and small skull. A larger than normal head circumference could be due to hydrocephalus, an enlargement of the head due to buildup of CSF in the brain.

The **chest circumference** should be less than the head circumference up to one year of age. After this age, the chest circumference should be larger than the head circumference. A smaller than average chest circumference can be due to prematurity.

Normal and Abnormal Findings During Physical Examination

Skin

The **color of skin** should be assessed for jaundice or cyanosis, especially apparent in the nose, external ear, lips, hands, and feet. Note any lesions. Birthmarks, freckles, and moles, flat or raised, are normal. **Eczema** is common in children; **erythema toxicum** (erythematous, maculopapular lesions) is also common in newborns, as well as stork bites on the back of the neck and diaper dermatitis. **Mongolian spots** (dark blue areas in the lumbar and sacral areas, buttocks, shoulders, or upper back) are normal in African, Latino, and Asian babies. One abnormal finding is a dimple or a dark patch of hair over the lumbosacral area (spina bifida occulta).

Skin temperature should be the same bilaterally. Very warm skin indicates fever, hyperthyroidism, or exercise. Hypothermia can be due to shock or a circulatory problem.

The skin should be soft and smooth. **Milia** (small white papules on the face) are common in newborns, as is **vernix caseosa** (a cheesy coating present at birth). Decreased skin turgor indicates dehydration. Edema is abnormal.

Head

The head should be symmetrical without bumps or depressions. The anterior fontanel may pulsate with the heartbeat. An occiput that is flattened with hair loss is caused by lying in the same position for long periods of time. Head lag after 4 months can be caused by prematurity, hydrocephalus, and developmental delays. Head lag remaining after 6 months can indicate brain damage. The fontanels should be flat and soft. Bulging, tense fontanels result from increased intracranial pressure and sunken fontanels from dehydration. Fontanels that fail to close or are larger than normal can indicate rickets or congenital hypothyroidism. Suture lines should line up, without gapping or overriding. Craniotabes (soft outer layers of the skull bones behind and above the ears that can be depressed) is abnormal, indicating rickets, hydrocephaly, syphilis, or hypervitaminosis. Cephalhematoma and caput succedaneum are abnormal findings resulting from pressure during delivery.

Ear and Nose

Hearing tests are usually performed starting at 3-4 years. The top of the ear should be level with or a little above the outer corner of the eye. If it is lower, it can indicate renal abnormalities or Down syndrome. When looking at the tympanic membrane, it should be pearly gray to light pink and transparent with a smooth membrane.

The **nose** should be symmetrical and centered. Congenital abnormalities may be present if the nose is short and small, flat, or large. Flaring can indicate respiratory distress, odor can indicate a foreign object stuck in the nasal canal, and discharge can indicate an infection. The mucous membrane should be pink and moist. The newborn should be assessed for patent nares. An obstruction indicates choanal atresia, a septum between the nose and pharynx.

Eyes

Upon physical assessment of the **eyes**, the sclera is normally bluish (newborns), white, or slightly darker in color (dark-skinned children). A yellow sclera indicates jaundice. The iris in newborns is blue or gray (light-skinned children) or brown (dark-skinned). The color may change up until 12 months. Brushfield's spots (small white spots around the edge of the iris) are abnormal and related to Down syndrome. Pupils should be equal size and react equally to light. If one or both pupils don't react to light, it can indicate a CNS abnormality. The newborn should exhibit the optical blink reflex. The red reflex should be assessed; black spots or opacities are abnormal (possible cataract resulting from eye trauma, infection during pregnancy or chromosomal disorders). A cat's eye reflex (yellow or white light) can indicate retinoblastoma, a malignant tumor of the eye. The retina is usually pink in color; red color is abnormal and usually indicates bleeding. The optic disc is examined for color and shape. If the margins are irregular or blurred, it can indicate papilledema or intracranial pressure.

Vision and Eyelids

A **vision test**, appropriate for age, should be done every 1-2 years through adolescence. Vision is abnormal if the child sees 20/40 or greater at 3 years of age or 20/30 or greater over 6 years of age (using the Snellen E chart). Congenital cataracts, tumors or retinal trauma can result in nearsightedness. Screening should be done for strabismus (eye muscle weakness), using an appropriate test. The **opening of the eyes** should be symmetrical, the upper lid should cover part of the iris and the lower lid should meet the iris. Asian children may have an epicanthal fold. Hydrocephalus can cause sunset eyes (part of the sclera is seen above the iris). Down syndrome children have a fold of skin covering the inner canthus and lacrimal caruncle. By 3 months, the lacrimal duct should be patent. Tearing and discharge from the eye can result from dacryocystitis (blockage of the lacrimal duct causes infection of the lacrimal sac.

Neck

Observe the **neck** for abnormal appearance, such as shortness, thickening, or swelling. Swelling of the parotid gland indicates mumps. The thyroid glands should be assessed for swelling, tenderness or masses, possibly indicative of hyperthyroidism. Lymph nodes can't normally be felt. Enlarged lymph nodes indicate infection; the site of which depends on which lymph nodes are affected. Bacterial infections of the pharynx are indicated by swelling of the anterior cervical nodes; tinea capitis and otitis media are indicated by swelling of the occipital or posterior cervical nodes. Small, cool nodes that are not fixed are common in children; these "shotty" nodes indicate a prior infection or allergies.

Mouth and Throat

The edges of the **lips** should meet. Cleft lip is present if there is a separation of the lip area. The mucosa of the mouth should be pink, smooth, and moist; a thick white coating can indicate thrush. The number of **teeth** should be noted and compared with normal teething guidelines. If normal teeth are not present and tooth buds are not noted on x-ray, genetic abnormalities may be present. Teeth should be without brown-black spots. These spots indicate cavities. The hard and soft **palates** should be continuous and have a slight arch. A separation of the palate indicates cleft palate. Epstein's pearls (small, white, hard cysts on the gums and hard palate) are abnormal. The **tonsils** are normally enlarged in early childhood, decreasing in size after age 10. The **uvula** should be pink and centered. The **mucosa** of the oropharynx should also be pink and smooth. Excess saliva production can be a sign of a tracheoesophageal fistula.

Heart

Abnormalities should be of primary concern when assessing the **heart**. Dextrocardia, when the apex of the heart points toward the right side of the chest, will affect the landmarks used in examining the heart. The apical pulse should be assessed for any deviation from its normal placement, indicating an enlarged heart or pneumothorax. The apical pulse is visible on the precordium, but no other movements should be seen. If the cardiac area heaves, or lifts, the left ventricle is working too hard and can indicate CHF or shunt defects. Septal defects will produce a thrill, a vibration of the chest similar to a purring cat. Peripheral pulses should be equal and simultaneous. If there is a lag or weakness in some pulses, consider heart defects, such as coarctation of the aorta. Some children have innocent murmurs and sinus arrhythmias, which are normal. Other abnormalities in heart sounds can indicate heart defects or CHF.

Respiratory Status

Assessment of respiratory status involves looking at the child's appearance, counting respirations, and listening to lung sounds. A child who is comfortable, breathing normally, and who has pink skin and a healthy appearance most likely has normal respiratory function. A child who is agitated, who appears pale or cyanotic, and who is breathing rapidly may be in respiratory distress. Other signs of respiratory distress include assuming a position of comfort to breathe, wheezes or stridor while breathing, and retractions noted above the sternum, between the ribs, or below the xiphoid process. Auscultation may result in lung sounds with rales or rhonchi, or breath sounds may be diminished or absent.

THORAX AND LUNGS

The **thorax** changes from rounded and boxy in shape during early childhood to longer and thinner at about age 6. An abnormal chest shape in the school age child can indicate cystic fibrosis. A funnel shaped chest (pectus excavatum) is progressive from birth and can affect heart function. Pigeon chest (pectus carinatum) is when the sternum sticks out from the body. It can be congenital in origin. Assess for retractions, which indicated respiratory distress, possibly resulting from pneumonia or asthma. Placing a hand on the chest, the nurse may feel a soft vibration which is normal. If the vibration is pronounced, it may indicate pneumonia. If the vibration is decreased, pulmonary edema or pleural effusion may exist. Percussion can reveal fluid or air trapped in the lungs. Upon auscultation, the lung sounds should be clear and equal. Crackles, wheezes, or rhonchi are abnormal signs of such conditions as bronchiolitis, cystic fibrosis, or asthma. Stridor, a high-pitched sound upon inspiration, can occur with croup and epiglottis.

MUSCULOSKELETAL SYSTEM

Muscles should be symmetrical and firm bilaterally. Spasticity, rigidity, or resistance can indicate cerebral palsy. Muscular dystrophy can cause decreased muscle strength, noted when the child cannot rise to a standing position without using the arms. Check for coordination in gross and fine motor skills. Observe for involuntary movements, such as tics, tremors, or jerking. Lordosis after age 6 is abnormal and can result from dislocation of the hips or congenital kyphosis. Scoliosis is abnormal. Polydactyly (extra digits) and syndactylism (fusion of digits) are signs of congenital syndromes. A knock knee appearance is normal until around 4-6 years of age. Bowlegs are normal until 2 years. If present later, it may indicate rickets. The joints should not be tender or swollen and should be flexible. Painful, swollen, warm joints are indicative of juvenile rheumatoid arthritis. Club foot is a turning in of the foot and toes and is abnormal. Dysplasia of the hips in the infant is abnormal and is associated with birth and familial factors.

ABDOMEN

Observe the child for crying and guarding of areas of the **abdomen** upon palpation, which indicates tenderness or pain. A separation of the rectus muscles in the midline (diastasis recti) is normal in infants. A vertical separation of the stomach muscle is abnormal. If peristalsis can be seen or an olive-shaped mass palpated in the upper right stomach area, pyloric stenosis should be considered. Hirschsprung's disease is indicated by distention of the abdomen by palpable stool and no stool in the rectum. Intussusception can cause pain associated with a sausage-shaped mass in the upper abdomen. Bowel sounds should not be heard in the thorax; this can indicate a diaphragmatic hernia in the newborn. The liver edge should be soft and smooth. If located more than 2 cm below the right rib cage, and hard with a firm border, hepatomegaly should be suspected. Causes can be cardiac failure, tumors, viruses, or bacteria.

GENITALIA

Assess females for discharge, bruising, or scarring of the **genitalia**. A small penis in the clitoral area of the female baby is abnormal. Blood in the diaper in the first two weeks of life are normal (maternal hormones are still present). In males, the urethral meatus should not be located behind or along the underside of the penis (hypospadias), or on the top side of the penis (epispadias). Two testes, round, smooth, and movable, should be felt, although the testes in infants can retract. Cryptorchidism is when the testes do not descend into the scrotal sac. A congenital hydrocele causes enlargement of the scrotum. Assess for inguinal hernias. Assess the anus for bleeding, fissures, skin tags, hemorrhoids, prolapse of the rectum and pinworms. Check for the anal wink (stroking area lightly should produce movement of the anus), the absence of which is abnormal and can result from spinal cord lesions, trauma, or tumors.

Customizing Assessment for Children with Special Needs

Children may present in the emergency department with a variety of special needs, so initial assessment should include determining what special needs a child may have and then addressing them.

- **Children with cognitive impairment** (e.g., Down syndrome): Ask the caregiver about the child's level of understanding and comfort measures that might distract or ease the child's anxiety. Talk to the child in a soothing manner.
- **Children with autism**: Ask the caregiver about the things that trigger anxiety/meltdown in the child and ask the caregiver to help support the child. Ask before touching, and touch only as necessary. Explain procedures, especially if the child is high functioning.
- **Children with impaired vision**: Maintain a dialogue explaining activities and procedures, such as "I'm going to feel your tummy." Allow the child to touch equipment, such as a stethoscope, when possible.
- **Children with impaired hearing**: Ask about the degree of hearing loss and methods the child uses to communicate. Use a sign language interpreter if appropriate or ensure hearing aids are in place and functioning. Use pictures of treatments or procedures if possible.

Hold Positions for Assessment and Procedures

Pediatric comfort holding positions for assessments and procedures include the following:

- **Hug hold**: Position an infant or small child facing the caregiver and straddling the caregiver's legs with the caregiver's arms securely hugging the child. Another person should distract the child or secure free arm(s). Good position for injections and venipuncture.
- **Side sitting**: Similar to a hug hold, with the child facing the caregiver, but legs to the side. Good position for older children who want less confinement.
- **Bracing**: Child is held in supine position in the caregiver's arms and braced against the chest or shoulder to prevent movement of the head. Good position for insertion of NG tubes or examination/treatment of mouth or other parts of face.
- **Sitting**: Child sits forward or sideways on caregiver's lap with caregiver's arms around child. Good position for children who want to watch or don't want to be more confined.
- **Supine**: Child lies on table with the caregiver lying behind the child so the child's head lies on the caregiver's lap while the caregiver holds the child or provides distraction.

Geriatric History and Physical Assessment

AGE CATEGORIES OF THE ELDERLY

The elderly population can be divided into three groups. The age group ranging from 65-74 years are considered the **young-old**, from 75-84 are considered the **middle-old**, and 85 and older are considered **old-old**. There are many physical and psychological changes that occur as someone moves through these age groups. As this population increases in size, so does the number of those with physical and mental illnesses.

FACTORS THAT INFLUENCE PRESENTATION OF ILLNESS IN OLDER ADULTS

There are three major factors that influence **how an illness will present in an older patient.** These factors, either alone or in combination with one another, have the potential to make an ordinarily standard clinical presentation confusing for the clinician.

- The first of these factors is **underreporting of illness or the symptoms associated** with illness. There are a number of reasons that illnesses are not reported: the patient may fear hospitalization, institutionalization, or loss of control, or the patient may be convinced that there really is no problem.
- Another factor is the **pattern of distribution of illness** amongst the elderly population. This affects presentation because there are a number of diseases and impairments that are prevalent among older adults, including congestive heart failure, arthritis, osteoporosis, and pneumonia; therefore, identifying and differentiating the primary diagnosis may be difficult.
- The last factor is an **altered response to illness**. This can make diagnosis and treatment very difficult because symptoms may be exaggerated by other problems, or they may be nonexistent.

AGE-RELATED CONSIDERATIONS WHEN EVALUATING ADULT PATIENTS

Because each individual patient is exposed to different environmental, psychological, and physical stressors that can affect the aging process, it is important to consider that some patients may experience adverse health impacts, while other patients of the same age may not be affected. As individuals age, the amount of wear on the body, as well as the likelihood of pathological changes, increases at different rates for every individual. Factors affecting the aging process include proper nutrition (or the lack thereof), level of physical activity, smoking, alcohol consumption, environmental or occupational exposures, and socioeconomic standing. Also, remember that as an individual ages, a disease or impairments with one organ or organ system will have a marked effect on other systems, because the body is not able to compensate as it once was. Symptoms may not be noticeable until other functions begin to decline. Most often, health issues manifest in the elderly as confusion, so close attention must be given to this symptom and investigated when present.

BASIC PATIENT SAFETY ASSESSMENTS WHEN EVALUATING A PATIENT

There are four basic assessments that the nurse should make when **assessing a patient's safety** and identifying possible safety concerns:

- The first of these is the **mobility assessment**; different safety risks apply to patients who are mobile as opposed to those who are not. An immobile patient, for example, has a tendency to form pressure injuries, or bedsores.
- The next assessment is the evaluation of the patient's **level of awareness**; is the patient able to communicate to the nursing staff when something is wrong? If not, certain measures should be undertaken to ensure that the nursing staff is aware of a change in the patient's condition.
- An extension of this assessment is determining whether the patient is in **critical condition**; these patients must be monitored more closely for changes.
- An assessment of the patient's **mental status** is also important because the patient may not be able to make safe decisions on his or her own.

FUNCTIONAL EVALUATION OF ELDERLY PATIENT

A functional evaluation of the elderly patient examines the patient's ability to carry out activities of daily living (ADL) that are critical in gauging the patient's ability to care for oneself without the need of assistance. Use the **Index of Independence in Activities of Daily Living Scale** to check foundational tasks such as taking a shower, getting dressed, eating, and going to the bathroom. Aged patients will be more likely to overstate what they are able to do and understate their limitations, while the patient's family will likely understate what the patient is able to handle. Assess mental ability with the following exams:

- Short Portable Mental Status Questionnaire (SPMSQ)
- Mini-Mental State Exam (MMSE)

The **Tinetti Balance and Gait Evaluation** exams are also important elements of the functional evaluation of an elderly patient. These tests, along with the simple **Up-and-Go test,** are used to assess the balance and gait issues that elderly patients have. The patient has to complete certain actions, such as sitting down and standing up from a chair, turning around, bending over, etc. The entire assessment takes approximately 15–20 minutes. The **Lawton and Brody: Instrumental Activities of Daily Learning** test is used to check whether the patient can do more complex activities important to daily living, second to the ADL's required for basic function. Examples of IADLs include the ability to go shopping, wash clothes, cook, etc. The **Index of Independence of Activities of Daily Living** is utilized to find what the patient is able do independently on a regular basis.

DEPRESSION AND SUICIDE IN THE ELDERLY

Depression commonly goes unidentified in an aging patient. Cognitive changes are often wrongly identified as dementia, confusion, or natural aging changes, rather than depression. It is important to be cognizant of the prevalence of this issue among the elderly, and treat appropriately.

Suicide rates for elderly patients are higher than any other age group. The compounding stress and emotional burden of losing loved ones, mobility, and independence often contribute to suicidal ideations. Other factors include seemingly unbearable psychological anguish, dissatisfaction, and unmet requirements. Suicide is more commonly seen in elderly males (seven times higher rate), Caucasians, unmarried individuals (divorced, separated, single), individuals who are poor and/or out of work, individuals with psychiatric or cognitive impairments, the very sick, individuals with substance additions, individuals that are grieving (particularly in the first year of loss or retirement), those without friends or community relationships, or those who have tried suicide before. Suicidal thoughts and attempts may be overt or covert.

As with patients of other age ranges, if an elderly patient hints at suicidal ideations or thoughts, this must be addressed directly by the nurse.

INDICATIONS AND ASSESSMENTS FOR DELIRIUM

Delirium (acute confusion) presents in a variety of indications. The patient may experience mental issues, including inattention or short attention span, difficulty remembering, trouble with perception, bafflement, and lack of decision-making. There may be changing moods, faulty ability to manage whims, stress, slight to moderate depression, visual or auditory hallucinations, confabulation, changing intellectual ability that worsens at night (sun-downing) and is more frequently seen in patients that have had prior dementia, psychomotor agitation including inability to sleep, tachycardia, enlarged pupils, and perspiration. The patient may appear restless, overcautious, not cautious enough, or appear lost/stunned. There may be tachycardia, high blood pressure, fever, rapid breathing, and there might be focal neurological indications.

Physical assessments include a complete history, physical examination, check of mind and neurological issues to determine what is causing the problem, foundation of lab work such as CBC, electrocardiogram, chest radiograph, urinalysis, urine toxicology, and other assessments that are deemed necessary, such as EED, CT, or blood work for drugs.

Changes Associated with Aging

Biological Changes

As people move from the young-old to the old-old, many **physical and biological changes** occur throughout their bodies. Organs and tissues such as the kidneys, liver, heart, GI tract, and brain begin to decline, and some, such as the ovaries and uterus, fall into disuse and atrophy. Dysfunction of the **kidneys and liver** is of particular importance because these organs are responsible for drug metabolism. This population may also experience peripheral neuropathy, decreased reaction times, and decreased balance due to changes in the nervous system. There can also be a decline in the five senses. Changes in vision and hearing can affect performance on many of the assessment tools used to evaluate this population for mental health issues such as depression, delirium, dementia, or anxiety.

Psychological Changes

Psychological changes can occur in cognition, learning capacity, and memory. These changes can lead to **decreased continued development** and can **change relationships** with family and friends. Many of the cognitive changes are brought about by a general atrophy of the brain. The aging process does not impair a person's state of consciousness, however, there can be a generalized decrease in concentration, attention span, and reaction times, leading to poor performance on many assessment tools. Learning may be diminished simply because the elderly person may lack motivation.

Memory loss does not go hand in hand with the aging process. Memory loss can occur for a variety of reasons such as disease processes, medications, substance abuse, or depression.

Sociocultural Changes

The elderly may experience many **social changes** such as change in functional independence, employment, and social experiences with groups and friends. As the individual moves from young-old to old-old, many of the things that they were able to **do for themselves** will diminish. This can range from fixing household problems to basic activities of daily living (ADLs) such as bathing and dressing. This population also enters retirement and daily life may become less organized and they may experience financial stress and anxiety. With retirement, this population may also have a reduction in healthcare benefits inhibiting them from seeking needed assistance. Debilitating medical conditions may also inhibit their social activities and they may experience feelings of isolation.

SOCIAL DETERMINANTS OF HEALTH

Social determinants of health, conditions that shape the health of the geriatric population, include the following:

- Socioeconomic status: Approximately 40% of the geriatric population have a low income, earning less than 200% of the poverty level, and approximately 10% live in poverty. This limits their ability to pay for medical care, medications, and living expenses.
- Food insecurity: Approximately 11% are unable to access enough nutritional food because of insufficient income or the unavailability of grocery stores and food markets in their area. Rates of food insecurity are especially high among racial and ethnic minorities.
- Housing: More than 20% of homeless individuals are older than age 55, and many are unsheltered. Rising housing costs, inadequate healthcare, financial insecurity, substance abuse, and a lack of affordable housing are all contributing factors.
- Support: Approximately 13% of adults older than 55 are sole family survivors with no family members left to provide support, increasing their isolation.
- Neighborhoods/exposure to violence and crime: Because many live in low-income areas, they are often exposed to an increased risk of violence and crime, resulting in a lower quality of life. Approximately 10% are victims of elder abuse, leading to impaired health and low self-esteem.
- Education/employment: Approximately 9% did not finish high school, and only 29% hold a bachelor's degree or higher, resulting in low-paying jobs with little in the way of retirement benefits.

Cardiovascular Assessment

ASSESSMENT OF THE CARDIOVASCULAR SYSTEM

Cardiovascular assessment includes questioning the patient for any family history of death at a young age or other cardiovascular diseases. Elderly African-American males are at highest risk for cardiovascular problems. One must question the patient about edema, chest pain, dyspnea, fatigue, vertigo, syncope or other changes in consciousness, weight gain, and leg cramps or pain. If chest pain is a symptom, one must ask about the intensity, timing, location, any radiation, quality, meaning to the patient, factors that aggravate or alleviate the pain, nausea, dyspnea, diaphoresis, or any other accompanying symptoms. Physical assessment includes assessment of vital signs, heart and lung sounds, skin assessment, radial, popliteal, and pedal pulses, circulation and sensation of extremities, and auscultation of the aorta, renal, iliac, and femoral arteries for bruits. Blood should be taken for a lipid profile and electrolytes. The patient must be helped to modify risk factors such as hypertension, smoking, diabetes, obesity, hyperlipidemia, inactivity, and stress.

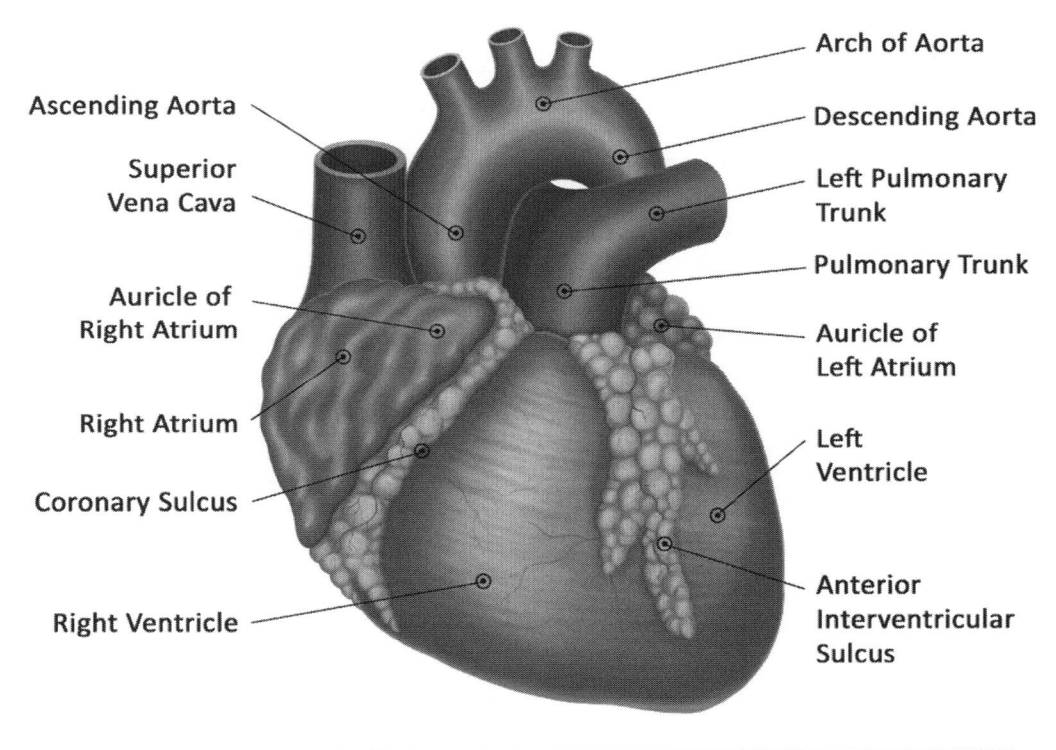

Review Video: Cardiovascular Assessment
Visit mometrix.com/academy and enter code: 323076

Review Video: Functions of the Circulatory System
Visit mometrix.com/academy and enter code: 376581

Review Video: Heart Blood Flow
Visit mometrix.com/academy and enter code: 783139

Review Video: Mnemonics for Heart Anatomy and Physiology
Visit mometrix.com/academy and enter code: 849489

ASSESSMENT OF HEART SOUNDS

Auscultation of heart sounds can help to diagnose different cardiac disorders. Areas to auscultate include the aortic area, pulmonary area, Erb's point, tricuspid area, and the apical area. The **normal heart sounds** represent closing of the valves.

> The **first heart sound** (S1) "lub" is closure of the mitral and tricuspid valves (heard at apex/left ventricular area of the heart).
> The **second heart sound** (S2) "dub" is closure of the aortic and pulmonic valves (heard at the base of the heart). There may be a slight splitting of the S2.

The time between S1 and S2 is systole and the time between S2 and the next S1 is diastole. Systole and diastole should be silent although ventricular disease can cause gallops, snaps, or clicks and stenosis of the valves or failure of the valves to close can cause murmurs. Pericarditis may cause a friction rub.

Additional heart sounds:

- **Gallop rhythms**: S3 commonly occurs after S2 in children and young adults but may indicate heart failure or left ventricular failure in older adults (when heard with patient lying on left side). S4 occurs before S1, during the contracting of the atria when there is ventricular hypertrophy, found in coronary artery disease, hypertension, or aortic valve stenosis.
- **Opening snap**: Unusual high-pitched sound occurring after S2 with stenosis of mitral valve from rheumatic heart disease
- **Ejection click**: Brief high-pitched sound after S1; aortic stenosis
- **Friction rub**: Harsh, grating holosystolic sound; pericarditis
- **Murmur**: Sound caused by turbulent blood flow from stenotic or malfunctioning valves, congenital defects, or increased blood flow. Murmurs are characterized by location, timing in the cardiac cycle, intensity (rated from Grade I to Grade VI), pitch (low to high-pitched), quality (rumbling, whistling, blowing) and radiation (to the carotids, axilla, neck, shoulder, or back).

> **Review Video: Diastolic vs Systolic**
> Visit mometrix.com/academy and enter code: 898934

CARDIAC MONITORING

Cardiac monitoring includes the evaluation of different intervals and segments on the electrocardiogram:

- **QT interval**: This is the complete time of ventricular depolarization and repolarization, which begins with the QRS segment and ends when the T wave is completed. Typically, duration usually ranges from 0.36–0.44 seconds, but this may vary depending on the heart rate. If the heat rate is rapid, the duration is shorter and vice versa. Certain medications can prolong the QT interval, in such cases monitoring this is critical. A prolonged QT interval puts the patient at risk for R-on-T phenomenon, which can result in dangerous arrhythmias.
- **ST segment**: This is an isoelectric period when the ventricles are in a plateau phase, completely depolarized and beginning recovery and repolarization. Deflection is usually isoelectric. If the ST segment is ≥0.5 mm below the baseline, it is considered depressed and may be an indication of myocardial ischemia. Depression may also indicate digitalis toxicity. If the ST segment is elevated ≥0.3 mm above baseline, this is an indication of myocardial injury.

MAP

The MAP **(mean arterial pressure)** is most commonly used to evaluate perfusion as it shows pressure throughout the cardiac cycle. Systole is one-third and diastole two-thirds of the normal cardiac cycle. The MAP for a blood pressure of 120/60 is calculated as follows:

$$\text{MAP} = \frac{\text{Diastole} \times 2 + \text{Systole}}{3} \frac{60 \times 2 + 120}{3} = \frac{240}{3} = 80$$

Normal range for mean arterial pressure is 70–100 mmHg. A MAP of greater than 60 mmHg is required to perfuse vital organs, including the heart, brain, and kidneys.

Oxygen Saturation as it Relates to Hemodynamic Status

Hemodynamic monitoring includes monitoring **oxygen saturation** levels, which must be maintained for proper cardiac function. The central venous catheter often has an oxygen sensor at the tip to monitor oxygen saturation in the right atrium.

- Increased oxygen saturation may result from left atrial to right atrial shunt, abnormal pulmonary venous return, increased delivery of oxygen or decrease in extraction of oxygen.
- Decreased oxygen saturation may be related to low cardiac output with an increase in oxygen extraction or decrease in arterial oxygen saturation with normal differences in the atrial and ventricular oxygen saturation.

Electrocardiogram

The electrocardiogram records and shows a graphic display of the electrical activity of the heart through a number of different waveforms, complexes, and intervals:

- **P wave**: Start of electrical impulse in the sinus node and spreading through the atria, muscle depolarization
- **QRS complex**: Ventricular muscle depolarization and atrial repolarization
- **T wave**: Ventricular muscle repolarization (resting state) as cells regain negative charge
- **U wave**: Repolarization of the Purkinje fibers

A modified lead II ECG is often used to monitor basic heart rhythms and dysrhythmias. Typical placement of leads for 2-lead ECG is 3–5 cm inferior to the right clavicle and left lower ribcage. Typical placement for a 3-lead ECG is (RA) right arm near shoulder, (LA) V_5 position over 5th intercostal space, and (LL) left upper leg near groin.

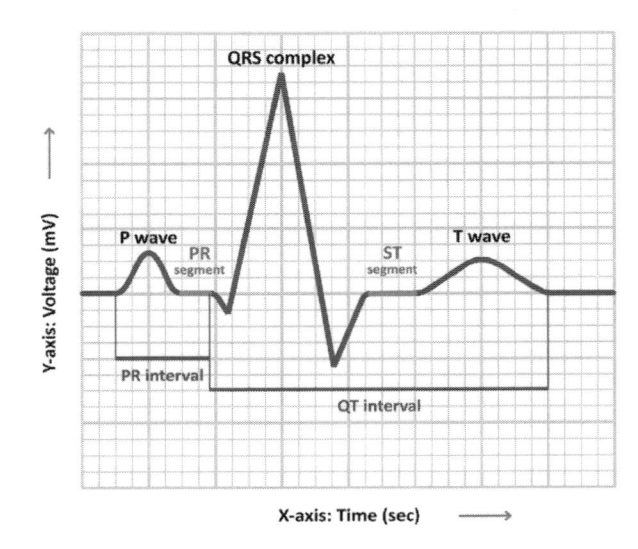

ADMINISTRATION OF 12-LEAD ECG

The electrocardiogram provides a graphic representation of the electrical activity of the heart. It is indicated for chest pain, dyspnea, syncope, acute coronary syndrome, pulmonary embolism, and possible MI. The standard **12 lead ECG** gives a picture of electrical activity from 12 perspectives through placement of 10 body leads:

- 4 limb leads are placed distally on the wrists and ankles (but may be placed more proximally if necessary).
- Precordial leads:
    - V1: Right sternal border at 4th intercostal space
    - V2: Left sternal border at 4th intercostal space
    - V3: Midway between V2 and V4
    - V4: Left midclavicular line at 5th intercostal space
    - V5: Horizontal to V4 at left anterior axillary line
    - V6: Horizontal to V5 at left midaxillary line

In some cases, additional leads may be used:

- Right-sided leads are placed on the right in a mirror image of the left leads, usually to diagnose right ventricular infarction through ST elevation.

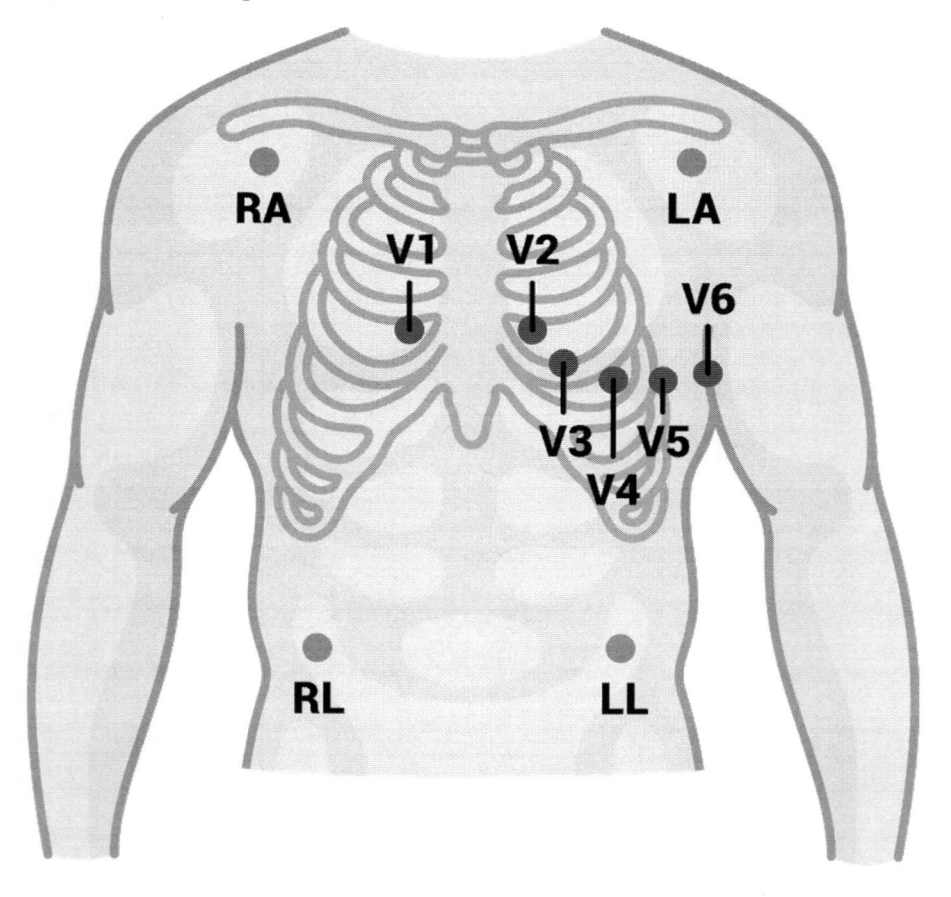

Assessing Jugular Venous Pressure

Jugular venous pressure (neck-vein) is used to assess the cardiac output and pressure in the right heart as the pulsations relate to changes in pressure in the right atrium. This procedure is usually not accurate if the pulse rate is >100. This is a non-invasive estimation of central venous pressure and waveform. Measurement should be done with the internal jugular if possible; if not, the external jugular may be used.

- **Elevate** the patient's head to 45° (and to 90° if necessary) with patient's head turned to the right.
- Position a **light** at an angle to illuminate veins and shadows.
- Measure the height of the **jugular vein pulsation** above the sternal joint, using a ruler.
    - Normal height is ≤4 cm above sternal angle.

Increased pressure (reflected in a height of >4 cm above the sternal angle) indicates increased pressure in the right atrium, and right heart failure. It may also indicate pericarditis or tricuspid stenosis. Laughing or coughing may trigger the Valsalva response and also cause an increase in pressure.

Additional Cardiac Assessments

The **stress test**, also called an exercise tolerance test, is a commonly used assessment to screen for ischemic heart disease. In this test, the patient is put through exercise with increasing rigor, generally on a treadmill, while attached to an ECG to monitor their heart's rhythm. The patient is assessed for chest pain and dizziness as the rigor level is increased, which is a reflection of the heart's capacity to handle increasing workloads effectively. The stress test is not diagnostic on its own, but provides feedback on the direction of additional testing.

Water-hammer pulse is characterized by the alternation between a bounding heartbeat that is strong and forceful, and then collapse. This could be the result of a heightened stroke volume, decreased peripheral resistance, or these two factors together. To assess for this pulse, the patient is seated and one arm is raised vertically. Upon palpation of the radial pulse in the raised arm, the pulse resembles a tapping in the muscles of the forearm. This is often an indication of aortic regurgitation.

Perfusion Pressure and Pulse Pressure

Coronary perfusion pressure directly affects coronary blood flow, and coronary perfusion occurs during diastole. Coronary artery perfusion pressure is equal to the diastolic blood pressure minus the pulmonary artery occlusion pressure. Normal values are 60–80 mmHg. Goal coronary perfusion when performing CPR to maintain enough perfusion necessary to achieve ROSC (return of spontaneous circulation) is thought to be 15 mmHg. During the cardiac cycle, *aortic pressure* causes the coronaries to be perfused, while *ventricular pressure* compresses the coronaries during systole, decreasing perfusion.

The **pulse pressure** is the difference between systolic and diastolic pressures, and this can be an important indicator. For example, with a decrease in cardiac output, vasoconstriction takes place in the body's attempt to maintain the blood pressure. In this case, the MAP may remain unchanged, but the pulse pressure narrows. Patients should be assessed for changes in pulse pressure that may be precipitated by medications, such as diuretics that alter fluid volume.

Assessment of Lower Extremities

Assessment of lower extremities includes a number of different elements:

- **Appearance** includes comparing limbs for obvious differences or changes in skin or nails as well as evaluating for edema, color changes in skin, such as pallor or rubor. Legs that are thin, pale, shiny, and hairless indicate peripheral arterial disease.
- **Perfusion** should be assessed by checking venous filling time and capillary refill, skin temperature (noting changes in one limb or between limbs), bruits (indicating arterial narrowing), pulses (comparing both sides in a proximal to distal progression), ankle-brachial index and toe-brachial index.
- **Sensory function** includes the ability to feel pain, temperature, and touch.
- **Range of motion** of the ankle must be assessed to determine if the joint flexes past 90° because this is necessary for unimpaired walking and aids venous return in the calf.
- **Pain** is an important diagnostic feature of peripheral arterial disease, so the location, intensity, duration, and characteristics of pain are important.

Assessment of Pulse and Bruit

Evaluation of the pulses of the **lower extremities** is an important part of assessment for peripheral arterial disease/trauma. Pulses should be first evaluated with the patient in supine position and then again with the legs dependent, checking bilaterally and proximal to distal to determine if intensity of pulse decreases distally. Pedal pulses should be examined at both the posterior tibialis and the dorsalis pedis. The pulse should be evaluated as to the rate, rhythm, and intensity, which is usually graded on a 0 to 4 scale:

$$0+= \text{pulse absent}$$
$$1+= \text{weak, difficult to palpate}$$
$$2+= \text{normal as expected}$$
$$3+= \text{full}$$
$$4+= \text{strong and bounding}$$

Pulses may be **palpable** or **absent** with peripheral arterial disease. Absence of pulse on both palpation and Doppler probe does indicate peripheral arterial disease.

Bruits may be noted by auscultating over major arteries, such as femoral, popliteal, peroneal, and dorsalis pedis, indicating peripheral arterial disease.

Assessing Perfusion of Lower Extremities

Assessment of perfusion can indicate venous or arterial abnormalities:

- **Venous refill time**: Begin with the patient lying supine for a few moments and then have the patient sit with the feet dependent. Observe the veins on the dorsum of the foot and count the seconds before normal filling. Venous occlusion is indicated with times greater than 20 seconds.
- **Capillary refill**: Grasp the toenail bed between the thumb and index finger and apply pressure for several seconds to cause blanching. Release the nail and count the seconds until the nail regains normal color. Arterial occlusion is indicated with times of more than 2–3 seconds. Check both feet and more than one nail bed.
- **Skin temperature**: Using the palm of the hand and fingers, gently palpate the skin, moving distally to proximally and comparing both legs. Arterial disease is indicated by decreased temperature (coolness) or a marked change from proximal to distal. Venous disease is indicated by increased temperature about the ankle.

ABI

PROCEDURE

The ankle-brachial index **(ABI) examination** is done to evaluate peripheral arterial disease of the lower extremities.

1. Apply BP cuff to one arm, palpate brachial pulse, and place conductivity gel over the artery.
2. Place the tip of a Doppler device at a 45-degree angle into the gel at the brachial artery and listen for the pulse sound.
3. Inflate the cuff until the pulse sound ceases and then inflate 20 mmHg above that point.
4. Release air and listen for the return of the pulse sound. This reading is the brachial systolic pressure.
5. Repeat the procedure on the other arm and use the higher reading for calculations.
6. Repeat the same procedure on each ankle with the cuff applied above the malleoli and the gel over the posterior tibial pulse to obtain the ankle systolic pressure.
7. Divide the ankle systolic pressure by the brachial systolic pressure to obtain the ABI.

Sometimes, readings are taken both before and after 5 minutes of walking on a treadmill.

INTERPRETING RESULTS

Once the ABI examination is completed, the ankle systolic pressure must be divided by the brachial systolic pressure. Ideally, the BP at the ankle should be equal to that of the arm or slightly higher. With peripheral arterial disease the ankle pressure falls, affecting the ABI. Additionally, some conditions that cause calcification of arteries, such as diabetes, can cause a false elevation.

Calculation is simple:

$$\text{ABI} = \frac{\text{Ankle systolic}}{\text{Brachial systolic}}$$

The degree of disease relates to the **score**:

- >1.4: Abnormally high, may indicate calcification of vessel wall
- 1.0–1.4: Normal reading, asymptomatic
- 0.9–1.0: Low reading, but acceptable unless there are other indications of PAD
- 0.8–0.9: Likely some arterial disease is present
- 0.5–0.8: Moderate arterial disease
- < 0.5: Severe arterial disease

PEDIATRIC CARDIOVASCULAR DYSFUNCTION SIGNS AND RISK FACTORS

The most apparent **clinical signs of cardiovascular dysfunction** will be poor feeding and weight gain, sweating and getting tired during feedings, signs of respiratory distress (rapid breathing, shortness of breath, and cyanosis), always feeling tired and inability to exercise. Children at risk are those whose mothers drank alcohol, smoked, or took medications, were exposed to radiation during pregnancy, had a viral illness during pregnancy, or were over 40 when pregnant. The child may have been premature or have autoimmune or chromosomal disorders. Smoking and alcohol use and medications can increase the risk. Family members who have had cardiovascular problems also increase the child's risk.

The following should be included in cardiac monitoring and maintenance of a child with cardiovascular disease or dysfunction:

- Cardiac monitoring and vital signs are essential.
- Watch for signs of inadequate oxygen intake, such as increased work of breathing, cyanosis, bradycardia or tachycardia, irritability, decreased muscle tone and syncope. Reposition to ease breathing and provide oxygen and medications as prescribed to manage respiratory distress.
- Monitor for respiratory distress (fast RR and HR, retracting, nasal flaring, grunting, coughing, and cyanosis). Thrombosis may present, along with edema, irritability, seizures, paralysis, coma, blood in urine, and decreased urine output.
- Maintain fluid and electrolyte balance.
- Encourage and promote rest.
- Monitor intake and output and provide nutritionally balanced diet with lots of iron and potassium and little sodium.
- Don't overtire with large feedings, and instead feed more often with smaller meals.
- Encourage infection control with hand washing, rest, good nutrition, administration of vaccines, and distancing people with infections from the cardiac patient. Prophylactic antibiotics should be administered before dental procedures to prevent bacterial endocarditis. This illness presents with fever, pale skin, petechiae, weight loss and fatigue.

NORMAL CARDIAC RATES IN THE PEDIATRIC POPULATION

Normal cardiac rates can vary widely from one child to another, so it's important to understand the normal range in order to determine if the child has an abnormal pulse. Rates will also vary depending upon whether the child is awake, asleep, or active. Pulse rate should be taken with a stethoscope because the pulse may be difficult to palpate or count accurately manually, especially for infants and small children. Additionally, this allows assessment for heart murmurs.

	At rest:	Asleep:	Active/sick:
Newborn infant	100–180	80–160	≤220
1–12 weeks	80–205	80–200	≤220
3–24 months	75–190	70–120	≤200
2–10 years	60–150	60–90	≤200
10–adulthood	55–100	50–90	≤200

RELATIONSHIP BETWEEN CO, HR, AND SV

In order to understand the hemodynamics of infants and children, it's important to understand the relationship between cardiac output, stroke volume, and heart rate as the child grows and cardiac size increases:

Age	CO	SV	HR
Newborn	800/mL/ min	5 mL	145
6 months	1,000–1,600 mL/min	10 mL	120
12 months	1,500 mL/min	13 mL	115
4 years	2,700 mL/min	26 mL	105
8 years	3,500 mL/min	42 mL	83
10 years	3,750 mL/min	50 mL	75
15 years (adult levels)	5,000–6,000 mL/min	85 mL	70

Endocrine Assessment

ASSESSING FOR ENDOCRINE DISORDERS

The **endocrine system** comprises organs that produce hormones that are critical to growth, sexual development, and metabolism, so changes in these areas are suggestive of endocrine disorders. While symptoms may vary widely, there are often generalized symptoms that can be associated with most endocrine disorders. One should question the patient about fatigue and ability to perform ADLs, heat or cold intolerance, changes in sexual libido, sexual functioning, and secondary sexual characteristics, weight fluctuation, sleep problems, decreased concentration and memory, and mood changes. During the physical exam, one should assess the patient for edema, "moon" face or "buffalo hump," exophthalmos, hair loss, female facial hair, enlarged trunk with thin extremities, and enlarged hands and feet. Vital signs should be assessed for hypo or hypertension, and one should assess for changes in skin appearance and vision.

THYROID IMAGING

Thyroid imaging plays a critical role in assessment of many thyroid diseases. This test may be used to determine the uptake characteristics of the thyroid gland in addition to the size and shape of the gland. In addition, **thyroid imaging** may determine how much iodine-131 is needed in order to safely ablate the gland when necessary. The radioactive iodine uptake scan (RAIU) is basically administration of iodine-123 with imaging performed 8 and 24 hours later:

Uptake of radioactive iodine is increased in disorders such as Graves' disease, "hot" nodules of various etiologies (including toxic multinodular goiter), TSH-secreting pituitary tumor, and iodine deficiency.

Uptake of radioactive iodine is decreased in the setting of thyroiditis and iodine excess.

Ultrasound imaging is used in thyroid disease to determine the size and structure of a thyroid nodule, such as to determine uniformity of shape, irregular contour, solid/cystic structure, and depth.

SIGNS/SYMPTOMS OF PEDIATRIC ENDOCRINE SYSTEM DISORDER

Endocrine disorders may be suspected in a child who is failing to stay within standard growth patterns. This could mean that height may be too tall or too short, that weight could be too heavy or too light, or even that puberty could start too early or too late.

Other signs/symptoms include:

- Developmentally behind peers
- More or less hungry or thirsty
- Vision problems
- Unusual tiredness
- Inability to sweat or too much sweating
- Inability to tolerate changes in temperature
- Behavior and mood swings
- Nausea
- Vomiting
- Sleep problems such as too much or too little sleep

Risk factors include maternal drug use, medication use, illness, or poor diet during pregnancy, prematurity, trauma involving the CNS, infections, chromosomal anomalies, medications, or a family history of endocrine disorders.

Physical Exam, Diagnostic Tests, and Nurse's Role with Suspected Endocrine Dysfunction

The physical exam should include assessing the head circumference in children less than 2 years of age, vital signs, mental functioning, skin disorders, vision, facial changes, oral problems or odor, neuromuscular functioning, sexual development, and heart murmurs. Thyroid function tests (thyroid disorders), growth hormone test (inadequate growth hormone), and blood glucose tests (diabetes) are used to diagnose specific disorders. Other tests done may include CBC, blood chemistry levels, urine analysis, x-rays, CT scan, MRI, ultrasound, and genetic studies. The nurse should counsel the family to continue with the treatment prescribed, including medication administration, dietary restrictions, and follow-up appointments.

Gastrointestinal Assessment

ASSESSMENT OF THE GASTROINTESTINAL SYSTEM

Assessment of the gastrointestinal system includes:

- Ask about personal and family history of gastrointestinal problems and risk factors, such as alcoholism, smoking, drug and medicine use, and poor dietary habits.
- Ask about symptoms, such as GI discomfort, flatus, nausea, vomiting, diarrhea, and abdominal pain.
- Determine the defecation pattern and ask about weight fluctuations.

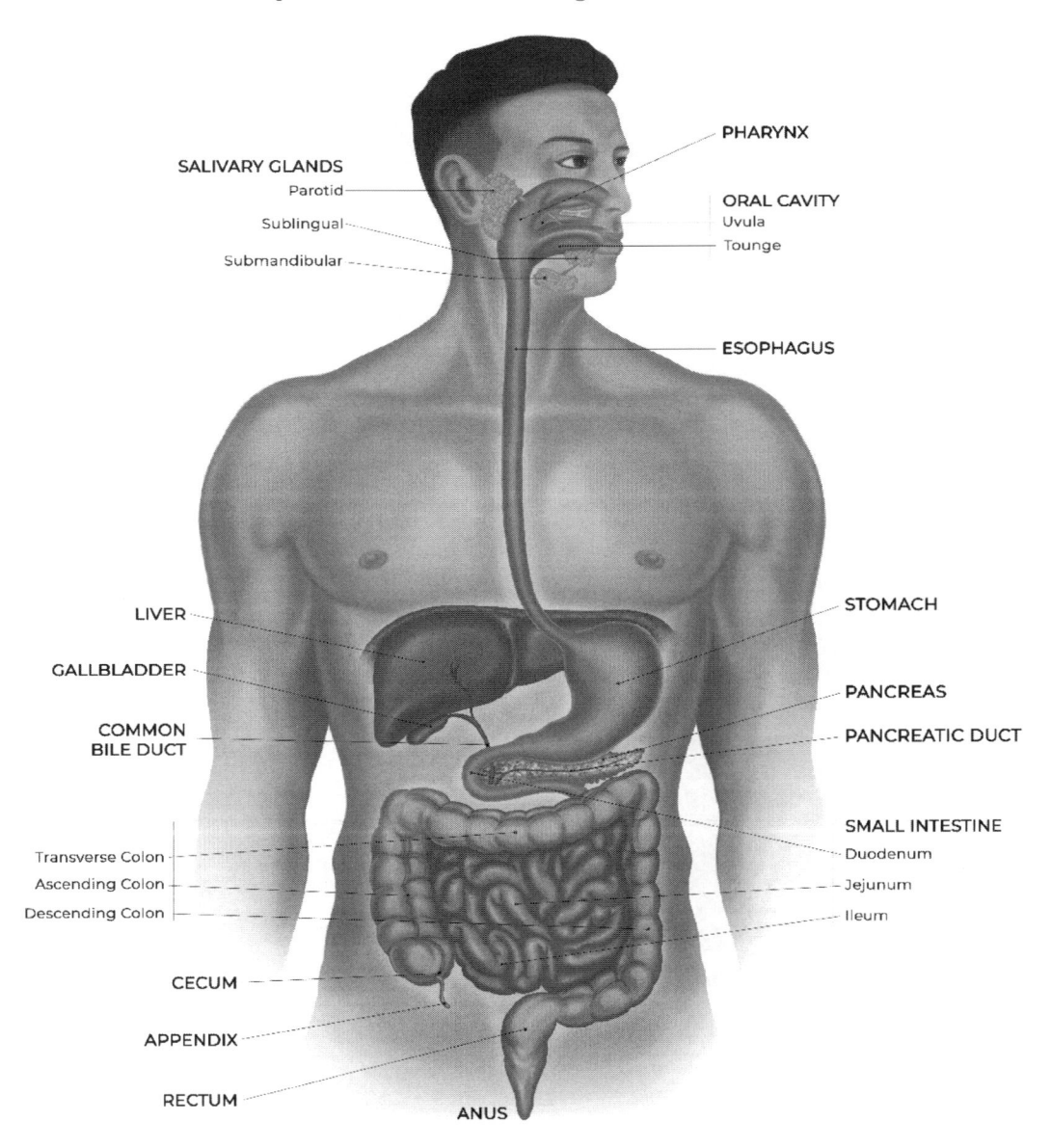

When performing a **physical assessment**, one must assess oral mucosa, tongue, teeth, pharynx, thyroid and parathyroid glands, skin color, moisture, turgor, nodules or lesions, bruises, scars, abdominal shape, and bowel sounds, assessing the abdomen in all 4 quadrants using the stethoscope diaphragm. The number of sounds heard determine if the intestines are functioning:

- **Absent**: no sounds in 3–5 minutes
- **Hypoactive**: only one sound in 2 minutes
- **Normal**: sounds heard every 5–20 seconds
- **Hyperactive**: 5–6 sounds in <30 seconds

One should examine the anal region for fissures, inflammation, tears, and dimples. Blood may be drawn for liver function studies, lipid profile, iron studies, CBC.

> **Review Video: Gastrointestinal System**
> Visit mometrix.com/academy and enter code: 378740

ASSESSMENT FOR GALLBLADDER AND PANCREATIC DISEASE

Gallbladder and pancreatic assessments are prompted by the appearance of symptoms. Symptoms of gallbladder disease include epigastric discomfort following fatty food intake, abdominal distension, right upper quadrant pain, which may be colicky, nausea, and vomiting. Pain may occur intermittently.

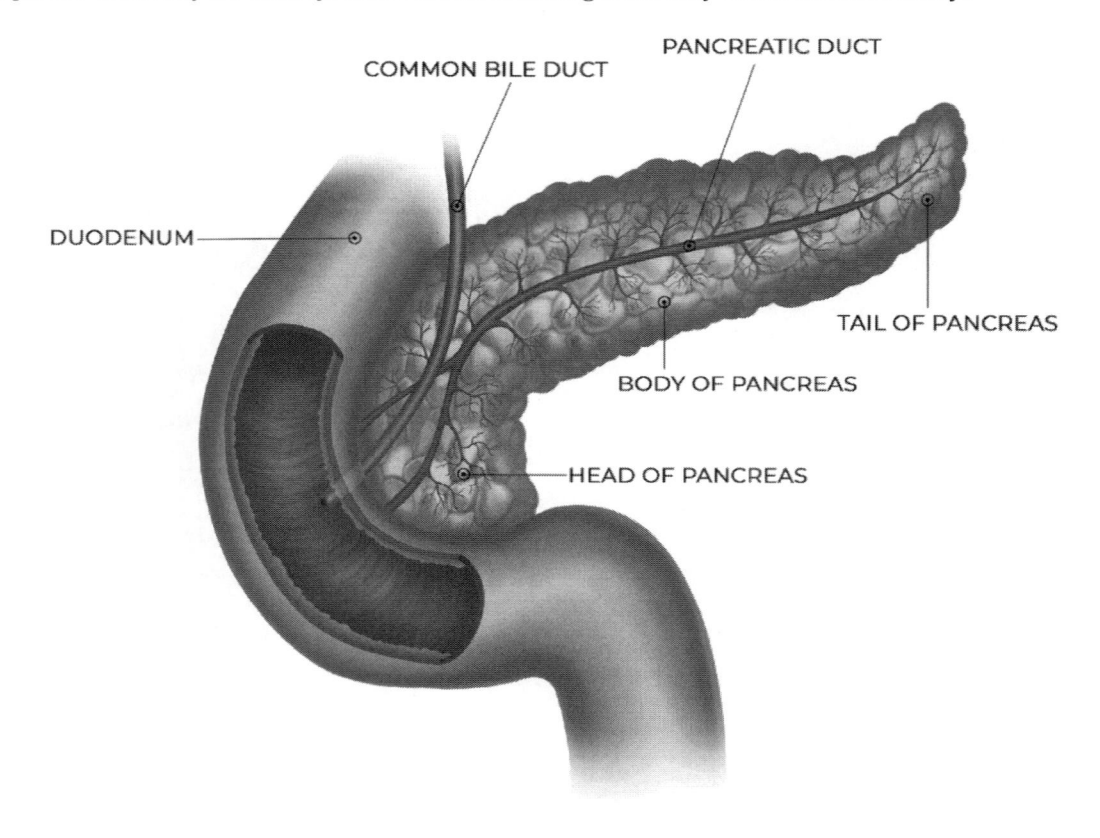

The patient with pancreatitis may have acute onset of severe abdominal pain, back pain, extensive vomiting, and dyspnea. Pancreatitis is most often related to gallstones or alcoholism, so history of alcohol use and examination for gallstones must be done:

- Assess for RUQ tenderness and mass, bowel sounds, and abdominal guarding.
- Assess the vital signs for hypotension, tachycardia, or fever and note any anxiety, agitation, or confusion.
- Note signs of hypoxia.
- Assess the skin for jaundice and bruising on the flanks and near the umbilicus.
- Blood is drawn to assess amylase and lipase, CBC, calcium, glucose, and bilirubin.

ASSESSMENT FOR LIVER DISEASE

The liver must be 70% damaged before lab tests show abnormalities. Assessment of risk factors and early symptoms are important to identify early disease. Risk factors for liver disease include alcoholism and drug abuse, risky sexual practices, exposure to infection or environmental toxins, and travel to countries with poor sanitation. One should question the patient about symptoms of liver disease, such as fatigue, itching, abdominal pain, anorexia, weight gain, fever, blood in stools or black stools, sleep problems, lack of menstruation, and lack of libido. Physical assessment includes checking vital signs and skin for scratches, pallor, jaundice, dryness, bruising, petechiae, abdominal veins and spider angiomas, and red palms:

- Assess for gynecomastia, abdominal distension, fluid waves, bowel sounds, liver margins, tenderness, consistency, and hardness and sharpness of the edge.
- Examine extremities for wasting, edema, and weakness.
- Assess neurological system for cognitive status, tremors, balance problems, slurred speech.
- Identify testicular atrophy.
- Blood should be drawn for serum enzymes and proteins, bilirubin, ammonia, clotting factors, and lipid profile.

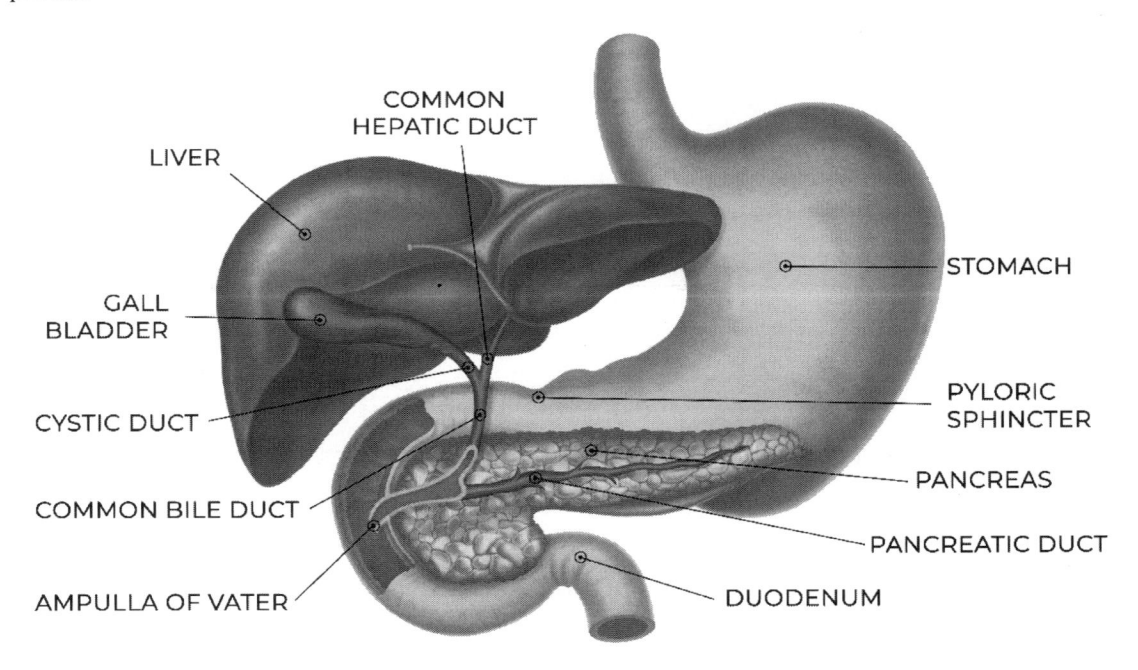

Assessment of Nutritional Status

Assessment of nutritional status begins with an assessment of the patient's intake. The patient is asked to report intake for the previous 24 hours. This may indicate the need for a **food diary** over a period of time:

- Compare the patient's nutritional intake with the requirements of the USDA's MyPlate.
- Measure height and weight and check against a BMI table to help determine nutritional status.
- Measure waist circumference.
- Assess the patient for physical signs of poor nutrition such as muscle wasting, obesity, hair breakage and loss, poor skin turgor, ulcers, bruising, and loss of subcutaneous tissue.
- Assess mucous membranes and condition of teeth, abdomen, extremities, and thyroid gland.

Nutritional status is connected to endocrine disease, infections, other acute and chronic diseases, digestion, absorption, excretion, and storage of nutrients, so these areas must also be assessed. Blood testing should include proteins, transferrin, electrolytes, vitamins A and C, carotene, and CBC. Test urine for creatinine, thiamine, riboflavin, niacin, albumin, and iodine.

Assessing Nutritional Status of Hospitalized Patients

Assessing the nutritional status of the hospital inpatient is an important part of forming a care plan. The two screening tools that are most commonly used are the **Subjective Global Assessment (SGA)** and the **Prognostic Nutritional Index (PNI)**. The SGA provides a nutritional assessment based on both the patient history and current symptoms. The patient is asked about any changes in weight and is also asked questions about his or her diet. The presence of symptoms that may lead to weight loss and poor nutritional status, such as diarrhea, nausea, and vomiting, as well as water retention (edema) and muscle wasting (cachexia), is also included in the SGA. The PNI is also used as an indicator of malnutrition and is especially helpful in determining how well a patient will recover from surgery. The PNI assesses nutritional status through the measurement of serum proteins such as albumin and transferrin combined with a skinfold measurement and a cutaneous hypersensitivity test as an indicator of immune function.

Gastrointestinal Abnormalities in Children

Abnormal GI findings would include the child who is anorexic or has a recent large weight gain or loss. Nausea, vomiting, diarrhea, constipation, pain in the abdomen, and blood in the stool are all cause for concern. Assess the family and child history for drugs or medications taken during pregnancy, any problems during or after birth, possible poisoning or drug use, or GI disorders. Assess the diet for deficiencies and assess growth for failure to thrive. Fever may reveal dehydration or infection. Assess the mouth for cavities, infection or cleft palate/lip. Palpate the palate for defects. The skin should not be pale, jaundiced, or orange (check the sclera). Assess the stomach for distention, masses, tenderness, rigidity, enlarged organs, umbilical hernia, or visible peristalsis. The bowel sounds should be audible without being excessive. The anus should be patent with no bleeding. Percuss for gas, fluid, and masses or enlarged organs.

Diagnostic Tests When Gastrointestinal Abnormality is Suspected

An ultrasound or CT scan can show cysts, tumors, abscesses, gallstones, biliary duct obstruction, and appendicitis. GI studies (upper, lower, esophagus, stomach, small bowel), such as a barium enema, help find lesions, obstructions and problems with movement of the system. Esophagogastroduodenoscopy, endoscopy, and gastroscopy examine the upper GI tract, detecting bleeding, ulcers, and tissue problems. Colonoscopy, proctoscopy, anoscopy, sigmoidoscopy, and proctosigmoidoscopy examine the lower GI tract, detecting bleeding, IBD, diarrhea, and allowing for biopsies.

STOOL COLLECTION

Collecting stool specimens may be indicated to identify what organisms are causing gastrointestinal disturbances or to assess for blood in the stool. Infants in diapers may need a urine bag to separate stool from urine. Toilet trained children can be told to urinate first, flush, and then helped to collect the stool in a bedpan or toilet. Plastic wrap can be placed over the toilet bowl to catch the stool. The specimen is collected and placed in the appropriate container, labeled, and delivered to the laboratory. If the sample cannot be delivered to the laboratory immediately, it may be refrigerated. Time limits for refrigeration exist and must be adhered to per laboratory orders. Take care not to contaminate the specimen.

PEDIATRIC ABDOMINAL PRESSURE MONITORING

Abdominal pressure monitoring is indicated for ascites, abdominal trauma, major fluid resuscitation, and abdominal/retroperitoneal bleeding. Intra-abdominal pressure is measured by attaching a pressure transducer or water-column manometer to a Foley catheter in the bladder, because bladder pressure correlates with abdominal pressure. The patient should be in supine flat position if possible. The bladder must be empty for accurate measurement. The catheter should be clamped, and the transducer should be zeroed at the iliac crest along the midaxillary line. Then, 1 mL/kg (usually about 10 mL for critically ill patients) of fluid is injected into the bladder and left in place for 30-60 seconds before reading the pressure following a patient expiration. Abdominal cavity pressure should be 0 mmHg in a well child, and 1-8 mmHg in a critically ill child. Intraabdominal pressure may also be checked with an indwelling NG tube. If risk for compartment syndrome exists, the wound should not be closed. Sudden release of pressure and reperfusion may cause acidosis, vasodilation, and cardiac arrest, so the patient should be given crystalloid solutions before decompression.

Hematologic Assessment

HEMATOLOGIC SYSTEM

The hematologic system comprises the blood and those areas involved in the production of blood, such as the bone marrow and the reticuloendothelial system. Blood is a tissue that circulates through the heart and vascular system. Blood consists of a serous liquid, plasma (78%) and solids (22%), such as platelets, red blood cells, and white blood cells. Blood has a number of functions:

- Transporting nutrients, ions, and hormones
- Providing a defense system (white blood cells)
- Transporting agents of immune responses
- Maintaining temperature
- Removing waste products such as urea and carbon dioxide

Blood cells are formed in the bone marrow. Bone marrow appears yellow in areas with fatty deposits but red in areas producing blood (hematopoiesis). In children, most of the marrow is red, but as bones age, more and more of the red marrow is replaced by yellow marrow. The health of the bone marrow is critical to blood production.

Blood cells are produced in the bone marrow from stem cells, which can replicate throughout life to produce new cells. Stem cells are stimulated, according to the needs of the body, to differentiate into 2 types of stem cells:

- **Lymphoid cells**, which produce T and B lymphocytes, which are integral to both the cell-mediated and the antibody-mediated immune response.
- **Myeloid cells**, which produce all other types of blood cells (RBCs, WBCs, and platelets).

Most blood cells have a life span that is relatively short, so there is a need for constant hematopoiesis to replenish the supply.

The reticuloendothelial system comprises tissue macrophages derived from monocytes, produced in the marrow. The monocytes circulate in the blood for the first 24 hours and then enter the tissues where they mature and differentiate into macrophages, which defend against pathogenic microorganisms through phagocytosis.

SPLEEN AND THYMUS

The spleen and the thymus are important to the reticuloendothelial system and the circulatory system:

- **Spleen:** This small organ contains small areas of white pulp (lymphoid tissue and B and T lymphocytes), red pulp (RBCs and macrophages), and cavities for storage of red blood cells (5%) and platelets (20-40%). Lymphocytes and other cells of the immune system are produced and stored in the spleen. The lymphoid tissue filters the blood as it circulates through, removing worn out cells and platelets and breaking down hemoglobin into bilirubin, which is then removed from circulation by the liver and kidneys. Blood circulating through the spleen can activate the lymphocytes. The spleen can produce some blood cells if the bone marrow malfunctions.
- **Thymus:** This organ is where T lymphocytes begin to mature. Then, they migrate to the spleen and lymph nodes where they continue to mature, after which they circulate between the lymph system and the blood.

Abnormally Functioning Hematologic System

Major symptoms of abnormal function of the hematologic system can include bone/joint pain, numerous infections, abnormal bleeding or bruising, weight loss, tiredness, headache, crankiness and dizziness. Assess for maternal-fetal blood incompatibility, prematurity, low birth weight, dietary factors (low iron intake, inadequate nutrition), or excess bleeding (menstruation). Increased heart rate or rapid breathing may be noted, along with blood spots on the skin, pallor or flushed skin, yellow sclera, retinal hemorrhage, blurry vision, pale mucus membranes, cyanosis, enlarged lymph nodes, apathy, swollen joints, blood in urine, or heavy menstrual bleeding. Abdominal organs may be enlarged. Small muscle mass and tenderness over joints or bones may be noted. Listen for heart murmurs and abnormal lung sounds. The following lab studies may be indicated (what they can detect): RBC count, WBC counts with differential (infection, deficiencies), Hgb (anemia), Hct (anemia), mean corpuscular volume (RBC size), Hgb, Hgb concentration, platelet count (bleeding disorders), retics (anemia), coagulation and hemostasis studies (hemorrhagic disorders), total iron-binding capacity, ferritin, iron, and transferring levels (anemia), and bone marrow aspiration (aplastic anemia, leukemia).

Monitor for infection (steroids increase risk of infection) and use precautions as needed. Adequate nutrition and rest can decrease risk of infection. Assess skin color and vital signs to monitor tissue oxygenation. Provide O_2 (severe tissue hypoxia) and blood transfusions as prescribed. Watch for signs of bleeding (petechiae, bruising, blood in stool or urine). If a bleeding problem exists, limit activities, do not give aspirin or take rectal temps, and avoid IM injections. Teach parents and patients the signs of bleeding: swelling, tingling, tenderness, pain, warmth, and petechiae. Teach the family ways to prevent bleeding: choose activities not likely to cause physical injury, avoid aspirin, tobacco, alcohol and drugs, and use protective gear for high-risk activities.

Pediatric White Blood Cell Count

White blood cell (leukocyte) count is used as an indicator of bacterial and viral infection. **WBC** is reported as the total number of all white blood cells.

- Neonate: 9000-30,000 per mm^3
- 1-2 months: 5000-19,500 per mm^3
- 3 months-1 year: 6000-17,500 per mm^3
- 1-2 years: 6000-17,000 per mm^3
- 2-6 years: 5500-15,500 per mm^3
- 6-18 years: 4500-10,800 per mm^3
- >18 years: 4500-10,500 per mm^3

The differential provides the percentage of each different type of leukocyte. An increase in the white blood cell count is usually related to an increase in one type of leukocyte and often an increase in immature neutrophils, known as bands, which is referred to as a "shift to the left," an indication of an infectious process.

Cells	Normal value	Changes
Immature neutrophils (bands)	0-5%	Increase with infection
Segmented neutrophils (segs)	40-60%	Increase with acute, localized, or systemic bacterial infections
Eosinophils	0-1%	Decrease with stress and acute infection
Basophils	0-1%	Decrease in acute stage of infection
Lymphocytes	20-40%	Increase in some viral and bacterial infections
Monocytes	0-2%	Increase in recovery stage of acute infection

Genitourinary Assessment

ASSESSMENT OF KIDNEYS AND URINARY TRACT

Assessment of kidneys and urinary tract includes:

- Assess the health history for family urinary system disease and risk factors, such as previous urinary disease, increased age, immobility, hypertension, diabetes, chemical exposure, chronic disease, radiation to the pelvis, STIs, alcohol or drug use, and complications of pregnancy and delivery.
- Determine daily fluid intake.
- Question symptoms such as flank or abdominal pain, hesitancy, urgency, difficulty or straining with voiding, difficulty emptying the bladder, urinary incontinence, fatigue, SOB, exercise intolerance from anemia, fever, chills, blood in the urine, and GI symptoms.

Physical assessment includes vital signs, kidney and bladder palpation, and percussion over the bladder after urination:

- Palpate for ascites and edema.
- Measure the DTRs and check gait and ability to walk heel-to-toe.
- Examine the genitalia and check the urethra and vagina for herniation, irritation, or tears.

Urine specimen is obtained via clean catch midstream technique for analysis and culture if indicated. Blood is taken for a CBC, and in males, prostate-specific antigen (PSA) levels will also be measured via blood specimen.

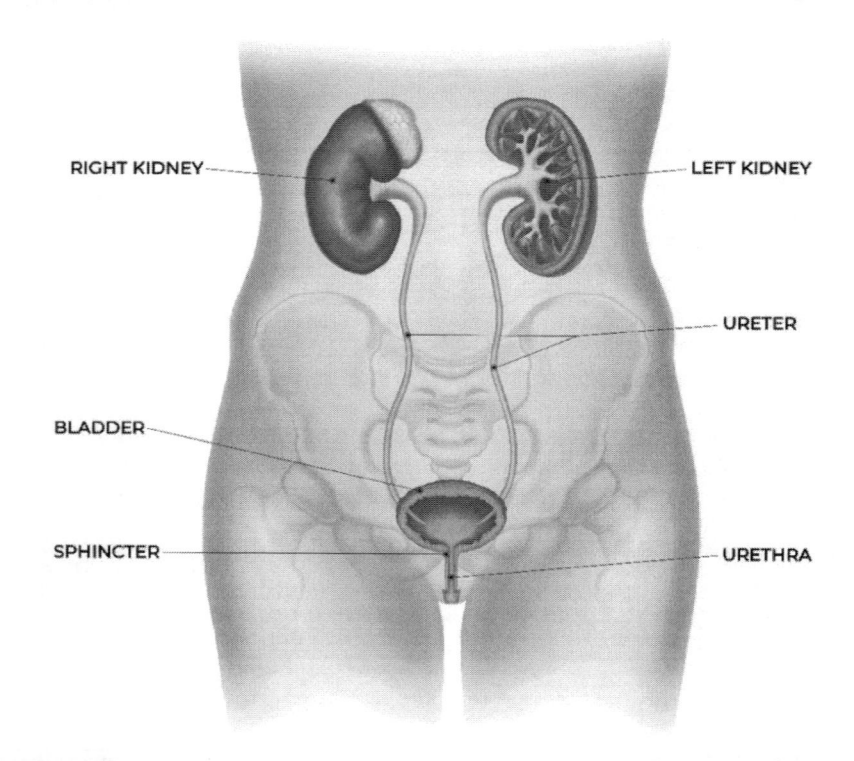

Review Video: Urinary System
Visit mometrix.com/academy and enter code: 601053

Kidney Regulatory Functions Regarding Fluid Balance

Kidney regulatory functions include maintaining **fluid balance**. Fluid excretion balances intake with output, so increased intake results in a large output and vice versa:

- **Osmolality** (the number of electrolytes and other molecules per kg/urine) measures the concentration or dilution. With dehydration, osmolality increases; with fluid retention, osmolality decreases. With kidney disease, urine is dilute and the osmolality is fixed.
- **Specific gravity** compares the weight of urine (weight of particles) to distilled water (1.000). Normal urine is 1.010–1.025 with normal intake. High intake lowers the specific gravity, and low intake raises it. In kidney disease, it often does not vary.
- **Antidiuretic hormone** (ADH/vasopressin) regulates the excretion of water and urine concentration in the renal tubule by varying water reabsorption. When fluid intake decreases, blood osmolality rises, and this stimulates the release of ADH, which increases reabsorption of fluid to return osmolality to normal levels. ADH is suppressed with increased fluid intake, so less fluid is reabsorbed.

Assessing Sexual Health and Preferences

Bringing up the topic of sex gives a patient permission to ask questions and openly discuss **sexual concerns**:

- Ask for permission to ask questions about sexual health and preferences during the gynecological/urological portion of the health history.
- If the patient refuses, go on with the rest of the health history, otherwise continue.
- Ask first if the person has sex with men, women, or both.
- Be nonjudgmental and do not assume that those who are elderly or disabled do not have sex. Use layman terms according to the patient's age and education level.
- Ask if the person is having any problems with relationships or sexual intercourse.
- Ask if the person has ever been forced to have sex or if is afraid of anyone close to them.
- End by asking if there are any questions about expression of sexual feelings, contraception, safe sex practices, or risky behavior.
- Refer those with problems to their doctor, or a gynecologist, urologist, or sex therapist.

Genitourinary System Dysfunction in Children

A newborn experiencing genitourinary system dysfunction may eat poorly, lose weight, excrete excess urine, cry when urinating, become dehydrated, possibly convulse, and develop a fever. An infant may strain while urinating, the urine may smell foul, and he may develop a diaper rash. The older child may complain of being thirsty and urinating all the time, incontinence, vomiting, bloody or foul-smelling urine, being tired, lack of appetite, fever, and pain in the side, stomach or back. Risk factors for a GU problem can include young or old maternal age during pregnancy, multiparity, frequent UTIs, catheterizations, problems with toilet training, diabetes, poor immune system, sexual activity, strep infections, and a family history of GU problems. Assess growth, temperature (elevated), BP (elevated or low), signs of respiratory distress (tachypnea, cyanosis, increased work of breathing, edema), abdomen (distention), any congenital abnormalities, bladder (distention), and kidneys (tender, enlarged).

Maintain strict I&O and daily weights. Provide fluids that the child likes to encourage intake. Avoid caffeine. Assess for dehydration. Assess for overhydration by checking BP frequently and monitoring respiratory status for signs of pulmonary edema. If prescribed, keep the child on a low-sodium diet. Offer meals with foods that are healthy and that the child likes to encourage adequate nutrition. Avoid infection with good hand washing, having the child avoid those with illnesses, making sure the child gets good nutrition and plenty of rest, and using good aseptic technique with invasive procedures.

Diagnostic Tools and Findings

The following are diagnostic tools used for a child with suspected genitourinary dysfunction and what the findings may show:

- **Urinalysis**: Assesses renal function
- **Urine culture and sensitivity**: Tests for the presence of bacteria (allowing for the provider to identify which antibiotic will work against it)
- **Blood urea nitrogen**: Will be elevated due to impaired renal filtration and rapid protein catabolism
- **Creatinine**: Will be elevated due to reduced creatinine excretion
- **Ultrasonography**: A noninvasive exam of the urinary tract
- **Voiding cystourethrography**: X-rays of the bladder and urethra with contrast medium
- **Computed tomography scan**: Visualizes cross sections of the kidney
- **Intravenous pyelography**: X-rays of the kidneys and ureters with contrast medium
- **Cystoscopy**: Visualizes the urinary tract through an inserted tube
- **Renal biopsy**: Removal of renal tissue that is then examined to determine types of nephrotic syndrome
- **Renal scan**: Serial films of the kidneys after injecting them with radioactive materials
- **Urodynamics**: Tests both bladder and urethral function and innervation

Urinalysis

Elements assessed in a **urinalysis** include the following:

- **Color**: Urine is normally a pale yellow/amber and darkens when urine is concentrated or other substances (such as blood or bile) are present.
- **Appearance**: Normally urine appears clear but may be slightly cloudy.
- **Odor**: Slight odor is normal. Bacteria may give urine a foul smell, depending upon the organism. Some foods, such as asparagus, change the odor of urine.
- **Specific gravity**: Normal range is 1.015–1.025. This may increase if protein levels increase or if there is fever, vomiting, or dehydration.
- **pH**: Normal range is 4.5–8.0 with an average of 5–6.
- **Sediment**: Sediment results from various casts. Red cell casts result from acute infections, broad casts from kidney disorders, and white cell casts from pyelonephritis. Leukocytes > 10 per mL^3 are present with urinary tract infections.
- **Glucose, ketones, protein, blood, bilirubin, and nitrate**: A negative result for these elements is normal. Urine glucose may increase with infection (with normal blood glucose). Frank blood may be caused by some parasites and diseases but also by drugs, smoking, excessive exercise, and menstrual fluids. Increased red blood cells may result from lower urinary tract infections.
- **Urobilinogen**: 0.1–1.0 units

Urine Collection in Infants

Obtaining **urine specimens** from infants requires a special collection bag. The perineal area is cleaned and dried, and then the bag, with an adhesive outer portion, is attached. Urine should be aspirated directly from the bag as soon as possible after voiding. Urine can also be obtained from disposable diapers if using a urine dipstick. If the urine must be saved, it requires refrigeration. Older children and adolescents can collect their urine in a cup, with help as needed. If it is a clean-catch specimen, they should be taught how to clean themselves (females wipe front to back three times with a separate wipe each time, males clean the tip of the penis) and then void a small amount into the toilet before collecting any urine in the cup. Answer any questions the school age child has and ask the adolescent female if she is menstruating (the collection may be delayed or documentation made about the presence of red blood cells). Toddlers may need support from parents and a "potty chair."

Catheterization and Suprapubic Aspiration of Pediatric Patients

When a urine specimen is needed quickly, the child cannot void, or if kidney failure or obstruction is suspected, **bladder catheterization** may be indicated. In seriously ill infants, suprapubic aspiration is used to confirm a diagnosis of urinary tract infection.

Some birth defects preclude the use of a catheter, and using **suprapubic aspiration** decreases the risk of contamination. The doctor will insert a needle above the pubic bone when the bladder is full. It is a painful procedure and pain management is essential, such as using lidocaine cream at the insertion site

Microscopic Analyses of Urine

Microscopic analyses of urine involve placing the urine specimen in a centrifuge to separate out the **sediment**, which is then examined under a microscope:

- **Erythrocytes** should not be in the urine and may indicate inflammation, injury, or slight bleeding from strenuous exercise.
- **Leukocytes** in the urine usually are indicative of infection, cancer, or kidney disorders.
- **Casts** are caused from kidney disease that causes tiny tube-like plugs of material (red or white cells, protein, fatty substances) to be flushed from the kidneys to the urine. The type of cast may help with diagnosis.
- **Crystals** should appear in small numbers. Some types of crystals or large numbers of crystals may be a sign of kidney stones or a metabolic disorder.
- **Bacteria** in the urine indicate an infection.
- **Fungi** in the urine indicate a yeast infection.
- **Parasites** may migrate to the urinary system in some types of infestation.

Voiding Cystourethrogram

A **voiding cystourethrogram (VCUG)** is a type of radiologic test, often with contrast, that is performed on the urinary system. The test takes a series of pictures of the child's bladder to determine how the contrast moves through the urinary system and to ensure that the bladder, ureters, and urethra are intact and that there are no blockages. When the child voids during the test, it also monitors the flow of urine exiting the body in a normal pattern. A VCUG can detect the presence of urinary reflux, or if a child is having frequent urinary tract infections, it may detect the presence of urinary abnormalities that are causing the condition.

Integumentary Assessment

GENERAL SKIN ASSESSMENT

Skin color varies according to ethnicity. Color changes should be assessed to determine if they are local or extend over the entire body, and if they are permanent or transient. Pallor may indicate stress, impaired oxygenation, and vasoconstriction. Erythema may indicate vasodilation, local inflammation, and blushing. Cyanosis indicates impaired oxygenation, and jaundice indicates increased bilirubin.

Temperature is typically assessed by touching the skin with the back of the hand. Skin should be warm and equal bilaterally. Hypothermia may indicate impaired circulation, intravenous infusion, and immobilized limb (such as in a cast). Hyperthermia may indicate fever, infection, and excessive exercise.

> **Review Video: Skin Assessment**
> Visit mometrix.com/academy and enter code: 794925

EFFECTS OF AGE ON SKIN

Age is an important consideration when evaluating the skin because the characteristics of the skin change as people age.

- An **infant's** skin is thinner than an adult's because, while the epidermis is developed, the dermis layer is only about 60% of that of an adult and continues to develop after birth. The skin of premature infants is especially friable, allowing for transepidermal water loss and evaporative heat loss.
- During **adolescence**, the hair follicles activate, the thickness of the dermis decreases about 20%, and epidermal turnover time increases, so healing slows.
- As people **continue to age**, Langerhans' cells decrease in number, making the skin more prone to cancer, and the inflammatory reactions decrease. The sweat glands, vascularity, and subcutaneous fat all decrease, interfering with thermoregulation and contributing to dryness and irritation of the skin. The epidermal-dermal junction flattens, resulting in skin that is prone to tearing. The elastin in the skin degrades with age and solar exposure. The thinning of the hypodermis can lead to pressure injuries.

> **Review Video: Integumentary System**
> Visit mometrix.com/academy and enter code: 655980

BRADEN SCALE

The Braden scale is a risk assessment tool that has been validated clinically as predictive of the risk of patient's developing pressure injuries. It was developed in 1988 by Barbara Braden and Nancy Bergstrom and is in wide use. The scale scores six different areas with five areas scored 1–4 points, and one area 1–3 points. The lower the score, the greater the risk.

Area	Score of 1	Score of 2	Score of 3	Score of 4
Sensory perception	Completely limited	Very limited	Slightly limited	No impairment
Moisture	Constantly moist	Very moist	Occasionally moist	Rarely moist
Activity	Bed	Chair	Occasional walk	Frequent walk
Mobility	Immobile	Limited	Slightly limited	No limitations
Nutritional pattern	Very poor	Inadequate	Adequate	Excellent
Friction and shear	Problem	Potential problem	No apparent problem	

EVALUATING WOUNDS FOR ETIOLOGY

Wounds should be evaluated for **etiology** during the initial assessment to ensure proper treatment. Wounds can arise from a number of different causes:

- **Pressure**: Wounds that occur over bony prominences, such as the heels and coccyx, may be related to pressure, shear, or friction. The skin should be carefully examined for discolorations or changes in texture that might indicate compromise.
- **Arterial**: Arterial insufficiency is associated with a decrease in pedal pulses, and cool atrophic (shiny, dry) skin. It may result in small punctate-type ulcers, frequently on the dorsum of foot.
- **Venous stasis**: A decrease in venous circulation often results in hemoglobin leaking into the tissues of the lower leg, giving a brown discoloration. Tissue is often edematous, and ulcers are most common near the medial malleolus.
- **Diabetic neuropathy/ischemia**: Neuropathy can result in a lack of sensation to pain so that injuries to the feet may go unnoticed. Diabetes may also cause damage to small vessels, resulting in ischemia that can lead to ulcerations.
- **Trauma**: Injuries resulting from accidents or other types of trauma may vary considerably with some resulting in extensive damage to bones, tissues, organs, and circulation. Additionally, the wounds may be contaminated. Each wound must be assessed individually for multiple factors.
- **Burns**: Burn wounds may be chemical or thermal and should be assessed according to the area, the percentage of the body burned, and the depth of the burn. First-degree burns are superficial and affect the epidermis only. Second-degree burns extend through the dermis. Third-degree burns affect underlying tissue, including vasculature, muscles, and nerves.
- **Infection**: An infected surgical or wound site can result in pain, edema, cellulitis, drainage, erosion of the sutures and ulceration of the tissue. Surgical sites must be assessed carefully and laboratory findings reviewed.

Elements of Wound Assessment

Location and Size

Wound location should be described in terms of anatomic position using landmarks (such as sternal notch, umbilicus, lateral malleolus), correct medical terminology, and directional terms:

- Anterior (in front)
- Posterior (behind)
- Superior (above)
- Inferior (below)

Wound size should be carefully described through actual measurement rather than association (the size of a dime). Measurements should be done with a disposable ruler in millimeters or centimeters. The current standard for measurement:

$$\text{length} \times \text{width} \times \text{depth} = \text{dimension}$$

However, a clear description requires more detail. The measurement should be done at the greatest width and greatest length. More than two measurements may be needed if the wound is very irregularly shaped. The depth of the wound should be measured by inserting a sterile applicator and grasping or marking the applicator at skin level and then measuring the length below. Ideally, the wound should be photographed as well, following protocols for photography.

Wound Bed Tissue

Wound bed tissue should be described as completely as possible, including color and general appearance:

- **Granulation tissue** is slightly granular in appearance and deep pink to bright red and moist, bleeding easily if disturbed.
- **Clean non-granular tissue** is smooth and deep pink or red and is not healing.
- **Hypergranulation** is excessive, soft, flaccid granulating tissue that is raised above the level of the periwound tissue, preventing proper epithelization, and may reflect excess moisture in the wound.
- **Epithelization** should appear at wound edges first and then eventually cover the wound. It is dry and light pink or violet in color.
- **Slough** is necrotic tissue that is viscous, soft, and yellow-gray in appearance and adheres to the wound.
- **Eschar** is hard dark brown or black leathery necrotic tissue that accumulates with death of the tissue.

Wound Margins

Wound margins and the tissue surrounding the wound should be described carefully and with correct terminology:

- **Color** should be described using color descriptions and such terms as blanched, erythematous (red), or ecchymosed (purple, green, yellow).
- **Skin texture** may be normal, indurated (hardened), or edematous (swollen). Note if there is cellulitis or maceration evident.
- **Wound edges** may be diffuse (without clear margins), well defined, or rolled. A healing ridge may be evident if granulation has begun. Note if the wound is closed (as with a surgical incision) or open (as with dehiscence or ulcerations). Note if wound edges are attached or unattached (indicating undermining or tunneling).
- **Tunneling or undermining** should be assessed by probing the wound margins with a moist sterile cotton applicator, using clock face locators (toward the head is 12 o'clock, for example). Tunneling may be described as extending from 3 o'clock to 4 o'clock. A large area is usually described as undermining. The size should be measured or estimated as closely as possible.

DISTRIBUTION, DRAINAGE, AND ODOR

Distribution of lesions should be clearly delineated if there is more than one lesion over an area. The arrangement of the lesions can be helpful for diagnosis and treatments.

- Linear (in a line)
- Satellites (small lesions around a larger one)
- Diffuse (scattered freely over an area)

Drainage may vary considerably from nothing at all to copious outpourings of discharge.

- Serous drainage is usually clear to slightly yellow.
- Serosanguineous drainage is a combination of serous drainage and blood.
- Sanguineous drainage is bloody.
- Purulent discharge may be thick and milky, yellow, brownish, or green, depending upon the infective agent.

Odor requires more subjective assessment, but the odor and type of discharge together can provide useful information. Some infective agents, such as *Pseudomonas*, produce distinctive odors, which may be described in various ways: musty, foul, sweet.

ASSESSMENT CHARACTERISTICS OF ARTERIAL, NEUROPATHIC, AND VENOUS ULCERS

The assessment process is important in delineating between the arterial, neuropathic, or venous origin of the ulcer. Characteristics of each must be known and closely examined:

Location

- **Arterial**: Ends of toes, pressure points, traumatic nonhealing wounds
- **Neuropathic**: Plantar surface, metatarsal heads, toes, and sides of feet
- **Venous**: Between knees and ankles, medial malleolus

Wound Bed

- **Arterial**: Pale, necrotic
- **Neuropathic**: Red (or ischemic)
- **Venous**: Dark red, fibrinous slough

Exudate

- **Arterial**: Slight amount, infection common
- **Neuropathic**: Moderate to large amounts, infection common
- **Venous**: Moderate to large amounts

Wound Perimeter

- **Arterial**: Circular, well-defined
- **Neuropathic**: Circular, well-defined, often with callous formation
- **Venous**: Irregular, poorly-defined

Pain

- **Arterial**: Very painful
- **Neuropathic**: Pain often absent because of reduced sensation
- **Venous**: Pain varies

Skin

- **Arterial**: Pale, friable, shiny, and hairless, with dependent rubor and elevational pallor
- **Neuropathic**: Ischemic signs (as in arterial) may be evident with comorbidity
- **Venous**: Brownish discoloration of ankles and shin, edema common

Pulses

- **Arterial**: Weak or absent
- **Neuropathic**: Present and palpable, diminished in neuroischemic ulcers
- **Venous**: Present and palpable

PEDIATRIC FLUORESCEIN STAINING

Fluorescein staining is used with a Wood's light, which converts ultraviolet light into visible light and is used to diagnose skin lesions and injuries to the eye. The procedure must be carried out in a room that can be darkened, and the procedure should be explained to the child and/or parent beforehand so that they are aware the room will be dark.

- **Skin**: The skin must be clean and dry prior to application of the dye. For the skin, the chemical is applied directly to the lesion and surrounding tissue or area of concern. The affected area will have a different color from the surrounding tissue although not all types of lesions fluoresce.
- **Eye**: A strip of blotting paper containing the fluorescein dye is touched lightly to the surface of the eye and the patient asked to blink in order to spread the dye about the corneal surface. Once the dye is applied, the room light is turned off, and the Wood's light is turned on and used to scan the area. If the cornea or sclera has been disrupted, this area will uptake more of the dye and the injured area will appear bright yellow-green.

Musculoskeletal Assessment

ASSESSING RISK OF FALLING

Many factors must be examined and combined to determine the **fall risk** status of a patient. They include age, sensory deficits, mobility problems, neurological disorders, past history of falling, cognitive impairment, and depression. Some medications, such as those associated with postural hypotension and psychotropic medications, may increase the danger of falls. The presence of dizziness, acute or chronic illness, poor physical status, elimination requirements, medications, and environmental concerns contribute to the risk for falls.

Multiple factors increase risk, so careful history and physical exam are necessary as part of assessment. When the presence of risk factors shows a risk for falls, this information should be communicated to other caregivers by wristband, colored markers on doors, care plans, or other effective means. The factors are then modified as much as possible. The patient should be re-evaluated as their condition changes or after a fall to determine the cause.

ASSESSING PATIENTS WITH DISABILITIES

A patient with **disabilities** may find it very difficult to obtain screening for health problems due to inaccessibility:

- Work with the patient to resolve barriers to obtain weight, mammography, bone density tests, and pap/pelvic exams on a regular basis.
- Ask how to best assist the patient during the assessment.
- Observe the patient carefully for nonverbal communication, such as grimacing.
- If sensation is affected, warn the patient before touching any part of the body.
- Always address all areas of the patient's history, including sexual history.
- Use an interpreter that is not a family member if needed.
- Give the patient extra time to respond to questions when there is aphasia or other communication problems.
- Address the impact of the disability on the ability to perform ADLs, health status in general, access to healthcare, financial status, emotional status, work, community roles, and family wellbeing.

MUSCULOSKELETAL DYSFUNCTION IN CHILDREN

The first sign of musculoskeletal dysfunction may be a delay in gross motor skills, such as walking. There may be limited range of motion, stiffness, or pain. The mother may have taken drugs or medications, experienced trauma, or had an infection during pregnancy. Other risk factors are hypoxia or a strange position in the womb, a multiple birth, breech delivery, or a genetic problem, obesity, sports, steroids, delayed development, or family history of skeletal or muscular disorders. Chart the height and weight of the child. Assess the child's walk, posture, spinal alignment (scoliosis), and any discrepancies in symmetry. Inspect for any deformities, masses, lesions, tenderness, or warmth. Assess joint range of motion, strength of muscles (symmetry), and any lack of muscle mass. Diagnostic tools that may be used include x-rays, ultrasound, arthroscopy (see inside the joints), arthrography, bone scans (find tumors and inflammation), CT scans, MRI (find tumors and assess muscles, ligaments, and bones), joint aspiration (aspirate excess fluid), and blood tests (check for certain enzymes that aid in the diagnosis).

Limb Assessment and Cast Care

If a limb is affected, assess the **vascular and nerve status**. Check the color, temperature, capillary refill, sensation, and if the child can move it. Help with physical therapy to maintain proper movement, muscle tone and bone health. Prevent injury and skin breakdown by turning the child frequently, using special mattresses, applying lotion to healthy skin, and protecting pressure points.

For **cast care**, assess the skin under the cast for odor and pain or warmth and keep the cast clean and dry. Use stool softeners, fluids, and a high fiber diet to help prevent constipation. Encourage frequent urination and a low calcium diet to prevent UTIs. Teach deep breathing techniques and assess for pulmonary or cardiac dysfunction related to bed rest. Give pain meds as needed, but use positioning and diversion to help with pain. Provide a proper diet and adequate fluids. Encourage as much physical activity as the child can tolerate and help the child to do as much as possible for herself.

Neurological Assessment

ASSESSMENT OF THE NEUROLOGICAL SYSTEM

Assessment of the neurological system includes:

- Assess the **health history** for any trauma, falls, alcoholism, drug abuse, medications taken, and family history of neurological problems.
- Ask about any presenting **neurological symptoms**, the circumstances in which they occur, whether they fluctuate, and any associated factors, such as seizures, pain, vertigo, weakness, abnormal sensations, visual problems, loss of consciousness, changes in cognition, and motor problems.

Assessment includes determining the level of consciousness and cognition. Posture and movements are assessed for abnormalities. Facial expression and movement are noted. Cranial nerve assessment is done. The patient is assessed for strength, coordination, and balance and the ability to perform ADLs. One should assess for clonus and test all reflexes, including Babinski, gag, blink, swallow, upper and lower abdominal, cremasteric in males, plantar, perianal, biceps, triceps, brachioradialis, patellar and ankle. Peripheral sensation is tested by touching the patient with cotton balls and the sharp and dull ends of a broken tongue blade.

> **Review Video: What is the Function of the Nervous System**
> Visit mometrix.com/academy and enter code: 708428

ASSESSING FUNCTIONAL STATUS

Functional abilities include the acts needed to meet basic needs and perform *activities of daily living* (ADLs), such as eating and elimination, as well as those *activities that are essential to independent living* (IADLs), such as shopping. A thorough assessment of the patient's functional abilities will identify areas that should be concentrated upon during rehabilitation. One should observe the patient as he/she performs these functions and record the following:

- Degree of independence shown
- Ability to complete activity without rest
- Nerve function
- Muscle function and strength
- Motion
- Coordination
- Cardiac status
- Respiratory status
- Assistance required to complete activity

The facility usually provides one of the tools available to record a functional assessment. The most common tool used is the Functional Independence Measure (FIM). Other tools available include the Barthel Index, the PULSES Profile, and the Patient Evaluation Conference System.

American Stroke Association Classification System for the Extent of Brain Attack Injury

The American Stroke Association developed a **brain attack outcome classification system** to standardize descriptions of stroke injuries:

- **Number of impaired domains** (Potentially affected neurological domains: motor, sensory, vision, language, cognition, and affect): Level 0: no domains impaired; Level 1: one domain impaired; Level 2: two domains impaired; Level 3: greater than 2 domains impaired.
- **Severity of impairment**: A (minimal or no neurological deficit due to stroke); B (mild/moderate deficit); or C (severe deficit). Note: When more than one domain is affected, severity is measured by the domain with the most impairment.

Assessment of function determines the ability to **live independently**:

- **I**: Independent in basic activities of daily living (BADL), such as bathing, eating, toileting, and walking; and instrumental activities of daily living (IADL), such as telephoning, shopping, maintaining a household, socializing, and using transportation
- **II**: Independent in BADL but partially dependent in IADL
- **III**: Partially dependent in BADL (less than 3 areas) and IADL
- **IV**: Partially dependent in BADL (3 or more areas)
- **V**: Completely dependent in BADL (5 or more areas) and IADL

Level III requires much assistance and Levels IV and V cannot live independently.

Administration of the NIHSS

The **National Institutes of Health Stroke Scale (NIHSS)** is administered with careful attention to directions. The examiner should record the answers and avoid coaching or repeating requests, although demonstration may be used with aphasic patients. The scale comprises 11 sections, with scores for each section ranging from 0 (normal) to 2, 3, or 4:

- **Level of consciousness**: Response to noxious stimulation (0–3), request for month and his/her age (0–2), request to open and close eyes, grip and release unaffected hand (0–2)
- **Best gaze**: Horizontal eye movement (0–2)
- **Visual**: Visual fields (0–3)
- **Facial palsy**: Symmetry when patient shows teeth, raises eyebrows, and closes eyes (0–3)
- **Motor, arm**: Drift while arm extended with palms down (0–4)
- **Motor, leg**: Leg drift at 30 degrees while patient supine (0–4)
- **Limb ataxia**: Finger-nose and heel-shin (0–2)
- **Sensory**: Grimace or withdrawal from pinprick (0–2)
- **Best language**: Describes action of pictures (0–3)
- **Dysarthria**: Reads or describes words on list (0–2)
- **Distinction and inattention**: Visual spatial neglect (0–2)

GLASGOW COMA SCALE

The Glasgow coma scale (GCS) measures the depth and duration of coma or impaired level of consciousness and is used for post-operative assessment. The GCS measures three parameters: best eye response, best verbal response, and best motor response, with a total possible score that ranges from 3 to 15:

Eye opening	4: Spontaneous
	3: To verbal stimuli
	2: To pain (not of face)
	1: No response
Verbal	5: Oriented
	4: Conversation confused, but can answer questions
	3: Uses inappropriate words
	2: Speech incomprehensible
	1: No response
Motor	6: Moves on command
	5: Moves purposefully respond pain
	4: Withdraws in response to pain
	3: Decorticate posturing (flexion) in response to pain
	2: Decerebrate posturing (extension) in response to pain
	1: No response

Injuries/conditions are classified according to the total score: 3–8 Coma; ≤8 Severe head injury likely requiring intubation; 9–12 Moderate head injury; 13–15 Mild head injury.

> **Review Video: Glasgow Coma Scale**
> Visit mometrix.com/academy and enter code: 133399

CRANIAL NERVES

	Name	Function	PE Test
I	Olfactory	Smell	Test olfaction
II	Optic	Visual acuity	Snellen eye chart; Accommodation
III	Oculomotor	Eye movement/pupil	Pupillary reflex; Eye/eyelid motion
IV	Trochlear	Eye movement	Eye moves down & out
V	Trigeminal	Facial motor/ sensory	Corneal reflex; Facial sensation; Mastication
VI	Abducens	Eye movement	Lateral eye motion
VII	Facial	Facial expression; Taste	Moves forehead, closes eyes, smile/frown, puffs cheeks; Taste
VIII	Vestibulo-cochlear (Acoustic)	Hearing; Balance	Hearing (Weber/Rinne tests); Nystagmus
IX	Glosso-pharyngeal	Pharynx motor/sensory	Gag reflex; Soft palate elevation
X	Vagus	Visceral sensory, motor	Gag, swallow, cough
XI	Accessory	Sternocleidomastoid and trapezius (motor)	Turns head & shrugs shoulders against resistance
XII	Hypoglossal	Tongue movement	Push out tongue; move tongue from side to side

Neurological Motor Testing and Testing for Nuchal Rigidity

Neurological motor testing requires careful observation for involuntary or spastic movements and examination of muscles for lack of symmetry or atrophy with observation of gait. Muscle tone is examined by flexing and extending the upper and lower extremities, observing for flaccid or spastic changes. Muscle strength is examined by having the patient press fingers, wrists, elbows, hips, knees, ankles, and plantar area against resistance, graded 0 (no movement) to 5 (normal).

Pronator drift is an indication of disease of the upper motor neurons. The patient stands with eyes closed and both arms extended horizontally in front with the palms facing upwards (supination). The patient should be told to hold the arms still and not move them while the examiner taps downward on the arm. If motor neuron disease is present, the patient's arms will drift downward and hands will drift toward pronation.

Nuchal rigidity is tested by placing the hands behind the patient's head and flexing the neck gently to determine if there is increased resistance.

Neurological Dysfunction Symptoms in Children

Abnormal neurological symptoms include headaches, dizziness or fainting, loss of consciousness, difficulty with movement or coordination, or delayed development. Factors that put the child at risk include maternal drug/alcohol use, maternal infection, poor maternal nutrition, prematurity, birth trauma, head injury, hypoxia, toxins, meningitis, drug use, chronic disease, child abuse, chromosomal abnormalities, or a family history of neurological disorders. The exam should consist of vital signs (suspect increased ICP if vital signs are abnormal), head circumference (suspect increased ICP if enlarged), level of consciousness (suspect neuro disorder if altered), development, cranial nerve function, senses, cerebellar function (altered gait, balance, or coordination), reflexes, and any abnormal movements. Full fontanels can result from increased ICP. Muscle tone, strength, and sense of position should be assessed. Blood studies will show any infection, toxins, and seizure med levels. UA will show drugs; X-rays will detect any skull fractures; an EEG can detect seizures; echoencephalography, CT scan, MRI, and nuclear brain scan can detect lesions and abnormalities of the brain. A lumbar puncture is used to collect CSF, which can show infection.

A complete neuro check should be done at least every 4 hours: vital signs, LOC, pupil size, equality and reaction to light, vision or reflex abnormalities, motor and sensory function, reflexes, head circumference, fontanels in infants. Assess for changes in developmental level. Provide for proper fluids and monitor I&O. Keep the head above the heart to decrease the ICP. Make sure emergency equipment is nearby. Use seizure precautions: Protective equipment to prevent injury during seizure, do not restrain the child who is seizing or place anything in the child's mouth, keep harmful objects away from the child, maintain a patent airway and turn the child to the side to allow fluids to drain. Note the time and length of the seizure. After the seizure, reorient the child to person, place, and time. Use infection precautions.

Cerebral Perfusion Pressure in Children

Normal values for cerebral perfusion pressure (CPP) varies based on age:

- Infants and toddlers: 40-50 mmHg
- Children: 50-60 mmHg
- 18 years: 60-100 mmHg

PERIPHERAL NERVE ASSESSMENT OF THE CHILD

A musculoskeletal evaluation should include **peripheral nerve assessment** to determine if injury has impaired nerve function. Nerve function should be assessed for both sensation and movement. Assessment of sensation is done with a sharp or pointed instrument, using care not to prick the skin. The child should feel a slight prick if the sensory function is intact:

- **Median**: The median nerve branches from the brachial plexus, which arises from C5, C6, C7, C8, and T1. The median nerve travels down the arm and forearm, through the carpal tunnel. Sensation is evaluated by pricking the top or distal surface of the index finger. Movement is evaluated by having the child touch the ends of the thumb and little finger together and having the child flex the wrist.
- **Peroneal**: The peroneal nerve branches from the sciatic nerve, which arises from the L4, L5, and S1, S2, and S3 dorsal nerves and travels down the leg. The peroneal nerve enervates the lower leg, foot, and toes. Evaluate sensation by pricking the webbed area between the great and second toe. Evaluate movement by having the child dorsiflex and extend the foot.
- **Radial**: The radial nerve branches from the brachial plexus and enervates the dorsal surface of the arm and hand, including the thumb and fingers 2, 3, and 4. Evaluate sensation by pricking skin in the webbed area between the thumb and the index finger. Evaluate movement by having the child extend the thumb, the wrist, and fingers at the metacarpal joint.
- **Tibial**: The tibial nerve branches from the sciatic nerve. The tibial nerve travels down the back of the leg, through the popliteal fossa at the back of the knee and terminates at the planter surface of the foot. Sensation is evaluated by pricking the medial and lateral aspects of the plantar surface of the foot. Movement is evaluated by having the child plantar-flex the toes and then the ankle.
- **Ulnar**: The ulnar nerve branches from the sciatic nerve and travels down the arm from the shoulder, traveling along the anterior forearm beside the ulna, to the palm of the hand. Sensation is evaluated by pricking the distal fat pad at the end of the small finger. Movement is evaluated by having the child extend and spread all fingers.

EXAMINATION OF THE PUPILS

Note size, shape, symmetry, reaction, and accommodation:

- **Benign anisocoria**: Slight inequality in size with no other abnormalities
- **Horner's syndrome** (impaired sympathetic nerve impulse): Pupil small, regular, reactive to light and accommodation, associated with ptosis
- **Ocular nerve paralysis**: Nonreactive dilated pupil, sometimes associated with lateral deviation and ptosis
- **Tonic pupil**: Large, regular with reduced or absent reaction to light and slow accommodation
- **Argyll Robertson** (usually associated with syphilis): Bilateral small, irregular pupils nonreactive to light but normal accommodation
- **Dilated, fixed**: Brain damage, hypoxia, anticholinergic agents and glutethimide poisoning
- **Small, fixed**: Pontine hemorrhage, glaucoma eye drops, and narcotic drugs
- **Surgical abnormalities**: Iridectomy

EENT Assessment

NORMAL HEARING DEVELOPMENTAL CHARACTERISTICS USED TO ASSESS HEARING DEFICITS IN INFANTS AND TODDLERS

Hearing deficits may be identified very early if developmental characteristics are carefully observed in infants and children. **Normal hearing** responses include:

- **≤3 months**: Positive Moro (startle) reflex to sound. Noise disturbs sleep and the infant reacts to sounds by opening eyes or blinking.
- **3-6 months**: The infant is comforted at the sound of their parent's voice and tries to emulate sounds. The infant looks in the direction of sound.
- **6-12 months**: The infant begins to vocalize more with cooing and gurgling with different inflections. The infant responds to their name and simple words and looks in the direction of sound.
- **12-18 months**: The toddler begins first words about 12-15 months and imitates sounds, follows vocal directions, and points to familiar items when asked.
- **18-24 months**: The toddler is more verbal with about half of vocabulary understandable and knows about 20-50 words. The toddler points to body parts of familiar objects with asked.

AUDIOMETRY

Audiometry is used to test hearing in pediatric patients 6 months or older. Testing requires an audiometry tool that tests for decibel frequencies between 500 and 4000 Hz and an earpiece in the appropriate size for the child so that it seals the opening of the ear canal. Impacted cerumen should be removed prior to testing, and testing should be done in a quiet area.

Procedure:

1. Position the child in a sitting position on the table or their mother's lap. If the child is able to cooperate, ask the child to raise a hand if hearing a sound or watch the child for a response.
2. Activate the probe and insert into the ear (procedure may vary depending on the type of audiometry). For handheld models, pull the pinna back for young children and up and back for adolescents when inserting the earpiece.
3. Test according to the procedure manual for the device.
4. Note the results for the different decibel settings.
5. Compare the child's results to those for normal hearing.
6. If the child's hearing is outside of normal limits, the test may be repeated at another time.
7. If the results show that the child's hearing is persistently outside the normal range after 2 or 3 tests, then the child should be referred to an audiologist for more comprehensive testing.

VISUAL ACUITY TESTING

Visual acuity testing uses the **Snellen eye chart**, which has various letters and numbers in decreasing sizes. The alternate **Illiterate/Tumbling Eye chart** with the letter E facing in various directions and in three different sizes can also be used. Testing is done with the child standing or sitting 20 feet from a chart, so charts are usually placed at the end of a long hallway, but lighting must be adequate. In some cases, mirrors are used to simulate 20 feet.

Procedure:

1. Place the child in the appropriate position and ask the child to cover one eye.
2. Ask the child to read the smallest line that the child is able to see well enough to read. If using the E chart, the child uses a finger to point in the direction the E is facing.
3. Repeat the test with the opposite eye and then both eyes.
4. Record the results. If there is a difference of 2 or more levels between the eyes, this may be an indication of amblyopia. The normal vision (20/20) line is usually considered the fourth line from the bottom of the Snellen chart.

Note: A measurement of 20/30 means that at 20 feet the person can read what a person with normal vision can read at 30 feet.

CERUMEN IMPACTION AND REMOVAL

Cerumen impaction may involve partial or complete obstruction of the ear canal and may cause pain, tinnitus, feeling of fullness, itching, loss of hearing, odor, and cough. Begin by examining the ear with an otoscope to determine the location and amount of cerumen. **Methods of removal** include:

- **Curettage:** A special loop instrument is used with an otoscope (for visualization) to scoop out cerumen, but this method may result in trauma. A lighted curette is also available.
- **Suction:** A special suction tube is used with an otoscope (for visualization) to remove the cerumen.
- **Cerumenolytic agent:** An agent (such as Cerumenex) is instilled into the ear with the child lying on the opposite side. An earplug is used to keep the solution in place for 15 to 30 minutes. This is followed by irrigation.
- **Irrigation:** With the child sitting upright or lying flat, hold an emesis basin below the ear to catch solution. Use an ear irrigating syringe with warm water and gently squirt water into the ear canal to loosen the cerumen. Check periodically with the otoscope and catch loose material with the loop instrument or crocodile forceps if necessary. The irrigation may be used with or without a cerumenolytic agent but is usually more effective if the cerumen has been softened.

Note that if the cerumen is very hard or thick, first softening may work best with all different approaches. In some cases, a combination of methods may be used.

Respiratory Assessment

ASSESSMENT OF THE RESPIRATORY SYSTEM

If significant respiratory distress is present, one must stabilize the patient before doing a **respiratory history** or ask family if available:

- Question the patient about risk factors, such as smoking, exposure to smoke or other inhaled toxins, past lung problems, and allergies.
- Ask the patient about symptoms of respiratory problems, such as dyspnea, cough, sputum production, fatigue, ability to do ADLs and IADLs, and chest pain.
- Determine how long symptoms have been present, the length of periods of dyspnea, aggravating and alleviating factors, and the severity of symptoms.

When performing a **physical assessment**, one should assess vital signs, posture, pulse oximetry, check nails for clubbing, do a skin assessment, listen to lung sounds via auscultation and percussion, and look for accessory muscle use, signs of anxiety, and edema. Depending on condition, blood may be drawn for arterial blood gases, electrolytes, and CBC. Sputum cultures may be obtained.

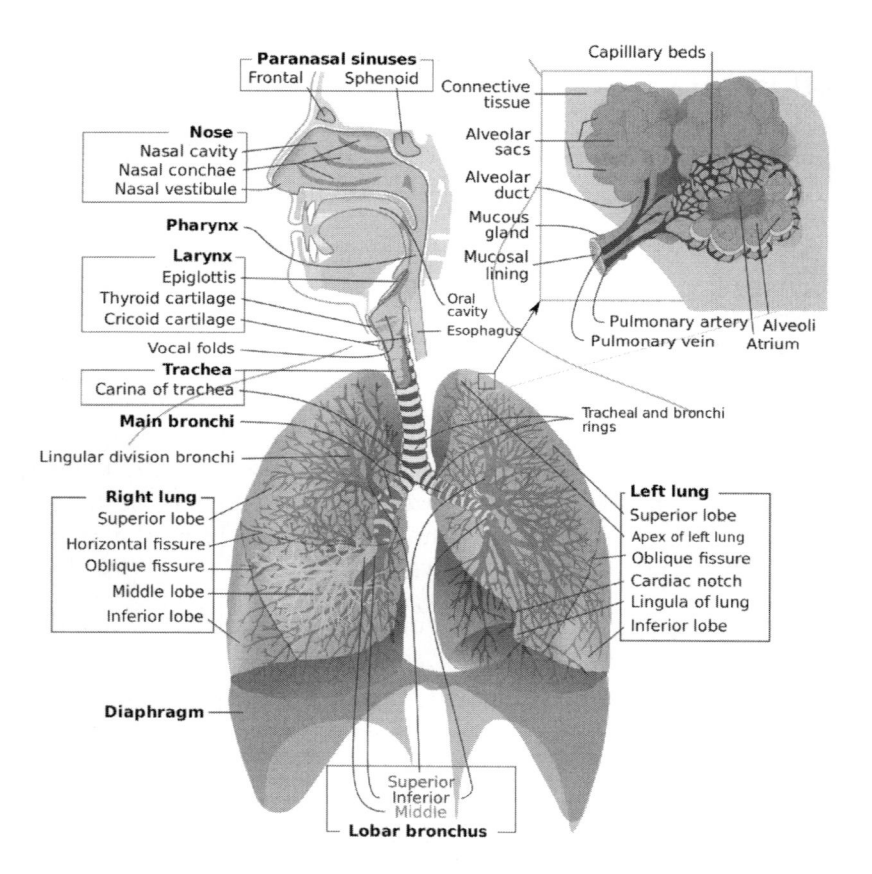

> **Review Video: Respiratory System**
> Visit mometrix.com/academy and enter code: 783075

Primary and Secondary Muscles Used for Breathing

Muscles used for breathing are separated into primary and secondary muscle groups.

- The **primary muscle groups** are those that are used in normal, quiet breathing. When patients are in respiratory distress and breathing is more difficult, secondary muscle groups become activated. The muscles considered primary for breathing are the diaphragm and the external intercostal muscles. These muscles act by changing the pressure gradient, allowing the lungs to expand and air to flow in and out.
- The **secondary muscle groups** include the sternocleidomastoid, scaleni, internal intercostals, obliques, and abdominal muscles. These secondary muscle groups work when breathing is difficult, both in inspiration and expiration, in cases such as obstructions or bronchoconstriction. Use of these secondary muscle groups can often be seen on exam and may be described as see-saw or abdominal breathing (when the abdominal muscles are being used during exhalation) or retractions as the muscles activate and can be seen between rigid structures such as bone.

Normal Physiological Airway Clearance

Normal airway clearance is caused by various aspects of the respiratory system. A thin layer of mucus lines the airways as a protective mechanism against debris and helps trap foreign objects before they enter the lower airways. Proper hydration keeps the mucosa adequately moist so it can trap foreign debris. As this debris lands in the mucus, the cilia in the respiratory tract act as an "elevator" to push the debris up to the larynx, where it can either be coughed up or swallowed and digested. An intact cough reflex is necessary for the debris to stimulate the cough, and normal muscle strength and nerve innervation of the diaphragm is required to produce a sufficiently forceful cough.

Ventilation/Perfusion Ratio

In order to maintain homeostasis, the respiratory and cardiac systems need to maintain a careful balance. The **ventilation/perfusion ratio** indicates that ventilation of the lungs and perfusion to the lungs are within a normal balance. A normal ventilation/perfusion ratio is equal to 0.8. A ventilation/perfusion ratio higher than normal is indicative of ventilation that is too high, perfusion that is too low, or some combination of the two. This can occur because of hyperventilation (either physiological or caused by healthcare practitioners due to incorrect ventilator settings), pulmonary embolism, or hypotension. Essentially, a high ventilation/perfusion ratio means that there is more ventilation than perfusion. If the ventilation/perfusion ratio is lower than normal, then ventilation is too low, perfusion is too high, or some combination of the two. This can be caused by atelectasis, pneumonia, or lung disease. Whatever the cause, a low ventilation/perfusion ratio indicates that there is more perfusion than ventilation.

Normal and Abnormal Breath Sound Terms

Normal breath sounds can be divided into three types. Vesicular breath sounds are low, soft sounds that can normally be heard over the peripheral lung space. Bronchovesicular breath sounds are moderate pitch breath sounds that are normally heard in the upper lung fields. Tracheal breath sounds are higher in pitch and heard over the trachea. Abnormal breath sounds are also known as adventitious lung sounds. Wheezes are high-pitched, expiratory sounds caused by air flowing through an obstructed airway. Stridor is also high-pitched, but is usually heard on inspiration in the upper airways. Coarse crackles are caused by an excessive amount of secretions in the airway and can be heard on inspiration and expiration. Fine crackles occur late in the expiratory phase and usually occur when the peripheral airways are being "popped" back open.

> **Review Video: Lung Sounds**
> Visit mometrix.com/academy and enter code: 765616

Diagnostics and Tools Used During Pulmonary/Thoracic Trauma Assessment

The diagnostic procedures and tools used during assessment of **pulmonary and thoracic trauma/disease** will vary according to the type and degree of injury/disease, but may include:

- **Thorough physical examination** including cardiac and pulmonary status, assessing for any abnormalities.
- **Electrocardiogram** to assess for cardiac arrhythmias.
- **Chest x-ray** should be done for all those with injuries to check for fractures, pneumothorax, major injuries, and placement of intubation tubes. X-rays can be taken quickly and with portable equipment so they can be completed quickly during the initial assessment.
- **Computerized tomography** may be indicated after initial assessment, especially if there is a possibility of damage to the parenchyma of the lungs.
- **Oximetry and atrial blood gases** as indicated.
- **12-lead electrocardiogram** may be needed if there are arrhythmias for more careful observation.
- **Echocardiogram** should be done if there is apparent cardiac damage.

Capnography with End-Tidal CO_2 Detector

Capnometry utilizes an **end-tidal CO_2 (ETCO) detector** that measures the concentration of CO_2 in expired air, usually through pH sensitive paper that changes color (commonly purple to yellow). Typically, the capnometer is attached to the ETT and a bag-valve-mask (BVM) ventilator. The capnogram provides data in the shape of a waveform that represents the partial pressure of exhaled gas. It is often used to confirm placement of endotracheal tubes as clinical assessment is not always sufficient, and it is a noninvasive mode of monitoring carbon dioxide in the respiratory cycle. Information provided by the capnogram includes:

- $PaCO_2$ level
- Type and degree of bronchial obstruction, such as COPD (waveform changes from rectangular to a fin-like)
- Air leaks in the ventilation system
- Rebreathing precipitated by need for new CO_2 absorber
- Cardiac arrest
- Hypothermia or reduced metabolism

The normal capnogram is a waveform that represents the varying CO_2 level throughout the breath cycle:

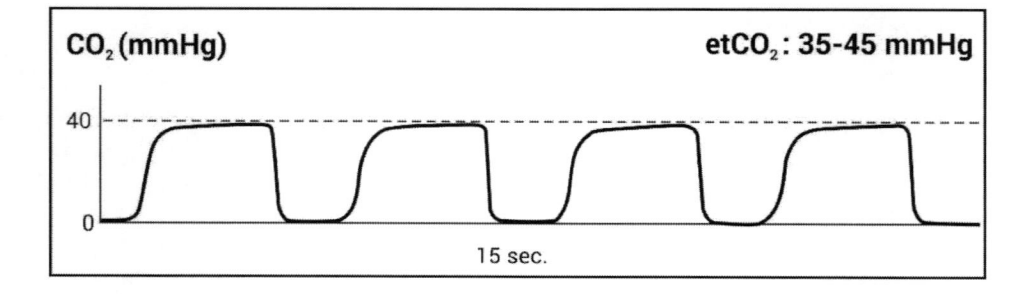

ARTERIAL BLOOD GASES

Arterial blood gases (ABGs) are monitored to assess effectiveness of oxygenation, ventilation, and acid-base status and to determine oxygen flow rates. Partial pressure of a gas is that exerted by each gas in a mixture of gases, proportional to its concentration, based on total atmospheric pressure of 760 mmHg at sea level. Normal values include:

- Acidity/alkalinity (pH): 7.35–7.45
- Partial pressure of carbon dioxide ($PaCO_2$): 35–45 mmHg
- Partial pressure of oxygen (PaO_2): ≥80 mmHg
- Bicarbonate concentration (HCO_3^-): 22–26 mEq/L
- Oxygen saturation (SaO_2): ≥95%

The relationship between these elements, particularly the $PaCO_2$ and the PaO_2 indicates respiratory status. For example, $PaCO_2$ >55 and the PaO_2 <60 in a patient previously in good health indicates respiratory failure. There are many issues to consider. Ventilator management may require a higher $PaCO_2$ to prevent barotrauma and a lower PaO_2 to reduce oxygen toxicity.

> **Review Video: Blood Gases**
> Visit mometrix.com/academy and enter code: 611909

NORMAL RESPIRATORY RATES IN INFANTS AND CHILDREN

Children's vital signs vary considerably according to age, height, and weight. **Normal respiratory rates** are as follows:

- Newborns breathe about 30-60 times per minute and then respirations begin to slow to 30 times per minute by age 1 month, dropping to 24-30 during ages 1-3, and 17-29 by age 6.
- Respiratory rates for children 6-12 are typically 13-23 and then decrease to a rate similar to adults (12-20) between ages 12 and 28.

RESPIRATORY MONITORING WITH PULSE OXIMETRY

Pulse oximetry, continuous or intermittent, utilizes an external oximeter that attaches to the child's foot, toe, or finger (depending on age) to indirectly estimate **arterial oxygen saturation (SPO_2)**, the percentage of hemoglobin that is saturated with oxygen. The oximeter also usually attaches to a machine that emits a beep with each heartbeat and indicates the current heart rate and BP. The oximeter uses light waves to determine oxygen saturation (SPO_2). Oxygen saturation should be maintained >95% although some patients with cardiovascular or pulmonary disorders may have lower SPO_2. Results may be compromised by impaired circulation, excessive light, poor positioning, and fingernail polish. If SPO_2 falls, the oximeter should be repositioned, as incorrect position is a common cause of inaccurate readings. Oximetry is often used post-surgically and when patients are on mechanical ventilation. Oximeters do not provide information about carbon dioxide levels, so they cannot monitor carbon dioxide retention. Oximeters cannot differentiate between different forms of hemoglobin, so if hemoglobin has picked up carbon monoxide, the oximeter will not recognize it.

SPIROMETRY/PULMONARY FUNCTION TEST

Spirometry, a form of pulmonary function testing, uses a device to measure the volume of gas and the flow rate. Spirometry measurements can include forced vital capacity (FVC), forced expiratory volume in 1 second (FEV1), multiple forced expiratory flow (FEF) values, forced inspiratory flow (FIFs), and the maximum voluntary ventilation (MVV). Procedure:

1. Explain the procedure and allow the patient to practice taking one or two deep breaths and then exhaling with lips sealed about the mouthpiece, so the patient understands what to do.
2. Gender, age, height, and weight is usually input into the device.
3. The patient should sit because sitting is safer as some may experience dizziness during the test.
4. Secure nose clips.
5. Ask the patient to take a deep breath and then to exhale through the mouthpiece as strongly as possible for as long as possible. (Some computerized devices provide feedback on a computer screen, such as candles that extinguish as the patient breathes out.)
6. Repeat at least 2 more times. The best score out of 3 or more is used.
7. If a patient is to be retested after a bronchodilator, the patient should wait for 15 minutes after receiving the medication before repeating the tests.

Psychological Assessment

ELEMENTS OF THE PSYCHOSOCIAL ASSESSMENT

A psychosocial assessment should provide additional information to the physical assessment to guide the patient's plan of care and should include:

- Previous hospitalizations and experience with healthcare
- Psychiatric history: Suicidal ideation, psychiatric disorders, family psychiatric history, history of violence and/or self-mutilation
- Chief complaint: Patient's perception
- Complementary therapies: Acupuncture, visualization, and meditation
- Occupational and educational background: Employment, retirement, and special skills
- Social patterns: Family and friends, living situation, typical activities, support system
- Sexual patterns: Orientation, problems, and sex practices
- Interests/abilities: Hobbies and sports
- Current or past substance abuse: Type, frequency, drinking pattern, use of recreational drugs, and overuse of prescription drugs
- Ability to cope: Stress reduction techniques
- Physical, sexual, emotional, and financial abuse: Older adults are especially vulnerable to abuse and may be reluctant to disclose out of shame or fear
- Spiritual/cultural assessment: Religious/spiritual importance, practices, restrictions (such as blood products or foods), and impact on health/health decisions

COGNITIVE ASSESSMENT

Individuals with evidence of dementia, delirium, or short-term memory loss should have cognition assessed. The **mini-mental state exam (MMSE)** or the **mini-cog test** are both commonly used. These tests require the individual to carry out specified tasks and are used as a baseline to determine change in mental status.

MMSE:

- Remembering and later repeating the names of 3 common objects
- Counting backward from 100 by 7s or spelling "world" backward
- Naming items as the examiner points to them
- Providing the location of the examiner's office, including city, state, and street address
- Repeating common phrases
- Copying a picture of interlocking shapes
- Following simple 3-part instructions, such as picking up a piece of paper, folding it in half, and placing it on the floor

A score of ≥24/30 is considered a normal functioning level.

Mini-cog:

- Remembering and later repeating the names of 3 common objects
- Drawing the face of a clock, including all 12 numbers and the hands, and indicating the time specified by the examiner

A score of 3–5 (out of 5) indicates a lower chance of dementia but does not rule it out.

Confusion Assessment Method

The Confusion Assessment Method is an assessment tool intended to be used by those without psychiatric training in order to assess the progression of delirium in patients. The tool covers 9 factors, some factors have a range of possibilities, and others are rated only as to whether the characteristic is present, not present, uncertain, or not applicable. The tool also provides room to describe abnormal behavior. Factors indicative of delirium include:

- **Onset**: Acute change in mental status
- **Attention**: Inattentive, stable, or fluctuating
- **Thinking**: Disorganized, rambling conversation, switching topics, illogical
- **Level of consciousness**: Altered, ranging from alert to coma
- **Orientation**: Disoriented (person, place, and time)
- **Memory**: Impaired
- **Perceptual disturbances**: Hallucinations, illusions
- **Psychomotor abnormalities**: Agitation (tapping, picking, moving) or retardation (staring, not moving)
- **Sleep-wake cycle**: Awake at night and sleepy in the daytime

The Confusion Assessment Method indicates delirium if there is an acute onset, fluctuating inattention, and disorganized thinking OR altered level of consciousness.

Hamilton Anxiety Scale

The Hamilton Anxiety Scale (HAS or HAMA) is utilized to evaluate the anxiety related symptomatology that may be present in adults as well as children. It provides an evaluation of overall **anxiety** and its degree of severity. This includes **somatic anxiety** (physical complaints) and **psychic anxiety** (mental agitation and distress). This scale consists of 14 items based on anxiety produced symptoms. Each item is ranked 0–4 with 0 indicating no symptoms present and 4 indicating severe symptoms present. This scale is frequently utilized in psychotropic drug evaluations. If performed before a particular medication has been started and then again at later visits, the HAS can be helpful in adjusting medication dosages based in part on the individual's score. It is often utilized as an outcome measure in clinical trials.

Beck Depression Inventory

The Beck Depression Inventory (BDI) is a widely utilized, self-reported, multiple-choice questionnaire consisting of 21 items, which measures the **degree of depression**. This tool is designed for use in adults ages 17–80. It evaluates physical symptoms such as weight loss, loss of sleep, loss of interest in sex, fatigue, and attitudinal symptoms such as irritability, guilt, and hopelessness. The items rank in four possible answer choices based on an increasing severity of symptoms. The test is scored with the answers ranging in value from 0–3. The total score is utilized to determine the degree of depression. The usual ranges include: 0–9 no signs of depression, 10–18 mild depression, 19–29 moderate depression, and 30–63 severe depression.

Evaluation for Suicidal or Homicidal Thoughts

During a risk assessment two of the most important areas to evaluate are the patient's **risk for self-harm or harm to others**. The staff member performing the assessment should very closely evaluate for any descriptions or thoughts the patient may have concerning these risks. Direct questioning on these subjects should be performed and documented. Close evaluation of any delusional thoughts the patient may be having should be carefully evaluated. Does the patient believe he or she is being instructed by others to perform either of these acts? Safety of the patient and others needs to be a top priority and carefully documented. If the patient indicates that they are having these thoughts or ideas, they must be placed in either suicidal or assault precautions with close monitoring per facility protocol.

SUICIDE RISK ASSESSMENT

A suicide risk assessment should be completed and documented upon admission, with each shift change, at discharge, or any time suicidal ideations are suggested by the patient. This risk assessment should evaluate some of the following criteria:

- Would the patient sign a contract for safety?
- Is there a suicide plan? How lethal is the plan?
- What is the elopement risk?
- How often are the suicidal thoughts, and have they attempted suicide before?

Any associated symptoms of hopelessness, guilt, anger, helplessness, impulsive behaviors, nightmares, obsessions with death, or altered judgment should also be assessed and documented. The higher the score the higher the risk for suicide.

ALCOHOL USE ASSESSMENT

The **Clinical Instrument for Withdrawal for Alcohol (CIWA)** is a tool used to assess the severity of alcohol withdraw. Each category is scored 0–7 points based on the severity of symptoms, except #10, which is scored 0–4. A score <5 indicates mild withdrawal without need for medications; for scores ranging 5–15, benzodiazepines are indicated to manage symptoms. A score >15 indicates severe withdrawal and the need for admission to the unit.

- Nausea/Vomiting
- Tremor
- Paroxysmal Sweats
- Anxiety
- Agitation
- Tactile Disturbances
- Auditory Disturbances
- Visual Disturbances
- Headache
- Disorientation or Clouding of Sensorium

The **CAGE** tool is used as a quick assessment to identify problem drinkers. Moderate drinking, (1–2 drinks daily or one drink a day for older adults) is usually not harmful to people in the absence of other medical conditions. However, drinking more can lead to serious psychosocial and physical problems. One drink is defined as 12 ounces of beer/wine cooler, 5 ounces of wine, or 1.5 ounces of liquor.

- **C** – *Cutting Down*: "Do you think about trying to cut down on drinking?"
- **A** – *Annoyed at Criticism*: "Are people starting to criticize your drinking?"
- **G** – *Guilty feeling*: "Do you feel guilty or try to hide your drinking?"
- **E** – *Eye opener*: "Do you increasingly need a drink earlier in the day?"

"Yes" on one question suggests the possibility of a drinking problem. "Yes" on ≥2 indicates a drinking problem

SCREENING FOR RISK-TAKING BEHAVIOR

The ability to assess outcomes and respond appropriately to risks are part of the decision-making process. Decision making can be impaired in patients with mental health disorders such as depression, anxiety, bipolar disorder, and personality disorders, as well as in patients who have experienced a brain injury or have a dependence on drugs or alcohol. Health care providers should screen patients for the presence of high-risk behaviors. This may be accomplished through a self-administered questionnaire or through a patient interview with a trained clinician. Examples of **high-risk behaviors** include substance use/abuse, high risk sexual behaviors, high risk driving behaviors such as drinking and driving, speeding or riding with a drunk driver, and violence related behaviors. Patients with an increased response to risk taking may exhibit signs of impulsivity and sensation seeking. Conversely, other patients may exhibit abnormally cautious behavior.

Pain Assessment

PATHOPHYSIOLOGY OF PAIN

NOCICEPTORS

Nociceptors are the primary neurons, or **sensory receptors**, responding to stimuli in the skin, muscle, and joints, as well as the stomach, bladder, and uterus. These neurons have specialized responses for mechanical, thermal, or chemical stimuli. The **neuron stimulation** is a direct result of tissue injury and follows four stages: **transduction** where a change occurs, **transmission** where the impulse is transferred along the neural path, **modulation** or translation of the signal, and **perception** by the patient. When injury occurs, the nociceptors initiate the process that begins **depolarization of the peripheral nerve**. Nociceptors may consist of either A-fiber axons or C-fiber axons. The message travels along the neural pathway and creates a perception of pain. A-fiber axons carry these pain messages at a much faster rate than C-fiber axons.

NOCICEPTIVE PAIN

Nociceptive pain is an umbrella term for pain caused by **stimulation of the neuroreceptor**. This stimulation is a direct result of tissue injury. The severity of pain is proportionate to the extent of the injury. Nociceptive pain can be subdivided into two classifications: somatic and visceral pain. **Somatic pain** is located in the cutaneous tissues, bone joints, and muscle tissues. **Visceral pain** is specific to internal organs protected by a layer of viscera, such as the cardiovascular, respiratory, gastrointestinal, or genitourinary systems. Both types are treatable with opioids.

VISCERAL PAIN

Visceral pain is associated with the internal organs. It can be very different depending on the affected organ. Not all internal organs are sensitive to pain (some lack **nociceptors**, such as the spleen, kidney, and pancreas), and may withstand a great deal of damage without causing pain. Other internal organs, such as the stomach, bladder, and ureters, can create significant pain from even the slightest damage. Visceral pain generally has a **poorly defined area**. It is also capable of referring pain to other remote locations away from the area of injury. It is described as a squeezing or cramping: a deep ache within the internal organs. The patient may complain of a generalized sick feeling or have nausea and vomiting. Visceral pain generally responds well to treatment with **opioids**.

> **Review Video: Visceral Pain**
> Visit mometrix.com/academy and enter code: 430402

SOMATIC PAIN

Somatic pain refers to messages from pain receptors located in the **cutaneous or musculoskeletal tissues**. When the pain occurs within the musculoskeletal tissue, it is referred to as **deep somatic pain**. Metastasizing cancers commonly cause deep somatic pain. **Surface pain** refers to pain concentrated in the **dermis and cutaneous layers** such as that caused by a surgical incision. Deep somatic pain is generally described as a dull, throbbing ache that is well focused on the area of trauma. It responds well to **opioids**. Surface somatic pain is also directly focused on the injury. It is frequently described as sharper than deep somatic pain. It may also present as a burning or pricking sensation.

> **Review Video: Somatic Pain**
> Visit mometrix.com/academy and enter code: 982772
>
> **Review Video: Somatic Nervous System**
> Visit mometrix.com/academy and enter code: 100382

Neuropathic Pain

Neuropathic pain results from injury to the **nervous system**. This can result from cancer cells compressing the nerves or spinal cord, from actual cancerous invasion into the nerves or spinal cord, or from chemical damage to the nerves caused by chemotherapy and radiation. Other causes include diabetes- and alcohol-related damage, trauma, neuralgias, or other illnesses affecting the neural path either centrally or peripherally. When the nerves become damaged, they are unable to carry accurate information. This results in more severe, distinct **pain messages**. The nerves may also relay pain messages long after the original cause of the pain is resolved. It can be described as sharp, burning, shooting, shocking, tingling, or electrical in nature. It may travel the length of the nerve path from the spine to a distal body part such as a hand, or down the buttocks to a foot. NSAIDs and opioids are generally ineffective against neuropathic pain, though adjuvants may enhance the therapeutic effect of opioids. Nerve blocks may also be used.

> **Review Video: Neuropathic Pain**
> Visit mometrix.com/academy and enter code: 780523

Adverse Systemic Effects of Pain

Acute pain causes adverse systemic effects that can negatively affect many body systems.

- **Cardiovascular**: Tachycardia and increased blood pressure is a common response to pain, causing increased cardiac output and systemic vascular resistance. In those with pre-existing cardiovascular disease, such as compromised ventricular function, cardiac output may decrease. The increased myocardial need for oxygen may cause or worsen myocardial ischemia.
- **Respiratory**: Increased need for oxygen causes an increase in minute ventilation and splinting due to pain, which may compromise pulmonary function. If the chest wall movement is constrained, tidal volume falls, impairing the ability to cough and clear secretions. Bed rest further compromises ventilation.
- **Gastrointestinal**: Sphincter tone increases and motility decreases, sometimes resulting in ileus. There may be an increased secretion of gastric acids, which irritates the gastric lining and can cause ulcerations. Nausea, vomiting, and constipation may occur. Reflux may result in aspiration pneumonia. Abdominal distension may occur.
- **Urinary**: Increased sphincter tone and decreased motility result in urinary retention.
- **Endocrine**: Hormone levels are affected by pain. Catabolic hormones such as catecholamine, cortisol, and glucagon increase, and anabolic hormones such as insulin and testosterone decrease. Lipolysis increases along with carbohydrate intolerance. Sodium retention can occur because of increased ADH, aldosterone, angiotensin, and cortisol. This in turn causes fluid retention and a shift to extracellular space.
- **Hematologic**: There may be reduced fibrinolysis, increased adhesiveness of platelets, and increased coagulation.
- **Immune**: Leukocytosis and lymphopenia may occur, increasing risk of infection.
- **Emotional**: Patients may experience depression, anxiety, anger, decreased appetite, and sleep deprivation. This type of response is most common in those with chronic pain, who usually have different systemic responses from those with acute pain.

CORE PRINCIPLES OF PAIN ASSESSMENT AND MANAGEMENT

According to the Joint Commission, assessing pain should be a priority in patient care, and organizations must establish **policies** for assessment and treatment of pain and must educate staff members about these policies. The Joint Commission considers a **plan of care** regarding pain control an essential patient right. Hospitals should be consistent in the use of the same assessment tools throughout the organization, specific to different patient populations (for example, pediatrics and geriatrics). The latest standards (2018) of evidence-based practice include the following:

- Organizations must establish a clinical leadership team to oversee pain management and safe prescription of opioids.
- Patients must be involved in planning and setting goals and should receive education regarding safe use of opioid and non-opioid medications.
- Patients should be screened for pain in all assessments, including visits to the emergency department.
- Patients at high risk for opioid misuse or adverse effects must be identified and monitored.
- Healthcare providers should have access to prescription drug monitoring safety databases, such as the prescription databases provided by most states.
- Organizations must provide performance improvement educational programs regarding pain assessment and management and must collect and analyze data on its pain assessment and management.

AREAS ADDRESSED WHEN ASSESSING PAIN

Information concerning a patient's pain can be gathered from a variety of sources, including observations, interviews with the patient and family, medical records, and observations of other health care providers. However, it is important to remember that each patient's pain is **subjective** and **personal**. Pain is defined as whatever the patient says it is. Having the patient give parameters of quality, location, duration, speed of onset, and intensity can all be beneficial in forming a treatment plan based on the patient's needs. Pain is also influenced by psychological, social, and spiritual factors. Behavioral, psychological, and subjective assessment information such as physical demeanor and vital signs can be helpful in further defining a patient's pain parameters.

PHYSICAL SIGNS OF PAIN

The best assessment of the patient's pain is **the patient's own report**. All other information is assessed as supporting this report. However, when this method is restricted or unavailable, **physical signs and symptoms** can help the nurse's assessment capabilities. It is important to be familiar with the patient's **baseline** or resting information to give a clear picture of the changes the body may go through when experiencing significant pain. Systolic blood pressure, heart rate, and respirations may all increase above the patient's normal parameters. Tightness or tension may be felt in major muscle groups. Posturing can also occur: the patient may guard areas of the body, curl themselves up into a fetal position, or hold only certain body portions rigid. Calling out, increased volume in speech, and moaning can also be indicators. Facial expressions, such as flat affect or grimacing, and distraction from their surroundings also indicate a significant increase in stressful stimuli.

IMPORTANCE OF PAIN ASSESSMENTS IN ADVANCED DISEASE

As many as 90% of all **advanced disease patients** will experience some level of pain. The hospice and palliative care philosophy focuses on the relief of pain and provision for comfort measures for all patients who desire it to improve quality of life. Each patient has the right to accept or refuse treatment for their pain. This becomes difficult when the patient is unable to **communicate** their desires and pain level. It can be assumed that if a patient was experiencing pain when able to communicate, they will continue to experience pain when the ability to communicate has been compromised—pain will be present even in an unconscious state. Changes from previous behavioral, psychological, and subjective and objective assessment data provide the supporting information for continued pain assessments in a nonverbal patient.

PAIN ASSESSMENT TOOLS
ABCDE MNEMONIC APPROACH TO PAIN ASSESSMENT
The Agency for Healthcare Policy and Research recommends use of the **ABCDE method** for assessing and managing pain:

- **Asking** the patient about the extent of pain and assessing systematically.
- **Believing** that the degree of pain the patient reports is accurate.
- **Choosing** the appropriate method of pain control for the patient and circumstances.
- **Delivering** pain interventions appropriately and in a timely, logical manner.
- **Empowering** patients and family by helping them to have control of the course of treatment.

The **5 key elements of pain assessment** include:

- **Quality**: Words are used to describe pain, such as *burning*, *stabbing*, *deep*, *shooting*, and *sharp*. Some may complain of pressure, squeezing, and discomfort rather than pain.
- **Intensity**: Use of a 0–10 scale or other appropriate scale to quantify the degree of pain.
- **Location**: Where does the patient indicate pain?
- **Duration**: Is it constant; does it come and go; is there breakthrough pain?
- **Aggravating/alleviating factors**: What increases the intensity of pain and what relieves the pain?

> **Review Video: Assessment Tools for Pain**
> Visit mometrix.com/academy and enter code: 634001
>
> **Review Video: How to Accurately Assess Pain**
> Visit mometrix.com/academy and enter code: 693250

UNIDIMENSIONAL TOOLS FOR PAIN ASSESSMENT
Unidimensional tools for pain assessment focus on one aspect only: the patient's level of pain. Tools include:

- **Visual analog/numeric rating scale**: A 1–10 rating scale presented visually or verbally from which the patient chooses a number to describe the degree of pain the patient is experiencing. Zero represents no pain, 1 very mild pain, and 10 the most severe pain the patient can imagine.
- **Descriptive**: Pain is described in simple terms that a patient can choose from: mild, moderate, or severe. This may be especially helpful for patients from other countries or cultures where the 1–10 scale is not generally used.
- **FACES**: A chart shows a facial expression scale of simple drawings showing faces with different emotions, such as happiness, fear, and pain. Used primarily for children over age 3 and for nonverbal adults, although both a child's and an adult's version are available. A revised version applies numeric values to expressions so that pain can be assessed according to a numeric rating scale as well.

MULTIDIMENSIONAL TOOLS FOR PAIN ASSESSMENT
Multidimensional tools used for pain assessment assess various aspects of pain in addition to its impact on mental health, sleep, and functional status. Tools include:

- **Multidimensional pain inventory**: The patient begins by identifying a significant other and then answering 20 questions (rating scale 0–6) about the current rate of pain, the degree of interference in daily life, the ability to work, satisfaction from social/recreational activities, support level of the significant other, mood, pain during the previous week, changes brought about by pain, concerns of the significant other, ability to deal with pain, irritability, and anxiety.

- **Brief pain inventory**: Patients are assessed on the severity of pain (on a 1–10 scale), location of pain, impact of pain on daily function, pain medication, and amount of pain relief in the past 24 hours or the past week. They are asked if the pain interferes with general activity, walking, normal work, mood, interpersonal relations, sleep, or enjoyment of life.
- **McGill pain questionnaire**: The patient marks areas of internal and external pain on body diagrams and selects appropriate adjectives for 20 different sections regarding sensory, affective, and evaluative perceptions. For example, the questionnaire allows the patient to indicate if the pain is "flickering, quivering, pulsing, throbbing, beating, or pounding." The patient also rates present pain intensity (PPI) from 0 (none) to 5 (excruciating).

ASSESSMENT TOOLS FOR COGNITIVELY IMPAIRED OR NONVERBAL PATIENTS

The following are types of assessment tools available for use with cognitively impaired or nonverbal patients:

- **Discomfort Scale for Dementia of the Alzheimer Type (DS-DAT)**: For use with elderly persons experiencing dementia, decreased cognition, and decreased verbalization
- **Assessment of Discomfort in Dementia Protocol (ADD)**: Particularly designed for use with patients exhibiting difficult behaviors
- **Checklist of Nonverbal Pain Indicators (CNPI)**: Pain measurement with cognitive impairment
- **Noncommunicative Patient's Pain Assessment Instrument (NOPPAIN)**: Specifically for use by nursing assistants
- **Pain Assessment for the Dementing Elderly (PADE)**: Assessing physical pain behaviors
- **Pain Assessment Tool in Confused Older Adults (PATCOA)**: Focuses on the observation of nonverbal cues
- **Pain Assessment in Advanced Dementia (PAINAD)**: Adapted from the DS-DAT
- **Pain Assessment Checklist for Seniors with Limited Ability to Communicate (PACSLAC)**: To assess common and subtle symptoms
- **Abbey Pain Scale**: For late-stage dementia in nursing home environments

NEUROPATHIC PAIN SCALE

The neuropathic pain scale (NPS) is the first tool designed specifically to assess the types of pain associated with neuropathy. The NPS comprises 10 sections with 9 assessed with a 0–10 (not unpleasant to intolerable) scale:

- Intensity of pain
- Sharpness of pain
- Heat of pain
- Dullness of pain
- Coldness of pain
- Skin sensitivity to touch, clothing
- Itchiness
- Overall unpleasantness of pain
- Intensity of deep and surface pain

The 10th section asks for narrative descriptions of the **time quality** of pain. The patient chooses from three options:

- Feeling background pain all of the time with occasional flare-ups
- Feeling a single type of pain all the time
- Feeling a single type of pain sometimes while having some pain-free periods. The patient then is asked to describe the pain experienced

PAIN ASSESSMENT OF NEONATES/INFANTS

Pain assessment of neonates and infants depends on careful observation of a number of characteristics. The Neonate/Infant Pain Scale (NIPS) assesses 6 areas with a score >3 indicating pain. Five areas are scored 0-1, depending upon the degree of stress. Crying, which is often the most indicative of pain, is scored 0-2:

Characteristic	0	1	2
Expression on face	Rested, normal	Negative, tightened muscles, grimace	
Crying	None	Intermittent, moaning, whimper	Loud, shrill continuous crying
Respiratory patterns	Relaxed, normal	Changes include irregular breathing, tachypnea, holding breath, gagging	
Upper extremities	Relaxed, random movement	Tense, rigid, or rapid extending and flexing.	
Lower extremities	Relaxed, random movement	Tense, rigid, or rapid extending and flexing.	
Arousal state	Quiet, awake or asleep with random leg movements	Restless, fussing, thrashing about.	

ASSESSING PAIN IN PEDIATRIC PATIENTS

When assessing the pediatric patient, the nurse must take into consideration the **chronological and developmental age** of the child. These factors help determine which measure the child might use to express pain, as well as treatments that might prove most successful. Assessment parameters must also include the presence of and parameters surrounding chronic illness, as well as neurological impairment. The nurse must identify the underlying cause of the pain, what nonpharmacological measures have been tried for pain control, and what methods can be used to deliver pharmacological interventions. The weight of the child in kilograms determines the appropriate dosages of medications. If the child is able to speak, do the child and the parents speak the same language as the health care provider, and are there any other obvious barriers to communication or pain relief measures?

> **Review Video: How to Properly Assess Pediatric Pain**
> Visit mometrix.com/academy and enter code: 264352

PRETEEN/ADOLESCENT PAIN SCALE

Pain is subjective and may be influenced by the individual's pain sensation threshold (the smallest stimulus that produces the sensation of pain) and tolerance threshold (the maximum degree of pain that a person can tolerate). The most common current pain assessment tool for preteens and adolescents is the 1-10 pain scale:

- 0 = no pain
- 1-2 = mild pain
- 3-5 = moderate pain
- 6-7 = severe pain
- 8-9 = very severe pain
- 10 = excruciating pain

However, assessment also includes information about onset, duration, and intensity. Identifying pain triggers and what relieves the pain is essential when developing a pain management plan. Children may show very different behaviors when they are in pain. Some may cry and moan with minor pain, and others may seem indifferent even when they are truly suffering. Thus, judging pain by behavior alone can lead to the wrong conclusions.

Non-Communicating Children's Pain Checklist

The **Non-Communicating Children's Pain Checklist** (NCCPC) is designed for children ages 3-8 who are cognitively impaired, but a modified version may be used for children recovering from anesthesia. The checklist contains 7 categories with sub-listings that are each scored: 0 (not occurring), 1 (occurring occasionally), 2 (occurring fairly often), 3 (occurring frequently), and NA (not applicable).

- **Vocal**: Moaning, whining, crying, screaming, yelling, or using a specific word for pain
- **Social**: Uncooperative, unhappy, withdrawn, seeking closeness, or can't be distracted
- **Facial**: Furrowed brow, eye changes, not smiling, lips tight or quivering, or clenching or grinding teeth.
- **Activity**: Not moving and quiet or agitated and fidgety.
- **Body and limbs**: Floppy, tense, rigid, spastic, pointing to a part of body that hurts, guarding part of the body, flinching, or positioning body to show pain.
- **Physiological**: Shivering, pallor, increased perspiration, tears, gasping, or holding breath
- **Eating and sleeping**: Eating less or sleeping significantly more or less than usual

The child is usually observed for 2 hours and then scored. All scores are then added together. A score of ≥7 indicates pain.

QUESTT Pediatric Pain Assessment Tool

QUESTT is designed to focus on assessment, action, and consequent reassessment for results.

- **Question** both the child and parent about the pain experience.
- **Use** assessment tools and rating scales that are appropriate to the developmental stage and situation and understanding of the child.
- **Evaluate** the patient for both behavioral and physiological changes.
- **Secure** the parent's participation in all stages of the pain evaluation and treatment process.
- **Take the cause of the pain into consideration** during the evaluation and choice of treatment methods.
- **Take action** to treat the pain appropriately, and then evaluate the results on a regular basis.

Barriers to Optimal Pain Assessments

Barriers to optimal pain assessments include:

- **Professional**: Health care providers may lack knowledge about pain assessment and management of different patient populations or may carry out assessments based on personal perceptions rather than validated pain assessment instruments. Some may be concerned about managing adverse effects or the patient's development of tolerance or addiction. In other cases, healthcare providers may lack empathy for patients' suffering. Lack of cultural awareness may affect interpretation of pain. For example, patients in cultures that encourage expression of pain may be assessed as having more pain than patients from cultures that value stoicism.
- **System**: The organization may lack clear policies regarding pain assessment and management, and may not have established clear guidelines for consistent use of pain assessment instruments. Additionally, supervision and accountability may be inadequate, and the organization may be concerned about costs and reimbursement for treatment.
- **Patient**: For personal or cultural reasons, patients may minimize or overstate the degree of pain, interfering with assessment. Some patients may be concerned about addiction or the effects of drugs on cognition (confusion, disorientation, lethargy) or other side effects (constipation, nausea, itching). Some may want to protect family from knowing the extent of pain.

- **Family**: Cultural biases may influence how the family responds to a patient's pain, and this can influence the patient's response as well. Families may lack understanding of the role of pain assessment and management. Some lack understanding about the difference between addiction and pain control at the end of life.
- **Society**: Concerns about drug abuse and addiction often permeate society and influence societal attitudes toward pain control and appropriate drugs to use. Laws and regulations may make access to certain drugs, such as those derived from marijuana, difficult or impossible to obtain.

INFLUENTIAL FACTORS IN PAIN PERCEPTION

Factors that can influence the perception of pain include:

- **Emotional state/attitude**: Patients who are extremely upset or anxious may be so overwhelmed they don't feel the pain, or they may experience pain as more severe than those who are relaxed and calm. If patients expect to suffer from pain, they are also more likely to report severe pain than patients who expect that their pain will be controlled.
- **Cultural expectations**: Perception may vary according to cultural beliefs about pain. For example, if a patient believes that pain is punishment, the patient may agonize over past sins. If a patient believes that pain is fate and reflects karma, then the patient may feel that bearing pain is necessary.
- **Pain threshold**: Different patients simply perceive and experience pain to different degrees. What may be a minor pain to one individual may be severe to another.

EFFECTS OF GENDER ON PAIN EXPERIENCE

Gender can affect pain sensitivity, tolerance, distress, and exaggeration of pain, and the patient's willingness to report pain, as well as displayed nonverbal cues concerning the pain experience. Studies indicate that women generally have **lower pain thresholds** and **less tolerance** for noxious stimuli or pain factors that hinder them from doing things they enjoy. Women seek help for pain-related problems sooner than men and respond better to therapy. Women also experience more **visceral pain** than men. Men are more prone to experience **somatic pain** and show more stoicism regarding pain experiences than women. **Neuropathic pain** seems to be experienced equally between men and women. Nurses need to be careful that biases concerning gender experiences with pain do not skew their assessments of pain. However, they need to be aware that pain experiences are always individual and may differ between the sexes.

PSYCHOLOGICAL FACTORS IN EXPERIENCE OF PAIN

Psychological factors that may influence a patient's experience of pain include:

- **Fear**: The fear of pain and the anticipation of having pain are factors in how much pain a person feels, because the fear stimulates areas of the brain that focus attention on the body so that the patient experiences an increased sensation of pain. Fear also causes muscles to tense, blood pressure to increase, and the heart rate to increase, and all of these can exacerbate the perception of pain. While pain medications may be necessary, practicing relaxation and mindfulness exercises may help to reduce anxiety and have a positive effect.
- **Depression**: The same neurotransmitters that transmit sensations of pain are also those that transmit moods, so many people with depression present first with complaints of pain or discomfort, and this can result in chronic pain if the depression is not resolved. In some cases, pain may lead to depression, but then the depression worsens the pain so it becomes a cycle of worsening discomfort. Patients may benefit from cognitive behavioral therapy or medication such as SSRIs.

PAIN DOCUMENTATION IN MEDICAL RECORDS

Recommendations for **pain documentation** in the medical record include:

- Describe the time of onset, the location of pain, the character of the pain, and the degree of pain, using a validated pain assessment instrument (either a self-reporting instrument, such as the visual analog scale, or one based on observation, such as PAINAD).
- Document all interventions, both pharmacological (opioids, adjuvants) and nonpharmacological (positioning, massage, relaxation exercises), including the time, the dosage, and the method of administration.
- Assess and document the initial response to the medication based on the expected response time. For example, an IV medication should take effect almost immediately, but oral medications may take up to 20 minutes to take effect.
- Assess and document the duration of response based on the expected duration of the medication. For example, if a medication response is expected to last for 6 hours, the patient's pain level should be assessed at least every 2 hours and more frequently if the rate of pain increases.
- Describe any adverse effects, such as itching or nausea.

> **Review Video: Pain Assessment Documentation**
> Visit mometrix.com/academy and enter code: 248521
>
> **Review Video: Documentation of Pain Management**
> Visit mometrix.com/academy and enter code: 760328

Functional Status and Rehabilitation

ADLs

Activities of daily living (ADLs) are a group of activities that are used to evaluate a patient's return to normal function; these are activities that the patient had performed on a daily basis before hospitalization, and will be expected to perform once he or she has completed rehabilitation. The **rate** at which the patient accomplishes these activities, in addition to the **level of independence** maintained by the patient when performing the activities, can help caregivers determine the amount of rehabilitation required, and can also be used to monitor the progress of the patient during the rehabilitation process. ADLs are grouped into 3 different areas: **personal or physical**, **instrumental**, and **occupational**.

GROUPING ADLS

The first group of ADLs, the **physical or personal group**, contains those daily activities that relate to the patient's ability to take care of him or herself. Included in this group are activities related to health management, nutritional needs, elimination of bladder and bowel contents, exercise, self-esteem, coping/stress management, cognitive abilities, communication, sexual health and ability, and relationship roles. The second group of ADLs, the **instrumental group**, contains activities such as shopping, answering the phone, and other activities that involve leaving home. The third group, **occupational activities**, includes activities that are required of being a parent, husband, or wife, as well as those required on the job.

REHABILITATION

Rehabilitation is an area of health care that is dedicated to helping patients improve and/or restore functions and abilities after a disease or injury. Although rehabilitation is usually thought of in relation to **physical therapy** (which is one of the many areas of rehabilitation), it also encompasses **drug and alcohol rehabilitation**, as well as **occupational therapy** for physically and mentally ill patients. The general goals of all types of rehabilitation include an improvement in overall function; the promotion of independence, satisfaction, and well-being; and the preservation of the individual's self-esteem in the face of illness or debilitating disease or injury.

ASSESSING POTENTIAL FOR REHABILITATION

There are various factors that are considered when assessing a patient to determine whether he or she will benefit from **rehabilitation**. A patient with the inability to perform any of the ADLs will automatically be considered for rehabilitation. At this point, however, other factors must be considered. First and foremost is whether or not the patient has a **desire to improve his or her functions** through rehabilitation; if the patient is not interested in improvement, the rehabilitation potential is poor. If the patient wants to improve function and increase independence, the potential for rehabilitation is greater. Another factor is whether or not the patient has **support at home**; even if the patient improves greatly during his or her rehabilitation stay, he or she will still most likely need some support at home. If the patient has no support at home, rehabilitation may eventually fail.

DISEASES AND ILLNESSES THAT COMMONLY REQUIRE REHABILITATION

There are some diseases, illnesses, and injuries that almost always require rehabilitation at some point during their course; in these cases, rehabilitation may be initiated before the patient even leaves the hospital to be transferred to a rehabilitation facility. It is important to know which diseases usually require rehabilitation, because the sooner evaluation and rehabilitation are initiated, the better the patient's chance of recovery. The following are diseases, illnesses, and injuries that **commonly require rehabilitation**: AIDS, amyotrophic lateral sclerosis (ALS), limb amputation, traumatic or ischemic brain injury, spinal cord injury, burns, Guillain-Barré syndrome, hip or knee replacement, multiple sclerosis (MS), and most types of cancer.

Rehabilitation Settings

There are various kinds of rehabilitation settings, depending on the needs of the patient. Once the need for rehabilitation has been determined and the patient has been evaluated regarding specific rehabilitation needs, he or she can be placed in an appropriate rehabilitation setting. A **long-term acute care hospital** is a rehabilitation facility that is best for patients who are physically and psychologically stable but are receiving medical treatment such as dialysis or ventilation and thus require medical support. A **subacute care unit** is appropriate for patients who require more limited treatment, such as cancer patients. A **comprehensive inpatient rehabilitation facility** is just what the name suggests; it addresses the needs of a broad range of different patients, from burn victims to amputees. The comprehensive rehabilitation center has a "team" of medical specialists that includes a rehabilitation medicine physician, nurses trained in rehabilitation, occupational therapists, physical therapists, social workers, and speech-language pathologists. **Outpatient rehab** is designed for the high-functioning patient who can return home after rehab sessions.

Interventions to Consider When Beginning Rehabilitation Process

When a patient is to be considered for rehabilitation, he or she must undergo a rather extensive **evaluation** in order to increase the likelihood that he or she will succeed during rehabilitation. This process of evaluation, which includes various interventions, should take place in the early stages of illness, when the patient is still in the hospital. The goal is to forestall any **secondary complications** that may inhibit the rehabilitation process. These **interventions** include health management, in which the patient and family are educated about his or her disease(s); nutritional status assessment and support; initiation of bowel and bladder management in order to prevent infection; exercises; assessment of cognitive function; and education involving self-esteem, relationship roles, sexual activity, and coping mechanisms.

Occupational Therapy

Occupational therapy is defined as the use of creative activities in the treatment of individuals with disabilities, whether physical or mental. The purpose of occupational therapy is to provide those individuals with the skills that are necessary to live life as fully and independently as possible; after completion of occupational therapy, the individual should be able to perform at his or her **maximum potential**. The occupational therapist will typically provide the patient with **interventions** tailored to his or her disability. The OT will also visit the patient's home and/or place of employment in order to assess potential problems and provide **adaptive solutions**. As part of occupational therapy, the patient will receive regular **assessments** of his or her skills, as well as specific training. The occupational therapist is also responsible for educating the patient's family, caretakers, friends, and coworkers.

The philosophy of occupational therapy is based on the idea that **occupation** (meaning, loosely, either an activity or activities in which an individual engages) is a **basic human need**, one that is important to an individual's health and overall well-being in that it is in and of itself therapeutic in nature. The basic assumptions of occupational therapy are based on the idea of occupational therapy as stated by its creator, **William Rush Dunton**. Dunton states that occupational therapy is a human need because an individual's occupation has an effect on his or her health and general well-being. It creates **structure** in the individual's life and allows for him or her to manage and organize time. Another assumption is that individuals have different sets of values and, therefore, will value different occupations; for each person, however, the occupation that he or she chooses is meaningful to him or her.

AREAS IN WHICH OCCUPATIONAL THERAPY MAY BE INSTITUTED AND PRACTICED

Although occupational therapy is an important part of the overall rehabilitation process for hospitalized individuals, it is also beneficial in other areas because occupational therapy deals not only with physical disabilities but with **emotional and cognitive disabilities** as well. Occupational therapy as related to **physical disabilities** may be practiced in outpatient clinics, pediatric hospitals or units, acute care rehabilitation facilities, and long-term, or comprehensive, inpatient rehabilitation centers. Occupational therapy as related to **mental disabilities** may be practiced in mental health clinics, acute and long-term psychiatric hospitals, prisons, and gateway or halfway houses. Occupational therapists may also work at schools, childcare facilities, workplaces, or shelters, or they may even work with individuals in their own homes.

ASSISTIVE DEVICES

Crutches should be properly fitted before client attempts ambulation. Correct height is one hand-width below axillae. The handgrips should be adjusted so the client supports the body weight comfortably with elbows slightly flexed rather than locked in place. The client should be cautioned not to bear weight under the axillae as this can cause nerve damage but to hold the crutches tight against the side of the chest wall. The type of gait used depends on the type of injury.

A **cane** should be held in the opposite hand of the side of injury. When holding the cane in neutral position, the elbow should be bent at about a 15-degree angle and if holding the cane straight down to the side of the body, the top of the cane should be in line with the crease of the wrist.

The same is true of a **walker**, the elbow should be bent at 15 degrees when standing up straight and grasping the handles, and the handle grasps should be in line with to the crease of the wrists. The client should be able to move the walker forward without leaning over.

Pediatric Growth and Development

PRINCIPLES OF HUMAN DEVELOPMENT

Principles of human development as they relate to the pediatric population are as follows:

- Development follows a basic sequence. Developmental changes will always occur in a specific order.
- Development follows a specific pathway. Development that progresses from the head downward through the body is termed cephalocaudal. Proximodistal denotes development that progresses from the inside to the outside of the body.
- Each child will progress through the developmental stages at their own pace.
- The different areas of development are dependent on each other.
- As the child develops, the responses of the systems become more specific.
- As the child grows, the skills learned will become more complex.
- From infancy, children have inborn survival tactics.
- While a new skill is being learned, that skill takes precedence over learning other new skills.

HUMAN DEVELOPMENT FROM INFANCY THROUGH ADOLESCENCE

The stages and characteristics of human development through adolescence are outlined below:

- **Infant stage**: From birth to 1 year: rapid growth occurs, bonding and development of trust with family members
- **Toddler stage**: From age 1-3: development of basic motor, sensory and coordination skills, beginning understanding of self, seeks autonomy
- **Preschool stage**: From age 3-6: continue to develop better motor, sensory and coordination skills, learning to dress self and take care of basic hygiene, plays with other children, increased understanding of who they are
- **School age stage**: Age 6-12 years: seek academic success, interests broaden to include activities outside the home, competitive
- **Adolescent stage**: Age 12-19: physical changes related to puberty, begin to question their own and their family's values and beliefs, transitioning between childhood and adulthood

PHYSICAL GROWTH AND DEVELOPMENT DURING INFANCY

The newborn sleeps about 16 hours/day during the **first month** and is growing and developing.

- **Growth**: Infant loses 5–7% of birth weight and then gains 4–7 ounces/week (about 2 lb/month). Head circumference increases 1.5 cm/month and length 1.5 cm.
- **Mobility**: The infant makes fists and flexes arms and legs. Reflexes such as Moro, sucking, grasping, startle, rooting, and asymmetric tonic neck are present.
- **Feeding**: About every 2–3 hours with breastfeeding.
- **Urine/feces**: Urination should occur about 8 times per day. Breastfed babies may have frequent loose stools or may skip 2–3 days. If bottle-fed, stools are usually firmer. Color varies (yellow, tan, green, brown).
- **Sensory**: Follows items in line of vision and often prefers faces and contrasting geometric designs. Vision is somewhat blurry with ability to focus at about 8–15 inches. Color distinction is poor. Babies hear well and respond with startle reflex. Sense of smell is strong.
- **Communication**: Infant signals distress with crying, gagging, and arching body and responds to comfort measures.

During **months 2-4**, the infant continues to sleep much of the time but is often awake for periods in the morning, afternoon, and evening.

- **Growth**: Gains 5-7 oz/wk and 1.5 cm length/month and 1.5 cm head circumference/month. Posterior fontanel closes.
- **Mobility**: Loses grasp reflex and hands start to stay open and grasp. Able to lift head while prone or supine and turn from side to side. Can roll stomach to back by 4 months. Moro reflex fades. Plays with hands. Can be pulled to standing position.
- **Feeding**: Needs about 2 oz/lb per 24 hours, usually feeding every 4 hours.
- **Urine/feces**: Urine is about 5-6 times/day. Stools vary from one each feeding to every 2-3 days, but usually are firmer and more regular.
- **Sensory**: Can focus at about 12 inches and follows objects 180° with eyes.
- **Communication**: Crying differentiates to show hunger, pain, frustration. Infant can smile indiscriminately by 2 months and socially responsive smile by 3 months. Child shows preference for mother and may turn from strangers.

During **4-6 months** the child sleeps about 10-11 hours at night, with 2-3 daytime naps (total 15 hours).

- **Growth**: Doubles weight by 5-6 months, gains 5-7 oz/week.
- **Mobility**: Infant can roll over and roll from back to side by 6 months; can hold head up at 90° and turn head in both directions when sitting or lying. Can sit with support for 10-15 minutes. Grasp improves and may hold bottle and play with feet. By 6 months, the infant can pick up items and move items from one hand to the other. Manipulates and mouths objects and watches objects fall.
- **Feeding**: Still having about 2 feedings at night and every 4 hours during the day, 1.5 oz/lb per 24 hours.
- **Urine/feces**: Urination and defecation are becoming regular.
- **Sensory**: Eyes focus well; the infant follows items/people with eyes.
- **Communication**: Vocalizes more and mimics tones. Squeals and laughs. Yells with anger. Vocalizes to get attention and recognizes family members.

During **6-8 months** the child begins to have more waking hours, sleeping 10-11 hours with 2 naps.

- **Growth**: Growth slows. Gains 3-5 oz/wk and 1 cm in length/month.
- **Mobility**: Can sit alone by 8 months. Can stand supported and bounces on legs. Starting to use pincer grasp. Easily manipulates and moves objects. Most birth reflexes have faded. Bangs objects together and mouths objects freely.
- **Feeding**: Starting to take solid foods (cereal, vegetables, and fruit) 2-3 times daily as well as breastfeeding/bottle-feeding 3-5 times daily. Teething biscuits, graham crackers, and Melba toast may be introduced.
- **Urine/feces**: Stool larger with solid foods. Urinating 5-6 times daily.
- **Sensory**: Watches and listens actively, turning head to sounds and to follow objects.
- **Communication**: Increased babbling and mimicking of sounds, including two syllable sounds and vowels, such as "mama" or "dada" but doesn't use intentionally. Has babbling conversations. May be fearful of strangers.

During **8-10 months,** the child continues to sleep about 10-11 hours at night and usually sleeps through the night, with 2 naps in the daytime.

- **Growth**: Gains 3-5 oz/wk and 1 cm in length/month.
- **Mobility**: Uses pincer grasp well and can pick up small objects. Crawls or creeps readily. Can sit up and by 10 months can pull to standing position by holding onto furniture.

- **Feeding**: Meat introduced. Breastfeeding or bottle-feeding 3–4 times daily with 3 meals. Eggs may be introduced, but must be cooked completely. Will enjoy finger foods, such as meat sticks.
- **Urine/feces**: Fairly regular.
- **Sensory**: Watches and listens freely, attentive.
- **Communication**: Babbles and may be able to say one or two words besides "mama" or "dada." Understands basic vocabulary, such as "no" and "cookie." Babbling follows speech-like rhythm when "talking."

During **10–12 months**, the child continues to sleep 10–11 hours at night with 2 naps in the daytime.

- **Growth**: Gains 3–5 oz/week and 1 cm/month. Head and chest circumference are equal. Birth weight tripled by 12 months.
- **Mobility**: Can make marks on paper with pens or crayons. Fits objects through holes. Can stand alone and walk holding onto furniture. Can sit from standing position.
- **Feeding**: Breastfeeding or bottle-feeding 3–4 times daily and starting with "sippy" cup. Eating solid foods, both prepared baby foods and soft home-cooked foods. Enjoys finger foods and may resist being fed.
- **Urine/feces**: May smear feces. Holding urine for longer periods of time, especially girls.
- **Sensory**: Watches and listens, engaging in activities.
- **Communication**: Understands many words. Uses "mama" and "dada" intentionally and may use a few other words. Plays patty-cake and peek-a-boo games. Enjoys repetition.

Between **1 and 2 years**, the child is growing in size and independence.

- **Growth**: Gains 8 oz/month and 3–5 in/year. Anterior fontanel closes.
- **Mobility**: Begins with first steps and by 2 walks and runs and can go up and down stairs. Scribbles on paper, throws toys, and learns to stack blocks. Begins independent exploration of environment.
- **Diet**: Child eats 3 meals and 2–3 snacks daily. Whole cow's milk can be taken after 1 year, 2–3 cups daily. Some may breastfeed. Child can consume a wide range of foods.
- **Toileting**: Between 18–24 months, some children show an interest in potty training.
- **Communication**: Begins with one word and grows. Learns names for common objects and begins trying to communicate with simple words leading to short sentences around 2 with vocabulary of 30–50 words. May show apprehension with strangers and anger with temper tantrums.

The **2- to 3-year-old** makes significant changes over the course of a year.

- **Growth**: Gains 3–5 lb/year and 3.5–5 in/year
- **Mobility**: Can run steadily, jump on two feet, and climb. Scribbling becomes more intentional and can draw simple shapes. Makes effort to color in the lines. Able to undress at 2 and dress at 3. Can throw a ball overhand. Plays side by side and begins to interact with others.
- **Diet**: Can switch to lowfat milk, 2–3 cups daily along with a regular well-balanced meal of meat, fruits, vegetables, and grains. Parents should limit fruit juice to 2–4 oz/day because of high sugar content. The child should not be receiving bottle feedings.
- **Toileting**: Most children become potty-trained sometime during this year.
- **Communication/cognition**: Begins to talk in short 3-word sentences and to understand rules. Begins to use pronouns (I, me, you) and can talk about feelings. Usually knows at least 5 body parts and colors and can categorize by size (big, little).

Language Milestones

While children develop at different rates, there are a number of **language milestones** of developmentally appropriate communication for infants and toddlers.

- **5–6 weeks**: Vocalizations usually small and throaty, sometimes during crying
- **2 months**: Single vowel sounds (ah, oh, oo, eh)
- **3 months**: Gurgling, laughing, and some consonant sounds (n, k, g, b, p)
- **8 months**: Add consonants (t, d, w) and may combine syllables ("mama") although may not attach meaning
- **10 months**: Understand simple words, such as "no" and "mama"
- **12 months**: Say a few words with comprehension, such as "mama," "dada," and can imitate some animal sounds
- **13–15 months**: Have a 4- to 6-word expressive vocabulary but understand many more words and can point to indicate a desire for something, such as a toy
- **16–18 months**: Use 7- to 20-word vocabulary and point to 5 body parts
- **20 months**: Can combine 2 words
- **24 months**: Understand 300 words and uses 2- to 3-word sentences

Physical Growth and Development During Preschool Years

At ages **3-6**, the child moves from being a toddler to a child.

- **Growth**: Gains 3–5 lb/yr and 1.5–2.5 in/yr. Most growth occurs in long bones as child increases in stature and proportionate head size decreases.
- **Mobility**: Becomes increasingly adept, drawing various shapes, coloring in the lines, using scissors to cut along lines. Can brush teeth. Can tie shoes by 6. Able to climb, run, jump, balance, and ride tricycle or bicycle with training wheels. Interacts with others.
- **Diet**: Eats 3 meals with snack and can manage spoon, fork, and knife independently by age 6.
- **Communication/cognition**: Becomes increasingly verbal and social and commands a large complex vocabulary by 6. Understands concepts of right and wrong, good and bad, and can lie. Learns letters and numbers and by age 6 is beginning to read. May focus on one thing to the exclusion of others.

Physical Growth and Development During School Age Years

During the school years **(ages 6-12)**, children go through many changes.

- **Dental**: Children lose deciduous teeth and begin acquiring permanent teeth.
- **Height and weight**: These should progress slowly and steadily, gaining an average of 2 inches each year, beginning at about 45 inches at 6 and attaining about 59 inches at 12. Weight usually doubles during this time from 46 pounds at 6 to 88 pounds at 12. Boys and girls are similar in size but by 12, some girls will be undergoing pubertal changes and may gain height and weight over boys.
- **Proportions**: The body becomes slimmer and better proportioned with an increase in muscle mass and decrease in fat. In relation to height, head circumference decreases, leg length increases, and waist circumference decreases. Facial characteristics change.
- **Body systems**: Systems mature with respirations and heart rate decreasing. Bladder capacity is usually better in girls than boys. Muscles strengthen and bones begin to ossify. Physical variation increases with age.

PHYSICAL GROWTH AND DEVELOPMENT PROBLEMS DURING SCHOOL-AGE YEARS

Routine health assessments should be done at ages 6, 8, 10, 11, and 12 to determine if there are developmental delays or problems, which may include:

- **6 years**: Peer problems, depression, cruelty to animals, poor academic progress, speech problems, lack of fine motor skills, and inability to catch a ball or state age.
- **8 years**: No close friends, depression, cruelty to animals, interest in fires, very poor academic progress with inability to do math, read, or write adequately and poor coordination.
- **10 years**: No team sports or extracurriculars and poor choices in peers (gangs), failure to follow rules, cruelty to animals, interest in fires, depression, failure to understand causal relationships, poor academic progress in reading, writing, math, and penmanship, and problems throwing or catching.
- **12 years**: Continuation of problems at 10 years with increasing risk-taking behaviors (drinking, drugs, sex) and continued poor academic progress in reading, following directions, doing homework, and organization.

PHYSICAL GROWTH AND DEVELOPMENT ISSUES FOR EARLY ADOLESCENCE

Early adolescence, ages **11-14,** is a transitional time for children as their hormones and their bodies go through changes. Children mature at varying rates, so there are wide differences. Emotions may be labile, and the child may feel isolated and confused at times, trying to find an identity. Peers take on more influence and the child may challenge the values of the family. Children may have much anxiety about their bodies and sexuality as secondary sexual characteristics develop. Developmental concerns include:

- Delayed maturation
- Short stature (female)
- Spinal curvature (females)
- Poor dental status (caries, malocclusion)
- Chronic illnesses, such as diabetes
- Lack of adequate physical activity
- Poor nutrition, anorexia, obesity
- Concerns about sexual identity
- Negative self-image, depression
- Lack of close friends, fighting or violent episodes, lack of impulse control
- Poor academic progress with truancy and failure to complete assignments

NORMAL GROWTH AND DEVELOPMENT ISSUES FOR MIDDLE ADOLESCENCE

In middle adolescence, ages **15-17**, most body changes have occurred, so there is less concern about this but more concern about the image they are projecting to others. Girls may worry about weight and boys about muscle development. Teenagers are interested in sexuality and many begin sexual experimentation. There is strong identification with peer groups, including codes of dress and behavior, often putting the individual at odds with family. **Developmental concerns** include:

- Spinal curvature (females) and short stature (males)
- Lack of testicular maturation/ persistent gynecomastia
- Acne
- Anorexia, obesity
- Sexual experimentation, multiple partners, and unprotected sex
- Sexual identification concerns
- Depression, poor self-image
- Lack of adequate exercise, poor nutrition, and poor dental health
- Chronic diseases

- Experimentation with drugs and alcohol and problems with authority figures
- Lack of peer group identification, gang association
- Poor academic progress, failing classes, truancy, attention deficits and disruptive class behavior, and poor judgment and impulse control

Normal Growth and Development Issues for Late Adolescence

Late adolescence, ages **18-21,** is the time when adolescents begin to take on more adult roles and responsibilities, entering the world of work or going to college. Most have come to terms with their sexuality and have a more mature understanding of people's motivations. Some young people will continue to engage in high-risk behaviors. Many of the problems associated with middle adolescence may continue if unresolved, interfering with the transition to adulthood. Developmental concerns include:

- Failure to take on adult roles, no life goals or future plans
- Low self-esteem, lack of impulse control
- Lack of intimate relationships, sexual identification concerns
- Gang association
- Continued identification with peer group or dependence on parents
- High-risk sexual behavior, multiple partners, and unprotected sex
- Poor academic progress or ability
- Psychosomatic complaints, depression
- Poor nutrition, obesity, anorexia
- Poor dental health
- Chronic disease
- Lack of exercise

Maturity Assessment

A maturity assessment should be part of the examination for children and adolescents to determine their level of sexual, dental, and skeletal maturity. **Skeletal maturity** is usually assessed by measurements of the hand and wrist as well as weight/height for age. Skeletal maturity and chronological age may differ. For example, if the chronological age is 14.3 and the skeletal age is 15.5, this would be expressed as 15.5–14.3 = SA +1.2. Another method is to divide the skeletal age by the chronological age: a score >1.0 equates with advanced skeletal maturity and <1.0 a delay in skeletal maturity.

The most common assessment tool for **sexual maturity** is Tanner's 5 stages of assessment. This tool assesses maturity for both males and females, based on direct observation of breasts and genitals.

- Females: Breast development, onset of menses, and pubic hair distribution
- Males: Penis and testes development and pubic hair distribution

Family Dynamics

FAMILY TYPES

A table of the different family types is provided below:

Family Type	Description
Nuclear	This husband-wife-children model was once the most common family type but is no longer the norm. In this model, the husband is the provider, and the mother stays home to care for the children. This makes up only about 7% of current American families.
Dual career/ dual earner	This model, where both parents work, is the most common in American society, affecting about 66% of two-parent families. One parent may work more than another, or both may work fulltime. There may be disparities in income that affect family dynamics.
Childless	10-15% of couples have no children because of infertility or choice.
Extended	These may include multigenerational families or shared households with friends, parents, or other relatives. Childcare responsibilities may be shared or primarily assumed by an extended family member, such as a grandparent.
Extended kin network	Two or more nuclear families live close together, share goods and services, and support each other, including sharing childcare. This model is common in the Hispanic community.
Single-parent	This is one of the fastest growing family models. Typically, the mother is the single parent, but in some cases, it is the father. The single parent may be widowed, divorced, or separated but more commonly has never married. In cases of divorce or abandonment, the child may have minimal or no contact with one parent, often the father. Single parents often face difficulties in trying to support and care for a child and may suffer economic hardship.
Stepparent	Because of the high rate of divorce, stepparent families are common. This can result in stress and conflict when a new child enters the picture. There may be jealousy and resentment on the part of siblings and estranged family members. In some cases, families can work together to achieve harmony and provide added support to children.
Binuclear/co-parenting	In this model, children share time between two primarily nuclear families because of joint custody agreements. While this may at times result in conflict, the child benefits from having a continued relationship with both parents.
Cohabiting	This model refers to unmarried heterosexual couples living together. The relationships within this model may vary, with some similar to the nuclear family. In some cases, people are in committed relationships and may avoid marriage because of economic or personal reasons. A planned child may strengthen the relationship, but an unplanned child may cause conflict.
Same sex	Whether those in same sex relationships marry or cohabit, they have the opportunity to create families using sperm donors, adoption, or surrogacy.

FAMILY THEORY

FAMILY DEVELOPMENTAL THEORY

According to the family developmental theory, families move through different developmental stages, which are accompanied by certain tasks:

- **Marriage**: Get to know significant other, establish good relationships with new kin, and discuss parenthood.
- **Birth of first child**: Adjust to and bond with new baby, maintain spousal relationship.

- **Preschool children**: Provide for different children's needs while family grows, teach socialization skills, maintain healthy relationships between immediate family and extended family, cope with decreased energy and privacy.
- **School-age children**: Encourage academic achievement and good relationships with peers and teachers.
- **Teenagers**: Help teens balance freedom and responsibility, maintain good communication between parents and teens, renewed focus on career and marital relations.
- **Launching adult children**: Allow children to start their own life, jobs, etc., welcome new family members by marriage, help with aging parents' needs, and work on marital relationship.
- **Empty nest**: Maintain relationships with children and aging parents, establish stronger marital relationship.
- **Aging family**: Adjust to health issues, reduced income and loss of spouse/family members/friends.

Limitation: The theory assumes a traditional, nuclear, middle-class family.

STRUCTURAL-FUNCTIONAL THEORY

According to the structural-functional theory, the family, a social system, serves society by performing functions needed for survival:

- **Affective**, or providing love and acceptance to each member
- **Socialization and social placement**, or teaching the children how to get along with others and fit into society as adults
- **Reproductive**, or producing of offspring to continue the family line
- **Economic**, or providing and distributing the necessary resources to the family members
- **Health care**, or providing basic necessities (food, clothing, shelter) and health care, as well as teaching basic hygiene to maintain good health

Limitation: The theory assumes the traditional definition of family and doesn't address the changes that a family encounters.

FAMILY SYSTEMS THEORY

According to the family systems theory, the family is a system where members can only be understood in relationship to other family members. They are interdependent, so that as one member experiences a change, other family members will change to maintain equilibrium. Each member has specific roles, with certain rules governing them.

Limitation: The theory is vague and therefore difficult to apply.

FAMILY STRESS THEORY

The stress theory has several different models. Most assume a stressor (sometimes more than one stressor can occur at the same time, termed **stressor pileup**), resources that are available to the family in coping with the stressor, and how the family perceives the stressor. These factors together will determine whether the family experiences stress or a crisis. Stress causes changes within the family, but it is usually short-lived. A crisis occurs when the family cannot recover from a stress using the resources at hand or the stress is too large for the family to handle.

RESILIENCY MODEL

The resiliency model assumes that some families develop strength over time by facing changes common to all families. These strengths, as well as strong resources and relationships, help protect against crises when uncommon stressors are present. Families respond to stressful events in two phases. The **adjustment phase** occurs when the family makes minor changes to its roles and routines. When the family moves into the **adaptation phase**, it makes major changes to its structure and functions.

Family Assessment and Factors that Influence Relationships and Parenting

Family assessment is the collection of data concerning the structure of the family and how family members relate to each other and society. It is an ongoing process, using assessment tools, such as a genogram (a map of a three generational family tree, including relationships and health histories), an ecomap (a chart depicting the relationships within and outside of the family and the support networks available to the family), interviews, questionnaires, and observations.

There are many factors that influence family relationships and parenting. These include: the type of family unit (nuclear, blended, single parent, gay, or lesbian), parental culture, parenting a foster child, adolescent parenting, parenting an adopted child, parenting by grandparents.

Family Functioning and Dynamics

Cultural/lifestyle factors that affect family integration include the following:

- **Values**: Values based on attitudes, ideas, and beliefs often connect family members to common goals. However, these values may be influenced by many external factors, such as education, social norms, and attitudes of peers, extended family, and coworkers, so values may change, which may affect family integration.
- **Roles**: In some families, roles are clearly defined by gender and task (homemaker and breadwinner), but the roles blur or are shared in many families, and in some cases the father becomes the primary caregiver while the mother works. Other common roles include peacemaker, nurturer, and social planner. How these roles are perceived and actualized affects the manner in which a child is integrated into the family and cared for.
- **Decision making**: Family power structures vary widely, but in many families, power rests with one person who makes ultimate decisions and whose opinions affect other family members. In many traditional cultures (Hispanic, Asian, Middle Eastern) power lies with the father, grandfather, or other male family member. However, in American society, this may vary because of diversity. Power may be shared or rest with the mother or the father.
- **Socioeconomic**: Employment trends, marriage rates, and economic trends all affect family integration. Many people have become unemployed and are unable to support their families, resulting in severe stress, which may be exacerbated by the arrival of a new child or illness. The divorce rate is high, leaving many parents with inadequate funds to support a child. Even if both parents are employed, the cost of living continues to escalate, including the cost of caring for a child.

Identifying Primary Caregiver

Identifying the primary caregiver is especially important in the emergency care of infants and children, as their ability to report is limited and may not be reliable, depending on age. With the diversity of family models, one cannot assume that the mother, father, or person accompanying the child is the primary caregiver. In some cases, custodial arrangements designate one parent as custodial and the other as non-custodial, and they may or may not share legal rights over medical care for the child. Therefore, the nurse should ask who is the primary caregiver in order to glean information about the child and ask who has the legal right to make medical decisions to determine who should sign consent forms and make decisions.

Impact and Complications When Patient Has Multiple Caregivers

Continuity of care is especially important for infants and young children, and the lack of stability in caregivers can lead to various problems. Even when children must have **multiple caregivers**, a primary care giver should be identified and should oversee care and ease the transitions whenever possible by introducing other caregivers and coordinating care activities. The greater the number of changes, the greater the impact on the child. The impacts/complications involved when a patient has multiple caregivers, either at the same time or sequentially, include:

- Inadequate communication of the patient's needs and condition
- Different approaches to caregiving, leading to confusion or discord
- Inability of the patient to adequately bond and form attachment with the caregivers
- Patient insecurity and impaired sociopsychological development
- Increased stress and anxiety
- Behavioral problems

Some children are able to adapt to multiple changes over time and can better handle the demands of change than others.

Functional Coping Strategies of Families

Some families utilize a number of functional coping strategies to deal with stress. These families exhibit resilience in difficult situations. Strategies include:

- The family gathers information, increases organization, discusses issues, and tries to jointly solve problems.
- Family members draw together as a strengthened family unit to deal with stressful situations.
- The family attempts to carry on as normal a routine as possible while making accommodations as needed for a child who is ill. This provides the child with a sense of security.
- The family accepts those things that cannot be changed rather than wasting energy trying to deny or alter reality.
- The family communicates openly and directly, avoiding family secrets and including the child in discussions as appropriate to the child's age.
- The family uses humor to deflect stress.
- The family uses resources outside of the immediate family for support, such as extended family, spiritual advisors, and community agencies.

Dysfunctional Coping Strategies of Families

Some families are not resilient when dealing with stressful situations and exhibit dysfunctional coping strategies, which include:

- Family members may resort to substance abuse, such as alcohol and/or drugs, rather than facing problems. This adds to the family dysfunction and negatively affects all members.
- The family may take out frustrations through domestic violence, aimed at the child or other family members. This can include physical, sexual, or mental abuse and can create an environment of fear within the family.
- The family denies problems and refuses to acknowledge that family dynamics have changed, attempting to carry on as usual.
- The family uses threats, aggression, and/or withholding of affection to retain control and maintain the family unit.
- The family may blame vulnerable members, such as the child, for the stressful situation, often scapegoating the member that they "blame" rather than dealing with the real problems.

Methods to Get Parents More Involved in Their Child's Health at School

Most children spend a great deal of time at school, and children with health conditions are often monitored and supported by school health staff, such as the school nurse, health aide, psychologist, or counselor. Parents can be involved with their child's health at school by maintaining communication with these professionals to provide the most comprehensive care for their child. This may mean partnering with school officials to develop a care plan to use at school, signing documents approving medication administration at school, and attending meetings to discuss the effects of their child's health on the classroom experience. Parents provide the health care providers in the school system with much of the information needed for their child to have a sufficient school experience without health issues standing in the way. School nurses can reinforce this behavior by keeping in frequent contact with parents about their child's health, communicating when the child receives health services at school, and keeping records updated and accurate.

Factors That Influence the Relationship Between the Child and Parents

Factors influencing parent-child relationships are cultural (some children consider themselves a part of the American culture, while their parents still hold true to the cultural practices of their home country), religious (some youth rebel against their religious upbringing, especially in the teen years), parenting style, and family structure (nuclear, extended, blended, gay/lesbian, single parent, adolescent parent, adoptive parenting, grandparents raising the children, and foster parenting).

Appropriate Disciplinary Practices for Families to Use

Appropriate discipline practices should be discussed with parents. These include:

- Make rules clear and appropriate for the age of the child.
- Set the consequences before the rule has been broken, making sure they are appropriate for the broken rule and age of the child. The consequence should be administered directly after the rule has been broken, with a calm attitude.
- Use lots of praise when the child behaves appropriately.

Temperament

Temperament is the way a person relates or responds to his environment and the people around him. Temperament is inborn, but it can be affected by how parents relate to the child/adolescent.

Attributes

The nine attributes of temperament are:

- **Activity**: How active is the child is during normal activities?
- **Rhythmicity**: How regular are the child's normal physiological activities, such as bowel movements, sleep cycle, and eating patterns?
- **Approach-withdrawal**: How does the child respond to different stimuli, such as being drawn readily to a new stuffed animal or withdrawing from the noise of fireworks?
- **Adaptability**: How does the child adapt to new circumstances?
- **Intensity of reaction**: How forcefully does the child respond to new circumstances?
- **Threshold of responsiveness**: How much stimulus is needed before the child responds?
- **Mood**: How much positive vs. negative behavior is exhibited in different situations?
- **Distractibility**: How easily can the child be distracted and the behavior changed?
- **Attention span and persistence**: How long will the child continue an activity and how much distraction is needed to pull the child away from the activity (persistence)?

TYPES

Types of temperament include:

- **Easy**: Easily adapts to new situations, gets along with others well, easy going behaviors
- **Difficult**: Responds negatively to new situations, behaviors are unpredictable, does well in highly structured environment
- **Slow-to-warm-up**: Moody, shy, slow to adapt to new situations, low activity level

EFFECTS OF PARENTING STYLES ON TEMPERAMENT OF CHILDREN

Although children are born with their own temperament, the parenting style they grow up with can influence how this temperament manifests over time.

- **Authoritarian (autocratic)** parents desire obedience without question. They tend toward harsh punishments, using their power to make their children obey. They are emotionally withdrawn from their children and enforce strict rules without discussing why the rules exist. These children tend to have low self-esteem, be more dependent, and are introverted with poor social skills.
- **Authoritative (democratic)** parents provide boundaries and expect obedience, but use love when they discipline. They involve their children in deciding rules and consequences, discussing reasons for their decisions, but will enforce the rules consistently. They encourage independence and take each child's unique position seriously. These children tend to have higher self-esteem, good social skills, and confidence in themselves.
- **Indulgent (permissive)** parents stay involved with their children, but have few rules in place to give the children boundaries. These children have a difficult time setting their own limits and are not responsible. They disrespect others and have trouble with authority figures.
- **Indifferent (uninvolved)** parents spend as little time as possible with their children. They are self-involved, with no time or patience for taking care of their children's needs. Guidance and discipline are lacking and inconsistent. These children tend toward delinquency, with a lack of respect for others.

Four Kinds of Parenting Styles

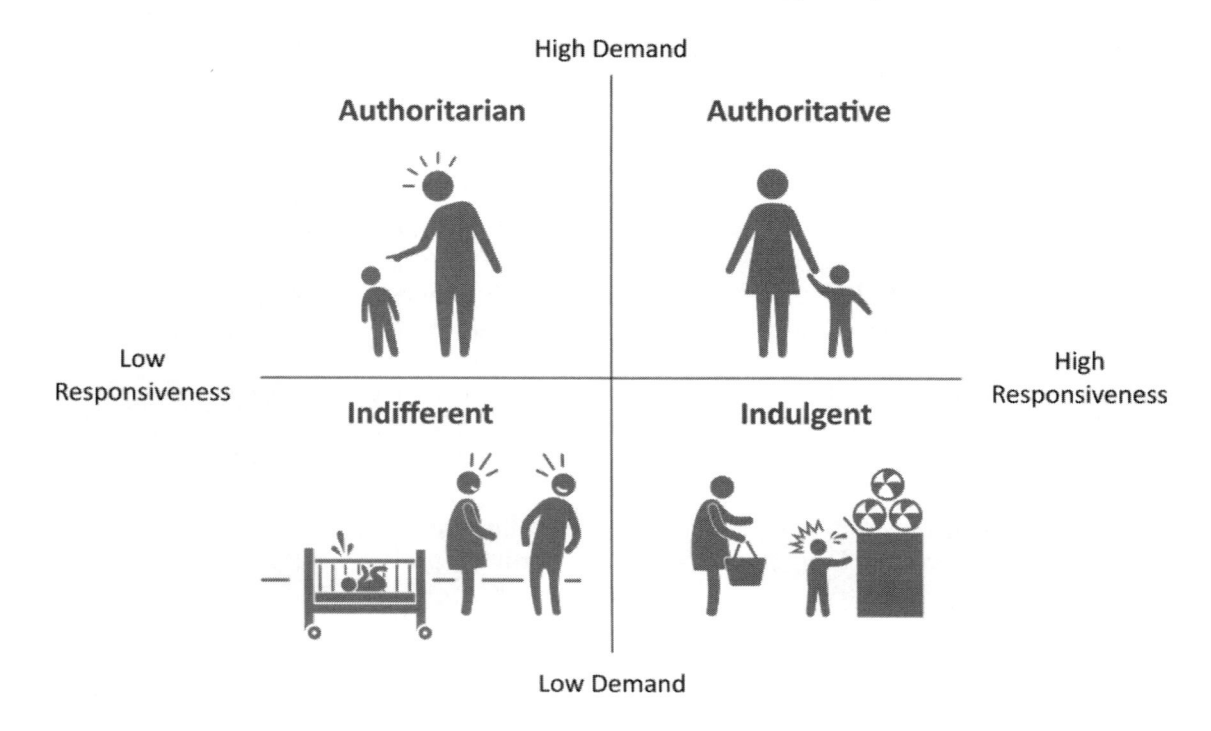

Abuse and Neglect

INDICATORS OF ABUSE THAT MAY BE IDENTIFIED IN THE PATIENT HISTORY

The healthcare provider should always be aware of the presence of any **indicators** that may present a potential for or an actual situation that involves **abuse**. These indicators may present in the **patient's history**. Some examples of indicators concerning their primary complaint may include the following: vague description about the cause of the problem, inconsistencies between physical findings and explanations, minimizing injuries, long period of time between injury and treatment, and over-reactions or under-reactions of family members to injuries. Other important information may be revealed in the family genome, such as family history of violence, time spent in jail or prison, and family history of violent deaths or substance abuse. The patient's health history may include previous injuries, spontaneous abortions, or history of pervious inpatient psychiatric treatment or substance abuse.

During the collection of the patient history, the financial history, the patient's family values, and the patient's relationships with family members can also reveal actual or potential **abuse indicators**.

- The **financial history** may indicate that the patient has little or no money or that they are not given access to money by a controlling family member. They may also be unemployed or utilizing an elderly family member's income for their own personal expenses.
- **Family values** may indicate strong beliefs in physical punishment, dictatorship within the home, inability to allow different opinions within the home, or lack of trust for anyone outside the family.
- **Relationships** within the family may be dysfunctional. Problems such as lack of affection between family members, co-dependency, frequent arguments, extramarital affairs, or extremely rigid beliefs about roles within the family may be present.

During the collection of the patient history, the sexual, social, and psychological history of the patient should be evaluated for any signs of actual or potential abuse.

- The **sexual history** may reveal problems such as previous sexual abuse, forced sexual acts, sexually transmitted infections (STIs), sexual knowledge beyond normal age-appropriate knowledge, or promiscuity.
- The **social history** may reveal unplanned pregnancies, social isolation as evidenced by lack of friends available to help the patient, unreasonable jealousy of significant other, verbal aggression, belief in physical punishment, or problems in school.
- During the **psychological assessment** the patient may express feelings of helplessness and being trapped. The patient may be unable to describe their future, become tearful, perform self-mutilation, have low self-esteem, and have had previous suicide attempts.

OBSERVATIONS THAT MAY INDICATE ABUSE

During the initial assessment, observations may also be made by the provider that can provide vital information about actual or potential abuse. **General observations** may include finding that the patient history is far different from what is objectively viewed by the provider or that there is a lack of proper clothing or lack of physical care provided. The home environment may include lack of heat, water, or food. It may also reveal inappropriate sleeping arrangements or lack of an environmentally safe housing situation. Observations concerning **family communications** may reveal that the abuser answers all the questions for the whole family or that others look to the controlling member for approval or seem fearful of others. Family members may frequently argue, interrupt each other, or act out negative nonverbal behaviors while others are speaking. They may avoid talking about certain subjects that they feel are secretive.

INDICATORS OF ABUSE THAT MAY BE EVIDENT DURING THE PHYSICAL ASSESSMENT

During the **physical assessment** the provider should always be aware of any **indicators of abuse**. These indicators may include increased anxiety about being examined or in the presence of the abuser; poor hygiene; looks to abuser to answer questions for them; flinching; over or underweight; presence of bruises, welts, scars or cigarette burns; bald patches on scalp for pulling out of hair; intracranial bleeding; subconjunctival hemorrhages; black eye(s); hearing loss from untreated infection or injury; poor dental hygiene; abdominal injuries; fractures; developmental delays; hyperactive reflexes; genital lacerations or ecchymosis; and presence of STIs, rectal bruising, bleeding, edema, or poor sphincter tone.

DOMESTIC VIOLENCE

Men, women, elderly, children, and the disabled may all be victims of **domestic violence**. The violent person harms physically or sexually and uses threats and fear to maintain control of the victim. The violence does not improve unless the abuser gets intensive counseling. The abuser may promise not to do it again, but the violence usually gets more frequent and worsens over time. The provider should ask all patients in private about abuse, neglect, and fear of a caretaker. If abuse is suspected or there are signs present, the state may require **reporting**:

- Give victims information about community hotlines, shelters, and resources.
- Urge them to set up a plan for escape for themselves and any children, complete with supplies in a location away from the home.
- Assure victims that they are not at fault and do not deserve the abuse.
- Try to empower them by helping them to realize that they do not have to take abuse and can find support to change the situation.

> **Review Video: Domestic Violence**
> Visit mometrix.com/academy and enter code: 530581

ASSESSMENT OF DOMESTIC VIOLENCE

According to the guidelines of the Family Violence Prevention Fund, **assessment** for domestic violence should be done for all adolescent and adult patients, regardless of background or signs of abuse. While females are the most common victims, there are increasing reports of male victims of domestic violence, both in heterosexual and homosexual relationships. The person doing the assessment should be informed about domestic violence and be aware of risk factors and danger signs. The interview should be conducted in private (special accommodations may need to be made for children <3 years old). The manager's office, bathrooms, and examining rooms should have information about domestic violence posted prominently. Brochures and information should be available to give to patients. Patients may present with a variety of physical complaints, such as headache, pain, palpitations, numbness, or pelvic pain. They are often depressed and may appear suicidal and may be isolated from friends and family. Victims of domestic violence often exhibit fear of spouse/partner, and may report injury inconsistent with symptoms.

STEPS TO IDENTIFYING VICTIMS OF DOMESTIC VIOLENCE

Identifying and assisting victims of domestic violence involves the following steps:

1. **Inquiry**: Non-judgmental questioning should begin with asking if the person has ever been abused—physically, sexually, or psychologically.
2. **Interview**: The person may exhibit signs of anxiety or fear and may blame himself or report that others believe he is abused. The person should be questioned if she is afraid for her life or for her children.
3. **Question**: If the person reports abuse, it's critical to ask if the person is in immediate danger or if the abuser is on the premises. The interviewer should ask if the person has been threatened. The history and pattern of abuse should be questioned, and if children are involved, whether the children are abused. Note: State laws vary, and in some states, it is mandatory to report if a child was present during an act of domestic violence as this is considered child abuse. The provider must be aware of state laws regarding domestic and child abuse, and all healthcare providers are mandatory reporters.
4. **Validate**: The interviewer should offer support and reassurance in a non-judgmental manner, telling the patient the abuse is not his or her fault.
5. **Give information**: While discussing facts about domestic violence and the tendency to escalate, the interviewer should provide brochures and information about safety planning. If the patient wants to file a complaint with the police, the interviewer should assist the person to place the call.
6. **Make referrals**: Information about state, local, and national organizations should be provided along with telephone numbers and contact numbers for domestic violence shelters.
7. **Document**: Record keeping should be legal, legible, and lengthy with a complete report and description of any traumatic injuries resulting from domestic violence. A body map may be used to indicate sites of injury, especially if there are multiple bruises or injuries.

INJURIES CONSISTENT WITH DOMESTIC VIOLENCE

There are a number of characteristic **injuries** that may indicate domestic violence, including ruptured eardrum; rectal/genital injury (burns, bites, or trauma); scrapes and bruises about the neck, face, head, trunk, arms; and cuts, bruises, and fractures of the face. The pattern of injuries associated with domestic violence is also often distinctive. The bathing-suit pattern involves injuries on parts of body that are usually covered with clothing as the perpetrator inflicts damage but hides evidence of abuse. Head and neck injuries (50%) are also common. Abusive injuries (rarely attributable to accidents) are common and include bites, bruises, rope and cigarette burns, and welts in the outline of weapons (belt marks). Bilateral injuries of arms/legs are often seen with domestic abuse. Defensive injuries are indicative of abuse.

Defensive injuries to the back of the body are often incurred as the victim crouches on the floor face down while being attacked. The soles of the feet may be injured from kicking at perpetrator. The ulnar aspect of hand or palm may be injured from blocking blows.

Identifying and Reporting Neglect of the Basic Needs of Adults

Neglect of the basic needs of adults is a common problem, especially among the elderly, adults with psychiatric or mental health problems, or those who live alone or with reluctant or incapable caregivers. In some cases, **passive neglect** may occur because an elderly or impaired spouse or partner is trying to take care of a patient and is unable to provide the care needed, but in other cases, **active neglect** reflects a lack of caring which may be considered negligence or abuse. Cases of neglect should be reported to the appropriate governmental agency, such as adult protective services. Indications of neglect include the following:

- Lack of assistive devices, such as a cane or walker, needed for mobility
- Misplaced or missing glasses or hearing aids
- Poor dental hygiene and dental care or missing dentures
- Patient left unattended for extended periods of time, sometimes confined to a bed or chair
- Patient left in soiled or urine- and feces-stained clothing
- Inadequate food, fluid, or nutrition, resulting in weight loss
- Inappropriate and unkempt clothing, such as no sweater or coat during the winter and dirty or torn clothing
- A dirty, messy environment

Identifying and Reporting Neglect or Lack of Supervision in Children

While some children may not be physically or sexually abused, they may suffer from profound **neglect** or **lack of supervision** that places them at risk. Indicators include the following:

- Appearing dirty and unkempt, sometimes with infestations of lice, and wearing ill-fitting or torn clothes and shoes
- Being tired and sleepy during the daytime
- Having untended medical or dental problems, such as dental caries
- Missing appointments and not receiving proper immunizations
- Being underweight for stage of development

Neglect can be difficult to assess, especially if the nurse is serving a homeless or very poor population. Home visits may be needed to ascertain if adequate food, clothing, or supervision is being provided; this may be beyond the care provided by the nurse, so suspicions should be reported to appropriate authorities, such as child protective services, so that social workers can assess the home environment.

Diagnosis

Cardiovascular Pathophysiology

ACUTE CORONARY SYNDROMES

Acute coronary syndrome (ACS) is the impairment of blood flow through the coronary arteries, leading to ischemia of the cardiac muscle. Angina frequently occurs in ACS, manifesting as crushing pain substernally, radiating down the left arm or both arms. However, in females, elderly, and diabetics, symptoms may appear less acute and include nausea, shortness of breath, fatigue, pain/weakness/numbness in arms, or no pain at all (*silent ischemia*). There are multiple **classifications of angina**:

- **Stable angina**: Exercise-induced, short lived, relieved by rest or nitroglycerin. Other precipitating events include decrease in environmental temperature, heavy eating, strong emotions (such as fright or anger), or exertion, including coitus.
- **Unstable angina** (preinfarction or crescendo angina): A change in the pattern of stable angina, characterized by an increase in pain, not responding to a single nitroglycerin or rest, and persisting for >5 minutes. May cause a change in EKG, or indicate rupture of an atherosclerotic plaque or the beginning of thrombus formation. Treat as a medical emergency, indicates impending MI.
- **Variant angina** (Prinzmetal's angina): Results from spasms of the coronary arteries. Associated with or without atherosclerotic plaques and is often related to smoking, alcohol, or illicit stimulants, but can occur cyclically and at rest. Elevation of ST segments usually occurs with variant angina. Treatment is nitroglycerin or calcium channel blockers.

> **Review Video: Coronary Artery Disease**
> Visit mometrix.com/academy and enter code: 950720

MYOCARDIAL INFARCTIONS
NSTEMI AND STEMI

Non–ST-segment elevation MI (NSTEMI): ST elevation on the electrocardiogram (ECG) occurs in response to myocardial damage resulting from infarction or severe ischemia. The absence of ST elevation may be diagnosed as unstable angina or NSTEMI, but cardiac enzyme levels increase with NSTEMI, indicating partial blockage of coronary arteries with some damage. Symptoms are consistent with unstable angina, with chest pain or tightness, pain radiating to the neck or arm, dyspnea, anxiety, weakness, dizziness, nausea, vomiting, and heartburn. Initial treatment may include nitroglycerin, β-blockers, antiplatelet agents, or antithrombotic agents. Ongoing treatment may include β-blockers, aspirin, statins, angiotensin-converting enzyme inhibitors, angiotensin-receptor blockers, and clopidogrel. Percutaneous coronary intervention is not recommended.

ST-segment elevation MI (STEMI): This more severe type of MI involves complete blockage of one or more coronary arteries with myocardial damage, resulting in ST elevation. Symptoms are those of acute MI. As necrosis occurs, Q waves often develop, indicating irreversible myocardial damage, which may result in death, so treatment involves immediate reperfusion before necrosis can occur.

> **Review Video: Myocardial Infarction**
> Visit mometrix.com/academy and enter code: 148923

Q-Wave and Non-Q-Wave Myocardial Infarctions

Formerly classified as transmural or non-transmural, myocardial infarctions are now classified as Q-wave or non-Q-wave:

- **Q-Wave**
  - Characterized by a series of abnormal Q waves (wider and deeper) on ECG, especially in the early morning (related to adrenergic activity).
  - Infarction is usually prolonged and results in necrosis.
  - Coronary occlusion is complete in 80–90% of cases.
  - Q-wave MI is often, but not always, transmural.
  - Peak CK levels occur in about 27 hours.
- **Non-Q-Wave**
  - Characterized by changes in ST-T wave with ST depression (usually reversible within a few days).
  - Usually reperfusion occurs spontaneously, so infarct size is smaller. Contraction necrosis related to reperfusion is common.
  - Non-Q-wave MI is usually non-transmural.
  - Coronary occlusion is complete in only 20–30%.
  - Peak CK levels occur in 12–13 hours.
  - Reinfarction is common.

Locations and Types

Myocardial infarctions are also classified according to their location and the extent of injury. Q-wave infarctions involve the full thickness of the heart muscle, often producing a series of Q waves on ECG. While an MI most frequently damages the left ventricle and the septum, the right ventricle may be damaged as well, depending upon the area of the occlusion:

- **Anterior** (V_2 to V_4): Occlusion in the proximal left anterior descending (LAD) or left coronary artery. Reciprocal changes found in leads II, III, aV_F.
- **Lateral** (I, aV_L, V_5, V_6): Occlusion of the circumflex coronary artery or branch of left coronary artery. Often causes damage to anterior wall as well. Reciprocal changes found in leads II, III, aV_F.
- **Inferior/diaphragmatic** (II, III, aV_F): Occlusion of the right coronary artery and causes conduction malfunctions. Reciprocal changes found in leads I and aV_L.
- **Right ventricular** (V_{4R}, V_{5R}, V_{6R}): Occlusion of the proximal section of the right coronary artery and damages in the right ventricle and the inferior wall. No reciprocal changes should be noted on an ECG.
- **Posterior** (V_1 to V_4): Occlusion in the right coronary artery or the left coronary artery or its circumflex branch and may be difficult to diagnose. Reciprocal changes found in V_1-V_4.
- **Septal** (V_1 and V_2): Occlusion of the left anterior descending (LAD) at the septal branch. T-wave inversion and absent R wave long with ST elevation.

Clinical Manifestations and Diagnosis

Clinical manifestations of myocardial infarction may vary considerably. More than half of all patients present with acute MIs with no prior history of cardiovascular disease.

Signs/symptoms: Angina with pain in chest that may radiate to neck or arms, palpitations, hypertension or hypotension, dyspnea, pulmonary edema, dependent edema, nausea/vomiting, pallor, skin cold and clammy, diaphoresis, decreased urinary output, neurological/psychological disturbances: anxiety, light-headedness, headache, visual abnormalities, slurred speech, and fear.

Diagnosis is based on the following:

- ECG obtained immediately to monitor heart changes over time. Typical changes include T-wave inversion, elevation of ST segment, abnormal Q waves, tachycardia, bradycardia, and dysrhythmias.

- Echocardiogram: decreased ventricular function is possible, especially for transmural MI.
- Labs:
  - **Troponin**: Increases within 3–6 hours, peaks 14–20; elevated for up to 1–2 weeks.
  - **Creatinine kinase (CK-MB)**: Increases 4–8 hours and peaks at about 24 hours (earlier with thrombolytic therapy or PTCA). (Not commonly used in the US)
  - **Ischemia modified albumin (IMA)**: Increase within minutes, peak 6 hours and return to baseline; verify with other labs.
  - **Myoglobin**: Increases in 0.5–4.0 hours, peaks 6–7 hours. While an increase is not specific to an MI, a failure to increase can be used to rule out an MI.

PAPILLARY MUSCLE RUPTURE

Papillary muscle rupture is a rare but often deadly complication of myocardial ischemia/infarct. It most commonly occurs with inferior infarcts. The papillary muscles are part of the cardiac wall structure. Attached to the lower portion of the ventricles, they are responsible for the opening and closing of the tricuspid and mitral valve and preventing prolapse during systole. Rupture of the papillary muscle can occur with myocardial infarct or ischemia in the area of the heart surrounding the papillary muscle. Since the papillary muscles support the mitral valve, rupture will cause severe mitral regurgitation that may result in cardiogenic shock and subsequent death. Rupture of the papillary muscle may be partial or complete and is considered a life-threatening emergency.

Signs/symptoms: Acute heart failure, pulmonary edema, and cardiogenic shock (tachycardia, diaphoresis, loss of consciousness, pallor, tachypnea, mental status changes, weak or thready pulse, and decreased urinary output).

Diagnosis: Transesophageal echocardiography (TEE) to visualize the papillary muscles, color flow Doppler, echocardiogram, and physical assessment. In patients with papillary muscle rupture, a holosystolic murmur starting at the apex and radiating to the axilla may be present.

Treatment: Emergent surgical intervention to repair the mitral valve.

In the cases of complete rupture, patients often experience the rapid development of cardiogenic shock and subsequent death.

AORTIC ANEURYSMS

TYPES

A **dissecting aortic aneurysm** occurs when the wall of the aorta is torn and blood flows between the layers of the wall, dilating and weakening it until it risks rupture (which has a 90% mortality). Aortic aneurysms are more than twice as common in males as females, but females have a higher mortality rate, possibly due to increased age at diagnosis.

Abdominal aortic aneurysms (AAA) are usually related to atherosclerosis, but may also result from Marfan syndrome, Ehlers-Danlos disease, and connective tissue disorders. Rupture usually does not allow time for emergent repair, so identifying and correcting before rupture is essential. Different classification systems are used to describe the type and degree of dissection. **DeBakey classification** uses anatomic location as the focal point:

- Type I (thoracic) begins in the ascending aorta but may spread to include the aortic arch and the descending aorta (60%). This is also considered a proximal lesion or Stanford type A.
- Type II (thoracic) is restricted to the ascending aorta (10–15%). This is also considered a proximal lesion or Stanford type A.
- Type III (abdominal) is restricted to the descending aorta (25–30%). This is considered a distal lesion or Stanford type B.

Diagnosis and Treatment

Aortic aneurysms are often asymptomatic, but when symptomatic, patients present with substernal pain, back pain, dyspnea and/or stridor (from pressure on trachea), cough, distention of neck veins, palpable and pulsating abdominal mass, edema of neck and arms.

Diagnosis: x-ray, CT, MRI, Cardiac catheterization, TEE/transthoracic echocardiogram.

Treatment includes:

- **Anti-hypertensives** to reduce systolic BP, such as β-blockers (esmolol) or Alpha-β-blocker combinations (labetalol) to reduce force of blood as it leaves the ventricle to reduce pressure against the aortic wall. IV vasodilators (sodium nitroprusside) may also be needed.
- **Intubation and ventilation** may be required if the patient is hemodynamically unstable.
- **Analgesia/sedation** to control anxiety and pain.
- **Surgical repair**: Types I and II are usually repaired surgically because of the danger of rupture and cardiac tamponade. Type III (abdominal) is often followed medically and surgically only if the aneurysm is >5.5cm or rapidly expanding. There are two types of surgical repair:
  - **Open**: Patient is placed on cardiopulmonary bypass, and through an abdominal incision the damaged portion is removed, and a graft is sutured in place.
  - **Endovascular**: A stent graft is fed through the arteries to line the aorta and exclude the aneurysm.

Complications: Myocardial infarction, renal injury, and GI hemorrhage/ischemic bowel, which may occur up to years after surgery. Endo-leaks can occur with a stent graft, increasing risk of rupture.

Aortic Rupture

Aortic rupture is a catastrophic breakage of the aorta, generally as the result of trauma or rupture of an aortic aneurysm. **Aortic rupture** (spontaneous) most commonly occurs in the abdominal aorta. The patient typically experiences a severe tearing pain and loses consciousness from hypovolemic shock as the blood pours out of the aorta. Tachycardia occurs and the patient may exhibit cyanosis. An ecchymotic area may appear in the flank area because of retroperitoneal pooling of blood. Diagnostic tests include ultrasound or CT. Survival depends on the size of the tear, the amount of blood loss, and the length of time until surgical repair. About 90% of patients die prior to surgery. An aortic occlusion balloon to stem bleeding may be placed temporarily in order to stabilize the patient. Surgical repair may be via an open procedure or endovascular therapy. Risk factors include male gender, older age, smoking, history of MI, family history of abdominal aortic aneurysm, peripheral arterial disease, and hypertension.

Cardiomyopathy
Dilated Cardiomyopathy

Dilated cardiomyopathy (DCM) occurs when some precipitating factor leads to decreased cardiac perfusion. The resulting ischemic cardiac tissue is replaced with scar tissue, and the healthy cells are forced to over-compensate, causing hypertrophy and over stretching. Eventually, the muscle cells become stretched beyond compensation, and dilated and weak chamber results, unable to properly contract. This causes a decrease in stroke volume and cardiac output, with the end result being enlargement of the mitral and tricuspid valves and severe valve regurgitation. While DCM is the most common form of cardiomyopathy, causes include:

- **Vascular**: Cardiac ischemia, hypertension, atherosclerosis
- **Metabolic**: Diabetes, uremia, thyrotoxicosis, and acromegaly, muscular dystrophy
- **Genetics** (familial DCM), and childbirth (peripartum DCM)
- **Viral infections**, particularly adenovirus, Varicella zoster, HIV, and Hepatitis C may cause DCM
- **Alcohol poisoning or cocaine addiction**
- **Radiation or heavy metal poisoning**, specifically cobalt

Signs/symptoms: Dyspnea, SOB, tachycardia, S3/S4 heart sounds, holosystolic murmur, wheezes/crackles, pleural effusions, edema, JVD, ascites

Diagnosis: EKG (tachycardia/T wave changes), chest x-ray (cardiomegaly), 2D Echocardiogram (valve regurgitation/EF).

Treatment includes:

- Treat underlying cause if possible; supportive care
- Heart transplant if patient is a candidate and damage is permanent

HYPERTROPHIC CARDIOMYOPATHY

Hypertrophic cardiomyopathy (HCM) is a genetic disorder that causes idiopathic thickening of the heart muscle, primarily involving the ventricular septum and portions of the left ventricle. Patients with HCM produce abnormal sarcomeres and misalignment of muscle cells (myocardial disarray). Basically, HCM is characterized by ventricular hypertrophy, an asymmetrical septum, forceful systole, cardiac dysrhythmias, and myocardial disarray. Because the abnormal cells develop over time, it is common for HCM to remain undiagnosed until middle or late adulthood.

Signs/symptoms: Exertional or atypical chest pain, dyspnea at rest, syncope, frequent palpitations (common due to reoccurring dysrhythmias).

Diagnosis: 2D echo (structure and EF), EKG (pathological Q waves and dysrhythmias), x-ray (cardiomegaly), Family history (especially cardiac death, reoccurring dysrhythmias, or myocardial hypertrophy).

Treatment for cases in which there is outflow tract obstruction includes the use of β-blockers and one of the following methods of septal reduction therapy:

- **Septal myectomy** (gold standard): high mortality (3–10%), but increases cardiac output and quality of life.
- **Alcohol-based septal ablation**: Ethanol 100% injected into a branch of the LAD, creating a controlled area of infarction and consequently thinning the septum.

RESTRICTIVE CARDIOMYOPATHY

Restrictive cardiomyopathy (RCM) occurs when the ventricles become stiff and noncompliant, resulting in decreased end-diastolic cardiac refill volume. The ventricular stiffening is caused by the infiltration of fibroelastic tissue into the cardiac muscle (such as in amyloidosis or sarcoidosis). Atrial enlargement can be seen in most cases of RCM as a result of the increased effort required to push blood from the atria into the ventricles. It is not uncommon for a patient to be in atrial fibrillation secondary to atrial enlargement. In advanced cases, ventricular dysrhythmias may also be seen.

Signs/symptoms: Exercise intolerance/fatigue, edema, crackles, elevated CVP, S3/S4, murmur, SOB at rest

Diagnosis: 2D echo (enlarged atria, decreased compliance of ventricle), hemodynamic monitoring (increased right atrial pressure and pulmonary wedge pressure, and SVR), x-ray (cardiomegaly), EKG (atrial fibrillation), endomyocardial biopsy (to differentiate from constrictive pericarditis).

Treatment includes:

- **Medications**: β-blockers increase ventricular filling; antiarrhythmics may be ordered
- **Surgical**: Heart transplant, if patient is a candidate

Stress (Takotsubo) Cardiomyopathy

Takotsubo cardiomyopathy, also referred to as stress cardiomyopathy or more casually as broken heart syndrome, is an acute weakening of the muscles of the heart secondary to an intensely stressful event. Stressors can be physical (extreme illness such as sepsis or shock) or emotional in nature and result in the release of stress hormones (epinephrine and norepinephrine) that are thought to be the major contributors to the ultimate weakening of the heart muscle. This produces symptoms that present similarly to a myocardial infarction (shortness of breath, chest pain, and EKG changes) without any ischemic event noted to contribute to these symptoms. Risk factors for takotsubo cardiomyopathy include:

- **Stressful events or conditions**
- **Sex**: Females have a higher risk for developing takotsubo cardiomyopathy
- **Endocrine disorders**: Pheochromocytoma and thyrotoxicosis

Treatment focuses on symptom management due to the risk for acute heart failure and cardiogenic shock. In severe cases, an intra-aortic balloon pump may be required for circulatory support until the patient is stabilized.

Dysrhythmias

Sinus Bradycardia

There are 3 primary types of **sinus node dysrhythmias**: sinus bradycardia, sinus tachycardia, and sinus arrhythmia. **Sinus bradycardia (SB)** is caused by a decreased rate of impulse from sinus node. The pulse and ECG usually appear normal except for a slower rate.

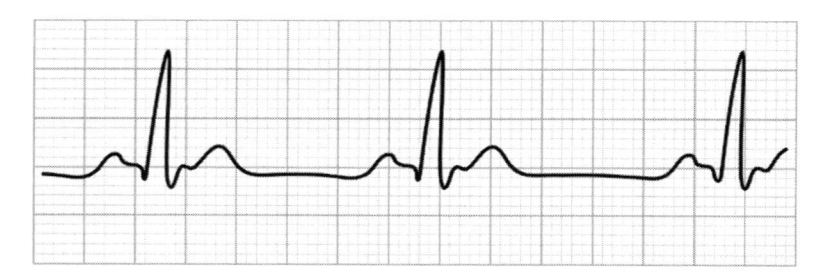

SB is characterized by a regular pulse <50–60 bpm with P waves in front of QRS, which are usually normal in shape and duration. PR interval is 0.12–0.20 seconds, QRS interval is 0.04–0.11 seconds, and P:QRS ratio of 1:1. SB may be caused by several factors:

- May be normal in athletes and older adults; generally not treated unless symptomatic
- Conditions that lower the body's metabolic needs, such as hypothermia or sleep
- Hypotension and decrease in oxygenation
- Medications such as calcium channel blockers and β-blockers
- Vagal stimulation that may result from vomiting, suctioning, defecating, or certain medical procedures (carotid stent placement, etc.)
- Increased intracranial pressure
- Myocardial infarction

Treatment: involves eliminating cause if possible, such as changing medications. Atropine 1 mg may be given IV to block vagal stimulation or increase rate if symptomatic.

Sinus Tachycardia

Sinus tachycardia (ST) occurs when the sinus node impulse increases in frequency. ST is characterized by a regular pulse >100 with P waves before QRS but sometimes part of the preceding T wave. QRS is usually of normal shape and duration (0.04–0.11 seconds) but may have consistent irregularity. PR interval is 0.12–0.20 seconds and P:QRS ratio of 1:1.

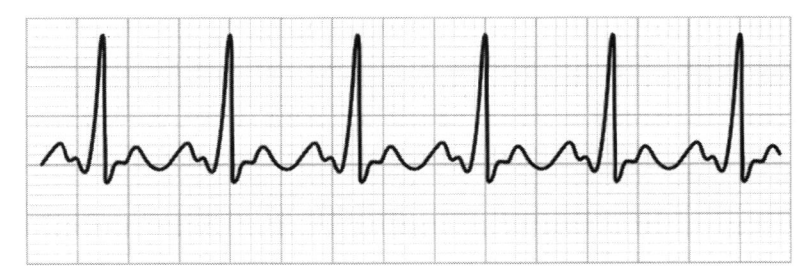

The rapid pulse decreases diastolic filling time and causes reduced cardiac output with resultant hypotension. Acute pulmonary edema may result from the decreased ventricular filling if untreated. ST may be **caused** by a number of factors:

- Acute blood loss, shock, hypovolemia, anemia
- Sinus arrhythmia, hypovolemic heart failure
- Hypermetabolic conditions, fever, infection
- Exertion/exercise, anxiety, stress
- Medications, such as sympathomimetic drugs

Treatment: eliminating precipitating factors, calcium channel blockers and β-blockers to reduce heart rate.

Supraventricular Tachycardia

Supraventricular tachycardia (SVT) (>100 BPM) may have a sudden onset and result in congestive heart failure. Rate may increase to 200–300 BPM, which will significantly decrease cardiac output due to decreased filling time. SVT originates in the atria rather than the ventricles but is controlled by the tissue in the area of the AV node rather than the SA node. Rhythm is usually rapid but regular. The P wave is present but may not be clearly defined as it may be obscured by the preceding T wave, and the QRS complex appears normal. The PR interval is 0.12–0.20 seconds and the QRS interval is 0.04–0.11 seconds with a P:QRS ratio of 1:1.

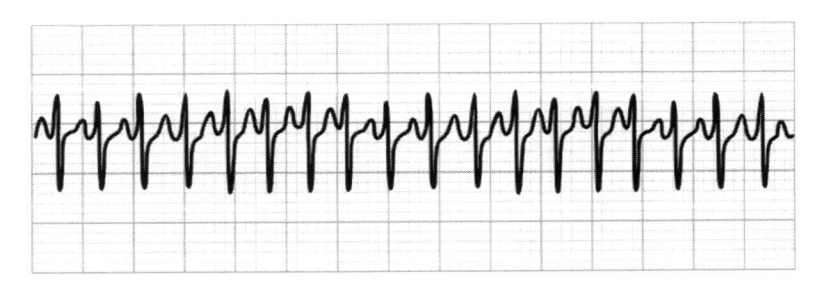

SVT may be episodic with periods of normal heart rate and rhythm between episodes of SVT, so it is often referred to as paroxysmal SVT (PSVT).

Treatment: Adenosine, digoxin, verapamil, vagal maneuvers, cardioversion.

SINUS ARRHYTHMIA

Sinus arrhythmia (SA) results from irregular impulses from the sinus node, often paradoxical (increasing with inspiration and decreasing with expiration) because of stimulation of the vagal nerve during inspiration and rarely causes a negative hemodynamic effect. These cyclic changes in the pulse during respiration are quite common in both children and young adults and often lesson with age but may persist in some adults. Sinus arrhythmia can, in some cases, relate to heart or valvular disease and may be increased with vagal stimulation for suctioning, vomiting, or defecating. Characteristics of SA include a regular pulse 50–100 BPM, P waves in front of QRS with duration (0.04–0.11 seconds) and shape of QRS usually normal, PR interval of 0.12–0.20 seconds, and P:QRS ratio of 1:1.

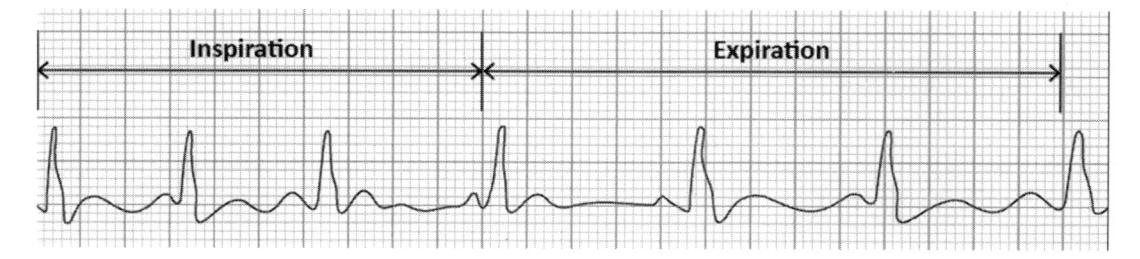

Treatment is usually not necessary unless it is associated with bradycardia.

PREMATURE ATRIAL CONTRACTION

There are 3 primary types of **atrial dysrhythmias**: premature atrial contraction, atrial flutter, and atrial fibrillation. Premature atrial contraction (PAC) is essentially an extra beat precipitated by an electrical impulse to the atrium before the sinus node impulse. The extra beat may be caused by alcohol, caffeine, nicotine, hypervolemia, hypokalemia, hypermetabolic conditions, atrial ischemia, or infarction. Characteristics include an irregular pulse because of extra P waves, the shape and duration of QRS is usually normal (0.04–0.11 seconds) but may be abnormal, PR interval remains between 0.12–0.20, and P:QRS ratio is 1:1. Rhythm is irregular with varying P-P and R-R intervals.

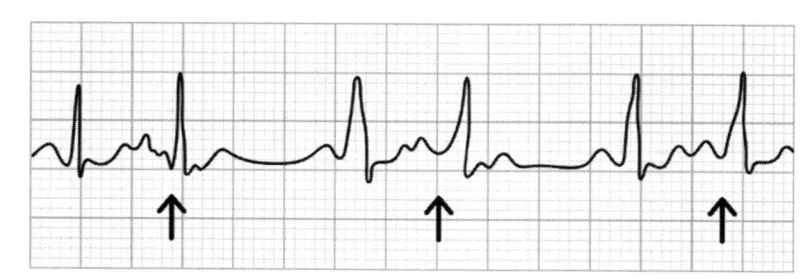

PACs can occur in an essentially healthy heart and are not usually cause for concern unless they are frequent (>6 per hr) and cause severe palpitations. In that case, atrial fibrillation should be suspected.

ATRIAL FLUTTER

Atrial flutter (AF) occurs when the atrial rate is faster, usually 250–400 beats per minute, than the AV node conduction rate so not all of the beats are conducted into the ventricles. The beats are effectively blocked at the AV node, preventing ventricular fibrillation although some extra ventricular impulses may pass through. AF is caused by the same conditions that cause A-fib: coronary artery disease, valvular disease, pulmonary disease, heavy alcohol ingestion, and cardiac surgery. AF is characterized by atrial rates of 250–400 with ventricular rates of 75–150, with ventricular rate usually being regular. P waves are saw-toothed (referred to as F waves), QRS shape and duration (0.04–0.11 seconds) are usually normal, PR interval may be hard to calculate because of F waves, and the P:QRS ratio is 2:1 to 4:1. Symptoms include chest pain, dyspnea, and hypotension.

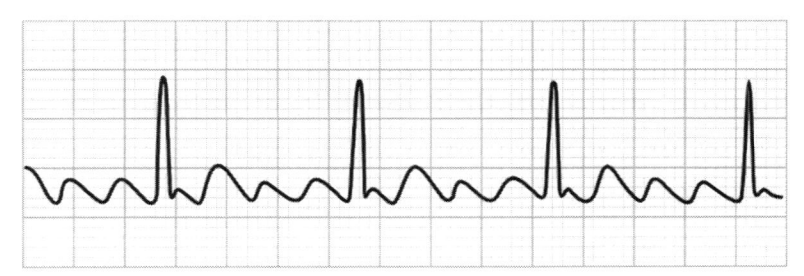

Treatment includes:

- Emergent cardioversion if condition is unstable
- Medications to slow ventricular rate and conduction through AV node: non-dihydropyridine calcium channel blockers (Cardizem, Calan) and beta blockers
- Medications to convert to sinus rhythm: ibutilide (Corvert), dofetilide (Tikosyn), amiodarone; also used in practice: quinidine, disopyramide (Norpace)

ATRIAL FIBRILLATION

Atrial fibrillation (A-fib) is rapid, disorganized atrial beats that are ineffective in emptying the atria, so that blood pools in the chambers. This can lead to thrombus formation and emboli. The ventricular rate increases with a decreased stroke volume, and cardiac output decreases with increased myocardial ischemia, resulting in palpitations and fatigue. A-fib is caused by coronary artery disease, valvular disease, pulmonary disease, heavy alcohol ingestion, infection, and cardiac surgery; however, it can also be idiopathic. A-fib is characterized by a very irregular pulse with atrial rate of 300–600 and ventricular rate of 120–200, shape and duration (0.04–0.11 seconds) of QRS is usually normal. Fibrillatory (F) waves are seen instead of P waves. The PR interval cannot be measured and the P:QRS ratio is highly variable.

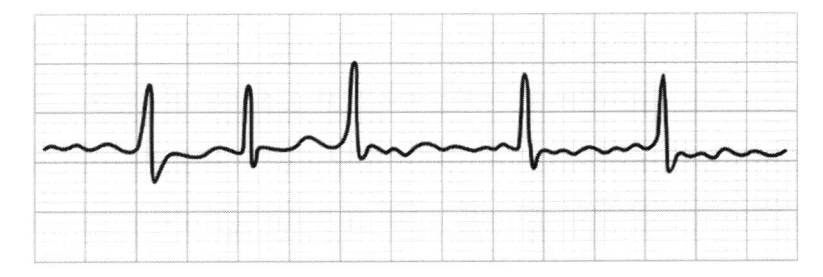

Treatment is the same as atrial flutter.

> **Review Video: Atrial Fibrillation and Atrial Flutter**
> Visit mometrix.com/academy and enter code: 263842

Premature Junctional Contraction

The area around the AV node is the junction, and dysrhythmias that arise from that area are called junctional dysrhythmias. Premature junctional contraction (PJC) occurs when a premature impulse starts at the AV node before the next normal sinus impulse reaches the AV node. PJC is similar to premature atrial contraction (PAC) and generally requires no treatment although it may be an indication of digoxin toxicity. The ECG may appear basically normal with an early QRS complex that is normal in shape and duration (0.04–0.11 seconds). The P wave may be absent or it may precede, be part of, or follow the QRS with a PR interval of 0.12 seconds. The P:QRS ratio may vary from <1:1 to 1:1 (with inverted P wave). The underlying rhythm is usually regular at a heart rate of 60–100. Significant symptoms related to PJC are rare.

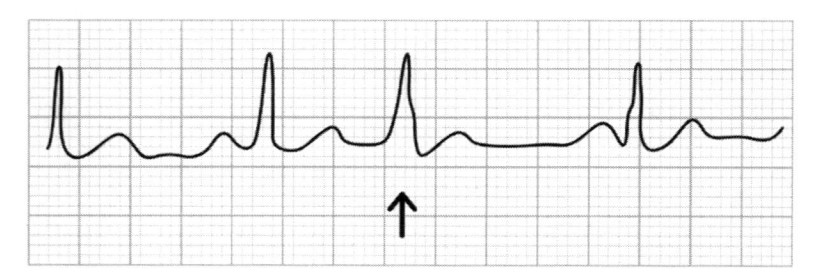

Junctional Rhythms

Junctional rhythms occur when the AV node becomes the pacemaker of the heart. This can happen because the sinus node is depressed from increased vagal tone or a block at the AV node prevents sinus node impulses from being transmitted. While the sinus node normally sends impulses 60–100 beats per minute, the AV node junction usually sends impulses at 40–60 beats per minute. The QRS complex is of usual shape and duration (0.04–0.11 seconds). The P wave may be inverted and may be absent, hidden or after the QRS. If the P wave precedes the QRS, the PR interval is <0.12 seconds. The P:QRS ratio is <1:1 or 1:1. The junctional escape rhythm is a protective mechanism preventing asystole with failure of the sinus node. An **accelerated junctional rhythm** is similar, but the heart rate is 60–100. **Junctional tachycardia** occurs with heart rate of >100.

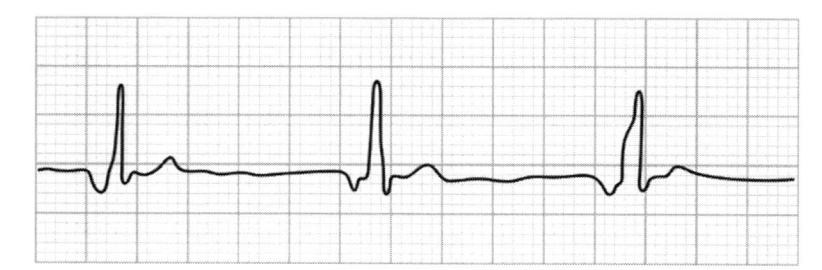

AV Nodal Reentry Tachycardia

AV nodal reentry tachycardia occurs when an impulse conducts to the area of the AV node and is then sent in a rapidly repeating cycle back to the same area and to the ventricles, resulting in a fast ventricular rate. The onset and cessation are usually rapid. AV nodal reentry tachycardia (also known as paroxysmal atrial tachycardia or supraventricular tachycardia if there are no P waves) is characterized by atrial rate of 150–250 with ventricular rate of 75–250, P wave that is difficult to see or absent, QRS complex that is usually normal and a PR interval of <0.12 if a P wave is present. The P:QRS ratio is 1–2:1. Precipitating factors include nicotine, caffeine, hypoxemia, anxiety, underlying coronary artery disease and cardiomyopathy. Cardiac output may be decreased with a rapid heart rate, causing dyspnea, chest pain, and hypotension.

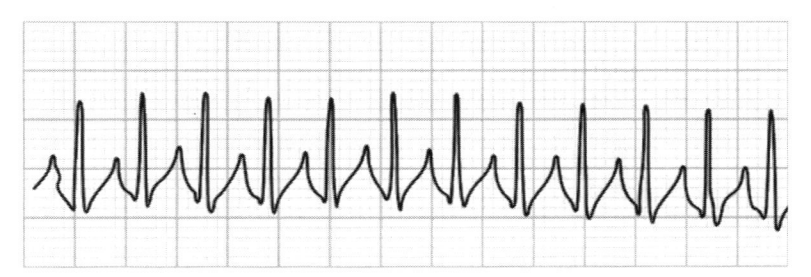

Treatment includes:

- Vagal maneuvers (carotid sinus massage, gag reflex, holding breath/bearing down)
- Medications (adenosine, verapamil, or diltiazem)
- Cardioversion if other methods unsuccessful

Premature Ventricular Contractions

Premature ventricular contractions (PVCs) are those in which the impulse begins in the ventricles and conducts through them prior to the next sinus impulse. The ectopic QRS complexes may vary in shape, depending upon whether there is one site (unifocal) or more (multifocal) that stimulates the ectopic beats. PVCs usually cause no morbidity unless there is underlying cardiac disease or an acute MI. PVCs are characterized by an irregular heartbeat, QRS that is ≥0.12 seconds and oddly shaped. PVCs are often not treated in otherwise healthy people. PVCs may be precipitated by electrolyte imbalances, caffeine, nicotine, or alcohol. Because PVCs may occur with any supraventricular dysrhythmia, the underlying rhythm must be noted as well as the PVCs. If there are more than six PVCs in an hour, that is a risk factor for developing ventricular tachycardia.

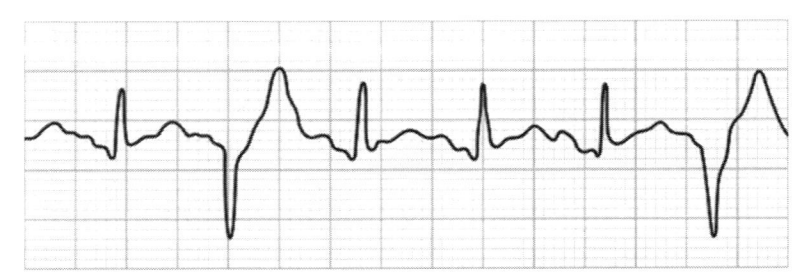

Bigeminy is a rhythm where every other beat is a PVC. **Trigeminy** is a rhythm where every third beat is a PVC.

Ventricular bigeminy is a rhythm where every other beat is a PVC. **Ventricular trigeminy** is a rhythm where every third beat is a PVC.

Treatment: Lidocaine (affects the ventricles, may cause CNS toxicity with nausea and vomiting), procainamide (affects the atria and ventricles and may cause decreased BP and widening of QRS and QT); treat underlying cause.

VENTRICULAR TACHYCARDIA

Ventricular tachycardia (VT) is greater than 3 PVCs in a row with a ventricular rate of 100–200 beats per minute. Ventricular tachycardia may be triggered by the same factors as PVCs and often is related to underlying coronary artery disease. The rapid rate of contractions makes VT dangerous as the ineffective beats may render the person unconscious with no palpable pulse. A detectable rate is usually regular and the QRS complex is ≥0.12 seconds and is usually abnormally shaped. The P wave may be undetectable with an irregular PR interval if P wave is present. The P:QRS ratio is often difficult to ascertain because of the absence of P waves.

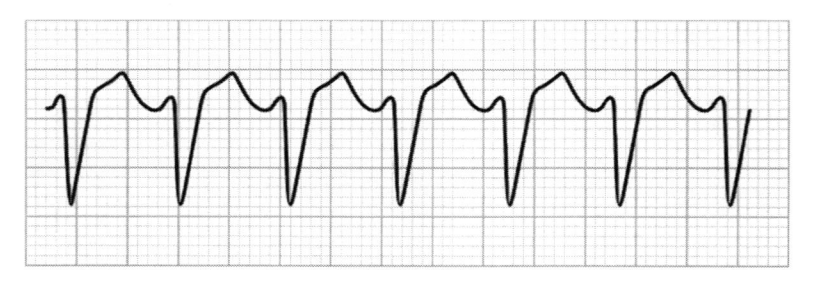

Treatment is as follows:

- With pulse: Synchronized cardioversion, adenosine
- No pulse: Same as ventricular fibrillation

NARROW COMPLEX AND WIDE COMPLEX TACHYCARDIAS

Tachycardias are classified as narrow complex or wide complex. Wide and narrow refer to the configuration of the QRS complex.

- **Wide complex tachycardia (WCT)**: About 80% of cases of WCT are caused by ventricular tachycardia. WCT originates at some point below the AV node and may be associated with palpitations, dyspnea, anxiety, diaphoresis, and cardiac arrest. Wide complex tachycardia is diagnosed with more than 3 consecutive beats at a heart rate >100 BPM and QRS duration ≥0.12 seconds.

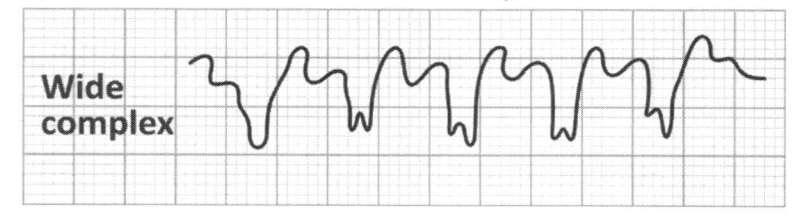

- **Narrow complex tachycardia (NCT)**: NCT is associated with palpitations, dyspnea, and peripheral edema. NCT is generally supraventricular in origin. Narrow complex tachycardia is diagnosed with ≥3 consecutive beats at heart rate of >100 BPM and QRS duration of <0.12 seconds.

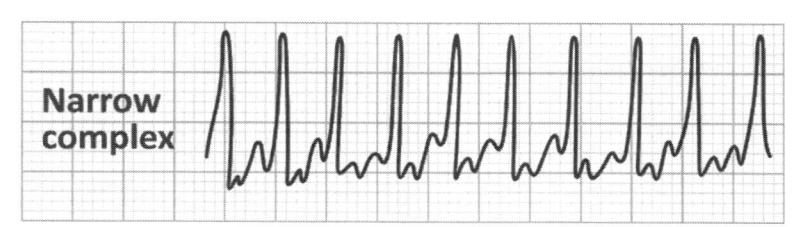

Ventricular Fibrillation

Ventricular fibrillation (VF) is a rapid, very irregular ventricular rate >300 beats per minute with no atrial activity observable on the ECG, caused by disorganized electrical activity in the ventricles. The QRS complex is not recognizable as ECG shows irregular undulations. The causes are the same as for ventricular tachycardia and asystole. VF is accompanied by lack of palpable pulse, audible pulse, and respirations and is immediately life threatening without defibrillation.

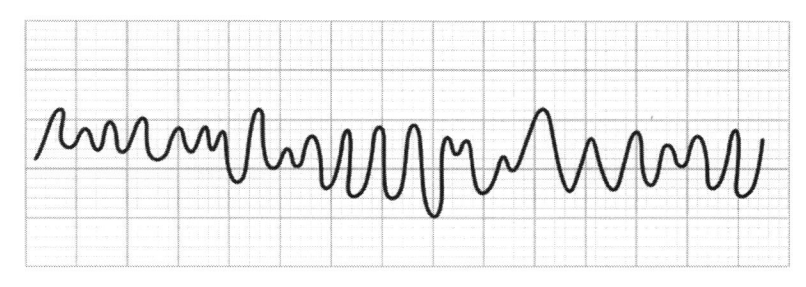

Treatment includes:

- Emergency defibrillation, the cause should be identified and treated
- Epinephrine 1 mg q 3–5 minutes then amiodarone 300 mg (2nd dose: 150 mg) IV push

> **Review Video: Ventricular Arrythmias**
> Visit mometrix.com/academy and enter code: 933152

Idioventricular Rhythm

Ventricular escape rhythm (idioventricular) occurs when the Purkinje fibers below the AV node create an impulse. This may occur if the sinus node fails to fire or if there is blockage at the AV node so that the impulse does not go through. Idioventricular rhythm is characterized by a regular ventricular rate of 20–40 BPM. Rates >40 BPM are called accelerated idioventricular rhythm. The P wave is missing and the QRS complex has a very bizarre and abnormal shape with duration of ≥0.12 seconds. The low ventricular rate may cause a decrease in cardiac output, often making the patient lose consciousness. In other patients, the idioventricular rhythm may not be associated with reduced cardiac output.

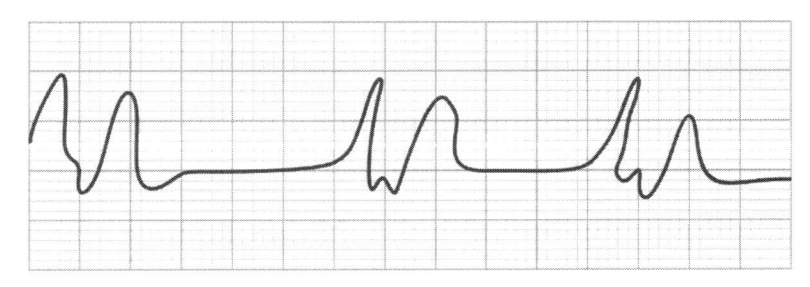

Ventricular Asystole

Ventricular asystole is the absence of audible heartbeat, palpable pulse, and respirations, a condition often referred to as "cardiac arrest." While the ECG may show some P waves initially, the QRS complex is absent although there may be an occasional QRS "escape beat" (agonal rhythm). Cardiopulmonary resuscitation is required with intubation for ventilation and establishment of an intravenous line for fluids. Without immediate treatment, the patient will suffer from severe hypoxia and brain death within minutes. Identifying the cause is critical for the patient's survival. Consider the "Hs & Ts": hypovolemia, hypoxia, hydrogen ions (acidosis), hypo/hyperkalemia, hypothermia, tension pneumothorax, tamponade (cardiac), toxins, and thrombosis (pulmonary or coronary). Even with immediate treatment, the prognosis is poor and ventricular asystole is often a sign of impending death.

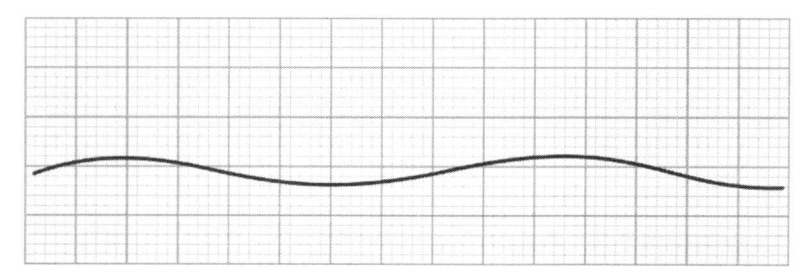

Treatment includes:

- CPR only; Asystole is not a shockable rhythm therefore defibrillation is not indicated
- Epinephrine 1 mg q 3–5 minutes

Sinus Pause

Sinus pause occurs when the sinus node fails to function properly to stimulate heart contractions, so there is a pause on the ECG recording that may persist for a few seconds to minutes, depending on the severity of the dysfunction. A prolonged pause may be difficult to differentiate from cardiac arrest. During the sinus pause, the P wave, QRS complex and PR and QRS intervals are all absent. P:QRS ratio is 1:1 and the rhythm is irregular. The pulse rate may vary widely, usually 60–100 BPM. Patients with frequent pauses may complain of dizziness or syncope. The patient may need to undergo an electrophysiology study and medication reconciliation to determine the cause. If measures such as decreasing medication are not effective, a pacemaker is usually indicated (if symptomatic).

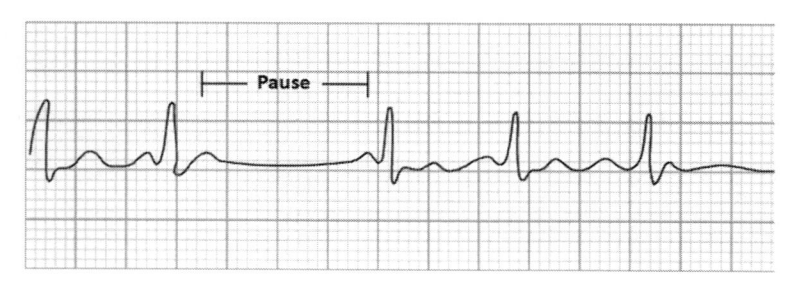

First-Degree AV Block

First-degree AV block occurs when the atrial impulses are conducted through the AV node to the ventricles at a rate that is slower than normal. While the P and QRS are usually normal, the PR interval is >0.20 seconds, and the P:QRS ratio is 1:1. A narrow QRS complex indicates a conduction abnormality only in the AV node, but a widened QRS indicates associated damage to the bundle branches as well. *Chronic* first-degree block may be caused by fibrosis/sclerosis of the conduction system related to coronary artery disease, valvular disease, cardiac myopathies and carries little morbidity, thus is often left untreated. *Acute* first-degree block, on the other hand, is of much more concern and may be related to digoxin toxicity, β-blockers, amiodarone, myocardial infarction, hyperkalemia, or edema related to valvular surgery.

Treatment: involves eliminating cause if possible, such as changing medications. Atropine 1 mg may be given IV if rate falls.

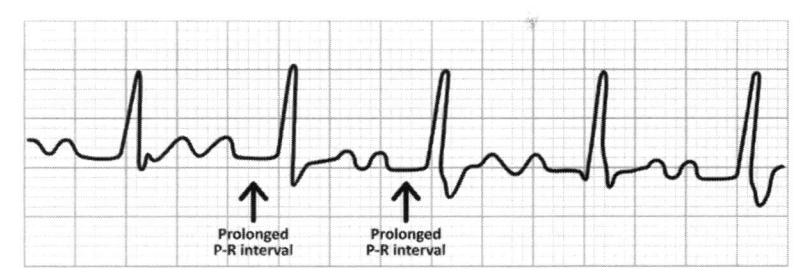

SECOND-DEGREE AV BLOCK

Second-degree AV block occurs when some of the atrial beats are blocked. Second-degree AV block is further subdivided according to the patterns of block.

TYPE I

Mobitz type I block (Wenckebach) occurs when each atrial impulse in a group of beats is conducted at a lengthened interval until one fails to conduct (the PR interval progressively increases), so there are more P waves than QRS complexes, but the QRS complex is usually of normal shape and duration. The sinus node functions at a regular rate, so the P-P interval is regular, but the R-R interval usually shortens with each impulse. The P:QRS ratio varies, such as 3:2, 4:3, 5:4. This type of block by itself usually does not cause significant morbidity unless associated with an inferior wall myocardial infarction.

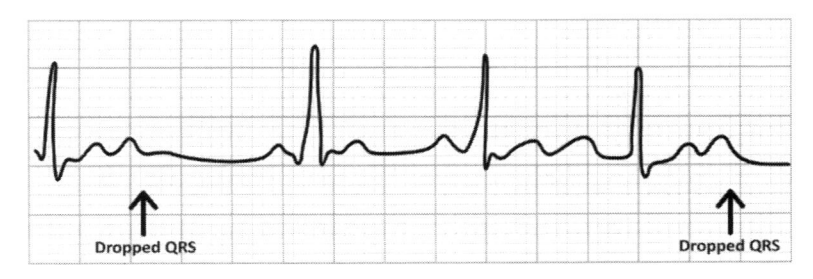

TYPE II

In Mobitz type II, only some of the atrial impulses are conducted unpredictably through the AV node to the ventricles, and the block always occurs below the AV node in the bundle of His, the bundle branches, or the Purkinje fibers. The PR intervals are the same if impulses are conducted, and the QRS complex is usually widened. The P:QRS ratio varies 2:1, 3:1, and 4:1. Type II block is more dangerous than Type I because it may progress to complete AV block and may produce Stokes-Adams syncope. Additionally, if the block is at the Purkinje fibers, there is no escape impulse. Usually, a transcutaneous cardiac pacemaker and defibrillator should be at the patient's bedside. **Symptoms** may include chest pain if the heart block is precipitated by myocarditis or myocardial ischemia.

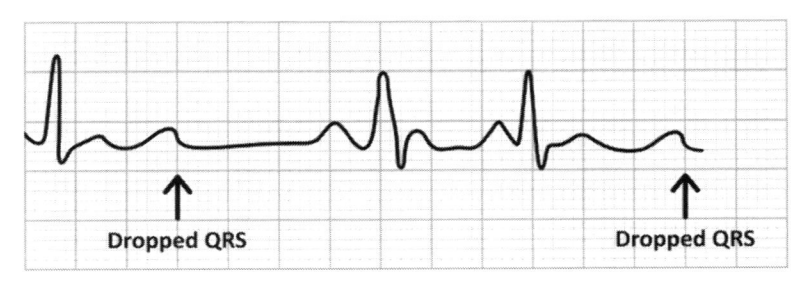

Third-Degree AV Block

With third-degree AV block, there are more P waves than QRS complexes, with no clear relationship between them. The atrial rate is 2–3 times the pulse rate, so the PR interval is irregular. If the SA node malfunctions, the AV node fires at a lower rate, and if the AV node malfunctions, the pacemaker site in the ventricles takes over at a bradycardic rate; thus, with complete AV block, the heart still contracts, but often ineffectually. With this type of block, the atrial P (sinus rhythm or atrial fibrillation) and the ventricular QRS (ventricular escape rhythm) are stimulated by different impulses, so there is AV dissociation.

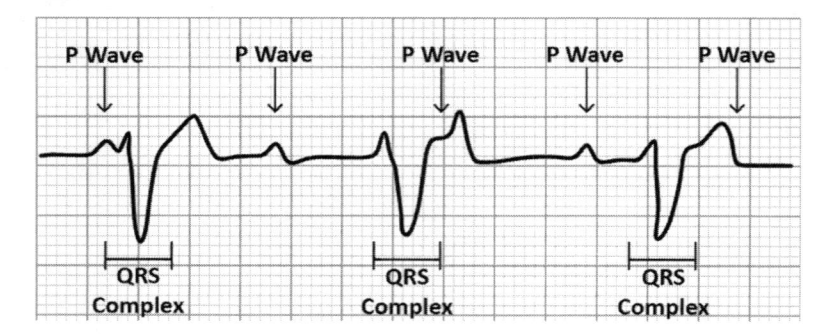

The heart may compensate at rest but can't keep pace with exertion. The resultant bradycardia may cause congestive heart failure, fainting, or even sudden death, and usually conduction abnormalities slowly worsen. **Symptoms** include dyspnea, chest pain, and hypotension, which are treated with IV atropine. Transcutaneous pacing may be needed. Complete persistent AV block normally requires implanted pacemakers, usually dual chamber.

> **Review Video: AV Heart Blocks**
> Visit mometrix.com/academy and enter code: 487004

Bundle Branch Blocks

A **right bundle branch block (RBBB)** occurs when conduction is blocked in the right bundle branch that carries impulses from the Bundle of His to the right ventricle. The impulse travels through the left ventricle instead, and then reaches the right ventricle, but this causes a slight delay in contraction of the right ventricle. A RBBB is characterized by normal P waves (as the right atrium still contracts appropriately), but the QRS complex is widened and notched (referred to as an "RSR pattern" that resembles the letter "M") in lead V1, which is a reflection of the asynchronous ventricular contraction. The PR interval is normal or prolonged, and the QRS interval is > 0.12 seconds. P:QRS ratio remains 1:1 with regular rhythms.

A **left bundle branch block (LBBB)** occurs when there is a delay in conduction between the left atrium and left ventricle. It is also characterized by normal or inverted P waves, but the QRS complex may be widened with a deep S wave and an interval of >0.12 seconds (in lead V1) that resembles a "W." The PR interval may be normal or prolonged. The P:QRS ratio is 1:1 and the rhythm is regular.

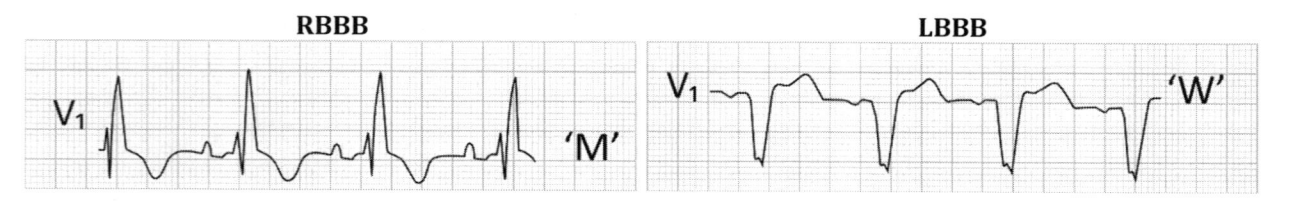

HEART FAILURE

Heart failure (formerly congestive heart failure) is a cardiac disease that includes disorders of contractions (systolic dysfunction) or filling (diastolic dysfunction) or both and may include pulmonary, peripheral, or systemic edema. The most common causes are coronary artery disease, systemic or pulmonary hypertension, cardiomyopathy, and valvular disorders. The incidence of chronic heart failure correlates with age. The 2 main types of HF are systolic and diastolic. HF is classified according to symptoms and prognosis:

- **Class I**: The patient is essentially asymptomatic during normal activities with no pulmonary congestion or peripheral hypotension. There is no restriction on activities, and prognosis is good.
- **Class II**: Symptoms appear with physical exertion but are usually absent at rest, resulting in some limitations of activities of daily living (ADLs). Slight pulmonary edema may be evident by basilar rales. Prognosis is good.
- **Class III**: Obvious limitations of ADLs and discomfort on any exertion. Prognosis is fair.
- **Class IV**: Symptoms at rest. Prognosis is poor.

Treatment may include:

- Careful monitoring of **fluid balance** and **weight** to determine changes in fluid retention
- **Low sodium diet**
- **Restriction of activity**
- **Medications** may include diuretics, vasodilators, or ACE inhibitors to decrease the heart's workload, digoxin may be given to increase contractibility
- **Anticoagulant therapy** if distended atria, enlarged ventricles, or atrial fibrillation to decrease the danger of thromboembolic

> **Review Video: Congestive Heart Failure**
> Visit mometrix.com/academy and enter code: 924118

SYSTOLIC HEART FAILURE

Systolic heart failure is the typical "left-sided" failure and reduces the amount of blood ejected from the ventricles during contraction (decreased ejection fraction). This stimulates the SNS to produce catecholamines to support the myocardium, which eventually causes down regulation, the destruction of beta and adrenergic receptor sites, and ultimately further myocardial damage. Because of reduced perfusion, the R-A-A pathway (renin, angiotensin I&II, aldosterone) is initiated by the kidneys, causing sodium and fluid retention. The end result of these processes is increased preload and afterload, thus increased workload on the ventricles. They begin to lose contractibility and blood begins to pool inside, stretching the myocardium (ventricular remodeling). The heart compensates by thickening the muscle (hypertrophy) without an adequate increase in capillary blood supply, leading to ischemia.

Symptoms: Activity intolerance, dyspnea/orthopnea (sleeping in a recliner is a classic symptom), cough (frothy sputum), edema, heart sounds S3 and S4, hepatomegaly, JVD, LOC changes, and tachycardia.

Treatment includes:

- Medication (most commonly β-blockers, diuretics, ACE inhibitors, or digoxin)
- **Surgery**: Heart transplant (if a candidate)
- **Lifestyle modification**: Low-sodium diet, supplemental oxygen, daily weights (report >3 lb/day or 5 lb/week weight gain to physician)

Diastolic Heart Failure

Diastolic heart failure may be difficult to differentiate from systolic heart failure based on clinical symptoms, which are similar. With diastolic heart failure, the myocardium is unable to sufficiently relax to facilitate filling of the ventricles. This may be the end result of systolic heart failure as myocardial hypertrophy stiffens the muscles, and the causes are similar. Diastolic heart failure is more common in females >75. Typically, intra-cardiac pressures at rest are within normal range but increase markedly on exertion. Because the relaxation of the heart is delayed, the ventricles do not expand enough for the fill-volume, and the heart cannot increase stroke volume during exercise, so symptoms (dyspnea, fatigue, pulmonary edema) are often pronounced on exertion. Ejection fractions are usually >40–50% with increase in left ventricular end-diastolic pressure (LVEDP) and decrease in left ventricular end-diastolic volume (LVEDV).

The major goal with all types of heart failure is to prevent further damage and remodeling, prevent exacerbations, and improve the patient's long-term prognosis.

Acute Heart Failure

Acute decompensated heart failure occurs when the body cannot compensate for the heart's inability to provide adequate perfusion. Cardiac output is no longer sufficient to meet the metabolic demands of the body. Acute heart failure occurs suddenly and can be precipitated by dysrhythmias, illness, noncompliance with medications, acute ischemia, fluid overload or hypertensive crisis. Acute heart failure is most commonly related to left ventricular systolic or diastolic dysfunction. It requires immediate treatment to restore adequate perfusion and is often life-threatening.

Signs/symptoms: Dyspnea, cough, edema, ascites and elevated jugular venous pressure, fatigue, cool extremities, hypotension and altered mental status

Diagnostic testing: Chest x-ray, electrocardiogram, physical exam; labs—basic metabolic panel, BUN, creatinine, and B-natriuretic peptide (BNP)

Treatment: Rapid assessment and stabilization of the patient. The physical assessment should include a thorough evaluation of the patient's respiratory status and supplemental oxygen and potentially ventilator support may be necessary. Medications: Diuretics to decrease fluid volume; vasodilators to decrease pulmonary congestion. Cardiac monitoring, urine output monitoring, sodium restriction, and venous thromboembolism prophylaxis may also be utilized.

Acute Cardiac-Related Pulmonary Edema

Acute cardiac-related pulmonary edema occurs when heart failure results in fluid overload, leading to third-spacing of fluid into the interstitial spaces of the lungs. Pulmonary edema may result from MI, chronic HF, volume overload, ischemia, or mitral stenosis.

Symptoms include severe dyspnea, cough with blood-tinged frothy sputum, wheezing/rales/crackles on auscultation, cyanosis, and diaphoresis.

Diagnosis: Auscultation, chest x-ray, and echocardiogram.

Treatment includes:

- Sitting position with 100% oxygen by mask to achieve PO_2 >60%
- Non-invasive pressure support ventilation (BiPAP) or endotracheal intubation and mechanical ventilation
- Morphine sulfate 2–8 mg (IV for severe cases), repeated every 2–4 hours as needed—decreases pre-load and anxiety
- IV diuretics (furosemide ≥40 mg or bumetanide ≥1 mg) to provide venous dilation and diuresis
- Nitrates as a bolus with an infusion—decreases pre-load
- Inhaled β-adrenergic agonists or aminophylline for bronchospasm
- Digoxin IV for tachycardia
- ACE inhibitors, nitroprusside to reduce afterload

ENDOCARDITIS

Endocarditis is an infection of the lining of the heart that covers the heart valves and contains Purkinje fibers, known as the endocardium. Risk factors include being over 60 years of age, being male, IV drug use, and dental infections. *Staphylococcal aureus* is the most common cause of infective endocarditis. Etiology includes subacute bacterial endocarditis (often related to dental procedures), prosthetic valvular endocarditis (following valve replacement), and right sided endocarditis (often related to catheter infections and IV drug use). Organisms enter the bloodstream from portals of entry (surgery, catheterization, IV drug abuse) and migrate to the heart, growing on the endothelial tissue and forming vegetations (verrucae), collagen deposits, and platelet thrombi. With endocarditis, the valves frequently become deformed, but the pathogenic agents may also invade other tissues, such as the chordae tendineae. The lesions may invade adjacent tissue and break off, becoming emboli. The mitral valve is the most common valve affected, followed by aortic, tricuspid, and the pulmonary valve being the least often affected. Positive blood cultures, widened pulse pressures, ECG, murmurs, and vegetations seen on a transesophageal echocardiogram are used to make the diagnosis. After diagnosis is made, antibiotics are used for treatment, and when unsuccessful or when heart failure is present, valve repair may be warranted. Serious complications from endocarditis include emboli, sepsis, and heart failure. Untreated endocarditis is fatal.

DIAGNOSIS AND TREATMENT

Diagnosis of endocarditis is made on the basis of clinical presentation and **diagnostic procedures** that may include:

- **Blood cultures** should be done with 3 sets for both aerobic and anaerobic bacteria. Diagnosis is definitive if 2 cultures are positive, but a negative culture does not preclude bacterial endocarditis.
- **Echocardiogram** may identify vegetation on valves or increasing heart failure
- **ECG** may demonstrate prolonged PR interval
- **Anemia** (normochromic, normocytic)
- Elevated **white blood cell count**
- Elevated **erythrocyte sedimentation rate** (ESR) and **C-reactive protein** (CRP)

Treatment includes general management of symptoms and the following:

- **Antimicrobials** specific to the pathogenic organism, usually administered IV for 4–6 weeks
- **Surgical replacement** of aortic and/or mitral valves may be necessary (in 30–40% of cases) if there is no response to treatment and/or after infection is controlled if there are severe symptoms related to valve damage

CLINICAL SYMPTOMS

Clinical symptoms of endocarditis usually relate to the response to infection, the underlying heart disease, emboli, or immunological response. Typical **symptoms** include:

- Slow onset with unexplained low-grade and often intermittent **fever**
- **Anorexia** and weight loss, difficulty feeding
- General **lassitude** and malaise
- **Splenomegaly** present in 60% of patients; **hepatomegaly** may also be present
- **Anemia** is present in almost all patients
- Sudden **aortic valve insufficiency** or mitral valve insufficiency
- **Cyanosis** with clubbing of fingers
- **Embolism** of other body organs (brain, liver, bones)
- **Congestive heart failure**
- **Dysrhythmias**
- New or change in **heart murmur**
- **Immunological responses**
- **Janeway lesions**: painless areas of hemorrhage on palms of hands and soles of feet
- **Splinter hemorrhages**: thin, brown-black lines on nails of fingers and toes
- **Petechiae**: pinpoint-sized hemorrhages on oral mucous membranes, as well as hands and trunk
- **Roth spots**: retinal hemorrhagic lesions caused by emboli on nerve fibers
- **Glomerulonephritis**: microscopic hematuria

MYOCARDITIS

Myocarditis is inflammation of the cardiac myocardium (muscle tissue), usually triggered by a viral infection, such as the influenza virus, Coxsackie virus, and HIV. Myocarditis can also be caused by bacteria, fungi, or parasites, or an allergic response to medications. In some cases, it is also a complication of endocarditis. It may also be triggered by chemotherapy drugs and some antibiotics. Myocarditis can result in dilation of the heart, development of thrombi on the heart walls (known as mural thrombi), and infiltration of blood cells around the coronary vessels and between muscle fibers, causing further degeneration of the muscle tissue. The heart may become enlarged and weak, as the ability to pump blood is impaired, leading to congestive heart failure. Symptoms depend upon the extent of damage but may include fatigue, dyspnea, pressure and discomfort in chest or epigastric area, and palpitations.

DIAGNOSIS AND TREATMENT

Diagnosis of myocarditis depends upon the clinical picture, as there is no test specific for myocarditis, although a number of tests may be done to verify the **clinical diagnosis**:

- **Chest radiograph** may indicate cardiomegaly or pulmonary edema.
- **ECG** may show nonspecific changes.
- **Echocardiogram** may indicate cardiomegaly and demonstrate defects in functioning.
- **Cardiac catheterization** and **cardiac biopsy** will yield confirmation in 65% of cases, but not all of the heart muscle may be affected, so a negative finding does not rule out myocarditis.
- **Viral cultures** of nasopharynx and rectal may help to identify organism.
- **Viral titers** may increase as disease progresses.
- **Polymerase chain reaction** (PCR) of biopsy specimen may be most effective for diagnosis.

Treatment:

- As indicated for underlying cause (such as antibiotics)
- Restriction of activities
- Careful **monitoring** for heart failure and medical treatment as indicated (e.g., diuretics, digoxin)
- **Oxygen** as needed to maintain normal oxygen saturation
- **IV gamma globulin** for acute stage

ACUTE PERICARDITIS

Pericarditis is inflammation of the pericardial sac with or without increased pericardial fluid. It may be an isolated process or the effect of an underlying disease. If the underlying cause is autoimmune or related to malignancy of some sort, the patient usually presents with symptoms that relate to that disorder. However, most cases are related to a viral etiology, and therefore usually present with flu-like symptoms. Patients that have idiopathic pericarditis or viral pericarditis have a good prognosis with medication alone.

Signs/symptoms: Sharp chest pain, worsened with inspiration and relieved by leaning forward or sitting up (most common symptom; "Mohammad's Sign"), pericardial effusion, respiratory distress, auscultated friction rub, ST elevation/PR depression (progresses to flattened T, inverted T, then return to normal); risk of pericardial effusion.

Diagnosis: Echocardiogram, ECG, pericardiocentesis or pericardial biopsy, cardiac enzymes (may be mildly elevated), WBC/ESR/CRP all elevated.

Treatment includes:

- **Medications**: NSAIDs for pain/inflammation, Colchicine 0.5 mg twice a day for six months is often prescribed in adjunct to NSAID therapy, as it decreases the incidence of recurrence
- **Surgery**: Pericardiectomy only in extreme cases

MITRAL STENOSIS

Mitral stenosis is a narrowing of the mitral valve that allows blood to flow from the left atrium to the left ventricle. Pressure in the left atrium increases to overcome resistance, resulting in enlargement of the left atrium and increased pressure in the pulmonary veins and capillaries of the lung (pulmonary hypertension). Mitral stenosis can be caused by infective endocarditis, calcifications, or tumors in the left atrium.

Signs/symptoms: Exertional dyspnea, orthopnea/nocturnal dyspnea, right-sided heart failure, loud S_1 and S_2, and mid-diastolic murmur.

Diagnosis: Cardiac catheterization, chest x-ray, echocardiogram, ECG.

Treatment includes:

- **Medications**: Antiarrhythmic, anticoagulant, and antihypertensive medications
- **Surgical**: Open/closed commissurotomy, balloon valvuloplasty, and mitral valve replacement

Mitral Valve Insufficiency

Mitral valve insufficiency occurs when the mitral valve fails to close completely so that there is backflow into the left atrium from the left ventricle during systole, decreasing cardiac output. It may occur with mitral stenosis or independently. Mitral valve insufficiency can result from damage caused by rheumatic fever, myxomatous degeneration, infective endocarditis, collagen vascular disease (Marfan's syndrome), or cardiomyopathy/left heart failure. There are **three phases** of the disease:

- **Acute**: May occur with rupture of a chordae tendineae or papillary muscle causing sudden left ventricular flooding and overload.
- **Chronic compensated**: Enlargement of the left atrium to decrease filling pressure, and hypertrophy of the left ventricle.
- **Chronic decompensated**: Left ventricle fails to compensate for the volume overload; decreased stroke volume and increased cardiac output.

Symptoms: Orthopnea/dyspnea, split S_2/S_3/S_4 heart sounds, systolic murmur, palpitations, right-sided heart failure, fatigue, angina (rare).

Diagnosis: Cardiac catheterization, chest x-ray, echocardiogram, ECG.

Treatment includes:

- **Medications**: Antiarrhythmic, anticoagulant, and antihypertensive medications.
- **Surgical**: Annuloplasty or valvuloplasty, and mitral valve replacement.

Aortic Stenosis

Aortic stenosis is a stricture (narrowing) of the aortic valve that controls the flow of blood from the left ventricle. This causes the left ventricular wall to thicken as it increases pressure to overcome the valvular resistance, increasing afterload and increasing the need for blood supply from the coronary arteries. This condition may result from a birth defect or childhood rheumatic fever, and tends to worsen over the years as the heart grows.

Symptoms: Angina, exercise intolerance, dyspnea, split S_1 and S_2, systolic murmur at base of carotids, hypotension on exertion, syncope, left-sided heart failure; sudden death can occur.

Diagnosis: Cardiac catheterization, chest x-ray, echocardiogram, ECG.

Treatment includes:

- **Medications**: Antiarrhythmic, anticoagulant, and antihypertensive medications
- **Surgical**: Balloon valvuloplasty, and aortic valve replacement

Pulmonic Stenosis

Pulmonic stenosis is a stricture of the pulmonary blood that controls the flow of blood from the right ventricle to the lungs, resulting in right ventricular hypertrophy as the pressure increases in the right ventricle and decreased pulmonary blood flow. The condition may be asymptomatic or symptoms may not be evident until adulthood, depending upon the severity of the defect. Pulmonic stenosis may be associated with a number of other heart defects.

Symptoms: May be asymptomatic; dyspnea on exertion, systolic heart murmur, right-sided heart failure.

Diagnosis: Cardiac catheterization, chest x-ray, echocardiogram, ECG.

Treatment includes:

- **Medications**: Antiarrhythmic, anticoagulant, and antihypertensive medications
- **Surgical**: Balloon valvuloplasty, valvotomy, valvectomy with or without transannular patch, and pulmonary valve replacement

HYPERTENSIVE CRISES

Hypertensive crises are marked elevations in blood pressure that can cause severe organ damage if left untreated. Hypertensive crises may be caused by endocrine/renal disorders (pheochromocytoma), dissection of an aortic aneurysm, pulmonary edema, subarachnoid hemorrhage, stroke, eclampsia, and medication noncompliance. There are two **classifications**:

- **Hypertensive emergency** occurs when acute hypertension, usually >220 systolic and 120 mmHg diastolic, must be treated immediately to lower blood pressure in order to prevent damage to vital organs.
- **Hypertensive urgency** occurs when acute hypertension must be treated within a few hours but the vital organs are not in immediate danger. Blood pressure is lowered more slowly to avoid hypotension, ischemia of vital organs, or failure of autoregulation.
    - 1/3 reduction in 6 hours
    - 1/3 reduction in next 24 hours
    - 1/3 reduction over days 2–4

Symptoms: Basilar HA, blurred vision, chest pain, N/V, SOB, seizures, ruddy pallor, and anxiety

Diagnostics: ECG, Chest x-ray, CBC, BMP, Urinalysis (+ blood and casts)

Treatment includes:

- Medications: Vasodilators (Cardene, Nitro, etc.) and diuretics
- Nursing Interventions: Raise HOB to 90°, supplemental O_2, frequent neuro checks, teach concerning medication compliance

CONGENITAL HEART DEFECTS SEEN IN ADULTHOOD

Congenital heart defects are often identified in infancy or early childhood; however, diagnosis may be delayed until adulthood due to the lack of signs and symptoms. Atrial septal and ventricular septal defects are common congenital anomalies that can present at any age. An atrial septal defect occurs when part of the atrial septum does not form properly, leaving a hole in the septum. A ventricular septal defect results from a hole in the septum separating the ventricles. Patent ductus arteriosus, coarctation of the aorta and Ebstein's anomaly are other types of congenital defects that are less commonly diagnosed in adulthood.

Signs/symptoms: Murmurs, cyanosis, clubbing of the fingernails, shortness of breath, fatigue, syncope, palpitations, and edema. Heart failure and endocarditis may also occur.

Diagnosis: Physical assessment, EKG, Chest x-ray, transesophageal echocardiogram, CT, and MRI.

Treatment: Treatment options depend on the size and location of the defect. Most commonly the anomaly will be corrected by open surgical repair; however percutaneous intervention may be an option in some patients.

Peripheral Arterial and Venous Insufficiency

Characteristics of peripheral arterial and venous insufficiency are listed below:

- **Arterial insufficiency**
    - **Pain**: Ranging from intermittent claudication to severe and constant shooting pain
    - **Pulses**: Weak or absent
    - **Skin**: Rubor on dependency, but pallor of foot on elevation; pale, shiny, and cool skin with loss of hair on toes and foot; nails thick and ridged
    - **Ulcers**: Painful, deep, circular, often necrotic ulcers on toe tips, toe webs, heels, or other pressure areas
    - **Edema**: Minimal
- **Venous insufficiency**
    - **Pain**: Aching/cramping
    - **Pulses**: Strong/present
    - **Skin**: Brownish discoloration around ankles and anterior tibial area
    - **Ulcers**: Varying degrees of pain in superficial, irregular ulcers on medial or lateral malleolus and sometimes the anterior tibial area
    - **Edema**: Moderate to severe

Acute Peripheral Vascular Insufficiency

Acute peripheral arterial insufficiency can occur when sudden occlusion of a blood vessel causes tissue ischemia, ultimately leading to cellular death and necrosis. This can occur as a result of traumatic injury or non-traumatic events such as arterial thrombus or embolism, vasospasm, or severe swelling (compartment syndrome). Risk factors for acute peripheral arterial insufficiency include age, tobacco use, diabetes mellitus, hyperlipidemia, and hypertension.

- **Signs/symptoms**: Classic 6 P's: Pain (extreme, unrelieved by narcotics), pallor, pulselessness, poikilothermia (the inability to regulate body temperature; extremity is room temperature), paresthesias, and paralysis (late).
- **Diagnosis**: Ultrasound, angiography, and physical exam; labs—coagulation studies, CBC, BMP, creatinine phosphokinase
- **Treatment**: Re-establishment of blood flow to the affected area
- **Arterial thrombus or embolism**: Mechanical thrombolysis may be performed to remove the clot occluding the vessel.
    - **Trauma**: Surgical repair of the severed/injured vessels. Fasciotomy may be performed in the event of compartment syndrome to relieve pressure.
    - **Other treatment options**: Hyperbaric oxygen therapy, anti-platelet therapy for the prevention of arterial thrombosis and anti-coagulant therapy for the prevention of venous thrombosis

Acute Venous Thromboembolism

Acute venous thromboembolism (VTE) is a condition that includes both deep vein thrombosis (DVT) and pulmonary emboli (PE). VTE may be precipitated by invasive procedures, lack of mobility, and inflammation, so it is a common complication in critical care units. **Virchow's triad** comprises common risk factors: blood stasis, injury to endothelium, and hypercoagulability. Some patients may be initially asymptomatic, but **symptoms** may include:

- Aching or throbbing pain
- Positive Homan's sign (pain in calf when foot is dorsiflexed)
- Unilateral erythema and edema
- Dilation of vessels
- Cyanosis

Diagnosis: ultrasound and/or D-dimer test, which tests the serum for cross-linked fibrin derivatives. A CT scan, pulmonary angiogram, and ventilation-perfusion lung scan may be used to diagnose pulmonary emboli.

Treatment includes:

- Medications: IV heparin, tPA, or other anticoagulation; analgesia for pain
- Surgical: May have to surgically remove clot if large
- Bed rest, elevation of affected limb; stockings on ambulation

Prevention: Use of sequential compression devices (SCDs) or foot pumps, routine anticoagulant use for those at highest risk (Heparin SQ), early and frequent ambulation

> **Review Video: DVT Prevention and Treatment**
> Visit mometrix.com/academy and enter code: 234086

CONGENITAL HEART DEFECTS IN CHILDREN

Congenital heart defects occur when the heart or great vessels develop with deformities in utero. Most cases have an unknown cause, but the following may contribute to the development of CHD: maternal infection during the first trimester, maternal alcohol or drug use during pregnancy, a mom who is over 40 years of age or who has insulin dependent diabetes, poor diet in pregnancy, an immediate family member has CHD, or the baby has a chromosomal disorder. CHD can include defects which lead to increased pulmonary blood flow (patent ductus arteriosus, atrial or ventricular septal defect, atrioventricular canal defect), defects which are obstructive (coarctation of aorta, aortic stenosis, pulmonic stenosis), defects that decrease pulmonary blood flow (tricuspid atresia, tetralogy of Fallot), and mixed defects (transposition of the great vessels, hypoplastic left heart syndrome, truncus arteriosus).

ACYANOTIC AND CYANOTIC CONGENITAL HEART DISEASE

Congenital heart disease is one of the leading causes of death in children within the first year of life. There are two main types of congenital heart disease: Acyanotic and cyanotic. They may also be classified according to hemodynamics related to the blood flow pattern.

ACYANOTIC

Increased pulmonary blood flow	Atrial septal defect
	Atrioventricular canal defect
	Patent ductus arteriosus
	Ventricular septal defect
Obstructed ventricular blood flow	Aortic stenosis
	Coarctation of aorta
	Pulmonic stenosis

CYANOTIC

Decreased pulmonary blood flow	Tetralogy of Fallot
	Tricuspid atresia
Mixed blood flow	Hypoplastic left heart syndrome
	Total anomalous pulmonary venous return
	Transposition of great arteries
	Truncus arteriosus.
	Ebstein's anomaly

ACYANOTIC CONGENITAL DEFECTS
ATRIAL SEPTAL DEFECT

An atrial septal defect (ASD) is an abnormal opening in the septum between the right and left atria. Because the left atrium has higher pressure than the right atrium, some of the oxygenated blood returning from the lungs to the left atrium is shunted back to the right atrium where it is again returned to the lungs, displacing deoxygenated blood.

Symptoms	Treatment
<ul><li>Asymptomatic (some infants)</li><li>Congestive heart failure</li><li>Heart murmur</li><li>Increased risk for dysrhythmias and pulmonary vascular obstructive disease over time</li></ul>	Treatment may not be necessary for small defects, but larger defects require closure:<ul><li>Open-heart surgical closure may be done.</li><li>Heart catheterization and placing of closure device across the atrial septal defect.</li></ul>

VENTRICULAR SEPTAL DEFECT

Ventricular septal defect is an abnormal opening in the septum between the right and left ventricles. If the opening is small, the child may be asymptomatic, but larger openings can result in a left to right shunt because of higher pressure in the left ventricle. This shunting increases over 6 weeks after birth with symptoms becoming more evident, but the defect may close within a few years.

Symptoms	Treatment
<ul><li>Congestive heart failure with peripheral edema</li><li>Tachycardia</li><li>Dyspnea</li><li>Difficulty feeding</li><li>Heart murmur</li><li>Recurrent pulmonary infections</li><li>Increased risk for bacterial endocarditis and pulmonary vascular obstructive disease</li></ul>	<ul><li>Diuretics, such as furosemide (Lasix) may be used for heart failure</li><li>Management of pulmonary hypertension</li><li>Surgical repair includes pulmonary banding or cardiopulmonary bypass repair of the opening with suturing or a patch, depending upon the size.</li></ul>

Atrioventricular Canal Defect

Atrioventricular canal defect is often associated with Down syndrome and involves a number of different defects, including openings between the atria and ventricles as well as abnormalities of the valves. In partial defects, there is an opening between the atria and mitral valve regurgitation. In complete defects, there is a large central hole in the heart and only one common valve between the atria and ventricles. The blood may flow freely about the heart, usually from left to right. Extra blood flow to the lungs causes enlargement of the heart. Partial defects may go undiagnosed for 20 years.

Symptoms	Treatment
Typical congestive heart failure signs: • Weakness and fatigue • Cough and/or wheezing with production of white or bloody sputum • Peripheral edema and ascites • Dysrhythmia and tachycardia • Dyspnea • Poor appetite • Failure to thrive, low weight • Cyanosis of skin and lips	• Symptom management as indicated. • Open-heart surgery to patch holes in the septum and valve repair or replacement.

PDA

Patent ductus arteriosus (PDA) is failure of the ductus arteriosus that connects the pulmonary artery and aorta to close after birth, resulting in left to right shunting of blood from the aorta back to the pulmonary artery. This increases the blood flow to the lung and causes an increase in pulmonary hypertension that can result in damage to the lung tissue.

Symptoms	Treatment
• Essentially asymptomatic (some infants) • Cyanosis • Congestive heart failure • Machinery-like murmur • Frequent respiratory infections and dyspnea, especially on exertion	• Indomethacin or ibuprofen given within 10 days of birth is successful in closing about 80% of defects • Surgical repair with ligation of the patent vessel

Coarctation of the Aorta

Coarctation of the aorta is a stricture of the aorta, proximal to the ductus arteriosus intersection. The increased blood pressure caused by the heart attempting to pump the blood past the stricture causes the heart to enlarge. Blood pressure to the head and upper extremities also increases, while blood pressure decreases to the lower body and extremities. With severe stricture, symptoms may not occur until the ductus arteriosus closes, causing sudden loss of blood supply to the lower body.

Symptoms	Treatment
• Difference in blood pressure between upper and lower extremities • Congestive heart failure symptoms in infants • Headaches, dizziness, and nosebleeds in older children • Increased risk of hypertension, ruptured aorta, aortic aneurysm, bacterial endocarditis, and brain attack	• Prostaglandin E1 (alprostadil) to reopen the ductus arteriosus for infants • Balloon angioplasty (sometimes followed by stent placement) • Surgical resection and anastomosis or graft replacement (usually at 3–5 years of age unless condition is severe). Infants who have surgery may need later repair.

Pulmonic Stenosis

Pulmonic stenosis is a stricture of the pulmonic valve that controls the flow of blood from the right ventricle to the lungs, resulting in right ventricular hypertrophy as the pressure increases in the right ventricle and resulting in decreased pulmonary blood flow. The condition may be asymptomatic, or symptoms may not be evident until the child enters adulthood, depending upon the severity of the defect. Pulmonic stenosis may be associated with a number of other heart defects.

Symptoms	Treatment
<ul><li>Loud heart murmur</li><li>Congestive heart murmur</li><li>Mild cyanosis</li><li>Cardiomegaly</li><li>Angina</li><li>Dyspnea</li><li>Fainting</li><li>Increased risk of bacterial endocarditis</li></ul>	<ul><li>Balloon valvuloplasty is used to separate the cusps of the valve for children.</li><li>Surgical repair includes the (closed) transventricular valvotomy (Brock) procedure for infants and the cardiopulmonary bypass pulmonary valvotomy for older children.</li></ul>

Aortic Stenosis

Aortic stenosis is a stricture (narrowing) of the aortic valve that controls the flow of blood from the left ventricle, causing the left ventricular wall to thicken as it increases pressure to overcome the valvular resistance, increasing afterload, and increasing the need for blood supply from the coronary arteries. This condition may result from a birth defect or childhood rheumatic fever and tends to worsen over the years as the heart grows. Treatment in children may be done before symptoms develop because of the danger of sudden death.

Symptoms	Treatment
<ul><li>Chest pain on exertion and intolerance of exercise.</li><li>Heart murmur</li><li>Hypotension on exertion may be associated with sudden fainting</li><li>Sudden death can occur</li><li>Tachycardia with faint pulse</li><li>Poor feeding</li><li>Increased risk for bacterial endocarditis and coronary insufficiency</li><li>Increases mitral regurgitation and secondary pulmonary hypertension</li></ul>	<ul><li>Balloon valvuloplasty is used to dilate the valve non-surgically</li><li>Surgical repair of the valve or replacement of the valve, depending upon the extent of stricture</li></ul>

Cyanotic Congenital Defects

Tricuspid Atresia

Tricuspid atresia is lack of tricuspid valve between the right atrium and right ventricle. This causes blood to flow through the foramen ovale or an atrial defect to the left atrium and then through a ventricular wall defect from the left ventricle to the right ventricle and out to the lungs, causing oxygenated and deoxygenated blood to mix. Pulmonic obstruction is common.

Symptoms	Treatment
- Postnatal cyanosis obvious - Tachycardia and dyspnea - Increasing hypoxemia and clubbing in older children - Increased risk for bacterial endocarditis, brain abscess, and stroke	- Prostaglandin (alprostadil) to keep the ductus arteriosus and foramen ovale open if there are no septal defects - Numerous surgical procedures may be required, including pulmonary artery banding, shunting from the aorta to the pulmonary arteries, Glenn procedure (connecting superior vena cava to pulmonary artery to allow deoxygenated blood to flow to the lungs), atrial septostomy to enlarge the opening between the atria, and the Fontan corrective procedure (usually done at 2–4 years after previous stabilizing procedures).

Transposition of the Great Vessels

Transposition of great arteries occurs when the aorta and pulmonary artery arise from the wrong ventricle (aorta from the right ventricle and pulmonary artery from the left). This means there is no connection between pulmonary and systemic circulation, with deoxygenated blood being pumped back to the body, and the oxygenated blood from the lungs is pumped back to the lungs. Septal defects may also occur, allowing some mixing of blood, and the ductus arteriosus allows mixing until it closes. Symptoms vary depending upon whether mixing of blood occurs.

Symptoms	Treatment
- Mild to severe cyanosis - Symptoms of congestive heart failure - Cardiomegaly develops in the weeks after birth - Heart sounds vary depending upon the severity of the defects	- Prostaglandin to keep the ductus arteriosus and foramen ovale open - Balloon atrial septostomy to increase size of foramen ovale - Surgical repair with cardiopulmonary bypass and aortic cross-clamping to transpose arteries to the normal position ("arterial switch") as well as repair septal defects and other abnormalities

Tetralogy of Fallot (TOF)

Tetralogy of Fallot (TOF) is a combination of four different defects:

- Ventricular septal defect (usually with a large opening)
- Pulmonic stenosis with decreased blood flow to lungs
- Overriding aorta (displacement to the right so that it appears to come from both ventricles, usually overriding the ventricular septal defect), resulting in mixing of oxygenated and deoxygenated blood
- Right ventricular hypertrophy

Infants are often acutely cyanotic immediately after birth while others with less severe defects may have increasing cyanosis over the first year.

Symptoms	Treatment
<ul><li>Intolerance to feeding or crying, resulting in increased cyanotic "blue spells" or "tet spells"</li><li>Failure to thrive with poor growth</li><li>Clubbing of fingers may occur over time</li><li>Intolerance to activity as child grows</li><li>Increased risk for emboli, brain attacks, brain abscess, seizures, fainting or sudden death</li></ul>	Total surgical repair at the age of one year or younger is now the preferred treatment rather than palliative procedures formerly used.

HYPOPLASTIC LEFT HEART SYNDROME

Hypoplastic left heart syndrome (HLHS) is underdevelopment of the left ventricle and ascending aortic atresia, causing inability of the heart to pump blood. Because of this, most blood flows from the left atrium through the foramen ovale to the right atrium and to the lungs, with the descending aorta receiving blood through the ductus arteriosus. There may be valvular abnormalities as well. Mortality rates are 100% without surgical correction and 25% with correction.

Symptoms may be mild until the ductus arteriosus closes at about 2 weeks, causing a marked increase in cyanosis and decreased cardiac output leading to cardiovascular collapse.

Treatment is through surgical procedures. These include a series of three staged operations:

1. The **Norwood procedure** connects the main pulmonary artery to the aorta, a shunt for pulmonary blood flow, and creates a large atrial septal defect.
2. The **Glenn procedure** then detaches the superior vena cava from the heart and to the pulmonary artery.
3. Finally, the **Fontan repair procedure** is used to detach the inferior vena cava from the heart and to the pulmonary artery.

Heart transplantation in infancy is preferred in many cases, but the shortage of hearts limits this option.

TRUNCUS ARTERIOSUS

Truncus arteriosus is the blood from both ventricles flowing into one large artery with one valve, with more blood flowing to the lower pressure pulmonary arteries than to the body, resulting in low oxygen saturation and hypoxemia. Usually, there is a ventricular septal defect so the blood in the ventricles mixes.

Symptoms	Treatment
<ul><li>Congestive heart failure with pulmonary edema because of increased blood flow to lungs</li><li>Typical symptoms of congestive heart failure</li><li>Cyanosis, especially about the face (mouth and nose)</li><li>Dyspnea, increasing on feeding or exertion</li><li>Poor feeding and failure to thrive</li><li>Heart murmur</li><li>Increased risk for brain abscess and bacterial endocarditis</li></ul>	<ul><li>Palliative banding of the pulmonary arteries to decrease the flow of blood to the lungs</li><li>Surgical repair with cardiopulmonary bypass includes closing the ventricular defect, utilizing the existing single artery as the aorta by separating the pulmonary arteries from it and creating a conduit between the pulmonary arteries and the right ventricle.</li></ul>

Ebstein Anomaly

Ebstein anomaly is an abnormality of the tricuspid valve separating the right atrium from the right ventricle with some valve leaflets displaced downward and one adhering to the wall so that there is backflow into the atrium when the ventricle contracts. This usually results in enlargement of the right atrium and congestive heart failure. As pressure increases in the right atrium, it usually forces the foramen ovale to stay open so that the blood is shunted to the left atrium, mixing the deoxygenated blood with oxygenated blood that then leaves through the aorta. Symptoms vary widely depending upon the degree of defect and range from asymptomatic to life threatening. Ebstein anomaly may occur with other cardiac defects. Many children are not diagnosed until their teens.

Symptoms	Treatment
<ul><li>Cyanosis with low oxygen saturation</li><li>Congestive heart failure</li><li>Palpitations, arrhythmias</li><li>Dyspnea on exertion</li><li>Increased risk for bacterial endocarditis</li></ul>	<ul><li>Milrinone, diuretics, and digoxin</li><li>Surgical repair of abnormalities with valve repair or replacement</li></ul>

Total Anomalous Pulmonary Venous Return

Total anomalous pulmonary venous return is a defect in which the four pulmonary veins connect to the right atrium by an anomalous connection rather than the left atrium, so there is no direct blood flow to the left side of the heart. This condition commonly occurs with an atrial septal defect, which allows for the mixed oxygenated and deoxygenated blood to shunt to the left and enter the aorta. There are four different types of anomalies, and in some cases pulmonary vein obstruction. If the pulmonary veins are not obstructed, children may be asymptomatic initially.

Symptoms	Treatment
<ul><li>Heart murmur</li><li>Severe post-natal cyanosis or mild cyanosis</li><li>Dyspnea with grunting and sternal retraction or dyspnea on exertion</li><li>Low oxygen saturation (in the 80s if there is no pulmonary obstruction)</li><li>Cardiomegaly (right-sided hypertrophy)</li></ul>	Surgical repair to attach the pulmonary veins to the left atrium and correct any other defects may be done immediately after birth or delayed for 1–2 months.

Congestive Heart Failure in Children

Congestive heart failure is a symptom rather than a disease. It results from the inability of the heart to adequately pump the blood that is needed for the body. In children (primarily infants) it most often occurs secondary to cardiac abnormalities with resultant increased blood volume and blood pressure:

- **Right-sided failure** occurs if the right ventricle cannot effectively contract to pump blood into the pulmonary artery, causing pressure to build in the right atrium and the venous circulation. This venous hypertension can result in peripheral edema or ascites and hepatosplenomegaly.
- **Left-sided failure** occurs if the left ventricle cannot effectively pump blood into the aorta and systemic circulation, increasing pressure in the left atrium and the pulmonary veins, with resultant pulmonary edema and increased pulmonary pressure.

Children often have some combination of both right and left-sided failure, depending on their cardiac defect.

Symptoms in Infants and Children

Congestive heart failure symptoms vary widely depending upon the type and degree, the primary cause, and the child's age. Because of increased pressure in the lungs after birth, symptoms may be delayed in infants for the first week or two:

- **Infants** with left failure typically suffer respiratory distress with tachypnea, grunting respirations, sternal retraction, and rales, but the most common symptom is failure to thrive and difficulty eating, often leaving the child exhausted and sweaty. Those with right-sided failure may have more generalized edema of lower extremities, distended abdomen from ascites, hepatomegaly, and jugular venous distension. Tachycardia and low cardiac output occur with both types of heart failure, resulting in sweating, pallor, and hypotension.
- **Older children** typically suffer from inability to tolerate activity or exercise, becoming short of breath on exertion. Appetite is often poor with weight loss.
- In **adolescents**, CHF may be caused by the use of illicit drugs if there is no structural or acquired heart disease.

Management in Infants and Children

Management of congestive heart failure (CHF) in infants and children can be difficult. It is extremely important to establish the etiology and to treat the underlying cause. For infants with structural cardiac abnormalities, surgical repair may be needed to resolve the CHF. There are some medical treatments that can relieve symptoms:

- **Diuretics**, such as furosemide (Lasix), metolazone, or hydrochlorothiazide, can reduce pulmonary and peripheral edema.
- **Antihypertensives**, such as ACE inhibitors or beta-blockers, can decrease heart workload.
- **Cardiac glycosides**, such as digoxin, may relieve symptoms if above medicines are not successful.
- **High caloric feedings**, either by bottle or nasogastric feeding, provide sufficient nutrients.
- **Oxygen** may be useful for some children with weak hearts.
- **Restriction of activities** reduces stress on the heart.
- **Dopamine or dobutamine** may be given to increase the contractibility of the heart.

Cardiac Hypertrophy

Cardiac hypertrophy occurs when the heart responds to stresses, such as an increase in blood pressure or structural abnormality that interferes with normal functioning, by adapting its size and shape according to the increased effort required to function. As the heart adapts, the heart muscle enlarges, but this change is not the result of proliferation of cells but an increase in the size of existing myocytes (muscles cells). Thus, the cells are not dividing and providing more cells but simply getting bigger, and sometimes crowding out and killing other cells, further increasing the stress on the heart and again causing the cells to enlarge in a cycle that progressively weakens the musculature or the heart. Recent studies show 12% of children with HIV demonstrate cardiac hypertrophy, and 55% of children with renal transplants showed left ventricular hypertrophy, suggesting that many of these children are at risk for congestive heart failure. Treating the cause of hypertrophy does not always reduce the hypertrophic changes.

Ear, Nose, and Throat Pathophysiology

PERITONSILLAR ABSCESS

Peritonsillar abscess (PTA), which usually derives from tonsillitis, progresses from cellulitis to abscess between the palatine tonsil and capsule. It is often polymicrobial. It usually occurs bilaterally between the ages of 20 and 30. Complications include obstruction of airway, rupture with aspiration of purulent material, septicemia, endocarditis, and epiglottitis. The infection is often polymicrobial. Symptoms include fever, pain, hoarseness, muffling of voice, dysphagia, tonsillar edema, erythema, exudate, and edema of palate with displacement of uvula.

Diagnosis:

- Aspiration of purulent material (usually diagnostic)
- CT with contrast, ultrasound
- On exam: Displacement of the uvula, with enlarged tonsils

Treatments include:

- Needle aspirations (often multiple) with needle penetrating 1 cm or less to avoid carotid artery
- Abscess incision and drainage if aspiration not successful
- IV volume replacement
- **Antibiotics**: IV ampicillin-sulbactam or clindamycin until culture results come back and in areas with high rates of CA-MRSA vancomycin may be added. Once the patient shows signs of clinical improvement, they may switch to oral antibiotics (needing 14 days total).

DENTAL AVULSIONS

Dental avulsions are the complete displacement of a tooth from its socket. The tooth may be reimplanted if done within one to two hours after displacement, although only permanent teeth are reimplanted, not primary.

Procedure:

1. Tooth can be **transported** from accident site to the emergency department in Hank solution, saline, or milk.
2. **Cleanse** tooth with sterile NS or Hank solution, handling only the crown and avoiding any disruption of fibers.
3. If tooth has been dry for 20-60 minutes, **soak** tooth in Hank solution for 30 minutes before reimplantation.
4. If tooth has been dry for more than 60 minutes, **soak** tooth in citric acid for 5 minutes, stannous fluoride 2% for 5 minutes, and doxycycline solution for 5 minutes prior to reimplantation.
5. Remove **clot** in socket and gently irrigate with NS.
6. Place tooth into **socket** firmly, cover with gauze, and have patient bite firmly on gauze until splinting can be applied.
7. Apply **splinting material and mold packing** over implanted tooth and 2 adjacent teeth on both sides (encompasses 5 teeth).

DENTAL FRACTURES

Dental fractures, most commonly of the maxillary teeth, may occur in association with other oral injuries and may be overlooked unless a careful dental examination is carried out. Fractures are classified according to severity of fracture with treatment to prevent further damage and necrosis.

- **Ellis I**: Chipping of enamel
  - Smoothen rough edges

- **Ellis II**: Fracture of enamel and dentin with pain on pressure and air sensitivity
    - Protect dentin with glass ionomer dental cement and refer to dentist within 24 hours
- **Ellis III**: Fracture of enamel, dentin, and pulp with pain on movement; air and temperature sensitivity; blood may be evident
    - Protect dentin with ionomer dental cement or calcium hydroxide base and refer to dentist for prompt treatment
    - Administer oral analgesics
- **Alveolar/root fracture:** Loose tooth and malocclusion, sensitivity to percussion
    - Prompt referral to dentist for splinting and/or root canal

> **Review Video: Anatomical and Clinical Parts of Teeth**
> Visit mometrix.com/academy and enter code: 683627

RECURRENT EPISTAXIS

Recurrent epistaxis is common in young children (2 to 10 years), especially boys, and is often related to nose picking, dry climate, or central heating in the winter. Incidence also increases between 50 and 80 years of age, and may be caused by NSAIDs and anticoagulants. Kiesselbach plexus in the anterior nares has plentiful vessels and bleeds easily. Bleeding in the posterior nares is more dangerous and can result in considerable blood loss. Bleeding from the anterior nares is usually confined to one nostril, but from the posterior nares, blood may flow through both nostrils or backward into the throat and the person may be observed swallowing. People abusing cocaine may suffer nosebleeds because of damage to the mucosa. Hematocrit and hemoglobin should be done to determine if blood loss is significant. Bleeding should stop within 20 minutes. Treatment:

- Upright position, leaning forward so blood does not flow down throat.
- Applying pressure below the nares or by pinching the nostrils firmly for 10 minutes.
- Severe bleeding: packing and/or topical vasoconstrictors.
- Humidifiers may decrease irritation.

BELL'S PALSY

Bell's palsy is caused by inflammation of cranial nerve VII, usually from a herpes simplex I or II infection, and generally affects only one side of the paired nerves. Onset is generally sudden, and symptoms peak by 48 hours with a wide range of presentation. **Symptoms** usually subside within two to six months but may persist one year:

- Mild weakness on one side of face to complete paralysis with distortion of features
- Drooping of eyelid and mouth
- Tearing in affected eye
- Taste impairment

Diagnosis includes:

- Neurological, eye, parotid gland, and ear exam to rule out other cranial nerve involvement or conditions.

Treatment includes:

- Artificial tears during daytime with lubricating ophthalmic ointment and patch at night to protect eye
- Prednisone 60 mg daily for 5 days with tapering over 5 days.
- For severe cases use prednisone AND valacyclovir 1000 mg 3 times daily for 7 days, with acyclovir as an alternative.

TEMPORAL ARTERITIS

Temporal arteritis (TA), also called giant cell arteritis, is inflammation of the blood vessels of the head, especially the temporal artery, and the thoracic aorta and branches. TA is commonly associated with polymyalgia rheumatica (30% or less of patients) but can occur with other systemic disorders such as lupus erythematous, Sjögren syndrome, and rheumatoid arthritis. TA is a progressive disorder that can result in blindness and is most common in those older than 50. **Symptoms** include:

- New onset of headaches
- Vision fluctuations, including decreased visual acuity and loss of vision
- Intermittent claudicating pain in jaw, tongue, and upper extremities
- Fever

Diagnosis includes:

- Temporal artery biopsy (definitive)
- ESR greater than 50 mm/hr (may be normal in about 20%)
- CRP greater than 2.45 mg/dL

Treatment should begin immediately if the diagnosis is suspected to prevent blindness:

- Prednisone 60 mg daily

TRIGEMINAL NEURALGIA

Trigeminal neuralgia (tic douloureux) is a neurological condition in which blood vessels press on the trigeminal nerve as it leaves the brainstem causing severe pain on one side of the face or jaw. The shock-like pains may involve a small area or half the face and in rare cases both sides of the face at different times. The pain lasts from seconds to two minutes and is extremely debilitating and may be precipitated by movement, vibration, or contact with the face or mouth. Trigeminal neuralgia is most common in women older than 50. Patients may go through periods of remission and recurrences. Diagnosis is by history and neurological exam.

Treatment is focused on symptom management and includes:

- **Carbamazepine** is the drug of choice and usually controls pain initially, but the effects may decrease over time.
- **Oxcarbazepine** may be used in place of carbamazepine.
- **Baclofen** (muscle relaxant) potentiates other drugs.
- **Surgical procedures** may be done if no response to medications.

FOREIGN BODIES

FOREIGN BODIES IN THE EAR

Foreign bodies in the ear (most often in children) can be organic or inorganic materials or insects. Careful history should be done to determine the type of foreign body before attempting removal. Children may require conscious sedation or general anesthesia for deep insertions. Irrigations should not be done if tympanic membrane is ruptured or cannot be visualized. Procedure:

1. Examine ear to determine if tympanic membrane is intact.
2. Drown insects with lidocaine 2% solution and then suction.
3. Irrigate small nonorganic particles with pulsatile flow aimed at wall of the canal.
4. Use cerumen loops, right-angle hooks, and/or alligator forceps to grasp and remove item.
5. Carefully examine the ear canal after removal of the item for lacerations or abrasions.
6. Topical antibiotic if extensive cutaneous abrasion or laceration or for organic material.

FOREIGN BODIES IN THE EYE

Foreign bodies in the eye should be assessed carefully with slit lamp with corneal examination using optical sectioning before attempting removal of the foreign body. Foreign bodies that penetrate the cornea full-thickness should not be removed in the ED, but superficial foreign bodies can safely be removed. Procedure:

1. Apply topical anesthetic to both eyes (to suppress blinking in the unaffected eye).
2. Eye held open by hand or with wire eyelid speculum.
3. Foreign body is carefully removed with small gauge needle or moistened cotton swab.
4. Rust ring from metallic objects should be removed with ophthalmic burr (if not over pupil), and patient referred to ophthalmologist for further rust ring removal within 24 hours.
5. Eyelid everted and examined carefully for further foreign bodies.
6. Abrasions treated as indicated.

FOREIGN BODIES IN THE NARES

Children may insert various organic and inorganic foreign bodies in the nose. In most cases, this is observed, but persistent unilateral obstruction of nose, foul discharge, or epistaxis is suggestive of foreign body. Small or uncooperative children may need to be restrained with conscious sedation or papoose board.

Procedure:

1. Vasoconstrictor/topical anesthetic applied: 1 mL of phenylephrine with 3 mL of lidocaine 4%.
2. Aerosolized racemic epinephrine may be used for decongestion, to loosen foreign body.
3. Examine nares with speculum.

Removal techniques:

- Positive pressure: Blowing nose on command. For small children, block opposite nares and have caregiver blow puff of air in mouth, forcing item out of nares.
- Suction with catheter.
- Use alligator or bayonet forceps to grasp item.
- Pass a curette behind item, rotate, and the use to pull item out.
- Pass Fogarty vascular catheter past item, inflate balloon, pull catheter back out.

LUDWIG ANGINA

Ludwig angina is cellulitis, usually caused by *Streptococcus* or *Staphylococcus,* of the submandibular spaces and lingual space that can result in obstruction of the airway as the swelling in the mouth floor pushes the tongue superior and posterior.

Symptoms include:

- Evidence of poor dental hygiene and odontogenic abscess (usually from lower third molars or surrounding gums) that has spread into soft tissue
- Dysphagia
- Odynophagia, trismus, edema of the upper neck (midline)
- Erythema, stridor, and cyanosis (late signs of obstruction)
- Changes in mental status

Diagnosis includes:

- Examination of the head and neck to observe for swelling of the upper neck, floor of mouth, and tongue
- CT scan
- Culture (treatment should, however, begin immediately)

Treatments include:

- Nasotracheal intubation (with fiberoptic tube if necessary) and ventilation if respiratory obstruction
- IV antibiotics, such as penicillin or clindamycin
- Referral to surgeon for incision and drainage as indicated

OTITIS EXTERNA

Otitis externa is infection of the external ear canal, either bacterial or mycotic. Common pathogens include bacteria, *Pseudomonas aeruginosa, Staphylococcus aureus,* and fungi, *Aspergillus* and *Candida.* OE is often caused by chlorine in swimming pools killing normal flora and allowing other bacteria to multiply. Fungal infections may be associated with immune disorders, diabetes, and steroid use.

Symptoms include:

- Pain, swelling, and exudate
- Itching (pronounced with fungal infections)
- Red pustular lesions
- Black spots over tympanic membrane (fungus)

Diagnosis: On exam, tenderness when touched on tragus or when the auricle is pulled, erythema, and history.

Treatment includes:

- Irrigate ear with Burow's solution or saline to clean and remove debris or foreign objects.
- **Bacteria**: Antibiotic ear drops, such as ciprofloxacin and ofloxacin. If impetigo, flush with hydrogen peroxide 1:1 solution and apply mupirocin twice daily for 5-7 days. Lance pointed furuncles.
- **Fungus**: Solution of boric acid 5% in ethanol; clotrimazole-miconazole solution with/without steroid for 5-7 days.
- Analgesics as needed.

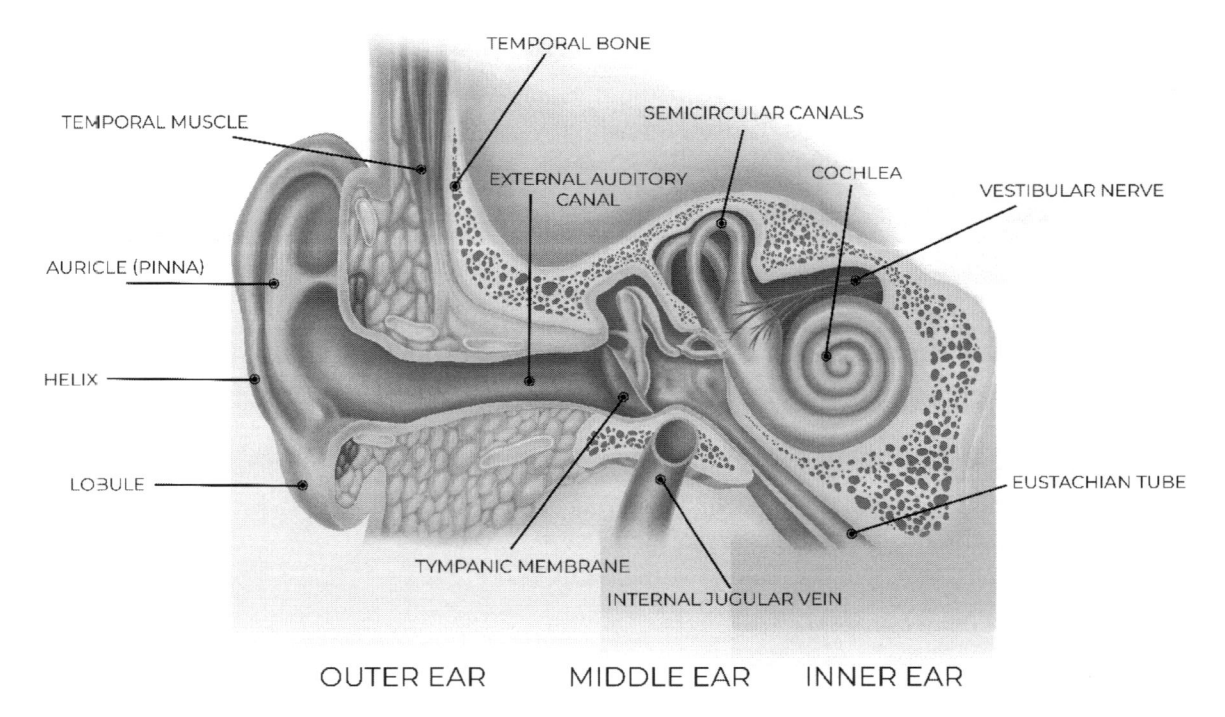

OTITIS MEDIA

Otitis media, inflammation of the middle ear, usually follows upper respiratory tract infections or allergic rhinitis. The eustachian tube swells and prevents the passage of air. Fluid from the mucous membrane pools in the middle ear, causing infection. Common pathogens include *Streptococcus pneumoniae, Haemophilus influenzae,* and *Moraxella catarrhalis*. Some genetic conditions, such as trisomy 21 and cleft palate, may include abnormalities of the eustachian tube, increasing risk. There are four forms:

- **Acute**: 1-3 weeks with swelling, redness, and possible rupture of the tympanic membrane, fever, pain (ear pulling), and hearing loss.
- **Recurrent**: 3 episodes in 6 six months or 4-6 in 12 months.
- **Bullous**: Acute infection with ear popping pressure in middle ear, pain, hearing loss, and bullae between layers of tympanic membrane, causing bulging.
- **Chronic**: Persists at least 3 months with thick retracted tympanic membrane, hearing loss, and drainage.

Diagnosis: Distinguishing features on assessment of acute otitis media include a bulging or perforated tympanic membrane, signs of inflammation, or purulent fluid present.

Treatment: 75-90% resolve spontaneously, so antibiotics are **withheld** for 2-3 days. Amoxicillin for 7-10 days. Referral for **tympanostomy and pressure-equalizing tubes** (PET) for severe chronic or recurrent infections.

> **Review Video: Otitis Media**
> Visit mometrix.com/academy and enter code: 328778

MASTOIDITIS

Mastoiditis usually results from extension of acute otitis media because the mucous membranes of the middle ear are continuous with the mastoid air cells in the temporal bone. All patients with otitis media should be considered at risk for mastoiditis. Patients with chronic otitis media also often develop chronic mastoiditis, which can result in formation of benign cholesteatoma. Signs and symptoms of mastoiditis include persistent fever, pain in or behind the ear (especially during the night), and hearing loss. Differential diagnoses may include Bell's palsy, otitis externa, and otitis media. **Diagnosis** is based on symptoms, CBC, audiometry, tympanocentesis or myringotomy with culture and sensitivities, and CT scan (definitive). Acute mastoiditis is treated with antibiotics, usually beginning with a 3rd generation cephalosporin or penicillin/aminoglycoside combination until culture and sensitivity results return. If spreading empyema or osteitis is present, then surgical mastoidectomy is required.

SINUSITIS

Sinusitis is inflammation of the nasal sinuses, of which there are two maxillary, two frontal, and one sphenoidal, as ethmoidal air cells. Inflammation causes obstruction of drainage with resultant discomfort.

Symptoms include:

- Frontal and maxillary presents with pain over sinuses
- Ethmoidal present with dull aching behind eye
- Tenderness to palpation and percussion of sinuses
- Mucosa of nasal cavity edematous and erythematous
- Purulent exudate

Diagnosis includes:

- Transillumination of sinus (diminished with inflammation)
- CT for those who are immunocompromised or if diagnosis is not clear
- Careful examination to rule out spreading infection, especially with signs of fever, altered mental status, or unstable vital signs

Treatment includes:

- Symptomatic relief with analgesia
- Topical decongestants and nasal irrigation
- Antimicrobial therapy if symptoms persist at least seven days or are severe (avoid routine use): Amoxicillin or TMP/SMX
- Steroid nasal spray twice daily

MENIERE'S DISEASE

Meniere's disease occurs when a blockage in the endolymphatic duct of the inner ear causes dilation of the endolymphatic space and abnormal fluid balance, which causes pressure or rupture of the inner ear membrane.

Symptoms include:

- Progressive fluctuating sensorineural hearing loss
- Tinnitus
- Pressure in the ear
- Severe vertigo that lasts minutes to hours
- Diaphoresis
- Poor balance
- Nausea and vomiting

Diagnosis includes:

- Complete physical exam and evaluation of cranial nerves
- Tuning fork sounds may lateralize to unaffected ear
- Assessment of hearing loss

Treatment:

- Low sodium diet
- Vestibular suppressant (antihistamine): Meclizine
- Benzodiazepine or SSRI for anxiety
- Antiemetics, such as promethazine suppositories
- Diuretics, such as hydrochlorothiazide
- Referral for surgical repair for persistent vertigo, but this will not correct other symptoms

Labyrinthitis

Labyrinthitis is a viral or bacterial inflammation of the inner ear, and it may occur secondary to bacterial otitis media. Viral labyrinthitis may be associated with mumps, rubella, rubeola, influenza, or other viral infections, such as upper respiratory tract infections. Because the labyrinth includes the vestibular system that is responsible for sensing head movement, labyrinthitis causes balance disorders. The condition often persists for 1 to 6 weeks with acute symptoms the first week and then decreasing symptoms. **Symptoms** include:

- Sudden onset of severe vertigo
- Hearing loss and sometimes tinnitus
- Nausea and vomiting
- Panic attacks from severe anxiety related to symptoms

Treatment includes:

- **Bacterial**: IV antibiotics
- **Viral**: Symptomatic as for bacterial (except for antibiotics)
- Volume replacement
- Antiemetics, such as promethazine suppositories
- Vestibular suppressant (antihistamine): Meclizine
- Benzodiazepine or SSRI for anxiety
- Referral to surgeon for I&D if necessary

TMD

Temporomandibular disorder (TMD) is jaw pain caused by dysfunction of the temporomandibular joint (TMJ) and the supporting muscles and ligaments. It may be precipitated by injury, such as whiplash, or grinding or clenching of the teeth, stress, or arthritis.

Symptoms include:

- Clicking or popping noises on jaw movement
- Limited jaw movement or "locked" jaw
- Acute pain on chewing or moving jaw
- Headaches and dizziness
- Toothaches

Diagnosis includes:

- Complete dental exam with x-rays to rule out other disorders
- MRI or CT may be needed

Treatment usually begins conservatively:

- Ice pack to jaw area for 10 minutes followed by jaw stretching exercises and warm compress for 5 minutes 3-4 times daily
- Avoidance of heavy chewing by eating soft foods and avoiding hard foods, such as raw carrots and nuts
- NSAIDs to relieve pain and inflammation
- Night mouthguard
- Referral for dental treatments to improve bite as necessary

Pediatric EENT Pathophysiology

INFECTIOUS CONJUNCTIVITIS

Infectious conjunctivitis (**pink eye**) is inflammation of the conjunctiva of the eye from bacteria or viruses. If it occurs less than 30 days after birth, it is referred to as **ophthalmia neonatorum** and is commonly acquired during delivery:

- Pathogenic agents include *Chlamydia trachomatis, Neisseria gonorrhea,* and herpesvirus.
- Antibiotic drops are applied to the newborn's eyes to prevent conjunctivitis. Intravenous acyclovir is given to infants exposed to herpes virus.

Infectious conjunctivitis in older children is usually caused by *Staphylococci, Streptococci, Pneumococci,* or viruses and is extremely contagious, so proper hand hygiene is essential. It is difficult to differentiate between bacterial and viral infections without cultures. The child should be kept from school and other children for 24 hours after starting treatment or until symptoms subside. **Symptoms** include:

- Red, swollen, itchy conjunctiva
- Eye pain
- Purulent discharge
- Scratchy feeling under eyelids
- Mild photophobia

Treatment is usually antibiotic drops or ointment and cool compresses although many cases are caused by viruses and the condition often disappears without treatment in 3-5 days.

STRABISMUS

Strabismus occurs when the muscles of the eyes are not coordinated so that one eye deviates from the axis of the other. Strabismus may be congenital or acquired or associated with other disorders, such as albinism. **Deviations** include:

- **Phoria** is intermittent deviation. The child can still focus eyes and maintain alignment for periods when looking at an object.
- **Tropia** is consistent or intermittent deviation in which the child is unable to maintain alignment of the eyes.
  - Both phorias and tropias may be *hyper* (up), *hypo* (down), *exo* (out), *eso* (in toward nose), or *cyclo* (rotational).

Esotropia is both eyes turning inwards (cross eyes) and **exotropia** is both eyes turning outward (wall eyes). Children often compensate by closing one eye or moving their head. They may have headaches or dizziness. **Treatment** before 24 months reduces **amblyopia** (reduced vision):

- Occlusion therapy: Patching or eye drops to blur vision in one eye
- Eye exercises
- Corrective lenses and/or prisms
- Surgical repair of rectus muscle

Retinopathy of Prematurity

Retinopathy of prematurity (ROP) occurs when small capillaries to the retina constrict, causing necrosis. ROP is associated with infants born ≤28 week and weighing <1600 g (3lb. 8 oz), especially those receiving oxygen therapy. It is also linked to respiratory distress, hypoxia, hypercarbia, acidosis, shock, blood transfusions, and systemic infection. In many cases, revascularization will occur, but ROP may result in myopia, retinal detachment, and blindness. Infants at risk for ROP should have regular evaluations for visual impairment:

- Infants may be unable to follow objects or lights with their eyes and may fail to make eye contact or imitate facial expressions. They may have a vacant stare.
- Toddlers and young children may thrust head forward, hold objects close to eyes, squint or blink frequently, rub or cover their eyes, and bump into objects.

Treatment:

- Corrective lenses
- Cryosurgery or laser surgery to stop disease progression
- Scleral buckle procedure or vitrectomy may be indicated for retinal detachment

Glaucoma

Glaucoma is an increase in intraocular pressure caused by abnormal circulation of fluid in the eyes. The ciliary body of the eyes produces aqueous fluid that flows between the iris and lens to the anterior chamber where it collects and increases pressure, which can result in blindness. Glaucoma may affect one eye or both. There are two **types**:

- **Congenital glaucoma** occurs before the age of 3 and includes an abnormality of structures that drain aqueous humor. Treatment is often unsuccessful. Symptoms include:
    - Photophobia
    - Tearing
    - Clouding of cornea
    - Eyelid spasms and enlargement of eyes
- **Secondary/juvenile glaucoma** occurs in children older than 3 and is caused by obstruction related to trauma, infection, tumors, or steroid use. Secondary glaucoma symptoms may be less specific; they include bumping into objects because of loss of visual field and seeing halos about objects.

Treatment:

- Eye drops used for adults are relatively ineffective for children.
- Surgical reduction of pressure is the treatment of choice, and the child may require multiple procedures.

Cataracts

Cataracts, partial or complete opacity of the lens of one or both eyes preventing refraction of light onto the retina, can be either congenital or acquired and is associated with prenatal infections, (such as rubella and CMV), hypocalcemia, or drug exposure. It can be related to trauma, systemic corticosteroids, genetic defects (albinism, Down syndrome), and prematurity. Clouding of the lens is not always obvious to the naked eye, so careful visual evaluations should be done for those children at risk. **Treatment** depends upon the extent of the cataracts and whether they are unilateral or bilateral. Early diagnosis is important because surgical repair before 2 months is the most successful, with visual acuity in 55% at 20/40. The opaque lens is removed, and the child uses corrective lenses or a lens is implanted. Antibiotic or steroid drops may be used after surgery.

NYSTAGMUS AND BLEPHAROPTOSIS

Nystagmus is involuntary rhythmic movements of one or both eyes, with horizontal, vertical, or circular movements, sometimes accompanied by rhythmic movements of the head. Nystagmus is common in neonates and should resolve in a few weeks but may indicate pathology if it persists. It is often associated with albinism, CNS abnormalities, or diseases of the ear or retina, and sudden onset is cause for concern. There is no specific treatment other than to identify and treat underlying causes.

Blepharoptosis is drooping of one or both upper eyelids and may be congenital (autosomal dominant), with defective development of the levator muscles or cranial nerve III, or acquired as the result of trauma or infection. If vision is affected, surgical repair is done early to avoid amblyopia. If vision is unaffected, surgical repair is deferred until the child is 3 or older.

HEARING LOSS

Identifying hearing loss early can facilitate treatment and prevent further deterioration, but most children are not diagnosed until 14-24 months even if hearing loss is profound. Diagnosis is delayed to at most 48 months for less severe hearing loss:

- **Mild hearing loss**: Pure-tone loss of ≥40 decibels at 500, 1000, and 2000 Hz in the better ear
- **Moderate hearing loss**: 40-60 decibel loss
- **Severe hearing loss**: 60-80 decibel loss
- **Profound hearing loss**: ≥80 decibel

There are three **types of hearing loss**:

- **Sensorineural hearing loss (SNHL)**: Damage occurs to the cochlear structure or nerve fibers. Hearing loss is permanent and associated with genetic disorders, birth injury, toxic drugs, head trauma, neoplasms, and viruses. A sub-form is noise-induced hearing loss (NIHL), which is preventable, but also permanent.
- **Conductive hearing loss (CHL)**: Transmission of sound is blocked by infection, foreign object, debris, impacted cerumen, and neoplasms. This type of hearing loss is usually reversible with medication or surgery.
- **Mixed hearing loss (MHL)**: Both conductive and sensorial loss.

COCHLEAR IMPLANTS

While there has been controversy in the deaf community about cochlear implants, by 2012, 38,000 children in the United States had received them. In 2020, the FDA approved lowering the age for cochlear implantation in children from 12 months to 9 months. A **cochlear implant** is an electronic device that provides sound, although not normal hearing, to those who have profound deafness. The person with the implant can often learn to understand speech and environmental sounds. Some use the sounds with lip-reading, but about half are able to understand speech by sound only, depending upon the degree of damage to the auditory nerve. A microphone by the ear picks up sounds that travels to an external speech processor and transmitter, which sends sounds to an implanted receiver where the sound is converted into electrical impulses sent to an internal electrode array implanted in the cochlea. The electrodes send the impulses to the auditory nerve, creating a perception of sound. Some children now receive bilateral cochlear implants. Studies show infants receiving the implant by age 2 acquire normal speech more rapidly than those implanted later.

Ocular Trauma

Orbital Fractures

Orbital fractures most often occur with blunt force against the globe causing a rupture through the floor of the orbital bone or a direct blow to the orbital rim, often related to an assault. Injuries are most common in adolescents and young adults. **Diagnosis** includes a complete eye (slit lamp) and vision examination, IOP measurement, and CT scan.

Signs and Symptoms	Treatment
<ul><li>Essentially asymptomatic</li><li>Ecchymosis and edema of eyelid</li><li>Infraorbital anesthesia from pressure or damage to infraorbital nerve</li><li>Decreased sensation of cheek and upper gum on injured side</li><li>Diplopia</li><li>Enophthalmos (sunken globe)</li></ul>	<ul><li>Usually supportive</li><li>Topical steroids for severe edema</li><li>The patient is advised not to blow nose for several weeks.</li><li>Surgical repair about 2 weeks after injury when edema has subsided for extensive fracture (≥33% of orbital floor) or enophthalmos >2 mm remaining 10–14 days post-injury.</li></ul>

Zygomatic Fractures

Zygomatic fracture involves the arch of bone that forms the lateral border of the eye orbit and the bony cheek prominence, most commonly associated with a blow to the lateral cheek from an altercation or accident. Fracture can result in a tilting of the eye and flattening of the cheek, which may be obscured by initial edema. Fracture may be only of the arch or may be a more extensive tripod fracture of the infraorbital rim, diastasis of the zygomaticofrontal suture, and disruption of the zygomaticotemporal arch junction. **Diagnosis** is by CT scan, which shows the extent of the fracture as well as the amount of displacement. **Treatment** for tripod fracture is referral to a surgeon for open reduction with fixation, exploration, and reconstruction of orbit as needed.

Traumatic Hyphema

Traumatic hyphema is characterized by blood coming into the anterior chamber, frequently because of eye injury. Most of the time, the blood will go out of the chamber with no consequences, but sometimes a problem does occur when heightened IOP or blood staining in the cornea results. 71-94% of hyphemas are due to tears in the front of the ciliary body, including disturbance in the primary arterial circle and the branches. It is frequently seen in physically energetic men and boys, and 70% of individuals are less than 20 in age. Ratio of boys to girls is 3:1. The consequences are contingent upon how much blood accumulates in the anterior chamber.

These **forms** of traumatic hyphema may be seen:

- **Microscopic**: Does not have layered blood; flowing red blood cells are seen
- **Grade I**: Affects less than a third of anterior chamber
- **Grade II**: One third to one half of anterior chamber affected
- **Grade III**: More than half of anterior chamber affected
- **Grade IV**: Complete hyphema

Assessments for another problem in the eye should be done, such as iridodialysis, cyclodialysis, lens subluxation, lacerations, detachment of the retina, decreased vision due to commotion in the retina, or fractures in the orbit. When the harm is broad or if there may be something inside the eye, utilize ultrasonography and radiologic imaging. If there may be sickle cell hemoglobinopathy, utilize sickle cell preparation.

CORNEAL ABRASIONS

Corneal abrasion results from direct scratching or scraping trauma to the eye, often involving contact lenses. This causes a defect in the epithelium of the cornea. Infection with corneal ulceration can occur with abrasions.

Symptoms:

- Pain
- Intense photophobia
- Tearing

Determining the **cause and source** of the abrasion is important for treatment, as organic sources pose the danger of fungal infection and soft contact lenses pose the danger of *Pseudomonas* infection.

Diagnosis	Treatment
- Topical anesthetic prior to testing for visual acuity. - Fluorescent staining and examination with cobalt blue light. - Eversion of eyelid to check for foreign body. - Examine cornea and assess anterior chamber with slit lamp.	- Cycloplegic agent to relieve spasm and pain: cyclopentolate 1%. - Erythromycin ophthalmic ointment 4 times daily with or without eye patch if not related to contact lens AND without eye patch if related to organic source. - Tobramycin ophthalmic ointment 4 times daily without eye patch if related to contact lens.

CHEMICAL EYE BURNS

Chemical burns are caused by splashing chemicals (solid, liquid, or fumes) into any part of the eye, often related to facial burns. Chemical burns may damage the cornea and conjunctiva, although other layers of the eye may also be damaged, depending upon the chemical and degree of saturation. Many injuries involve alkali (greater than 7 pH), acid (less than 7 pH; often muriatic acid or sulfuric acid), or other irritants (neutral pH) such as pepper spray. Alkali chemicals (such as ammonia, lime, and lye) usually cause the most serious injuries.

Symptoms	Diagnosis	Treatment
- Pain - Blurring of vision - Tearing - Edema of eyelids	- History of event - Eye exam showing corneal irritation	- Irrigate the eye and other areas of contact with copious amounts of water or normal saline. - Litmus paper exam of the eye to determine residual pH and continue irrigation until pH returns to neutral. - Apply cycloplegic agent to relieve spasm and pain (cyclopentolate 1%). - Apply antibiotic ointment to prevent infection.

Endocrine Pathophysiology

DIABETES MELLITUS TYPES 1 AND 2

Diabetes mellitus is the most common metabolic disorder. Over 6% of adults have diabetes, but only 4% of adults are diagnosed. Insulin resistance tends to increase in older adults, so there is less ability to handle glucose. Type II is more common in older adults, with incidence increasing with age.

- **Type I:** Immune-mediated form with insufficient insulin production because of the destruction of pancreatic beta cells
    - **Symptoms** include pronounced polyuria and polydipsia, short onset, obesity or recent weight loss, and ketoacidosis present on diagnosis.
    - **Treatment** includes insulin as needed to control blood sugar, glucose monitoring 1–4 times daily, diet with carbohydrate control, and exercise.
- **Type II:** Insulin resistant form with defect in insulin secretion
    - **Symptoms** include long onset, obesity with no weight loss or significant weight loss, mild or absent polyuria and polydipsia, ketoacidosis or glycosuria without ketonuria, androgen-mediated problems such as hirsutism and acne (adolescents), and hypertension.
    - **Treatment** includes diet and exercise, glucose monitoring, and oral medications.

> **Review Video: Diabetes Mellitus**
> Visit mometrix.com/academy and enter code: 501396
>
> **Review Video: Diet, Exercise, and Medications for Diabetes**
> Visit mometrix.com/academy and enter code: 774388
>
> **Review Video: Complications of Diabetes**
> Visit mometrix.com/academy and enter code: 996788

DIABETIC KETOACIDOSIS

Diabetic ketoacidosis is a complication of type 1 diabetes mellitus, usually related to noncompliance with treatment, stress, illness, or lack of awareness of having diabetes (this event often being the first time that diabetes is diagnosed). Inadequate production of insulin results in glucose being unavailable for metabolism, so lipolysis (breakdown of fat) produces free fatty acids (FFAs) as an alternate fuel source. Glycerol is converted to ketone bodies which are used for cellular metabolism less efficiently than glucose. Excess ketone bodies are excreted in the urine (ketonuria) or exhalations. Acidosis of any type causes potassium in cells to shift to the serum. The ketone bodies lower serum pH, leading to ketoacidosis.

Symptoms include:

- Kussmaul respirations: "Ketone breath," or fruity smelling breath; progresses to CNS depression with loss of airway
- Fluid imbalance, including loss of potassium and other electrolytes from cellular death resulting in dehydration and diuresis with excess thirst
- Dangerous cardiac arrhythmias, related to potassium loss; hypotension, chest pain, tachycardia
- GI: Nausea/vomiting, abdominal pain, loss of appetite
- Neurological: malaise, confusion/lethargy progressing to coma

Diagnosis is based on:

- Labs: Blood glucose >250 mg/dL, lower Na and elevated K (switches after treatment), elevated beta-hydroxybutyrate (byproduct of ketones)
- ABG: pH <7.3, HCO$_3$ <18 mEq/L
- Urine: positive for glucose and ketones

TREATMENT AND POTENTIAL COMPLICATIONS

Treatment of DKA:

- **Fluids**: Priority is fluid resuscitation with 1–2 liters of isotonic fluids given in the first hour, up to 8 liters in the first 24 hours. Potassium will be added to the fluids when levels begin to fall.
- **Insulin**: Continuous drip IV, with/without loading dose. Will usually begin at 0.1 unit/kg/ hour (5–7 units an hour generally), with a goal of decreasing blood glucose 50–75 mg/dL an hour. Blood glucose is checked every hour, and when levels are < 200 mg/dL, add dextrose to IV fluids to prevent rebound hypoglycemia.
- **Potassium**: Watch carefully, as fluids and insulin will cause rapid fall in serum levels. When K <5 mEq/L, it should be added to the IV fluids (Per liter: 20 mEq for K 4–5, 40 mEq for K 3–4). If potassium falls below 3, stop insulin drip and give 10–20 an hour until >3.5.
- **Sodium and Magnesium**: Na has an inverse relationship with potassium, and will increase as potassium falls. If sodium levels rise above 150 mEq, switch fluids to 0.45 NS. Low magnesium levels prevent potassium uptake, so replace as necessary.
- **Electrolytes**: Continue to monitor electrolytes and anion gap during ICU stay. When ABG and electrolytes normalized, transition to SQ insulin.

Potential complications include:

- Sudden electrolyte shifts (potassium) leading to catastrophic arrythmias, cerebral edema, and other complications
- Vomiting and decreased LOC leading to aspiration/ARDS
- Mechanical ventilation stops respiratory alkalosis and increases acidosis

HHNK

Hyperglycemic hyperosmolar nonketotic syndrome (HHNK) occurs in people without history of diabetes or with mild type 2 diabetes, resulting in persistent hyperglycemia leading to osmotic diuresis. Fluid shifts from intracellular to extracellular spaces to maintain osmotic equilibrium, but the increased glucosuria and dehydration results in hypernatremia and increased osmolarity. This condition is most common in those 50–70 years old and often is precipitated by an acute illness, such as a stroke, medications (thiazides), or dialysis treatments. HHNK differs from ketoacidosis because, while the insulin level is not adequate, it is high enough to prevent the breakdown of fat. Onset of symptoms often occurs over a few days. Glucose levels are often higher than those in DKA due to the gradual increase over time (often greater than 600), and the body living in a state of hyperglycemia, therefore the individual is not symptomatic until the blood glucose level is at an extreme high.

Symptoms: Polyuria, dehydration, hypotension, tachycardia, changes in mental status, seizures, hemiparesis.

Diagnosis: Increased glucose, Na, osmolality (urine and serum), BUN/Creatinine.

Treatment is similar to that for ketoacidosis:

- Insulin drip with frequent (hourly) blood sugar monitoring.
- Intravenous fluids and electrolytes.
- Correct blood glucose and other labs.

ACUTE HYPOGLYCEMIA

Acute hypoglycemia (hyperinsulinism) may result from pancreatic islet tumors or hyperplasia, increasing insulin production, or from the use of insulin to control diabetes mellitus. Hyperinsulinism can cause damage to the central nervous and cardiopulmonary systems, interfering with functioning of the brain and causing neurological impairment. Other causes may include: genetic defects (chromosome 11: short arm), severe infections, and toxic ingestion of alcohol or drugs (salicylates).

Symptoms include:

- Blood glucose <50–60 mg/dL
- Central nervous system: seizures, altered consciousness, lethargy, and poor feeding with vomiting, myoclonus, respiratory distress, diaphoresis, hypothermia, and cyanosis
- Adrenergic system: diaphoresis, tremor, tachycardia, palpitation, hunger, and anxiety

Diagnosis: Blood work, patient history, presentation.

Treatment depends on underlying cause:

- Glucose/Glucagon administration to elevate blood glucose levels
- Diazoxide to inhibit release of insulin
- Somatostatin to suppress insulin production
- Careful monitoring

DIABETES INSIPIDUS

Diabetes insipidus (DI) is caused by a deficiency of the antidiuretic hormone (ADH), or vasopressin. DI may develop secondary to head trauma, primary brain tumor, meningitis, encephalitis, or surgical ablation or irradiation of the pituitary gland, or metastatic tumors. This is different from congenital nephrogenic diabetes insipidus, in which production of ADH is normal but the renal tubules do not respond.

Symptoms:

- Polydipsia—enormous quantities of fluid may be ingested (3–30 L/day)
- Polyuria—large volumes of very dilute urine is excreted (3–30 L/day); nocturia almost always occurs
- Dehydration and hypovolemia can develop quickly if urinary losses are not continuously replaced

Diagnosis: A water deprivation test is the most reliable diagnostic test, but should only be done while the patient is under constant supervision. The test measures urine production, blood electrolyte levels, and weight over about 12 hours, during which the person is not allowed to drink. At the end of the 12 hours, vasopressin is given and a diagnosis of DI is confirmed if the person's excessive urination stops, BP rises to normal, and HR is normal.

Treatment includes:

- **Hormonal drugs**—Desmopressin, a synthetic analog of vasopressin, has prolonged antidiuretic activity, lasting 12–24 hours in most patients, and may be given intranasally, SQ, IV, or orally. Overdosage can lead to water intoxication, so monitor neurological status.
- **Nonhormonal drugs**—Three groups of nonhormonal drugs can reduce polyuria:
    - Diuretics, primarily thiazides (hydrochlorothiazide)
    - Vasopressin-releasing drugs (chlorpropamide or carbamazepine)
    - Prostaglandin inhibitors (indomethacin)

SIADH

Syndrome of inappropriate secretion of antidiuretic hormone (SIADH) is related to hypersecretion of the posterior pituitary gland. This causes the kidneys to reabsorb fluids, resulting in fluid retention, and triggers a decrease in sodium levels (dilutional hyponatremia), resulting in production of only concentrated urine. This syndrome may result from central nervous system disorders, such as brain trauma, surgery, or tumors. It may also be triggered by other disorders, such as tumors of various organs, pneumothorax, acute pneumonia, and other lung disorders. Some medications (vincristine, phenothiazines, tricyclic antidepressants, and thiazide diuretics) may also trigger SIADH.

Symptoms: Edema, dyspnea, crackles on auscultation, anorexia with nausea and vomiting, irritability, stomach cramps, alterations of personality, stupor, and seizures (related to progressive sodium depletion).

Diagnosis: Increased urine specific gravity, decreased Na and serum osmolality.

Treatment includes: (treat underlying cause)

- Correct fluid volume excess and electrolytes.
- Monitor urine output continuously: <0.5 mL/kg/hour is cause for concern.
- Seizure precautions.
- With SIADH expect low serum sodium and serum osmolality with high urine osmolality.

CHRONIC ADRENAL INSUFFICIENCY (ADDISON DISEASE)

Adrenal/Adrenocortical insufficiency (Addison disease) is caused by damage to the adrenal cortex related to a variety of causes, such as autoimmune disease or genetic disorders, but it may relate to destructive lesions or neoplasms. Without treatment the condition is life threatening.

Symptoms may be vague and the condition undiagnosed until 80–90% of the adrenal cortex has been destroyed:

- Chronic weakness and fatigue
- Abdominal distress with nausea and vomiting
- Salt or licorice craving as a result of aldosterone deficiency
- Pigmentary changes in skin and mucous membranes, hyperpigmentation
- Hypotension
- Hypoglycemia
- Recurrent seizures (more common in children)

Treatment includes hormone replacement therapy with glucocorticoids (cortisol) and mineralocorticoids (aldosterone), which may be taken orally or by monthly parenteral injections. Androgen replacement is sometimes recommended for women.

Note: During times of stress or illness, the demand for glucocorticoids may increase, and dosages up to 3 times the normal dosage may be needed to prevent an acute crisis.

> **Review Video: Addison Disease**
> Visit mometrix.com/academy and enter code: 813552

ACUTE ADRENAL INSUFFICIENCY (ADRENAL CRISIS)

Acute adrenal insufficiency (adrenal crisis) is a sudden, life-threatening condition resulting from an exacerbation of primary chronic adrenal insufficiency (Addison disease), often precipitated by sepsis, surgical stress, adrenal hemorrhage related to septicemia, anticoagulation complications, and cortisone withdrawal related to a decreased or inadequate dose to compensate for stress. Acute adrenal insufficiency may occur in those who do not have Addison disease, such as those who have received cortisone for various reasons, usually a minimum of 20 mg daily for at least 5 days.

Symptoms:

- Fever
- Nausea and vomiting
- Abdominal pain
- Weakness and general fatigue
- Disorientation, confusion
- Hypotensive shock
- Dehydration
- Electrolyte imbalance with hyperkalemia, hypercalcemia, hypoglycemia, and hyponatremia

Treatment:

- IV fluids in large volume
- Glucocorticoid
- 50% dextrose if indicated (hypoglycemia)
- Mineralocorticoid may be needed after intravenous solutions
- The precipitating cause must be identified and treated as well

HYPERTHYROIDISM

Hyperthyroidism (thyrotoxicosis) usually results from excess production of thyroid hormones (Graves' disease) from immunoglobulins providing abnormal stimulation of the thyroid gland. Other causes include thyroiditis and excess thyroid medications.

> **Review Video: Hyperthyroidism**
> Visit mometrix.com/academy and enter code: 923159
>
> **Review Video: Graves' Disease**
> Visit mometrix.com/academy and enter code: 516655
>
> **Review Video: An Overview of Thyroid and Antithyroid Drugs**
> Visit mometrix.com/academy and enter code: 666133

Symptoms vary and may be non-specific, especially in the elderly:

- Hyperexcitability
- Tachycardia (100–160) and atrial fibrillation
- Increased systolic (but not diastolic) BP
- Poor heat tolerance, skin flushed and diaphoretic
- Dry skin and pruritus (especially in the elderly)
- Hand tremor, progressive muscular weakness
- Exophthalmos (bulging eyes)
- Increased appetite and intake but weight loss

Treatment includes:

- Radioactive iodine to destroy the thyroid gland. Propranolol may be used to prevent thyroid storm. Thyroid hormones are given for resultant hypothyroidism.
- Antithyroid medications, such as Propacil or Tapazole to block conversion of T4 to T3.
- Surgical removal of thyroid is used if patients cannot tolerate other treatments or in special circumstances, such as large goiter. Usually one-sixth of the thyroid is left in place and antithyroid medications are given before surgery.

THYROTOXIC STORM

Thyrotoxic storm is a severe type of hyperthyroidism with sudden onset, precipitated by stress such as injury or surgery, in those un-treated or inadequately treated for hyperthyroidism. If not promptly diagnosed and treated, it is fatal. Incidence has decreased with the use of antithyroid medications but can still occur with medical emergencies or pregnancy. Diagnostic findings are similar to hyperthyroidism and include increased T3 uptake and decreased TSH.

Symptoms:

- Increase in symptoms of hyperthyroidism
- Increased temperature >38.5 °C
- Tachycardia >130 with atrial fibrillation and heart failure
- Gastrointestinal disorders such as nausea, vomiting, diarrhea, and abdominal discomfort
- Altered mental status with delirium progressing to coma

Treatment:

- Controlling production of thyroid hormone through antithyroid medications such as propylthiouracil and methimazole
- Inhibiting release of thyroid hormone with iodine therapy (or lithium)
- Controlling peripheral activity of thyroid hormone with propranolol
- Fluid and electrolyte replacement
- Glucocorticoids, such as dexamethasone
- Cooling blankets
- Treatment of arrhythmias as needed with antiarrhythmics and anticoagulation

HYPOTHYROIDISM

Hypothyroidism occurs when the thyroid produces inadequate levels of thyroid hormones. Conditions may range from mild to severe myxedema. There are a number of **causes**:

- Chronic lymphocytic thyroiditis (Hashimoto's thyroiditis)
- Excessive treatment for hyperthyroidism
- Atrophy of thyroid
- Medications such as lithium and iodine compounds
- Radiation to the area of the thyroid
- Diseases that affect the thyroid such as scleroderma
- Iodine imbalances

Symptoms may include chronic fatigue, menstrual disturbances, hoarseness, subnormal temperature, low pulse rate, weight gain, thinning hair, thickening skin. Some dementia may occur with advanced conditions. Clinical findings may include increased cholesterol with associated atherosclerosis and coronary artery disease. Myxedema may be characterized by changes in respiration with hypoventilation and CO_2 retention resulting in coma.

Treatment involves hormone replacement with synthetic levothyroxine (Synthroid) based on TSH levels, but this increases the oxygen demand of the body, so careful monitoring of cardiac status must be done during early treatment to avoid myocardial infarction while reaching euthyroid (normal) level.

HYPERPARATHYROIDISM

Hyperparathyroidism occurs when there is **overproduction of parathyroid hormone (PTH)**. Normal range is 10–55 pg/mL. This occurs more often in women and those over 50 years old. Hypercalcemia (total Ca^{++} >10.4 mg/dL) is the most common finding in hyperparathyroidism. Patients may complain about signs of hypercalcemia which can be easily remembered with bones, stones, groans, and moans. This includes **bone pain** due to demineralization, **kidney stones**, **abdominal groans** (nausea, vomiting, constipation, loss of appetite), and **psychiatric moans** (nervous system issues: muscle weakness, fatigue, lethargy, depression, confusion). Polyuria can occur with renal failure. Cardiac arrhythmias, hypertension, and even coma can occur. Ca^{++} levels >12 mg/dL may be due to cancer, and therefore cancer must be ruled out, especially if Ca^{++} levels rise rapidly. Hyperparathyroidism is treated with parathyroidectomy of affected glands.

HYPOPARATHYROIDISM

Hypoparathyroidism is the **deficiency of PTH**. This is more common in women and is usually due to accidental damage during thyroid/neck surgery, radioactive iodine treatment for hyperthyroidism, radiation, or due to autoimmune causes. As Ca^{++} levels drop, patients may complain of paresthesia of the fingers, toes, and perioral area. Patients will show other signs of neuromuscular irritability with muscle aches, hyperreflexia, carpopedal spasm (tetany), laryngospasm, and facial grimacing. A positive Chvostek sign (unilateral spasm of the facial muscles when the facial nerve is tapped) and a positive Trousseau sign (carpal spasm when upper arm is compressed with a blood pressure cuff) may be present. Irritability, confusion, fatigue, seizures, brittle hair and nails, and personality changes may occur. Diagnose with an ionized Ca^{++} level (<4.7 mg/dL), reduced PTH, and elevated phosphate. Treat with Ca^{++} and vitamin D supplements. Patients with renal failure must also reduce the amount of phosphate in their diet. Patients with tetany are treated with IV calcium gluconate.

CUSHING SYNDROME AND CUSHING'S DISEASE

Cushing syndrome results when **cortisol levels** are increased. Most commonly, this is due to steroid treatment with **prednisone**. Endogenous causes include a pituitary adenoma producing excess amounts of adrenocorticotropic hormone (ACTH) which leads to elevated cortisol (termed **Cushing's disease**) or a primary tumor of the adrenal gland causing increased cortisol secretion. Forms of cancer (e.g., lung, carcinoid) can present with ectopic sources of ACTH secretion. Patients will develop proximal muscle weakness, muscular atrophy, truncal obesity with thin arms and legs, round facies, buffalo hump, and purple striae usually across the abdomen. Patients may bruise easily, have non-healing sores, and women may be affected with hirsutism and oligomenorrhea/amenorrhea. Osteoporosis can occur as can glucose intolerance. For diagnosis a patient should be screened with one of the following: 24-hour urine free cortisol x3, low dose (1 mg) dexamethasone suppression test, midnight serum or salivary cortisol. Once Cushing syndrome is established, determine the cause using an ACTH and simultaneous cortisol measurement (elevated = adrenal adenoma or carcinoma) or a high-dose (8 mg overnight, or 2-day) dexamethasone suppression test (differentiates between pituitary cause and ectopic ACTH cause). Patients should be weaned off prednisone if possible. Removal of a pituitary adenoma can decrease ACTH production. Removal of an adrenal adenoma or other ectopic source of hormone secretion can decrease cortisol levels. Complications include hypertension, CV disease, DM, osteoporosis, risk of adrenal crisis, and psychosis.

HYPERALDOSTERONISM

Hyperaldosteronism leads to hypokalemia and hypernatremia (and often resulting hypertension). In fact, patients with untreated hypertension and potassium <2.8meq/dL often have primary hyperaldosteronism:

- **Aldosterone-producing adenoma** (Conn's syndrome) accounts for most primary hyperaldosteronism and affects women more often than men.
- **Idiopathic hyperaldosteronism** accounts for about 30% of primary hyperaldosteronism and has no identifiable changes on imaging.
- **Glucocorticoid suppressible hyperaldosteronism** is familial and rare.
- **Aldosterone-producing adrenocortical carcinoma** is another rare cause and presents with hyperandrogenism.

Diagnosis of hyperaldosteronism requires diastolic hypertension without edema, low renin levels that do not respond to volume depletion, and high aldosterone levels that fail to drop with saline boluses. An adrenal CT scan is performed to distinguish between Conn's syndrome and idiopathic hyperaldosteronism. **Treatment** includes spironolactone or eplerenone to block the mineralocorticoid receptor, normalizing potassium and improving blood pressure. Adrenalectomy is indicated for unilateral hyperplasia or Conn's syndrome.

PHEOCHROMOCYTOMA

Pheochromocytoma is a rare tumor of chromaffin tissue. Ninety percent of these occur in the adrenal medulla, 10% are bilateral, and 10% are malignant. These tumors produce epinephrine and norepinephrine, leading to episodic symptoms of headaches, chest pain, palpitations, diaphoresis, tremor, nausea, vomiting, weight loss, and constipation. Initial diagnosis requires a 24-hour urine test to check for metanephrine, VMA, and catecholamines. These are always elevated with pheochromocytoma. If associated with a multiple endocrine neoplasia (MEN) syndrome, then one must check serum free metanephrine. Then one should begin imaging with CT or MRI scanning of the adrenals. If the adrenals appear normal, a radiolabeled iodine (called MIBG-metaiodobenzylguanidine scintigraphy) scan can localize extra-adrenal pheochromocytoma tissue or metastases. This scan uses a compound that concentrates in the adrenals to highlight the pheochromocytoma tissue. **Treatment** is surgical. But first, phenoxybenzamines are used to block the catecholamines, and then beta-blockers are used to control heart rate. Surgery has a 90% cure rate. Urinary catecholamines should be followed for at least 10 years.

PAGET'S DISEASE

Paget's disease is a disease of high bone turnover and disorganized osteoid formation. It is most prevalent in patients in the northeast US or of European descent and in older patients. The disease is usually asymptomatic, being detected on radiographs. However, it may present with bone pain, fractures, and bony deformities. Commonly involved bones include the skull, femur, tibia, pelvis, and humerus. Specifically, with skull involvement, the patient may note frequent headaches and increasing hat size, sometimes associated with deafness. Examination findings include frontal bossing, bowed legs, and superficial erythema and warmth, due to the increased vascularity of the bones. This disease is **diagnosed** with increased alkaline phosphatase, and elevated urinary hydroxyproline. Calcium and phosphorous are often normal. Imaging reveals hyperdense and enlarged bones in some regions and erosions in others. Bone scanning reveals increased uptake in certain areas. **Treatment** includes bisphosphonate and management of complications, including CHF, spinal cord compression, or nerve entrapment.

Hypopituitarism Related to Deficient Growth Hormone

Hypopituitarism may affect production of one or multiple hormones because of organic defects or idiopathic ideology, but deficiency in somatotropin, or growth hormone, (GH) is the primary disorder, which may be associated with other disorders. A decrease in GH causes a condition known as hypopituitary dwarfism, with **symptoms** characterized by:

- Normal growth in the first year but below 5th percentile in year 2
- Height retarded to a greater extent than weight
- Well-nourished with proportional skeleton
- Inactive as infants and children
- Primary teeth normal but permanent teeth delayed and overcrowded because of lack of adequate development of the jaw
- Sexual development delayed

Treatment:

- Identify any organic causes, such as tumors, and treat them accordingly.
- Biosynthetic GH administration can more than double growth rate, but the degree of benefit depends upon the age the treatments are started and the individual response.
- Provide sex hormone therapy during adolescence.

Congenital and Juvenile Hypothyroidism

Hypothyroidism is caused by a deficiency in production of the thyroid hormones (TH) T4 and T3. It may be congenital or acquired from a lack of adequate dietary iodine, rare in the United States because salt is iodized. A number of disorders can cause hypothyroidism: congenital hypoplasia, partial or complete thyroidectomy, irradiation for Hodgkin's disease or other cancers, and infections. **Congenital hypothyroidism** (formerly called cretinism) may manifest at birth or be delayed for years, but severe early onset can result in profound neurological deficit and intellectual disability if undiagnosed and treated:

- **Neonates**: Widened posterior fontanel, hypothermia ≤95 °F, edema, respiratory distress, feeding difficulties, lethargy, delayed passage of meconium, prolonged physiologic jaundice, and vomiting
- **≤3 months of age**: Umbilical hernia, dry skin, constipation, enlarged tongue, lethargy, and minimal crying
- **Childhood**: Short stature with infantile proportions of trunk relative to legs, obesity, short forehead, broad nose, enlarged protruding tongue, dry skin and hair, and intellectual deficit

The brain is developed by age 2-3, and the onset of symptoms with **juvenile hypothyroidism** usually occurs after this time, so the condition is not associated with intellectual disability or neurological impairment. This form of hypothyroidism is most commonly caused by Hashimoto's thyroiditis, an autoimmune disease in which the immune system attacks the thyroid. **Symptoms** vary according to age of onset and include:

- Deceleration of growth
- Sensitivity to cold
- Constipation
- Muscle cramps
- Lethargy
- Mental decline
- Dry skin, thinning hair, and puffy face
- Goiter (swelling of the thyroid gland) may occur in some

Treatment for all types of hypothyroidism includes:

- Oral TH replacement therapy. Prompt initiation of therapy is critical for congenital hypothyroidism in order to prevent developmental abnormalities. If symptoms of hypothyroidism are severe, therapy to reach appropriate levels of TH is initially given gradually over 3-4 weeks to avoid hyperthyroidism.

PRECOCIOUS PUBERTY

Precocious puberty is the onset of puberty before age 7 in girls and 9 in boys. It can result from disorders of the gonads, the adrenal gland, or the hypothalamic-pituitary-gonad axis, producing gonadotropin hormones (GH) that cause early maturing of secondary sexual characteristics. It is much more common in girls than boys. Symptoms of **complete precocious puberty** include:

- Breast development and menstruation in girls
- Enlargement of testes and penis in boys with deepening of voice
- Development of pubic and axillary hair in both and facial hair in boys
- Acne
- Rapid increase in height for age
- Production of perspiration and odor

Partial precocious puberty presents similarly but results from overproduction of sex hormones, often because of a tumor of the ovary or testes, hyperplasia of the adrenal gland, or exogenous sources of hormones.

Treatment:

- Identifying and treating underlying causes
- If caused by GH, parenteral synthetic analog of luteinizing hormone-releasing hormone until puberty to slow development

INBORN ERRORS OF METABOLISM

Inborn errors of metabolism comprise a wide range of genetic metabolic disorders, usually related to defects in gene coding for enzymes, resulting in toxic accumulations that interfere with metabolism. Disorders are **classified** according to the type of metabolic disorder and include:

- Carbohydrate (glycogen storage disease, fructose intolerance)
- Proteins (clotting defects, sickle cell, thalassemia, osteogenesis imperfecta, Marfan)
- Amino acids (phenylketonuria, hyperammonemia)
- Organic acid (alcaptonuria)
- Cholesterol/lipoprotein (hyperlipoproteinemia, hypoproteinemia)
- Mitochondrial (Kearns-Sayre syndrome)
- Porphyrin (porphyria)
- Defective DNA repair (xeroderma pigmentosum)

Symptoms relate to the specific defect. Some symptoms are present in the neonate but others appear in childhood or adulthood. Some diseases are life-threatening, and others slowly progress. **Symptoms** common to many metabolic disorders may include:

- Encephalopathy with poor feeding, lethargy, tachypnea
- Metabolic acidosis and/or hyperammonemia
- Hypoglycemia
- Hepatic dysfunctions with jaundice
- Dysmorphism (structural anomalies)
- Abnormal body odor or urine odor

Fever and Fibromyalgia

FEBRILE SEIZURE

Febrile seizure is a generalized seizure associated with high fever (usually more than 38°C [100.4°F]) from any type of infection (upper respiratory tract, urinary) but without intracranial infection or other cause, occurring between six months and five years of age. Careful clinical examination must be conducted to rule out more serious disorders. Laboratory tests are conducted in relation to symptoms. Lumbar puncture is not usually indicated unless intracranial infection is suspected. Seizures usually last less than 15 minutes and are without subsequent neurological deficit.

Treatment includes:

- Fever control: Acetaminophen 10-15 mg/kg every 4-6 hours OR ibuprofen 10 mg/kg every 6-8 hours. Antipyretics are NOT recommended as prophylaxis for recurrent febrile seizures.
- Tepid water bath.
- Antiepileptic drugs (AEDs) are usually not advised unless seizures are complex or continuous, child is younger than 6 months, or there is a preexisting neurological disorder: IV diazepam 0.1-0.2 mg/kg or IV lorazepam 0.05-0.1 mg/kg. (May cause lethargy.)

FIBROMYALGIA

Fibromyalgia is a complex syndrome of disorders that include fatigue, chronic generalized muscle pain, and focal areas of tenderness persisting for at least three months. The cause of fibromyalgia is not clear and has only recently been recognized as a distinct disorder. Diagnosis is by clinical exam and ruling out joint and muscle inflammation that could be cause of the pain. On clinical exam there are specific points of tenderness, usually in multiple areas of the body.

Symptoms:

- Fatigue.
- Pain and stiffness unresponsive to treatment, persisting for months.
- Sleep disorders.
- Irritable bowel syndrome.
- Stiffness in neck and shoulders associated with headache and pain in face.
- Sensitivity to odor, noises, and lights.
- Mood disorders, such as depression, anxiety.
- Dysmenorrhea.
- Paresthesia in hands and feet.

Treatment:

- **Analgesia**: Acetaminophen, tramadol, or NSAIDs.
- **Antidepressants**, such as amitriptyline, nortriptyline, or fluoxetine. Duloxetine and venlafaxine have been shown to reduce pain.
- **Antiseizure medication**: Pregabalin is the first FDA-approved treatment for the pain of fibromyalgia.
- **Referral** for physical therapy and/or cognitive therapy.

Gastrointestinal Pathophysiology

PERITONITIS

Peritonitis (inflammation of the peritoneum) may be primary (from infection of blood or lymph) or, more commonly, secondary, related to perforation or trauma of the gastrointestinal tract. Common causes include perforated bowel, ruptured appendix, abdominal trauma, abdominal surgery, peritoneal dialysis or chemotherapy, or leakage of sterile fluids, such as blood, into the peritoneum.

Symptoms: Diffuse abdominal pain with rebound tenderness (Blumberg's sign), abdominal rigidity, paralytic ileus, fever (with infection), nausea and vomiting, and sinus tachycardia.

Diagnosis: Increased WBC (>15,000), abdominal x-ray/CT, paracentesis, blood and peritoneal fluid culture.

Treatment includes:

- Intravenous fluids and electrolytes
- Broad-spectrum antibiotics
- Laparoscopy as indicated to determine cause of peritonitis and effect repair

APPENDICITIS

Appendicitis is inflammation of the appendix often caused by luminal obstruction and pressure within the lumen; secretions build up and can eventually perforate the appendix. Diagnosis can be made difficult by the fact that there is some variation in the exact location of the appendix in some patients. Appendicitis can occur in all ages, but children younger than 2 years usually present with peritonitis or sepsis because of difficulty in early diagnosis. **Symptoms** include:

- Acute abdominal pain, which may be epigastric, periumbilical, right lower quadrant, or right flank with rebound tenderness
- Anorexia
- Nausea and vomiting
- Positive psoas and obturator signs
- Fever may develop after 24 hours
- Malaise
- Bowel irregularity and flatulence

Diagnosis is based on clinical presentation, CBC (although leukocytosis may not be present), urinalysis, and imaging studies (usually an abdominal CT with contrast).

CHOLECYSTITIS

Cholecystitis can result in obstruction of the bile duct related to calculi as well as pancreatitis from obstruction of the pancreatic duct. In acute cholecystitis, there is fever, leukocytosis, right upper quadrant abdominal pain, and inflammation of the gallbladder. The disease is most common in overweight women 20–40 years of age, but can occur in pregnant women and people of all ages, especially those who are diabetic or elderly. Cholecystitis may develop secondary to cystic fibrosis, obesity, or total parenteral nutrition. Many times, cholecystitis may resolve in about 7–10 days on its own, but acute cholecystitis may need surgical intervention to prevent complications such as gangrene in the gallbladder or perforation. Diagnosis is confirmed by ultrasound of gallbladder showing thickening of gallbladder walls or positive Murphy's sign, or a HIDA scan showing failure to fill.

Symptoms:

- Severe right upper quadrant or epigastric pain (ranging from 2–6 hours per episode)
- Nausea and vomiting
- Jaundice
- Altered mental status
- Positive Murphy's sign

Treatment:

- Antibiotics for sepsis/ascending cholangitis
- Antispasmodic agents (glycopyrrolate) for biliary colic and vomiting
- Analgesics (note that opioids result in increased sphincter of Oddi pressure)
- Antiemetics
- Surgical consultation for possible laparoscopic or open cholecystectomy

EROSIVE VS. NONEROSIVE GASTRITIS

Gastritis is inflammation of the epithelium or endothelium of the stomach. Types include:

- **Erosive**: Typically caused by alcohol, NSAIDs, illness, portal hypertension, and/or stress. Risk factors include severe illness, mechanical ventilation, trauma, sepsis, organ failure, and burns. Patients may be essentially asymptomatic but may have hematemesis or "coffee ground" emesis. Treatment depends on cause and severity but often includes a proton pump inhibitor (such as omeprazole 20–40 mg per day). Some may receive an H2-rceptor (such as famotidine). Those with portal hypertension may respond to propranolol or nadolol or portal decompression.
- **Nonerosive**: Typically caused by Helicobacter pylori infection or pernicious anemia. H. pylori infection can lead to gastric and duodenal ulcers. Treatment for H. pylori is per antibiotics and proton pump inhibitors with standard triple or standard quadruple therapy. Pernicious anemia is treated with vitamin B-12. Gastritis may also be caused by a wide range of pathogens, including parasites, so treatment depends on the causative agent.

> **Review Video: Pernicious Anemia**
> Visit mometrix.com/academy and enter code: 353419

GASTROENTERITIS

VIRAL GASTROENTERITIS

Viral gastroenteritis (commonly referred to as stomach flu) is characterized by nausea, vomiting, abdominal cramping, watery (may become bloody) diarrhea, headache, muscle aches, and fever. Viral gastroenteritis is spread through the fecal-oral route. Common **causes** include:

- **Norovirus**: Symptoms generally include diarrhea and vomiting with symptoms persisting for 1–3 days. Most people do not require treatment, but if diarrhea or vomiting is severe, an antiemetic or antidiarrheal may be prescribed if the patient is younger than 65. If severe dehydration occurs, the patient may require intravenous fluids until she is able to resume adequate oral intake.
- **Rotavirus**: Symptoms include watery diarrhea, nausea, vomiting, abdominal pain and cramping, lack of appetite and fever. Patients may become easily dehydrated and require rehydration with Pedialyte or Rice-Lyte or IV fluids. Medications are usually not needed but the rotavirus vaccine prevents severe rotavirus-related diarrhea and is given in 3 doses (2 months, 4 months, and 6 months).

BACTERIAL GASTROENTERITIS

Bacterial gastroenteritis generally results in cramping, nausea, and severe diarrhea. Some bacteria cause gastroenteritis because of enterotoxins that adhere to the mucosa of the intestines and others because of exotoxins that remain in contaminated food. Some bacteria directly invade the intestinal mucosa. Bacterial gastroenteritis is commonly **caused** by:

- *Salmonella*: Sudden onset of bloody diarrhea, abdominal cramping, nausea, and vomiting, leading to dehydration. Infection may become systemic and life-threatening. Treatment is supportive although antibiotics may be administered to those at risk.
- *Campylobacter*: Bloody diarrhea, cramping, fever, for up to 7 days that usually resolves but may become systemic in those who are immunocompromised. Treatment is primarily supportive with antibiotics only for those at risk.
- *Shigella* spp.: Most common in children <5 and presents with fever, abdominal cramping, and bloody diarrhea, persisting 5–7 days. Treatment is primarily supportive (rehydration) although those at risk (very young, old, immunocompromised) may receive antibiotics because the disease may become systemic.
- *Escherichia coli*: Different strains are associated with traveler's diarrhea and food-borne illnesses, and severity varies. Most result in diarrhea, nausea, vomiting, and cramping, but some strains (O157) may develop into life-threatening hemolytic uremic syndrome (HUS). Treatment is supportive. Antibiotics increase risk of developing HUS.

PARASITIC GASTROENTERITIS

Parasitic gastroenteritis is generally caused by infection with protozoa (one-celled pathogens):

- *Giardia intestinalis*: Common cause of waterborne (drinking and recreational) disease and non-bacterial diarrhea, resulting from fecal contamination. Symptoms include diarrhea, abdominal cramping, flatulence, greasy floating stools, nausea and vomiting as well as weight loss. Symptoms usually persist for up to 3 weeks although some develop chronic disease. Metronidazole is the drug of choice: Adults, 250 mg TID for 5–7 days. Pediatrics, 15 mg/kg/day in 3 doses for 5–7 days.
- *Cryptosporidium parvum*: About 10,000 cases occur in the US each year, usually from contact with fecal-contaminated water. Symptoms include watery diarrhea, abdominal pain, nausea, vomiting, weight loss, and fever and persist for up to 2 weeks although a severe chronic infection may occur in those who are immunocompromised. Treatment for non-HIV-infected patients (medications ineffective for HIV patients): Adults and children >11, Nitazoxanide 500 mg BID for 3 days. Pediatrics, 1–3 years 100 mg BID for 3 days; 4–11 years 200 mg BID for 3 days.

CONSTIPATION AND IMPACTION

Constipation is a condition with bowel movements less frequent than normal for a person, or hard, small stool that is evacuated fewer than 3 times weekly. Food moves through the GI from the small intestine to the colon in semi-liquid form. Constipation results from the colon, where fluid is absorbed. If too much fluid is absorbed, the stool can become too dry. People may have abdominal distension and cramps and need to strain for defecation.

Fecal impaction occurs when the hard stool moves into the rectum and becomes a large, dense, immovable mass that cannot be evacuated even with straining, usually as a result of chronic constipation. In addition to abdominal cramps and distention, the person may feel intense rectal pressure and pain accompanied by a sense of urgency to defecate. Nausea and vomiting may also occur. Hemorrhoids will often become engorged. Fecal incontinence, with liquid stool leaking about the impaction, is common.

Medical Procedures to Evaluate Causes of Constipation

Medical procedures to evaluate causes of constipation should be preceded by a careful history as this may help to define the type and guide the choice of diagnostic procedures. Most tests are necessary only for severe constipation that does not respond to treatment. Medical **diagnostic procedures** may include the following:

- **Physical exam** should include rectal exam and abdominal palpation to assess for obvious hard stool or impaction.
- **Blood tests** can identify hypothyroidism and excess parathyroid hormone.
- **Abdominal x-ray** may show large amounts of stool in the colon.
- **Barium enema** can indicate tumors or strictures causing obstruction.
- **Colonic transit studies** can show defects of the neuromuscular system.
- **Defecography** shows the defecation process and abnormalities of anatomy.
- **Anorectal manometry studies** show malfunction of anorectal muscles.
- **Colonic motility studies** measure the pattern of colonic pressure.
- **Colonoscope** allows direct visualization of the lumen of the rectum and colon.

Bowel Obstructions

Bowel obstruction occurs when there is a mechanical obstruction of the passage of intestinal contents because of constriction of the lumen, occlusion of the lumen, adhesion formation, or lack of muscular contractions (paralytic ileus). **Symptoms** include abdominal pain, rigidity, and distention, n/v, dehydration, constipation, respiratory distress from the diaphragm pushing against the pleural cavity, sepsis, and shock. **Treatment** includes strict NPO, insertion of naso/orogastric tube, IV fluids and careful monitoring; may correct spontaneously, severe obstruction requires surgery.

Bowel Infarctions

Bowel infarction is ischemia of the intestines related to severely restricted blood supply. It can be the result of a number of different conditions, such as strangulated bowel or occlusion of arteries of the mesentery, and may follow untreated bowel obstruction. Patients present with acute abdomen and shock, and mortality rates are very high even with resection of infarcted bowel. **Treatment** includes replacing volume, correcting the underlying issue, improving blood flow to the mesentery, insertion of NGT, and/or surgery.

Intestinal Perforation

Intestinal perforation is a partial or complete tear in the intestinal wall, leaking intestinal contents into the peritoneum. Causes include trauma, NSAIDs (elderly, patients with diverticulitis), acute appendicitis, PUD, iatrogenic (laparoscopy, endoscopy, colonoscopy, radiotherapy), bacterial infections, IBS, and ingestion of toxic substances (acids) or foreign bodies (toothpicks). The danger posed by infection after perforation varies depending upon the site. The stomach and proximal portions of the small intestine have little bacteria, but the distal portion of the small intestine contains aerobic bacteria, such as *E. coli,* as well as anaerobic bacteria.

Signs/symptoms: (appear within 24–48 hours): Abdominal pain and distention and rigidity, fever, guarding and rebound tenderness, tachycardia, dyspnea, absent bowel sounds/paralytic ileus with nausea and vomiting; Sepsis and abscess or fistula formation can occur.

Diagnosis: Labs: elevated WBC; lactic acid and pH change as late signs. X-ray and CT will show free air in abdominal cavity.

Treatment includes:

- Prompt antibiotic therapy and surgical repair with peritoneal lavage
- The abdominal wound may be left open to heal by secondary intention and to prevent compartment syndrome

Gastroesophageal Reflux

Gastroesophageal reflux (GER) occurs when the lower esophageal sphincter fails to remain closed, allowing the contents of the stomach to back into the esophagus. This reflux of the acid containing contents of the stomach may cause irritation of the lining of the esophagus. Over time, damage to the lining of the esophagus can occur. In some patients, this may lead to the formation of Barrett's esophagus. In Barrett's esophagus, the lining of the esophagus begins to resemble the tissue lining the intestine. Patients with Barrett's esophagus have an increased risk of developing esophageal adenocarcinoma.

Signs/symptoms: Heartburn, dysphagia, belching, water brash, sore throat, hoarseness, and chest pain.

Diagnosis: Clinical signs/symptoms, ambulatory esophageal reflux monitoring (this test uses a thin pH probe that is placed in the esophagus). Data is collected on the amount of acid entering the esophagus along with the presence of clinical symptoms. Endoscopy may be used in the diagnosis of GERD in patients with persistent or progressive symptoms.

Treatment: GER is often treated with proton pump inhibitors (inhibit gastric acid secretion). Surgical therapy may be utilized if medical management is unsuccessful. Patients are taught to eliminate foods that trigger symptoms (chocolate, caffeine, alcohol, and highly acidic foods). In addition, patients with GERD should avoid meals 2–3 hours before bed and may find it helpful to sleep with the head of the bed elevated to alleviate symptoms.

> **Review Video: GERD**
> Visit mometrix.com/academy and enter code: 294757

Peptic Ulcer Disease

Peptic ulcer disease (PUD) includes both ulcerations of the duodenum and stomach. They may be primary (usually duodenal) or secondary (usually gastric). Gastric ulcers are commonly associated with **H. pylori** infections (80%) but may be caused by aspirin and NSAIDs. *H. pylori* are spread in the fecal-oral route from person to person or contaminated water and cause a chronic inflammation and ulcerations of the gastric mucosa. PUD is 2–3 times more common in males and is associated with poor economic status that results in a crowded, unhygienic environment, although it can occur in others. Usually, other family members have a history of ulcers as well.

Symptoms include abdominal pain, nausea, vomiting, and GI bleeding in children younger than 6 years with epigastric and postprandial pain and indigestion in older children and adults.

Treatment includes:

- Antibiotics for *H. pylori*: amoxicillin, clarithromycin, metronidazole
- Proton pump inhibitors: lansoprazole or omeprazole
- Bismuth
- Histamine-receptor antagonists: cimetidine or famotidine

> **Review Video: Peptic Ulcers and GERD**
> Visit mometrix.com/academy and enter code: 184332

Inflammatory Bowel Disease

Ulcerative Colitis

Ulcerative colitis is superficial inflammation of the mucosa of the colon and rectum, causing ulcerations in the areas where inflammation has destroyed cells. These ulcerations, ranging from pinpoint to extensive, may bleed and produce purulent material. The mucosa of the bowel becomes swollen, erythematous, and granular. Patients may present emergently with **severe ulcerative colitis** (having >6 blood stools a day, fever, tachycardia, anemia) or with **fulminant colitis** (>10 blood stools per day, severe bleeding, and toxic symptoms) These patients are at high risk for megacolon and perforation. For patients with severe and fulminant ulcerative colitis:

Symptoms:

- Abdominal pain
- Anemia
- F&E depletion
- Bloody diarrhea/rectal bleeding
- Diarrhea
- Fecal urgency
- Tenesmus
- Anorexia
- Weight loss
- Fatigue
- Systemic disorders: Eye inflammation, arthritis, liver disease, and osteoporosis as immune system triggers generalized inflammation

Treatment:

- Glucocorticoids
- Aminosalicylates
- Antibiotics if signs/symptoms of toxicity
- D/C anticholinergics, NSAIDS, and antidiarrheals
- If fulminant: Admitted & monitored for deterioration. Kept NPO, and given IV F&E replacement. NGT for decompression if intestinal dilation is present. Knee-elbow position to reposition gas in bowel. Colectomy for those with megacolon or who are unresponsive to therapy.

> **Review Video: Ulcerative Colitis**
> Visit mometrix.com/academy and enter code: 584881

CROHN'S DISEASE

Crohn's disease manifests with inflammation of the GI system. Inflammation is transmural (often leading to intestinal stenosis and fistulas), focal, and discontinuous with aphthous ulcerations progressing to linear and irregular-shaped ulcerations. Granulomas may be present. Common sites of inflammation are the terminal ileum and cecum. The condition is chronic, but patients with severe or fulminant disease (fevers, persistent vomiting, abscess, obstruction) often present emergently for treatment.

Symptoms:

- Perirectal abscess/fistula in advanced disease
- Diarrhea
- Watery stools
- Rectal hemorrhage
- Anemia
- Abdominal pain (commonly RLQ)
- Cramping
- Weight loss
- Nausea and vomiting
- Fever
- Night sweats

Treatment:

- Triamcinolone for oral lesions, aminosalicylates, glucocorticoids, antidiarrheals, probiotics, avoid lactose, and identify and eliminate food triggers.
- For patients who present with toxic symptoms: hospitalization for careful monitoring, IV glucocorticoids, aminosalicylates, antibiotics, and bowel rest. Parenteral nutrition for the malnourished.
- For repeated relapses (refractory):
    - Immunomodulatory agents (azathioprine, mercaptopurine, methotrexate) or Biologic therapies (infliximab). Bowel resection if unresponsive to all treatment or with ischemic bowel.

DIVERTICULAR DISEASE

Diverticular disease is a condition in which diverticula (saclike pouchings of the bowel lining that extend through a defect in the muscle layer) occur anywhere within the GI tract. About 20% of patients with diverticular disease will develop acute diverticulitis, which occurs as diverticula become inflamed when food or bacteria are retained within the diverticula. This may result in abscess, obstruction, perforation, bleeding, or fistula. Diagnosis is best confirmed by abdominal CT with contrast (showing a localized thickening of the bowel wall, increased density of soft tissue, and diverticula in the colon). Many patients have normal lab studies, but some present with leukocytosis, elevated serum amylase, and pyuria on urinalysis.

Symptoms (similar to appendicitis):

- Steady pain in left lower quadrant
- Change in bowel habits
- Tenesmus
- Dysuria from irritation
- Recurrent urinary infections from fistula
- Paralytic ileus from peritonitis or intra-abdominal irritation
- Toxic reactions: fever, severe pain, leukocytosis

Treatment:

- Rehydration and electrolytes per IV fluids
- Nothing by mouth initially
- Antibiotics, broad spectrum (IV if toxic reactions)
- NG suction if necessary, for obstruction
- Careful observation for signs of perforation or obstruction

HEPATIC CIRRHOSIS
COMPENSATED

Cirrhosis is a chronic hepatic disease in which normal liver tissue is replaced by the fibrotic tissue that impairs liver function. There are three **types**:

- **Alcoholic** (from chronic alcoholism) is the most common type and results in fibrosis about the portal areas. The liver cells become necrotic, replaced by fibrotic tissue, with areas of normal tissue projecting in between, giving the liver a hobnail appearance.
- **Post-necrotic** with broad bands of fibrotic tissue is the result of acute viral hepatitis.
- **Biliary**, the least common type, is caused by chronic biliary obstruction and cholangitis, with resulting fibrotic tissue about the bile ducts.

Cirrhosis may be either compensated or decompensated. **Compensated** cirrhosis usually involves non-specific symptoms, such as intermittent fever, epistaxis, ankle edema, indigestion, abdominal pain, and palmar erythema. Hepatomegaly and splenomegaly may also be present.

DECOMPENSATED

Decompensated cirrhosis occurs when the liver can no longer adequately synthesize proteins, clotting factors, and other substances so that portal hypertension occurs.

Symptoms:

- Hepatomegaly
- Chronic elevated temperature
- Clubbing of fingers
- Purpura resulting from thrombocytopenia, with bruising and epistaxis
- Portal obstruction resulting in jaundice and ascites
- Bacterial peritonitis with ascites
- Esophageal varices
- Edema of extremities and presacral area resulting from reduced albumin in the plasma. Vitamin deficiency from interference with formation, use, and storage of vitamins, such as A, C, and K
- Anemia from chronic gastritis and decreased dietary intake
- Hepatic encephalopathy with alterations in mentation
- Hypotension
- Atrophy of gonads

Treatment varies according to the symptoms and is supportive rather than curative as the fibrotic changes in the liver cannot be reversed:

- Dietary supplements and vitamins
- Diuretics (potassium sparing), such as Aldactone and Dyrenium, to decrease ascites
- Colchicine to reduce fibrotic changes
- Liver transplant (the definitive treatment)

FULMINANT HEPATITIS

Fulminant hepatitis is a severe acute infection of the liver that can result in hepatic necrosis, encephalopathy, and death within 1–2 weeks. Most hepatitis is caused by infection with hepatitis viruses A, B, C, D, or E, but it can also be caused by numerous viruses, toxic chemicals (carbon tetrachloride), metabolic diseases (Wilson disease), and drugs, such as acetaminophen. Fulminant hepatitis can result from any of these factors. Fulminant hepatitis can be divided into three stages according to the duration from jaundice to encephalopathy:

$$0-7 \text{ days} = \text{Hyperacute liver failure}$$
$$7-28 \text{ days} = \text{Acute liver failure}$$
$$28-72 \text{ days} = \text{Subacute liver failure}$$

Symptoms:

- Poor feeding/anorexia
- Increased intracranial pressure with cerebral edema and encephalopathy
- Coagulopathies
- Renal failure
- Electrolyte imbalances

Treatment:

- Identify and treat underlying cause
- Intracranial pressure monitoring and treatment
- Diuresis; liver transplantation may be necessary
- Survival rates vary from 50–85%

PORTAL HYPERTENSION

Portal hypertension occurs when obstructed blood flow increases blood pressure throughout the portal venous system, preventing the liver from filtering blood and causing the development of collateral blood vessels that return unfiltered blood to the systemic circulation. Increasing serum aldosterone levels cause sodium and fluid retention in the kidneys, resulting in hypervolemia, ascites and esophageal varices. Portal hypertension can be caused by any liver disease, especially cirrhosis and inherited or acquired coagulopathies that cause thrombosis of the portal vein.

Symptoms: Ascites with distended abdomen, esophageal varices with bleeding, dyspnea, abdominal discomfort, fluid/electrolyte imbalances.

Diagnosis: Labs (CBC, BMP, liver panel, Hep B &C), abdominal ultrasound or CT/MRI, EGD, Hemodynamic measurement of the hepatic venous pressure gradient (HVPG)

Treatment includes:

- Restricted sodium intake & use diuretics as needed
- Endoscopic treatment of obstruction
- Portal vein shunting redirecting blood from the portal vein to the vena cava
- Liver transplant in severe cases
- These patients are at high risk for esophageal varices, which, if they rupture, can cause instantaneous hemorrhage and death

ESOPHAGEAL VARICES

Esophageal varices are torturous, dilated veins in the submucosa of the esophagus (usually the distal portion). They are a complication of cirrhosis of the liver, in which obstruction of the portal vein causes an increase in collateral vessels and resulting decrease in circulation to the liver, increasing the pressure in the collateral vessels. This causes the vessels to dilate. Because they tend to be fragile and inelastic, they tear easily, causing sudden, massive esophageal hemorrhage.

Signs/symptoms: Usually asymptomatic until rupture; projectile vomiting bright red blood, dark stools, and shock.

Diagnosis: EGD, capsule endoscopy, CT, and MRI.

Treatment (in the case of rupture) includes:

- Emergent fluid and blood replacement
- IV vasopressin, somatostatin, and octreotide to decrease venous pressure and provide vasoconstriction/clotting
- Endoscopic injection with sclerosing agents and band ligation
- Esophagogastric balloon tamponade using Sengstaken-Blakemore and Minnesota tubes (Note: always inflate gastric balloon first, keep scissors nearby in case of balloon migration, do not use longer than 24 hrs as there is increased risk of ulceration from pressure.)
- Transjugular intrahepatic portosystemic shunting (TIPS) creates a channel between systemic and portal venous systems to reduce portal hypertension

Hepatic Coma

Hepatic coma or hepatic encephalopathy occurs when the liver's inability to remove ammonia and other toxins from the bloodstream causes a decrease in neurologic function. Hepatic encephalopathy often occurs in patients with severe liver disease, most commonly in patients diagnosed with cirrhosis of the liver. The fibrous tissue that forms in cirrhosis affects the liver structure and impedes the blood flow to the liver, ultimately causing the liver to fail. There are four stages of hepatic encephalopathy ranging from grade 0 to grade 4. Grade 4 encephalopathy is defined as hepatic coma. Neurologic alterations may progress slowly and if left untreated may result in irreversible neurologic damage.

Signs/symptoms: Altered mental status, personality or mood changes, poor judgment, and poor concentration. As symptoms progress, patients may experience agitation, disorientation, drowsiness, increasing confusion, lethargy, slurred speech, tremors, and seizures. In grade 4 encephalopathy, patients become unresponsive and ultimately comatose.

Diagnosis: Physical assessment, lab tests including a complete blood count, liver function tests, serum ammonia levels, BUN, creatinine and electrolyte levels, CT or MRI of the brain, and electroencephalogram may be used to diagnose hepatic encephalopathy.

Treatment: Address precipitating factors such as infection, gastrointestinal bleeding, dehydration, hypotension, or alcohol use. Other treatment options may include limiting protein intake, administration of lactulose to prevent the absorption of ammonia, and the administration of an antibiotic such as neomycin, rifaximin, or metronidazole (Flagyl) to reduce the serum ammonia level.

Acute Pancreatitis

Acute pancreatitis is related to chronic alcoholism or cholelithiasis in 90% of patients, but may have unknown etiology. It may also be triggered by a variety of drugs (tetracycline, thiazides, acetaminophen, and oral contraceptives). Complications may include shock, acute respiratory distress syndrome, and MODs.

Signs/symptoms: acute pain (mid-epigastric, LUQ, or generalized), nausea and vomiting, Abdominal distension.

Diagnosis: Serum lipase (>2x normal), amylase (less accurate), CT with contrast, abdominal U/S, MRI cholangiopancreatography, ERCP.

Treatment (supportive) includes:

- **Medications**: IV fluids, antiemetics, antibiotics (if necrosis is secondary to infection), and analgesia. NOTE: do not give morphine, can cause spasms in sphincter of Oddi, making pain worse.
- **TPN, NPO, or restricted to clear liquids** may help manage vomiting, ileus, and aspiration.
- **Surgical**: may remove gallbladder and biliary duct obstructions if cause of recurrent pancreatitis.

Prevention: Avoid smoking and alcohol consumption; limit fat intake and increase fresh fruits/vegetables and water.

Hernias

Hernias are protrusions into or through the abdominal wall and may occur in children and adults. Hernias may contain fat, tissue, or bowel. There are a number of **types**:

- **Direct inguinal hernias** occur primarily in adults and rarely incarcerate.
- **Indirect inguinal hernias** related to congenital defect is most common on the right in males and can incarcerate, especially during the first year and in females.
- **Femoral hernias** occur primarily in women and may incarcerate.

- **Umbilical hernias** occur in children, especially those of African-American descent, and rarely incarcerate. They may also occur in adults, primarily women, and may incarcerate.
- **Incisional hernias** are usually related to obesity or wound infections, and may incarcerate.

Hernias are evident on clinical examination.

Symptoms of incarceration include:

- Severe pain
- Nausea and vomiting
- Soft mass at hernia site
- Tachycardia
- Temperature

Treatment for hernias includes:

- Reduction if incarceration is very recent with patient in Trendelenburg position and gentle compression
- Surgical excision and fixation
- Broad-spectrum antibiotics

BILIARY ATRESIA

Biliary atresia is a rare life-threatening condition that occurs in infancy of unknown cause. Bile ducts are tubes that transport bile from the liver to the gallbladder (where it is stored) and the small intestine (where it aids in digestion). Biliary atresia occurs when the bile ducts (either inside or outside of the liver) become inflamed, causing damage to the ducts and an impedance of bile flow. Without treatment, the trapped bile causes damage to the liver eventually causing it to fail. The life expectancy for infants with untreated biliary atresia is approximately 2 years.

Signs/symptoms: Early identification is key in successfully treating biliary atresia. Signs and symptoms include dark urine, gray or white stools, slow weight gain and delayed growth, jaundice, abdominal swelling, and itching.

Diagnosis: Physical assessment, abdominal films, ultrasound, lab tests including bilirubin levels, and liver biopsy.

Treatment: The only treatment options for biliary atresia are liver transplant or the Kasai procedure. Named after the surgeon who invented it, the Kasai procedure involves using a loop of intestine to act as a new bile duct and removing the damaged ducts. Flow of bile is then restored to the small intestine. The Kasai procedure is most successful when performed on younger infants (less than 3 months old).

HYPERTROPHIC PYLORIC STENOSIS

Hypertrophic pyloric stenosis (PS) is obstruction of the pyloric sphincter between the gastric pylorus and small intestine, caused by hypertrophy and hyperplasia of the circular muscle of the pylorus so the enlarged tissue obstructs the sphincter. PS is more common in boys than girls and has a genetic predisposition. Onset of **symptoms** is usually >3 weeks:

- Projectile vomiting, usually shortly after eating but may be delayed for a few hours (Emesis may be blood-tinged but non-bilious.)
- Child hungry and eats readily but shows weight loss and signs of dehydration
- Upper abdominal distention with palpable mass in epigastrium (to right of umbilicus)
- Visible left to right peristaltic waves

Diagnosis is based on ultrasound. Decreased sodium and potassium levels may not be evident with dehydration.

Treatment includes:

- Intravenous fluids to restore hydration and electrolyte balance
- Surgical pyloromyotomy: Longitudinal incisions through the circular muscle fibers down to the submucosa to release the restriction and allow the muscle to expand

MALROTATION/VOLVULUS

Malrotation is a congenital defect in which the intestines are attached to the back of the abdominal wall by one single attachment rather than a broad band of attachments across the abdomen, essentially suspending the bowels so that they can easily twist, resulting in a **volvulus** (twisted bowel), cutting off blood supply. It may untwist but can lead to bowel infarction. Some children with malrotation have no symptoms, but most develop **symptoms** by 1 year:

- Cycles of cramping pain about every 15–30 minutes that cause the child to cry and pull knees to chest
- Distended painful abdomen
- Diarrhea, bloody stools, or no stools
- Vomiting (occurring soon after crying begins usually indicates small intestine obstruction; later vomiting usually indicated large intestine blockage)
- Tachycardia and tachypnea
- Decreased urinary output
- Fever

Treatment:

- Surgical repair (Ladd procedure) is indicated immediately if there is volvulus. Most malrotations require surgical repair even with less severe symptoms.

INTUSSUSCEPTION

Intussusception is a telescoping of one portion of the intestine into another, usually at the ileocecal valve, causing an obstruction. As the walls of the intestine come in contact, inflammation and edema cause decreased perfusion, which can result in infarction with peritonitis and death. Fecal material cannot move past the obstruction. It is most common between 3–12 months but can occur until 6 years and may relate to viral infections.

Symptoms	Treatment
- "Currant jelly stool" composed of blood and mucous (occurs with 60%) - Sudden acute episodes of severe abdominal pain during which child pulls knees to chest - Vomiting - Lethargy and weakness - Distended abdomen, painful to palpation - Sausage-shaped mass in RUQ of abdomen - Progressive fever and prostration if peritonitis occurs	- Barium or air enema to diagnose and apply pressure that may resolve the intussusception (nonoperative reduction) - Surgical repair if there is shock, peritonitis, intestinal perforation, or failure to resolve with barium/air enema

Hirschsprung's Disease

Hirschsprung's disease (congenital aganglionic megacolon) is failure of ganglion nerve cells to migrate to part of the bowel (usually the distal colon), so that part of the bowel lacks enervation and peristalsis, causing stool to accumulate and leading to distention and megacolon. There is a genetic predisposition to the disease that affects more males than females and is associated with trisomy 21 (Down syndrome). **Symptoms** include:

- Failure to pass meconium in 24-48 hours
- Poor feeding
- Bilious vomitus
- Abdominal distension

Delayed diagnosis:

- Chronic constipation
- Failure to thrive
- Periods of diarrhea and vomiting
- (With infection) Severe prostration with watery diarrhea, fever, and hypotension

Childhood symptoms:

- Chronic constipation with ribbon-like stools.
- Abdominal distension with visible peristalsis and palpable fecal mass. Poorly-nourished, anemic, child.

Treatment:

- Resection of aganglionic section and colorectal anastomosis. There are a number of procedures (Swenson, Duhamel, and Soave) but recently laparoscopic or trans-anal minimally-invasive approaches have proven successful.

Abdominal Wall Malrotation Defect
Incarcerated Hernia

Hernias are protrusions into or through the abdominal wall and may occur in children and adults. Hernias may contain fat, tissue, or bowel. There are a number of types that are common in children. Hernias are evident on clinical examination. Incarceration (strangulation of an organ in the hole of the hernia) is a life-threatening condition that requires immediate surgical repair.

- **Indirect inguinal hernias** related to congenital defect are most common on the right in males and can incarcerate, especially during the first year and in females.
- **Umbilical hernias** occur in children, especially African American children, and rarely incarcerate.
- **Incisional hernias** occur, usually related to obesity or wound infections, and may incarcerate.

Symptoms	Treatment
<ul><li>Severe abdominal pain</li><li>Nausea and vomiting</li><li>Soft mass at hernia site</li><li>Tachycardia</li><li>Fever</li></ul>	<ul><li>Intravenous fluids</li><li>Immediate surgical excision and fixation</li><li>Broad-spectrum antibiotics</li></ul>

Umbilical Hernia

Umbilical hernia is a skin-covered herniation of intestine and omentum through an abdominal wall defect near the umbilicus caused by an incomplete closure of the umbilical ring. The herniation may range from 1-5 cm in size and may be obvious on physical examination or felt on palpation. It may appear flat when the child is supine but protrude when the child is upright or crying. Approximately 1 in 6 infants are born with umbilical hernias. **Symptoms** are usually absent unless strangulation of the hernia occurs, and then the infant may cry with pain, feed poorly, vomit, and have an increase in temperature. The abdomen may become distended. In this case, emergency surgical repair must be done. **Treatment** usually involves just observing the hernia for complications as, in most cases, it will reduce on its own. If the hernia is still present at 3-4 years, a simple surgical repair of the hernia may be done.

Congenital Diaphragmatic Hernia

Congenital diaphragmatic hernia is herniation of abdominal contents into chest cavity. During fetal development, a hole in the diaphragm that should close at about 3 months stays open, allowing loops of the intestine or the stomach to herniate into the chest and preventing adequate development of the lungs (pulmonary hypoplasia) and/or heart. The infants are usually very dyspneic at birth and may need to be ventilated. They may need temporary heart/bypass as well. The kidneys are often enlarged. Radiographic studies are done to show the extent of the abnormality, usually showing a high gastrointestinal obstruction, often at the duodenum. A nasogastric feeding tube is inserted, and an intravenous line is inserted as well. Supportive treatment is given for dyspnea as well as correction of acidosis. Surgical repair may be done after birth or delayed for weeks until the child stabilizes. Surgical repair may be done in one stage or more, depending upon the degree of abnormality.

Encopresis and Fecal Incontinence

Encopresis is the voluntary or involuntary passage of stool in places or manners that are inappropriate for a child. 80% of children with encopresis are male, 4 years or older. There are two types: retentive encopresis, which accounts for about 80% of those affected, and non-retentive, which accounts for the other 20%. Retentive encopresis is characterized by a history of long term, painful constipation and the development of overflow diarrhea. The chronic constipation causes distention of the rectum and stretching of both the internal and external anal sphincters. As a result, the child may no longer feel the urge to defecate, so stool eventually leaks from the rectum, causing **chronic fecal incontinence**. Non-retentive encopresis, usually involving passage of normally formed stools on a daily basis, does not involve constipation or bowel abnormalities, except in a small subset that may have irritable bowel syndrome. It is generally a behavioral/psychological problem.

Diarrhea

Diarrhea is common in infants and children and can be caused by a variety of different infections and conditions. Diarrhea accounts for about 20% of hospitalizations of children <2 and causes about 500 deaths in children <4 in the United States each year. Because of the potential for loss of fluids, electrolytes, and nutrition, and the danger of ulceration and bleeding, diarrhea should be monitored carefully to determine the **cause**:

- **Osmotic**: Increased fluid in the stool and may be related to lactose intolerance and overfeeding.
- **Secretory**: Inhibited electrolyte (ion) absorption or increased electrolyte secretion related to bacterial endotoxins.
- **Motility disorders**: Interfere with absorption of fluids, including bile salt or pancreatic enzyme deficiencies.
- **Inflammatory**: Related to Crohn's disease or ulcerative colitis.
- **Viral/bacterial**: The most common cause of diarrhea in children. A wide range of viral and bacterial pathogens can cause mild to severe life-threatening diarrhea.

Bacterial Causes

A wide range of bacterial and viral pathogens can cause mild to severe life-threatening diarrhea:

- ***Campylobacter jejuni*** transmitted from pets to children <7 through contaminated food and water, usually in the summer. Diarrhea with fever, vomiting, and abdominal pain persists for 7–12 days. **Treatment**: Erythromycin (40 mg/kg/day) in 3 doses daily for 5–7 days.

- **Clostridioides difficile** occurs secondary to antibiotic use. Some children are asymptomatic carriers, but severe illness is life threatening with bloody diarrhea and abdominal pain leading to megacolon. **Treatment**: Metronidazole 30 mg/kg/day in 4 doses or Vancomycin 40 mg/kg/day in 4 doses for 7–10 days.
- **Yersinia enterocolitica** found in uncooked pork or unpasteurized milk causes secretory diarrhea in all ages with fever, foul, green and bloody stool, and pain in right lower abdomen. Usually resolves in 3–4 days.
- **Shigella** is transmitted by the fecal-oral route from contaminated food and water and occurs from 6–36 months. Characterized by bloody diarrhea, abdominal pain, and fever. **Treatment**: TMP-SMZ 8 mg TMP/kg/day in 2 doses for 7–10 days.

SALMONELLA

Salmonella causes up to 4 million infections in the United States, resulting in 500 deaths, primarily of young children. *Salmonella* is spread by the fecal-oral route through ingestion of contaminated food or water, including all meats, milk, eggs, and vegetables. Raw or undercooked meat, unpasteurized milk, and unwashed produce are high-risk. *Salmonella* may be found in the feces of pets, particularly reptiles such as snakes and turtles. Small children should not have reptiles as pets. **Symptoms** appear 12–72 hours after infection and include bloody diarrhea with abdominal pain, fever, and vomiting. Most cases resolve within 7–10 days, but in some cases, life-threatening sepsis may occur, requiring **treatment** with antibiotics. For mild cases in children, oral azithromycin may be administered, and for more severe cases in children, IV ceftriaxone may be necessary. In adolescents, oral ciprofloxacin or levofloxacin may be administered for mild infection, and IV ceftriaxone or cefotaxime for serious cases. Antibiotic prophylaxis is usually contraindicated except in children <1 year that are at risk for bacteremia or those who are immunocompromised.

ESCHERICHIA COLI

Escherichia coli is part of the normal flora of the intestines and serves to inhibit other bacteria, but 5 serotypes can cause intestinal disease and severe diarrhea. Some types are more common in developing countries and may occur in children who are traveling in areas where feces have contaminated food supplies and water. Severe outbreaks of *E. coli* infection have occurred in the United States with a toxic strain, O157:H7, which produces a toxin that can cause damage to the intestinal lining, including blood vessels, resulting in hemorrhage and watery diarrhea that becomes bloody. This hemorrhagic colitis usually clears with supportive treatment after 10 days. However, about 15% of children develop sepsis and hemolytic uremic syndrome with kidney failure, hemolytic anemia, and thrombocytopenia. Death rates are 3–5%, but residual renal and neurological damage may result. **Treatment** is supportive with intravenous therapy, blood transfusions, and kidney dialysis. Antibiotics and antidiarrheals are contraindicated as they may worsen *E. coli* infections.

SHORT GUT SYNDROME

Short gut (bowel) syndrome occurs when removal of part of the small intestine results in a malabsorptive condition. **Symptoms** relate to the amount of bowel removed and the area of resection:

- Resection of the terminal ileum interferes with absorption of bile salts and vitamin B_{12}. If <100 cm removed, malabsorption of bile salts causes watery diarrhea. Treatment includes salt binding resins (cholestyramine 2-4 g three times daily). If >100 cm removed, steatorrhea with resultant malabsorption of fat-soluble vitamins occurs. Additional treatment includes a low-fat diet, vitamins, and calcium supplements to prevent oxalate kidney stone.
- Resection of >40-50% of small bowel results in weight loss, diarrhea, and electrolyte imbalance. If colon and 100 cm of proximal jejunum are retained, a low fat, high complex carbohydrate diet, and electrolytes may maintain nutrition, but if the colon is removed, 200 cm of jejunum is required for adequate nutrition. Otherwise, parenteral nutrition is required, and this can lead to liver failure and death or liver/intestine transplantation.

Imperforate Anus

Imperforate anus (anorectal malfunction) is a congenital abnormality where the rectum is absent, malformed, or displaced from normal position. It may include disorders of the urinary tract. Imperforate anus occurs in 1 in 5000 births, more commonly in males than females. Imperforate anus may include stenosis or atresia of anus. There are three main **categories**, classified according to relationship of rectum to puborectalis musculature:

- **Low anomalies:** No external opening, but rectum is otherwise in normal position through the puborectalis muscle, with normal function, and no connection to the genitourinary tract.
- **Intermediate anomalies:** Rectum is at or below the level of puborectalis muscle and an anal dimple is evident. The external sphincter is in normal position.
- **High anomalies:** Rectum ends above the puborectalis muscles, and internal sphincter is absent. Frequently, there is a rectourethral fistula in males or a rectovaginal fistula in females. There may be fistulas to the bladder or perineum.

Symptoms	Diagnosis	Treatment
Absence of anal opening: There is no meconium in 24-48 hours, abdominal distention, and vomiting. **Rectovaginal fistula or rectourethral fistula:** Symptoms may not be evident at first because stool passes through the fistula. **Fistula between the rectum and the bladder:** Gas or fecal material may be expelled per the urethra. **Displacement of the anus:** Chronic constipation develops over time.	Physical examination. Digital or endoscopic examination. Contrast radiography with the infant inverted and an opaque marker at the anal dimple will outline the location of a pouch in relation to the normal position of the anus.	Most forms of imperforate anus require treatment by surgery. The type depends on the extent of the abnormality: Simple excision of anal opening may suffice. 2-3 step procedures for higher anomalies in which a colostomy is first performed with later reconstruction of the anus in the proper position, involving anoplasty and pull through procedures. Manual dilation may treat stenosis.

Cystic Fibrosis

Cystic fibrosis (CF) is a genetic disease. It affects the respiratory, gastrointestinal, reproductive and cardiovascular systems. The body produces excess secretions that are thick; these secretions build up in the respiratory system, resulting in obstructions which contribute to respiratory infections, which lead to fibrosis and bronchiectasis.

- **Respiratory symptoms** include shortness of breath, cyanosis, wheezing, cough, atelectasis, emphysema, and chronic infections such as sinusitis, bronchitis, and pneumonia.
- **GI symptoms** include thick meconium trapped in the ileus at birth, rectal prolapse, stools that are fatty, loose, and frothy, big appetite while losing weight, vitamin deficiencies, and intestinal obstruction.
- **Reproductive problems** include delayed puberty and decreased fertility in females, and males are usually not fertile.
- **Cardiovascular issues** include the right side of the heart becoming enlarged and failing, blood sodium levels drop, and sodium and chloride are excreted in the sweat of the child (tastes excessively salty). A sweat test will show chloride levels greater than 60 mEq/L, the stool will have excess fat in it, and a chest x-ray will reveal atelectasis and obstructive emphysema.

Genitourinary Pathophysiology

URINARY INCONTINENCE

Urinary incontinence occurs more commonly in women than men and can range from an intermittent leaking of urine to a full loss of bladder control. Causes of urinary incontinence may include neurologic injury (including cerebral vascular accidents), infections, weakness of the muscles of the bladder, and certain medications, including diuretics, antihistamines, and antidepressants. **Stress incontinence** is defined as an involuntary leakage of urine with sneezing, coughing, laughing, lifting, or exercising. **Urge incontinence** is defined as an uncontrollable need to urinate on a frequent basis. **Total incontinence** is the full loss of bladder control.

Signs/symptoms: Urinary frequency and urgency may accompany the inability to control urine. If urinary incontinence is severe, incontinence-associated dermatitis may occur, predisposing the patient to skin breakdown and the development of pressure injuries.

Diagnosis: Physical assessment and presence of symptoms. Ultrasound, urinalysis, urodynamic testing, and cystoscopy may be used to determine the underlying cause.

Treatment: Treatment options are dependent on the type of urinary incontinence and the severity. Bladder training and pelvic muscle exercises may be utilized to strengthen muscles to control leakage of urine. In female patients with stress incontinence, a vaginal pessary may be inserted into the vagina to help support the bladder. Suburethral slings may also be surgically implanted to support the urethra. Anticholinergics, antispasmodics, and tricyclic antidepressants may also be used in the treatment of urinary incontinence.

HYDRONEPHROSIS

Hydronephrosis is a symptom of a disease involving swelling of the kidney pelvises and calyces because of an obstruction that causes urine to be retained in the kidney. In chronic conditions, symptoms may be delayed until severe kidney damage has occurred. Over time, the kidney begins to atrophy. The primary conditions that predispose to hydronephrosis include:

- Vesicoureteral reflux
- Obstruction at the ureteropelvic junction
- Renal edema (non-obstructive)
- Any condition that impairs drainage of the ureters can cause backup of the urine

Symptoms vary widely depending upon cause and whether the condition is acute or chronic.

- Acute episodes are usually characterized by flank pain, abnormal creatinine and electrolyte levels, and increased pH.
- The enlarged kidney may be palpable as a soft mass.

Treatment includes:

- Identifying the cause of obstruction and correcting it to ensure adequate drainage.
- A nephrostomy tube, ureteral stent or pyeloplasty may be done surgically in some cases.
- A urinary catheter may be inserted if there is outflow obstruction from the bladder.

RENAL AND URETERAL CALCULI

Renal and urinary calculi occur frequently, more commonly in males, and can relate to diseases (hyperparathyroidism, renal tubular acidosis, gout) and lifestyle factors, such as sedentary work. Calculi can form at any age, most composed of calcium, and can range in size from very tiny to larger than 6 mm. Those smaller than 4 mm can usually pass in the urine easily.

Diagnostic studies include clinical findings, UA, pregnancy test to rule out ectopic pregnancy, BUN and creatinine if indicated, ultrasound (for pregnant women and children), IV urography. Helical CT (non-contrast) is diagnostic.

Symptoms occur with obstruction and are usually of sudden onset and acute:

- Severe flank pain radiating to abdomen and ipsilateral testicle or labium majus, abdominal or pelvic pain (young children)
- Nausea and vomiting
- Diaphoresis
- Hematuria

Treatment includes:

- Instructions and equipment for straining urine
- Antibiotics if concurrent infection
- Extracorporeal shock-wave lithotripsy
- Surgical removal: percutaneous/standard nephrolithotomy
- Analgesia: opiates and NSAIDs

CHRONIC KIDNEY DISEASE

Chronic kidney disease (CKD) occurs when the kidneys are unable to filter and excrete wastes, concentrate urine, and maintain electrolyte balance because of hypoxic conditions, kidney disease, or obstruction in the urinary tract. It results first in azotemia (increase in nitrogenous waste in the blood) and then in uremia (nitrogenous wastes cause toxic symptoms). When >50% of the functional renal capacity is destroyed, the kidneys can no longer carry out necessary functions, and progressive deterioration begins over months or years. Symptoms are often non-specific in the beginning, with loss of appetite and energy.

Symptoms and complications are as follows:

- Weight loss
- Headaches, muscle cramping, general malaise
- Increased bruising and dry or itchy skin
- Increased BUN and creatinine
- Sodium and fluid retention with edema
- Hyperkalemia
- Metabolic acidosis
- Calcium and phosphorus depletion, resulting in altered bone metabolism, pain, and retarded growth
- Anemia with decreased production on RBCs. Increased risk of infection
- Uremic syndrome

Treatment includes:

- Supportive/symptomatic therapy
- Dialysis and transplantation
- Diet control: low protein, salt, potassium, and phosphorus
- Fluid limitations
- Calcium and vitamin supplementation
- Phosphate binders

UREMIC SYNDROME

Uremic syndrome is a number of disorders that can occur with end-stage renal disease and renal failure, usually after multiple metabolic failures and decrease in creatinine clearance to <10 mL/min. There is compromise of all normal functions of the kidney: fluid balance, electrolyte balance, acid-base homeostasis, hormone production, and elimination of wastes. Metabolic abnormalities related to uremia include:

- **Decreased RBC production**: The kidney is unable to produce adequate erythropoietin in the peritubular cells, resulting in anemia, which is usually normocytic and normochromic. Parathyroid hormone levels may increase, causing calcification of the bone marrow, causing hypoproliferative anemia as RBC production is suppressed.
- **Platelet abnormalities**: Decreased platelet count, increased turnover, and reduced adhesion leads to bleeding disorders.
- **Metabolic acidosis**: The tubular cells are unable to regulate acid-base metabolism, and phosphate, sulfuric, hippuric, and lactic acids increase, leading to congestive heart failure and weakness.
- **Hyperkalemia**: The nephrons cannot excrete adequate amounts of potassium. Some drugs, such as diuretics that spare potassium may aggravate the condition.
- **Renal bone disease**: Decreased calcium, elevated phosphate, elevated parathyroid hormone, decreased utilization of vitamin D lead to demineralization. In some cases, calcium and phosphate are deposited in other tissues (metastatic calcification).
- **Multiple endocrine disorders**: Thyroid hormone production is decreased and abnormalities in reproductive hormones may result in infertility/impotence. Males have decreased testosterone but elevated estrogen and LH. Females experience irregular cycles, lack of ovulation and menses. Insulin production may increase but with decreased clearance, resulting in episodes of hypoglycemia or decreased hyperglycemia in those who are diabetic.
- **Cardiovascular disorders**: Left ventricular hypertrophy is most common, but fluid retention may cause congestive heart failure and electrolyte imbalances, dysrhythmias. Pericarditis, exacerbation of valvular disorders, and pericardial effusions may occur.
- **Anorexia and malnutrition**: Nausea and poor appetite contribute to hypoalbuminemia, sometimes exacerbated by restrictive diets.

PYELONEPHRITIS

Pyelonephritis is a potentially organ-damaging bacterial infection of the parenchyma of the kidney. Pyelonephritis can result in abscess formation, sepsis, and kidney failure. Pyelonephritis is especially dangerous for those who are immunocompromised, pregnant, or diabetic. Most infections are caused by *Escherichia coli*. **Diagnostic studies** include urinalysis, and blood and urine cultures. Patients may require hospitalization or careful follow-up.

Symptoms vary widely but can include:

- Dysuria and frequency, hematuria, flank and/or low back pain
- Fever and chills
- Costovertebral angle tenderness
- Change in feeding habits (infants)
- Change in mental status (geriatric)
- Young women often exhibit symptoms more associated with lower urinary infection, so the condition may be overlooked.

Treatment includes:

- Analgesia
- Antipyretics
- Intravenous fluids

- Antibiotics: started but may be changed based on cultures
    - IV ceftriaxone with fluoroquinolone orally for 14 days
    - Monitor BUN. Normal 7–8 mg/dL (8–20 mg/dL >age 60). Increase indicates impaired renal function, as urea is end product of protein metabolism.

CYSTITIS

Cystitis is a common and often-chronic low-grade kidney infection that develops over time, so observing for symptoms of urinary infections and treating promptly are very important.

Changes in **character of urine**:

- **Appearance**: The urine may become cloudy from mucus or purulent material. Hematuria may be present.
- **Color**: Urine usually becomes concentrated and may be dark yellow/orange or brownish in color.
- **Odor**: Urine may have a very strong or foul odor.
- **Output**: Urinary output may decrease markedly.

Pain: There may be lower back or flank pain from inflammation of the kidneys.

Symptoms: Fever, chills, headache, and general malaise often accompany urine infections. Some people suffer a lack of appetite as well as nausea and vomiting. Fever usually indicates that the infection has affected the kidneys. Children may develop incontinence or loose stools and cry excessively.

Treatment:

- Increased fluid intake
- Antibiotics

NEPHROTOXIC AGENTS

Medications are a common cause of renal damage, especially among older patients. The **nephrotoxic effects** may be reversible if the drug is discontinued before permanent damage occurs. Those at increased risk include patients who are older than 60, have a history of renal insufficiency, suffer from volume depletion, or have diabetes mellitus, sepsis, or heart failure. Initial signs may be quite subtle. Preventive measures include baseline renal function tests and monitoring of renal function and vital signs during treatment. The following are some common effects, and the drugs that may cause them:

- **Chronic interstitial nephritis**: Acetaminophen, lithium, carmustine, cisplatin, cyclosporine.
- **Acute interstitial nephritis**: NSAIDs, acyclovir, beta-lactams, rifampin, quinolones, sulfonamides, vancomycin, indinavir, loop/thiazide diuretics, lansoprazole, allopurinol, phenytoin.
- **Rhabdomyolysis**: Amitriptyline, diphenhydramine, doxylamine, benzodiazepines, haloperidol, lithium, ketamine, methadone, methamphetamine, statins.
- **Crystal nephropathy**: Acyclovir, foscarnet, ganciclovir, quinolones, sulfonamides, indinavir, methotrexate, triamterene.
- **Tubular cell toxicity**: Aminoglycosides, amphotericin B, pentamidine, adefovir, tenofovir, contrast dye, zoledronate.
- **Thrombotic microangiopathy**: Cyclosporine, clopidogrel, mitomycin-C, quinine.
- **Impaired intraglomerular hemodynamics**: NSAIDs, cyclosporine, tacrolimus, ACE inhibitors.
- **Glomerulonephritis**: NSAIDs, lithium, beta-lactams, interferon-alpha, gold therapy, pamidronate.

PHIMOSIS AND PARAPHIMOSIS

Phimosis and paraphimosis are both restrictive disorders of the penis that occur in males who are uncircumcised or incorrectly circumcised. **Phimosis** is the inability to retract the foreskin proximal to the glans penis, sometimes resulting in urinary retention or hematuria. **Treatments** include:

- Dilating the foreskin with a hemostat (temporary solution)
- Circumcision
- Application of topical steroids (triamcinolone 0.025% twice daily) from end of foreskin to glans corona for 4–6 weeks

Paraphimosis occurs when the foreskin tightens above the glans penis and cannot be extended to normal positioning. This results in edema of the foreskin and circulatory impairment of the glans penis, sometimes progressing to gangrene, so immediate treatment is critical. **Symptoms** include pain, swelling, and inability to urinate. **Treatments** include:

- Compression of the glans to reduce edema (wrapping tightly with 2-inch elastic bandage for 5 minutes)
- Reducing edema by making several puncture wounds with 22- to 25-gauge needle
- Local anesthetic and dorsal incision to relieve pressure

TESTICULAR TORSION

Testicular torsion is a twisting of the spermatic cord within or below the inguinal canal, causing constriction of blood supply to the testis. Testicular torsion is most common at puberty but can occur at any age, sometimes precipitated by strenuous athletic participation or trauma, but it can also occur during sleep.

Symptoms include acute onset of severe testicular pain and edema, although children may present with nonspecific abdominal discomfort initially.

Diagnosis is based on clinical examination that demonstrates a firm scrotal mass. Color-flow duplex Doppler ultrasound may be helpful if diagnosis is not clear.

Treatment includes:

- **Manual detorsion** (usually 1.5 rotations) with elective surgical repair. Right testicle is usually rotated counterclockwise and left, clockwise. Reduction of pain should occur. If pain increases with rotation, then rotation should be done in the opposite direction.
- **Emergency surgical repair** (if manual detorsion not successful)

EPIDIDYMITIS AND ORCHITIS

Epididymitis, infection of the epididymis, is often associated with infection in a testis (epididymo-orchitis). In children, infection may be related to congenital anomalies that allow reflux of urine. In sexually active males 35 years or younger, it is usually related to STDs. In men older than 40, it is often related to urinary infections or benign prostatic hypertrophy with urethral obstruction.

Symptoms include progressive pain in lower abdomen, scrotum, and/or testicle. Late symptoms include large tender scrotal mass.

Diagnosis includes: Clinical examination. Pyuria. Urethral culture for STDs. Sonography.

Orchitis alone is rare but occurs with mumps, other viral infections, and epididymitis. Ultrasound may be needed to rule out testicular torsion.

Treatment for both conditions depends upon the cause, but epididymitis usually resolves with antibiotics:

- Younger than 40, associated with STDs:
  - Ceftriaxone 500 mg IM and doxycycline 100 mg twice daily for 10 days
- Older than 35, associated with other bacteria:
  - Levofloxacin 500 mg daily for 10–14 days
  - TMP/SMS DS twice daily for 10–14 days

PROSTATITIS

Prostatitis is an acute infection of the prostate gland, commonly caused by *Escherichia coli, Pseudomonas aeruginosa, Staphylococcus aureus,* or other bacteria. *Symptoms* include fever, chills, lower back pain, urinary frequency, dysuria, painful ejaculation, and perineal discomfort. PSA will often be elevated in this patient population, unrelated to prostate cancer. *Diagnosis* is based on clinical findings of perineal tenderness and spasm of rectal sphincter. *Treatments* include Ciprofloxacin 500 mg orally twice daily for 1 month **or** TMP/SMX DS twice daily for 1 month. Most patients also have a urethral culture to check for STDs. Patients with suspected bacteremia should be admitted for monitoring.

BENIGN PROSTATIC HYPERTROPHY

Benign prostatic hypertrophy/hyperplasia usually develops after age 40. The prostate may slowly enlarge, but the surrounding tissue restrains outward growth, so the gland compresses the urethra. The bladder wall also goes through changes, becoming thicker and irritated, so that it begins to spasm, causing frequent urinations. The bladder muscle eventually weakens and the bladder fails to empty completely.

Symptoms include urgency, dribbling, frequency, nocturia, incontinence, retention, and bladder distention.

Diagnosis may include IVP, cystogram, and PSA.

Treatment includes: Catheterization for urinary retention/bladder distention. Surgical excision. Avoid fluids close to bedtime, double void, avoid caffeine and alcohol, alpha-adrenergic antagonists, and 5-alpha-reductase inhibitors.

PID

Pelvic inflammatory disease (PID) comprises infections of the upper reproductive system, often ascending from vagina and cervix, and includes salpingitis, endometritis, tubo-ovarian abscess, peritonitis, and perihepatitis. *Neisseria gonorrhoeae* and *Chlamydia trachomatis* are implicated in most cases but some infections are polymicrobial. Complications include increase in ectopic pregnancy and tubal factor infertility. *Symptoms* include lower abdominal pain, vaginal pain, discharge, or bleeding, dyspareunia, dysuria, fever, and nausea and vomiting.

Diagnostic studies include:

- Pregnancy test
- Vaginal secretion testing, endocervical culture
- CBC
- Syphilis, HIV, and hepatitis testing
- Transvaginal pelvic ultrasound
- Endometrial biopsy
- Laparoscopy for definitive diagnosis

Treatments include:

- Broad spectrum antibiotics:
  - (Inpatient) Cefotetan 2 g IV every 12 hours or cefoxitin 2 g IV every 6 hours with doxycycline 100 mg every 12 hours
  - (Outpatient) Ceftriaxone 250 mg IM x 1 dose with doxycycline 100 mg orally every 12 hours for 14 days with metronidazole 500 mg twice daily for 2 weeks for patients who had gynecological procedures recently
- Laparoscopy to drain abscesses if symptoms do not improve in 72 hours or less
- Treatment specific to associated disorders (such as HIV or hepatitis)

VULVOVAGINITIS

Vulvovaginitis is inflammation of vulvar and vaginal tissues:

- **Bacterial vaginosis** (Gardnerella vaginalis or other bacteria)
- **Fungal infections** (usually Candida albicans)
- **Parasitic infections** (Trichomonas vaginalis)
- **Allergic contact vaginitis** (from soaps or other irritants)
- **Atrophic vaginitis** (postmenopause)

Symptoms include vaginal odor, swelling, discharge, or bleeding, pain and discomfort, or severe itching (common with *C. albicans*).

Diagnostic studies include:

- Physical exam and culture of discharge, pH testing with nitrazine paper: Greater than 4.5 is typical of bacterial and trichomonas infections. Less than 4.5 is typical of fungal infections.

Treatment includes:

- **Bacterial infections**: Metronidazole 500 mg orally twice daily for 7 days AND Metronidazole 0.75% gel intravaginally twice daily for 5 days AND Clindamycin 2% cream intravaginally at bedtime for 7 days
- **Fungal infections**: Fluconazole 150 mg tablet in 1 dose OR vaginal creams, tablets, or suppositories, such as butoconazole 2% cream for 3 days or tioconazole 6.5% ointment for 1 dose
- **Parasitic (trichomonas)**: Metronidazole 2 g orally in 1 dose

OVARIAN CYSTS

Ovarian cysts can grow within or on the ovaries. When a normal monthly follicle continues to grow, this is known as a functional cyst, of which there are two types:

- A follicular cyst begins when the follicle doesn't rupture or release its egg, but continues to grow.
- A corpus luteum cyst develops when fluid accumulates inside the follicle after it releases its egg.

Functional cysts are usually harmless, rarely cause pain, and often resolve on their own within 2–3 months. Other types of ovarian cyst include the following:

- **Cystadenomas** form on the exterior of an ovary and may enlarge and cause pain.
- **Endometriomas** develop as a result of endometriosis, where some of the tissue attaches to the ovary and causes pain during menses and sexual activity.
- **Dermoid cysts**, also called teratomas, can contain tissue, such as skin or teeth, because they from embryonic cells. They may enlarge and cause pain but are rarely cancerous.

Polycystic ovaries have multiple cysts. Ovarian cysts may cause problems if they rupture or hemorrhage and if they twist or become infected. Presenting symptoms include **hypotension** and **hypovolemia** if hemorrhage occurs, pain (often acute) and tenderness in the lower abdomen on the affected side, lower back pain, dysuria, and weight gain.

Diagnostic studies include a pregnancy test to rule out ectopic pregnancy, ultrasound with Doppler flow.

Treatment depends upon the type of cyst and complications:

- Emergency surgery for torsion
- Antibiotics for infection
- Hormone therapy may be useful for endometrioma

BARTHOLIN CYSTS

The Bartholin glands are small glands located on both sides of the vagina in the lips of the *labia minora*. The glands help to lubricate the vulvar area. A Bartholin cyst occurs when a duct to one gland becomes obstructed, usually because of infection or trauma, resulting in swelling and formation of a cyst (usually 1–3 cm but may be much larger with infection). Bartholin cyst is most common in women in their 20s. Blockage may result from tumors as well, but usually in women older than 40.

Symptoms of a Bartholin cyst include:

- Palpable mass on one side of the vagina (usually painless)
- Pain and tenderness and increasing size of lesion if infection and abscess occurs

Treatment includes:

- Warm, moist compresses or sitz baths
- Antibiotics for infection
- Surgical incision and drainage may be necessary in some cases

URINARY TRACT INFECTION

A urinary tract infection (UTI) is an inflammation of the urethra, bladder, ureters and/or kidneys. If it only involves the lower tract, it is considered uncomplicated. A kidney infection (pyelonephritis) or recurrent infections can cause chronic problems. Usually caused by bacteria (mostly E. coli), UTIs occur mostly in girls, primarily between the ages of 2 and 6. The following can contribute to the development of a UTI:

- Obstructed flow of urine
- Reflux of urine
- Poor fluid intake
- Improper perineal cleansing
- Constipation
- Uncircumcised male
- Catheterization (indwelling)
- Antibiotic use
- Tight underwear
- Perineal infection
- Sexual activity
- Bubble baths

Babies may be irritable, have fever (or hypothermia), be jaundiced, have vomiting, diarrhea and a diaper rash, and poor feeding with weight loss. The older child may have urine that smells bad, blood in urine, frequency, urgency, burning with urination, and stomach pain; if involving the kidneys, the symptoms may include flank pain, fever, and chills.

DIAGNOSTIC TOOLS AND NURSING CARE

Diagnosis is assisted by a urinalysis (blood, protein, or pus in urine), visually assessing the urine (foul odor, cloudy, mucus), a urine culture (detect bacteria), ureteral catheterization, bladder washout or renography (determine where the infection is located), and/or renal ultrasound, IVP, and VCU (assess for structural abnormalities). The nurse should assess the urine appearance, color and odor. Take note of any symptoms the child is having. Give antibiotics as ordered. Use aseptic technique to avoid infection. The child should increase fluid intake, rest, take tub baths to help with burning pain, and take meds as prescribed for pain and fever.

BLADDER EXSTROPHY

Bladder exstrophy is eversion of the posterior wall of the bladder through the anterior wall of the bladder and through the lower abdominal wall with bladder and urethra exposed, a wide pubic arch, anterior displacement of the anus, renal disorders, and abnormalities of reproductive organs in both males and females. Symptoms include urinary and bowel problems related to specific anomalies. **Diagnosis** is by physical examination to assess abnormalities. Renal ultrasound is done to determine the number of kidneys and presence of hydroureteronephrosis.

Treatment is as follows:

First stage:

- **Primary closure of bladder**: No ostomy is necessary if done within 72 hours of birth. Procedures include ureteral stents and suprapubic urinary drainage.
- **Bilateral iliac ostomies**: Necessary after 72 hours because pelvic ring is not malleable.
- **Epispadias repair**: May be done in the first or second stage.

Second stage:

- **Epispadias repair**: Usually done between 6-12 months

Final stage:

- **Bladder neck reconstruction and reimplantation of ureters**
- **Permanent urinary diversion**: Required by 10-15% of individuals with bladder exstrophy

POSTERIOR URETHRAL VALVES

Posterior urethral valves are a urethral abnormality in males where urethral valves have narrow slit-like openings that impede flow and allow reverse flow, damaging urinary organs, which swell and become engorged with urine. 30% will develop long-term kidney failure. **Symptoms** vary, depending upon severity:

- Dysuria: Pain, weak stream, frequency
- Hematuria
- Urinary retention
- Incontinence
- Enlarged bladder palpable as abdominal mass
- Urinary infection (most common after 1 year of age)
- Possible sepsis, metabolic acidosis, and azotemia (increased blood levels of urea and other nitrogenous compounds)

Diagnosis includes the following:

- **Fetal ultrasound**
- **Voiding cystourethrogram (VCUG)**: Evaluate extent of valvular abnormality and other urinary defects
- **Endoscopy**: Examine inside of urinary tract/take tissue samples
- **Blood tests**: Assess kidney function and electrolytes

Treatment includes the following:

- **Medical management**: Supportive care, antibiotics, electrolytes, Foley catheter
- **Urinary diversion**: Usually closed after valve repair
- **Endoscopic ablation/resection**: Examine obstruction and remove valve leaflets

ENURESIS

Enuresis is repeated involuntary urinary incontinence in children old enough to have bladder control, usually about 5-6 years old. Diabetes and other disorders should be ruled out although 95% of enuresis cases are not associated with structural or neurological disorders. There are three **types**:

- **Primary**: The child has never been dry at night, and incontinence is associated with delay in maturation and small functional bladder rather than stress or psychiatric disorders.
- **Intermittent**: The child stays dry part of the time with episodes of incontinence at night.
- **Secondary**: The child has had long periods (6-12 months) staying dry and then is incontinent because of infection, stress, or a sleep disorder.

Treatment includes:

- Laboratory assessment and examination to rule out primary causes
- Fluid restriction
- Bladder training and enuresis alarms
- Imipramine (tricyclic antidepressant) is used with many children younger than 6 years of age but requires close monitoring
- Desmopressin nasal spray may be used for short-term control
- Support and acceptance

PRUNE BELLY (EAGLE-BARRETT) SYNDROME

Prune belly (Eagle-Barrett) syndrome is a group of abnormalities involving lack of developed abdominal muscles, undescended testicles, and urinary tract problems. Urinary abnormalities may include large, hypotonic bladder, dilated ureters, and prostatic urethra. Males comprise 96-99% of cases. It may include anomalies of the pulmonary, cardiac, skeletal, and GI tracts. **Symptoms** vary widely, frequently including cardio-pulmonary complications:

- **Prune-like appearance of abdomen** due to fetal abdominal distention. After birth, abdominal fluid is lost, and the abdomen develops a wrinkled "prune" appearance, noticeable because of undeveloped abdominal muscles.
- **Undescended testicles** bilaterally.
- **Urinary tract abnormalities** such as urinary infections, obstruction, and chronic renal failure.

Diagnosis is by physical examination, chest x-rays to evaluate pulmonary problems, renal ultrasound to evaluate kidneys, and voiding cystourethrogram (VCUG) to evaluate urinary defects.

Treatment: Monitor the condition and provide antibiotics, both therapeutic and prophylactic. Intermittent catheterization is needed.

Surgical repair to correct genitourinary defects varies according to abnormality. Procedures may include a vesicostomy, ureterostomy, or pyelostomy; reduction cystoplasty; urethroplasty; or abdominoplasty.

MEGAURETER

Megaureter is dilation of ureters from the normal 3-5 mm to more than 10 mm in diameter with or without obstruction and/or reflux from abnormality of ureters or secondary causes:

- **Primary obstruction**: At point where ureter joins bladder; can cause kidney damage
    - Refluxing: Backward flow of urine from bladder to ureters.
    - Non-obstructing/non-refluxing: Dilated ureters without blockage may resolve over time
    - Obstructed/ refluxing: Ureters continue to dilate with blockage
- **Secondary**: Ureters enlarge because of other conditions, such as neurogenic bladder

Symptoms include urinary tract infection, dysuria, back/flank pain, and fever.

Diagnosis is by:

- Fetal ultrasound: in utero diagnosis
- Ultrasound: To evaluate appearance of the urinary tract
- Voiding cystourethrogram (VCUG): To check for reflux
- Diuretic renal scan: To check for obstruction
- Intravenous pyelogram: To view the urinary system

Treatment includes:

- Antibiotic prophylaxis until surgery
- Ureteral implantation: Trimming the widened portion of the ureter, removing the obstruction, and reattaching

URETEROPELVIC JUNCTION OBSTRUCTION

Ureteropelvic junction (UPJ) obstruction is congenital obstruction at the point where the ureter connects to the renal pelvis, unilaterally or bilaterally, causing inadequate urinary flow and hydronephrosis. Some children improve markedly within first 18 months, but others require surgery.

Symptoms include:

- Urinary tract infections
- Abdominal or flank pain
- Palpable mass from hydronephrosis
- Vomiting

Diagnosis is by:

- Fetal ultrasound: For in utero diagnosis
- Renal ultrasound: To show dilation of renal pelvis
- Intravenous pyelogram (IVP): To identify obstruction
- Renal isotope scan: To evaluate and measure kidney function

Treatment includes:

- Fetal urinary diversion: Remains controversial
- Pyeloplasty: Open surgical procedure where ureteropelvic junction is excised and the ureter is reattached to the renal pelvis with wide junction, allowing adequate drainage
- Laparoscopic pyeloplasty: Through the abdominal wall and abdominal cavity with internal excision of ureteropelvic junction
- Insertion of wire through ureter: To cut the ureteropelvic junction from inside with a ureteral drain left in place for a few weeks

NEUROGENIC BLADDER

Neurogenic bladder is bladder dysfunction from lesions in the peripheral or central nervous system that are related to traumatic or congenital etiologies or that developed from cerebrovascular accident or diabetic neuropathy. Nerve damage can cause an under-active bladder that is unable to contract to effectively empty or an overactive bladder that contracts frequently and ineffectually.

Symptoms include:

- Underactive: Incontinence, dribbling, straining or inability to urinate, retention
- Overactive: Frequency, urgency, dysuria, urinary tract infection, fever

Diagnosis is by:

- Neurological testing (x-rays, MRI, and EEGs): To determine etiology
- 24-hour urine collection: To determine volume and urine patterns
- Bladder stress test: To determine reaction to full bladder while bending over, coughing, walking, or doing other activities

Treatment includes:

- Antibiotics: To control infections
- Clean intermittent catheterization (CIC): To empty bladder
- Endoscopy: Combined with cutting of external sphincter or injecting sphincter with paralytic agents to allow urination
- Surgical repair: Placing of permanent stents at bladder neck, bladder augmentation to increase bladder size, repair of vesicoureteral reflux, or urinary diversion

VESICOURETERAL REFLUX

Vesicoureteral reflux is an abnormality where urine flows from the bladder back up the ureters. Reflux is graded on the international scale of 1 to 5, depending upon degree of dilation of the ureters and renal pelvis.

- **Primary**: Congenital defect with impaired valve where ureter opens to bladder. The ureter may be too short so the valve doesn't close properly.
- **Secondary**: Caused by infection or other cause of obstruction

Symptoms include:

- Neonates: Fever, irritability, lethargy, emesis
- Older infants, children: Abdominal pain, emesis, diarrhea, fever, dysuria with enuresis, frequency, urgency, cloudy/foul urine
- Late symptoms: Hypertension, dysuria with difficulty urinating, proteinuria, chronic renal insufficiency

Diagnosis is by:

- Ultrasound: Evaluate appearance of urinary system
- Voiding cystourethrogram (VCUG): Identify reflux (after infection has cleared)
- Intravenous pyelogram: Reveal obstructions
- Nuclear scans: Show urinary functioning
- Cystoscopy: View bladder interior

Treatment includes:

- Antibiotics: For infection
- Surgical repair or reconstruction: Usually involves severing ureter from bladder and reattaching at a different angle to prevent reflux

RENAL TRAUMA

Most renal trauma in children is the result of blunt trauma associated with motor vehicle accidents, falls, sports injuries, and child abuse, although gunshot wounds and stabbings also occur with increasing frequency. Various staging systems are used, but overall injuries are **graded by severity**:

- Grade A: Contusion of cortex with fracture (tear) of small confined area
- Grade B: Major fracture with peri-renal hematoma and/or extravasation of urine
- Grade C: Multiple fractures with extensive bleeding
- Grade D: Severe vascular disruption decreasing perfusion of kidney

Kidney injuries are often accompanied by other trauma (75%) so **symptoms** may be complex:

- Pain in abdominal or flank area
- Hematuria
- Abrasions or contusions in flank or abdominal area
- Shock
- Delayed symptoms include hypertension, hydronephrosis

Treatment includes:

- Treatment is usually non-operative if the child is hemodynamically stable, based on evaluation by CT, especially for blunt trauma.
- Bed rest is required.

POLYCYSTIC KIDNEY DISEASE

Polycystic kidney disease (PK) is caused by renal cysts (fluid-filled sacs in renal tissue), which may be genetic or acquired. The cysts develop from nephrons and can cause gross enlargement of kidneys. Cysts may be single or multiple (polycystic) and may involve one or both kidneys. PK is often associated with cystic disease in other organs as well.

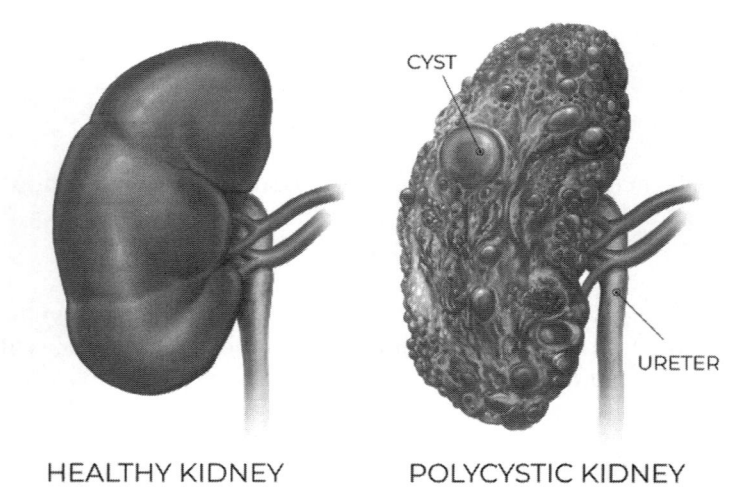

HEALTHY KIDNEY   POLYCYSTIC KIDNEY

There are three **types** of PK:

- **Autosomal dominant** is the most common (90%), but symptoms are usually delayed until adulthood although they can occur in childhood. However, it may progress to ESRD over time. Symptoms include urinary and cyst infections, rupture of cysts with hematuria, hypertension, and renal calculi.
- **Autosomal recessive** is rarer and symptoms arise much earlier, sometimes in the fetus.
- **Acquired** usually does not affect children because it develops from long-term kidney disease or dialysis.

Treatment cannot cure but can delay effects:

- Antihypertensives
- Antibiotics for infections
- Analgesia
- Growth hormone (autosomal recessive)
- Long-term: dialysis and transplantation

OBSTRUCTIVE UROPATHY WITH NEPHROSIS

Obstructive uropathy with nephrosis may present with a variety of **symptoms** depending upon the underlying cause, but most include:

- Pain in flank area
- Recurrent urinary infections with associated pain and fever
- Dysuria decreased urinary output, foul urine, and/or hematuria
- Edema
- Renal failure

Sometimes obstructions will resolve over time and may not constitute medical emergencies, especially if only one side is involved. However, if blockage is causing severe symptoms or does not resolve, various **treatments** may be used:

- Prenatal shunts may be done if the condition is identified through ultrasound. The procedure carries risk, so it is done primarily if the life of the fetus is threatened.
- A ureteral/urethral stent may be inserted to maintain patency of ureter.
- Urinary diversions, such as ileal conduit or cutaneous ureterostomy may be indicated in cases of severe obstruction, especially those associated with congenital abnormalities.
- Antibiotics are given for infections.

PERSISTENT CLOACA

Persistent cloaca is a condition in females with an imperforate anus and the rectum, vagina, and urethra forming a single channel with a rectal fistula attached to the posterior wall of the channel. **Diagnosis** is made with a physical exam showing a single perineal opening. An abdominal mass (hydrocolpos—distended bladder) may occur. A voiding cystourethrogram (VCUG) will show bladder abnormalities if catheterization is possible.

Treatment includes the following:

- **Colostomy**: Fecal diversion in neonate prevents fecal material from entering urinary system and causing infection.
- **Decompression of vagina**: Prevents infection and scarring and relieves obstruction of urinary tract.
- **Posterior sagittal anorectovagino-urethroplasty (PSARVUP)**: (Usually two months after colostomy.) The rectum is separated from the vagina, and the vagina is separated from the urethra. The urethra is reconstructed, the vagina is reconstructed, and the rectum is reconstructed with anoplasty
- **Postoperative anal dilation**: Two weeks after surgery until the final size is reached
- **Cystoscopy/vaginoscopy**: Checks for urethrovaginal fistula
- **Colostomy removal**: Anastomosis of colon and rectum and colostomy is removed

ADOLESCENT MENSTRUAL DISORDERS

Menarche occurs between 9-15 years of age in most girls, preceded by development of secondary sexual characteristics. The usual menstrual cycle is every 21-35 days, lasting 2-7 days with blood loss of 35-150 mL per monthly cycle. **Menstrual disorders** may cause considerable discomfort:

- **Dysmenorrhea** is pain associated with menses, usually 6-24 months after menarche. Pain usually lasts about 2 days and is accompanied by mild to severe cramping in the supra-pubic area, lumbar back, and labia. **Treatment** includes:
    - NSAIDs (ibuprofen) 400-900 mg up to 4 times daily
    - Naproxen 250-500 mg every 6-12 hours
- **Endometriosis** occurs when endometrial tissue outside of the pelvic area irritates nerve endings and causes severe pain and uterine cramping during periods, usually preceded by a few days of increasing dysmenorrhea. **Treatment** consists of the following:
    - Referral to gynecologist
    - NSAIDs
    - Oral contraceptives to reduce shedding
    - Gonadotropin-releasing hormone to reduce estrogen and androgen levels
    - Laparoscopy to remove extrauterine endometrial tissue.
- **Dysfunctional uterine bleeding** results from an abnormality in hormones so that shedding of the endometrium is irregular, resulting in excessive bleeding or irregular periods. **Treatment** includes:
    - Hgb >12: NSAIDs with iron supplementation
    - Hgb 10-12 add folic acid supplement
    - Hgb <10 may require hospitalization or referral to gynecologist
- **Mittelschmerz** is pain in the middle of the menstrual cycle, usually dull in the lower abdomen and lasting for minutes to hours, and probably related to enlargement of follicle before rupture. **Treatment** includes the following:
    - Heating pad may relieve discomfort
    - NSAIDs
- **Amenorrhea** may be primary (absence at ≤16 years old) with normal pubertal development (within 3 years) or with no pubertal development. It may also be secondary (no periods for 3 cycles or 6 months), related to excessive exercise or dieting. Primary and secondary amenorrhea requires testing to determine if there are abnormalities in hormones, genetic disorders, obstructive disorders, or other causes. **Treatment** depends on the underlying cause.

Hematologic Pathophysiology

ANEMIA

Anemia occurs when there is an insufficient number of red blood cells to sufficiently oxygenate the body. As a result of the decreased level of oxygen being supplied to the organs, the body will attempt to compensate by increasing cardiac output and redistributing blood to the brain and heart. In return, the blood supply to the skin, abdominal organs, and kidneys is decreased. Anemia can occur from blood loss, increased destruction of red blood cells (hemolytic anemia), or as a result of a decreased production in red blood cells.

Signs/symptoms: Pallor, fatigue, hypotension, weakness, and mental status changes. As perfusion decreases and the body attempts to compensate for the lack of oxygenation, tachycardia, chest pain, and shortness of breath may occur. In hemolytic anemias, jaundice and splenomegaly may occur as the result of the breakdown of red blood cells and the excretion of bilirubin.

Diagnosis: A complete blood count, reticulocyte count, and iron studies may be used to diagnose anemia.

Treatment: The treatment of anemia is focused on treating the underlying cause. Parenteral iron may be given for patients with iron deficiency anemias caused from chronic blood loss, or inadequate iron intake or absorption. Blood transfusions are used to treat patients with active bleeding as well as those patients who are displaying significant clinical symptoms. Erythropoietin stimulating proteins may also be utilized to decrease the need for a transfusion.

SICKLE CELL DISEASE

Sickle cell disease is a recessive genetic disorder of chromosome 11, causing hemoglobin to be defective so that red blood cells (RBCs) are sickle-shaped and inflexible, resulting in their accumulating in small vessels and causing painful blockage. While normal RBCs survive 120 days, sickled cells may survive only 10–20 days, stressing the bone marrow that cannot produce fast enough and resulting in severe anemia. There are 5 variations of sickle cell disease, with sickle cell anemia the most severe. Different types of crises occur (aplastic, hemolytic, vaso-occlusive, and sequestrating), which can cause infarctions in organs, severe pain, damage to organs, and rapid enlargement of liver and spleen. Complications include anemia, acute chest syndrome, congestive heart failure, strokes, delayed growth, infections, pulmonary hypertension, liver and kidney disorders, retinopathy, seizures, and osteonecrosis. Sickle cell disease occurs almost exclusively in African Americans in the United States, with 8–10% carriers.

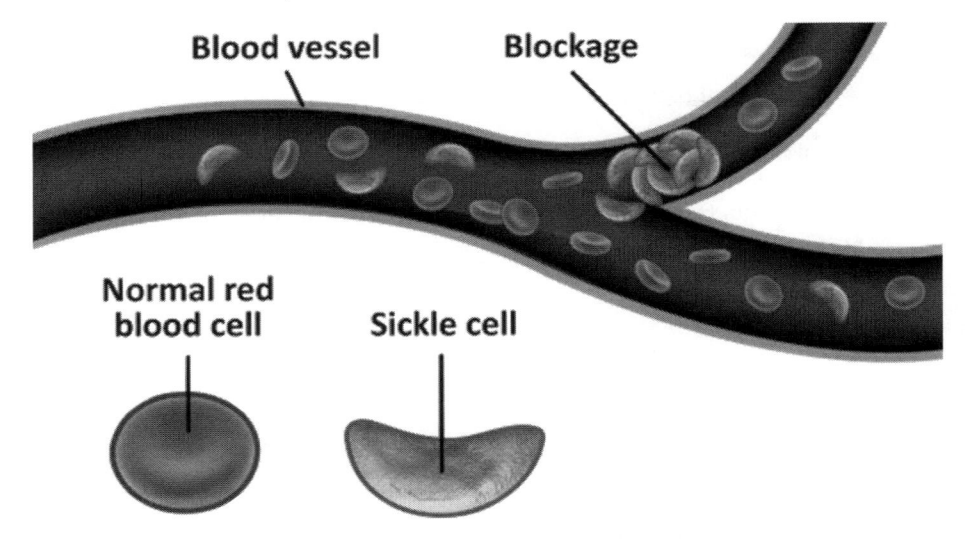

Review Video: Sickle Cell Disease
Visit mometrix.com/academy and enter code: 603869

TREATMENT

Treatment for sickle cell disease includes:

- **Prophylactic penicillin** for children from 2 months to 5 years to prevent pneumonia
- **Hydroxyurea** for long-term management of sickle cell disease in individuals ages 6 months and older. This medication has been shown to decrease the complications from sickle cell disease, increase life expectancy, and improve overall quality of life.
- **IV fluids** to prevent dehydration
- **Analgesics** (morphine) during painful crises
- **Folic acid** for anemia
- **Oxygen** for congestive heart failure or pulmonary disease
- **Blood transfusions** with chelation therapy to remove excess iron OR erythropheresis, in which red cells are removed and replaced with healthy cells, either autologous or from a donor
- **Hematopoietic stem cells transplantation** is the only curative treatment, but immunosuppressive drugs must be used and success rates are only about 85%, so the procedure is only used on those at high risk. It requires ablation of bone marrow, placing the patient at increased risk.
- **Partial chimerism** uses a mixture of the donor and the recipient's bone marrow stem cells and does not require ablation of bone marrow. It is showing good success.

THROMBOCYTOPENIA

Thrombocytopenia is a deficiency of circulating platelets in the blood. It can be caused by a decrease in the production of platelets from the bone marrow or an increase in destruction of platelets. Thrombocytopenia may also be caused from the use of heparin. Heparin induced thrombocytopenia can occur after heparin therapy (average 4–14 days post therapy) and is characterized by a decrease in platelet count to less than 50% of baseline or the occurrence of an unexplained thrombolytic event. A decreased production of platelets within the bone marrow can occur as a result of malignancy, bone marrow failure, infection, alcohol abuse, or a nutritional deficiency. An increase in the destruction of platelets may occur in disseminated intravascular coagulation, vasculitis, thrombotic thrombocytopenic purpura, sepsis, or idiopathic thrombocytopenic purpura.

Signs/symptoms: Petechiae, ecchymosis, bleeding from the mouth or gums, epistaxis, pallor, weakness, fatigue, splenomegaly, blood in the urine or stool, and jaundice.

Diagnosis: Physical exam and lab studies including complete blood count, partial thromboplastin time and prothrombin time may be used to diagnosis thrombocytopenia. A bone marrow biopsy may be indicated to determine the cause of the decreased production of platelets.

Treatment: Treatment of thrombocytopenia involves identifying and treating the underlying cause. Medications that decrease the platelet count should be held. Platelet transfusions may be administered to patients with extremely low counts (less than 50,000) or if spontaneous bleeding occurs. Platelet transfusions are contraindicated in patients with thrombotic thrombocytopenia purpura.

ITP

The autoimmune disorder **idiopathic thrombocytopenic purpura (ITP)** causes an immune response to platelets, resulting in decreased platelet counts. ITP affects primarily children and young women although it can occur at any age. The acute form primarily occurs in children, but the chronic form affects primarily adults. Platelet counts are usually 150,000–400,000 per mcL. With ITP, platelet levels are less than 100,000. Maintaining a platelet count of at least 30,000 is necessary to prevent intracranial hemorrhage, the primary concern. The cause of ITP is unclear and may be precipitated by viral infection, sulfa drugs, and conditions, such as lupus erythematosus. ITP is usually not life threatening and can be controlled. **Symptoms** include:

- Bruising and petechiae with hematoma in some cases
- Epistaxis
- Increased menstrual flow in post-puberty females

Treatment includes:

- Corticosteroids to depress immune response and increase platelet count
- Splenectomy may be indicated for chronic conditions
- Platelet transfusions
- Avoiding aspirin, ibuprofen, or other NSAIDs

HITTS

Heparin-induced thrombocytopenia and thrombosis syndrome (HITTS) occurs in patients receiving heparin for anticoagulation. There are two types:

- **Type I** is a transient condition occurring within a few days and causing depletion of platelets (<100,000 mm³), but heparin may be continued as the condition usually resolves without intervention.
- **Type II** is an autoimmune reaction to heparin that occurs in 3–5% of those receiving unfractionated heparin and also occurs with low-molecular-weight heparin. It is characterized by low platelets (<50,000 mm³) that are ≥50% below baseline. Onset is 5–14 days but can occur within hours of heparinization. Death rates are <30%. Heparin-antibody complexes form and release platelet factor 4 (PF4), which attracts heparin molecules and adheres to platelets and endothelial lining, stimulating thrombin and platelet clumping. This puts the patient at risk for thrombosis and vessel occlusion rather than hemorrhage, causing stroke, myocardial infarction, and limb ischemia with symptoms associated with the site of thrombosis. Treatment includes:
    - Discontinuation of heparin
    - Direct thrombin inhibitors (lepirudin, argatroban)
    - Monitor for signs/symptoms of thrombus/embolus

THALASSEMIA

Thalassemia refers to a group of inherited blood disorders in which hemoglobin production is increased, resulting in destruction of RBCs. **Thalassemia minor** usually produces no symptoms and results in slight anemia. **Thalassemia major** produces symptoms starting at about 6 months of age, such as anemia, fever, loss of appetite and weight, and enlarged spleen. These symptoms are followed by hypoxia, damage to some major organs, jaundice, slow growth, thickened cranial bones and delayed sexual maturation. Over time, complications can include skeletal deformities of the face and head, fractures, splenomegaly, heart problems, enlarged liver and cirrhosis, gallstones, jaundice, growth delays and endocrine system abnormalities (diabetes). Hgb and Hct will be decreased. A complete blood count will show small red blood cells with varying sizes and shapes, spotted staining, nonspecific enlarged RBCs, and decreased reticulocytes.

Hyperbilirubinemia

Hyperbilirubinemia, excess of bilirubin in the blood, is characterized by jaundice. There are four basic types:

- **Physiologic**: Common in newborns and usually benign, resulting from immature hepatic function and increased RBC hemolysis. Onset is usually within 24–48 hours, peaking in 72 hours and declining within a week. Phototherapy is the indicated treatment.
- **Breast-feeding associated**: Relates to inadequate calories during early breast-feeding with onset in the first 2–3 days. More frequent feeding with caloric supplements is usually sufficient, but phototherapy may be used for bilirubin 18–20 mg/dL.
- **Breast milk jaundice**: May result from breast milk breaking down bilirubin and its being reabsorbed in the gut. Jaundice is characterized by less frequent stools and onset in the 4th or 5th day, peaking in 10–15 days, but it may persist for a number of weeks. Treatment involves discontinuing breastfeeding for 24 hours.
- **Hemolytic**: Caused by blood/antigen (Rh) incompatibility with onset in the first 24 hours. Preventive treatment is RhoGAM prenatally or post-natal exchange transfusion.

SCID

Severe combined immunodeficiency (SCID) ("bubble boy disorder") is a genetic disorder characterized by dysfunction of one or both of the T- and B-lymphocytes, essentially crippling the immune system so that the child has no immune response to pathogenic microorganisms. Many different molecular variations occur, but all have the lack of antibody formation. The disorder may be X-linked (50%) or autosomal recessive. Onset of **symptoms** is usually within the first 2 months of life and includes:

- Severe infection, especially pneumonia or sepsis from bacterial, herpetic, or fungal infections with associated fever, tachypnea, dyspnea, tachycardia
- Marked failure to thrive with retarded growth
- Chronic diarrhea and dehydration
- Fever, tachypnea

Without diagnosis and treatment, most children will die before 2 years of age.

Treatment:

- Prophylactic antibiotics: often trimethoprim-sulfamethoxazole (Bactrim)
- Bone marrow/stem cell transplant
- Intravenous immunoglobulin replacement therapy (if B cells fail to graft)
- Gene therapy (experimental)

Immunologic Pathophysiology

IMMUNE DEFICIENCIES

There are multiple disorders that fall into the category of **primary immunodeficiency diseases.** These disorders are genetic or inherited disorders in which the body's immune system does not function properly. These disorders may involve low levels of antibodies, defects in the antibodies, or defects in cells that make up the immune system (T-cells, B-cells). Common variable immune deficiency is a common immune deficiency diagnosed in adulthood. This disorder is characterized by low levels of serum immunoglobins and antibodies, which substantially increases the risk of infection.

- **Signs/symptoms**: Recurrent infections are the hallmark sign of immune deficiency disorders. Recurrent infections most often involve the ears, sinuses, bronchi, and lungs. Lymphadenopathy may occur as well as splenomegaly. GI symptoms may include abdominal pain, nausea, vomiting, diarrhea, and weight loss. Some patients may experience polyarthritis. Granulomas are also common and may occur in the lungs, lymph nodes, liver, and skin.
- **Diagnosis**: A physical assessment and patient history are used to diagnose immune deficiency disorders. Since immune deficiency disorders are genetic or inherited, family history should also be evaluated. Lab tests such as serum antibodies, serum immunoglobin levels and a complete blood count may also be used to assist in the diagnosis of immune deficiency disorders.
- **Treatment**: Patients with immune deficiency disorders often receive immunoglobulin replacement. Long term antibiotics may also be administered for recurrent infections. Educate patients to frequently wash hands, cook foods thoroughly, avoid large crowds, and other infection prevention techniques.

CONGENITAL IMMUNODEFICIENCIES

Congenital immunodeficiencies include:

- **Common variable immunodeficiency** is primarily an IgG deficiency due to absent plasma cells and B cell differentiation. These patients have increased susceptibility to encapsulated organisms and are more likely to develop bronchiectasis from the recurrent damage. They are also at higher risk for B cell neoplasms, GI malignancy, and autoimmune disease. Test is with functional antibody response and treatment with IVIG.
- **Congenital Agammaglobulinemia** (Bruton's, x-linked) usually leads to a susceptibility to recurrent pyogenic infections and low IgG and no IgA, IgM, IgE, IgD, or B cells.
- **Selective IgA deficiency** is the most common Ig deficiency and leads to recurrent sinopulmonary infections. It has association with recurrent giardiasis, GI malignancy, and autoimmune disorders, including celiac sprue. One should withhold IVIG due to possible anaphylactic reaction to IgA.
- **Wiskott-Aldrich syndrome** is the combination of thrombocytopenia, eczema, and immunodeficiency. It has associated low IgM and elevated IgA and IgE. BMT treats this successfully.

COMPLEMENT DEFICIENCIES

There are deficiencies of all parts of the complement pathway, including the following:

- **Classical deficiency** may include C1 (q, r, s), C2, and C4. This leads to immune complex syndromes and pyogenic infection, such as recurrent sinopulmonary infections with encapsulated bacteria. There is an association with SLE and other rheumatoid diseases. C2 is the most common deficiency in Caucasians in the US.
- **C3 and alternative complement deficiency** may lead to immune complex syndromes and recurrent infections, such as severe pyogenic infections. It may also be associated with HUS.
- **Membrane attack complex (MAC) deficiency** is also known as terminal complement deficiency. This is associated with recurrent Neisseria infections (which can cause meningitis and sepsis) and immune complex diseases. The CH50 assay must be checked to determine the activity of the classical pathway. CH50 may also be used to follow disease activity in SLE.

Autoimmune System Disorders

Allergic interstitial/tubulointerstitial nephritis is inflammation and edema of the interstitial areas of the kidneys. Up to 92% of cases caused by allergic reaction to medications, such as antibiotics (B-lactams, fluoroquinolones, macrolides, and anti-tuberculin drugs), antivirals, NSAIDs, PPIs, antiepileptics, diuretics, chemotherapy, and allopurinol. **Symptoms** include fever, rash, and renal enlargement as well as fatigue, nausea, vomiting, and weight loss. **Diagnosis** is by renal biopsy. Urine tests may show eosinophils, blood, RBC casts and sterile pyuria. Increased protein may be seen in response to NSAIDs. **Treatment** is primarily supportive but requires stopping the triggering medication.

Eosinophilic esophagitis is the accumulation of eosinophils in the esophagus, resulting in chronic inflammation. Damage from proteins produced in esophageal tissue causes scarring and narrowing, resulting in dysphagia, vomiting, choking, GERD, upper abdominal pain, heartburn, and regurgitation. **Causes** include allergic reaction to pollens or foods. **Risk factors** include cold/dry climate, male gender, family history, allergies, and asthma. **Diagnosis** is per endoscopy with biopsy. Blood tests may help confirm allergic reactions. **Treatment** may include dietary limitations, PPIs, and topical steroids. Some may require dilation of the esophagus.

Churg-Strauss syndrome (AKA **eosinophilic granulomatosis with polyangiitis**) is an idiopathic form of pulmonary vasculitis that can affect multiple systems (skin and lungs most often) as well as affecting small- and medium-sized arteries in those with asthma. **Symptoms** include dyspnea, chest pain, skin rash, myopathy, arthropathy, rhinitis, sinusitis, abdominal pain, blood in stools, and paresthesia (from the involvement of nerves). The syndrome is characterized by eosinophilia >1500 cells/mcL or >10% of peripheral total WBC count. X-rays or CTs may show transient opacities or multiple nodules. Tissue biopsies typically show allergic granulomas. **Treatment** usually begins with corticosteroids but other immunosuppressive drugs (cyclophosphamide, methotrexate, azathioprine) may be used, especially if critical organs are involved. The goal of treatment is remission, but patients usually need to take drugs at least 2 years before they are tapered off of the drugs. Up to 50% of patients have relapses.

Neutropenia

Neutropenia is identified as a **polymorphonuclear neutrophil count** equal to or less than 500/mL. **Chronic neutropenia** is a sustained condition of minimal neutrophils lasting 3 or more months. Neutropenia may occur from a decreased production of **white blood cells** (e.g., from chemotherapy or radiation therapy). It may also occur from a loss of white blood cells from autoimmune disease processes. Neutropenia is silent but dangerous. It leaves essentially no neutrophils to fight any threat of infection. Neutrophils make up as much as 70% of the white blood cells circulating in the blood. Neutropenia can be the cause of a septic situation, which can be life-threatening. Up to 70% of patients experiencing a fever while in a neutropenic state will die within 48 hours if not treated aggressively.

Leukopenia

Leukopenia is defined as a decrease in white blood cells. Neutropenia is defined as a low number of neutrophils and is often used interchangeably with the term leukopenia. With a decrease in the number of circulating white blood cells, the patient is at an increased risk for the development of an infection. Leukopenia and neutropenia can occur from either a decrease in the production of white blood cells or an increase in their destruction. Infections, malignancy, autoimmune disorders, medications (including chemotherapy) and a history of radiation therapy may contribute to the development of leukopenia/neutropenia.

Signs/symptoms: Malaise, fever, chills, night sweats, shortness of breath, headache, cough, abdominal pain, tachycardia, and hypotension. A patient with neutropenia/leukopenia is at risk for the development of infections including pneumonia, skin infections, urinary tract infections and gastrointestinal infections. In addition, the patient is at an increased risk for sepsis.

Diagnosis: Complete blood count including an absolute neutrophil count. In addition, a bone marrow biopsy may be performed to determine the cause of the decrease in neutrophils.

Treatment: Supportive therapy is used in the treatment of leukopenia including the aggressive treatment of infections that may develop. Precautions should be taken to protect the patient from additional infections, including strict adherence to sterile technique and infection control procedures. Hematopoietic growth factors may also be given to stimulate the production of neutrophils.

LYMPHEDEMA

Lymphedema results from untreated or incurable **edema**. It is a chronic condition marked by swelling and accumulated fluids within the tissue. This accumulation is a result of lymphatic drainage failure, inadequate lymph transport capacity, an increased lymph production, or a combination of these. Primary disease is a result of **inadequately developed lymphatic pathways**, while the secondary disease process is due to **damage outside of the pathways**. The process is worsened and complicated as **macrophages** are released to control inflammation caused by the increased release of fibroblasts and keratinocytes. There is a gradual increase in adipose tissue and leakage of lymph through the skin. The skin and tissues gradually thicken and change in color, texture, tone, and temperature. It begins to blister and produce hyperkeratosis, warts, papillomatosis, and elephantiasis. There is an ever-increasing risk of infection and further complications.

HIV/AIDS

AIDS is a progression of infection with **human immunodeficiency virus** (HIV). AIDS is diagnosed when the following criteria are met:

- HIV infection
- CD4 count less than 200 cells/mm^3
- AIDS defining condition, such as opportunistic infections (cytomegalovirus, tuberculosis), wasting syndrome, neoplasms (Kaposi sarcoma), or AIDS dementia complex

Because there is such a wide range of AIDS defining conditions, the patient may present with many types of **symptoms**, depending upon the diagnosis, but more than half of AIDS patients exhibit:

- Fever
- Lymphadenopathy
- Pharyngitis
- Rash
- Myalgia/arthralgia
- It is important to review the following:
    - CD4 counts to determine immune status
    - WBC and differential for signs of infection
    - Cultures to help identify any infective agents
    - CBC to evaluate for signs of bleeding or thrombocytopenia

Treatment aims to cure or manage opportunistic conditions and control underlying HIV infection through highly active anti-retroviral therapy (HAART), 3 or more drugs used concurrently.

Integumentary Pathophysiology

CELLULITIS

Cellulitis occurs when an area of the skin becomes infected, usually following injury or trauma to the skin. Cellulitis is most likely to be caused by staphylococcus or streptococcus bacteria. Patients with peripheral vascular disease, diabetes mellitus, and immunosuppression are at a higher risk for the development of cellulitis. **Signs and symptoms** include pain, erythema, and warmth at the affected site that progresses rapidly. In addition, the patient may experience fever, chills, fatigue, and malaise. **Diagnosis** is made by physical exam. Labs include complete blood count, culture of the involved area and blood. **Treatment** for cellulitis is the administration of antibiotics. Surgical irrigation and debridement may be indicated in severe cases.

EXTRAVASATION

Extravasation occurs when an intravenously infused vesicant medication or fluid leaks from the vein and into the subcutaneous space. Vesicant medications are those that cause tissue injury if extravasated and that may ultimately lead to tissue necrosis. Extravasation and infiltration are similar in nature, with infiltration occurring when the infusate is a non-vesicant solution or medication. Extravasation occurs more commonly in peripheral IVs; however, it can also occur with central venous catheters. Common vesicant agents include several chemotherapeutic agents, vancomycin, electrolytes, dobutamine, norepinephrine, phenytoin, promethazine, propofol, and vasopressin.

Signs/symptoms: Pain, burning, erythema, and edema at the site of the extravasation. Oftentimes, a blood return from the peripheral IV or central venous catheter is not present. Long term complications include complex regional pain syndrome, tissue necrosis, and nerve or tendon damage.

Diagnosis: Physical assessment and review of patient symptoms and medications/infusions administered.

Treatment: Early recognition is key to the successful treatment of an extravasation. When an extravasation is suspected, the IV infusion should be immediately stopped and the infusion site assessed. For some medications, antidotes may be available to minimize the damage caused by the extravasation. Heat or cold therapy may also be utilized depending on the medication. In cases of severe damage, debridement, skin grafting, and even amputation may result.

TISSUE DAMAGE RELATED TO ALLERGIC CONTACT DERMATITIS

Contact dermatitis is a localized response to contact with an allergen, resulting in a rash that may blister and itch. Common allergens include poison oak, poison ivy, latex, benzocaine, nickel, and preservatives, but there is a wide range of items, preparations, and products to which people may react.

Treatment includes:

- Identifying the causative agent through evaluating the area of the body affected, careful history, or skin patch testing to determine allergic responses
- Corticosteroids to control inflammation and itching
- Soothing oatmeal baths
- Pramoxine lotion to relieve itching
- Antihistamines to reduce allergic response
- Lesions should be gently cleansed and observed for signs of secondary infection
- Antibiotics are used only for secondary infections as indicated
- Rash is usually left open to dry
- Avoidance of allergen to prevent recurrence

PRESSURE INJURIES

Pressure injuries occur when pressure from the weight of the body causes a decrease in perfusion, affecting arterial and capillary blood flow and resulting in ischemia. These tissue injuries may then develop from pressure, shearing, and friction. Common pressure points include the occiput, scapula, sacrum, buttocks, ischium, and heels. Patients with a decreased level of consciousness, brain/spinal cord injuries, peripheral neuropathies, malnutrition, dehydration, PVD, or impaired mobility are at a higher risk for pressure-related injuries. Critically ill patients are at an increased risk due to prolonged immobility, sedation, and often incontinence of urine and stool. In addition, patients on vasopressors are at a higher risk due to the constriction of the peripheral circulation.

Signs/symptoms: Early stages include redness, tenderness, and firmness at the site of the injury. Once the injury progresses to severe tissue injury, bone, muscle, or tendons may be exposed, and there may be a yellow or black wound base in addition to pain and drainage at the site.

Diagnostics: Skin and wound assessment, including staging of the pressure injury.

Treatment: Wet-to-dry dressings, Wound VAC therapy, and hyperbaric oxygen may be used; a wound care consult is often advised.

Prevention: Begins with a risk assessment; the Braden scale is a commonly used scale. A score of 16 or below indicates that the patient is at risk. At-risk patients or patients with active pressure-related injuries should be placed on a turning and positioning schedule or on a specialty bed to relieve pressure. Moisture barriers and skin protectants may also be utilized.

NATIONAL PRESSURE INJURY ADVISORY PANEL STAGING

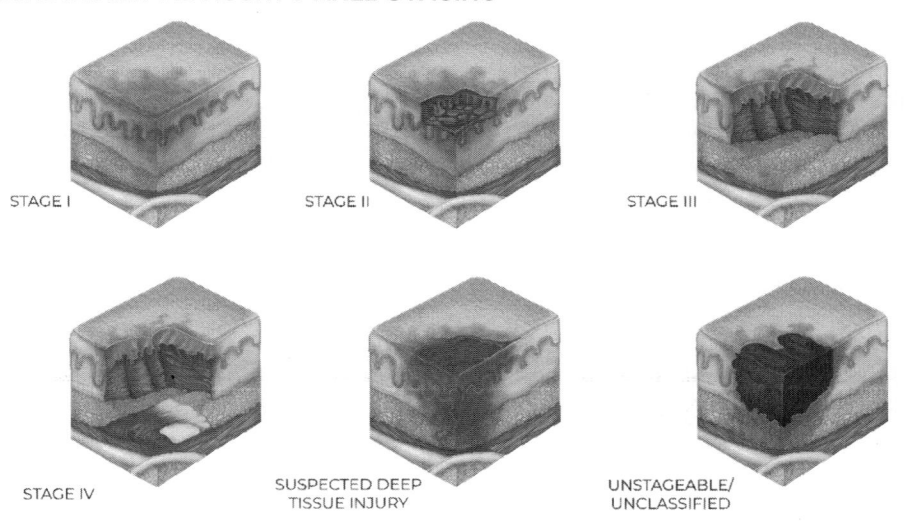

Pressure-related injuries result from pressure with or without shear and/or friction over bony prominences. The National Pressure Injury Advisory Panel developed a staging system to ensure that definitions for pressure injuries were standardized:

- **Suspected deep tissue injury**: Skin discolored, intact or blood blister
- **Stage I**: Intact skin with non-blanching reddened area
- **Stage II**: Abrasion or blistered area without slough but with partial-thickness skin loss
- **Stage III**: Deep tissue injury with exposed subcutaneous tissue; tunneling or undermining may be evident with or without slough or epibole (rolling inward of wound edge)
- **Stage IV**: Deep tissue injury, full thickness, with necrosis into muscle, bone, tendons, and/or joints
- **Unstageable**: Eschar and/or slough prevents staging prior to debridement

Patients should be placed on pressure-reducing support surfaces and turned at least every two hours, avoiding the area(s) with a pressure injury. Wound care depends on the stage of the wound and the amount of drainage but includes irrigation, debridement when necessary, antibiotics for infection, and appropriate dressing. Patients should be encouraged to have adequate protein and iron in their diets to promote healing and to maintain adequate hydration.

INFECTIOUS WOUNDS

All types of wounds have the potential to become infected. Infectious wounds are commonly health care acquired. Wound infections increase a patient's risk of sepsis, multisystem organ failure and death. Trauma patients are at an increased risk of developing an infected wound due to exposure to various contaminants that they may have encountered during their injury (e.g., dirt from a motor vehicle accident).

Signs/symptoms: Erythema, edema, induration, drainage, increasing pain and tenderness, fever, leukocytosis, and lymphangitis.

Diagnosis: Wound infections are diagnosed by wound cultures (anaerobic and aerobic). Fluid or tissue biopsy may also be performed.

Treatment: Wound infections are treated with antibiotics and a wound care regimen that includes routine cleaning and dressing of the wound. Wound care treatment is based on the type and severity of the wound. Surgical irrigation and debridement may also be indicated. For deep, complex wounds, a wound-care consult is often indicated.

> **Review Video: Treating Wound Infections**
> Visit mometrix.com/academy and enter code: 761736

NECROTIZING FASCIITIS

Necrotizing fasciitis is an infection that develops deep within the fascia, causing a rapidly developing tissue necrosis resulting in destruction and death of the soft tissue and nerves. Complications of necrotizing fasciitis may include the loss of the affected limb, sepsis, and death. Group A *Streptococcus*, *Klebsiella*, *Clostridioides*, *Escherichia coli*, *Staphylococcus aureus*, and *Aeromonas hydrophila* are organisms that have the potential to cause necrotizing fasciitis.

Signs/symptoms: Edema, erythema, and pain at the affected site. Nausea, vomiting, fatigue, malaise, fever, and chills may also occur.

Diagnosis: Diagnosis is based on physical assessment and patient history. In addition, excisional deep skin biopsy and gram staining may be performed to determine the causative organism. CT/MRI may also be utilized to assess the extent of the infection.

Treatment: Treatment options for necrotizing fasciitis include antibiotics and fasciotomy with radical debridement. Hyperbaric oxygen therapy may also be utilized.

SURGICAL WOUNDS

Surgical wounds or incisions are made during a surgical procedure in a sterile, controlled environment. The American College of Surgeons has defined four classes of surgical wound types. This classification can help to predict how the wound will heal and the risk of infection.

- **Class I** is defined as clean (e.g., laparoscopic surgeries and biopsies).
- **Class II** is defined as clean contaminated (e.g., GI and GU surgeries).
- **Class III** is defined as contaminated (e.g., traumatic wounds such as a gunshot wound).
- **Class IV** is defined as dirty (e.g., traumatic wound from a dirty source).

Surgical wounds should be assessed for signs and symptoms of infection including erythema, edema, fever, increasing pain, and drainage. Surgical drains are commonly placed near the surgical incision to promote drainage—inspect drains for patency, amount, and characteristics of drainage. Patients are often treated with antibiotics prophylactically to help prevent a surgical site infection. Wound vacuum assisted closure devices may also be utilized to remove blood or serous fluid from the surgical wound/incision site.

MANAGEMENT OF INFLAMMATION RESULTING FROM TATTOOS AND PIERCING

Tattoos and piercing have both been implicated in **MRSA infections**. Tattooing uses needles that inject dye, sometimes resulting in local infection with erythema, edema, and purulent discharge. Body piercing for insertion of jewelry carries similar risks. Piercings of concern include the upper ear cartilage, nipples, navel, tongue, lip, penis, and nose. Some people who do piercings use reusable piercing equipment that is difficult to adequately clean and sterilize. Infections resulting from piercing in cartilage are often resistant to antibiotics because of lack of blood supply.

Treatment includes:

- **Cleansing wounds**. Jewelry may need to be removed in some cases.
- **Antibiotics**: Culture should be obtained, but medications for community-acquired MRSA should be started immediately:
  - **Mupirocin** may be used topically 3 times daily for 7–10 days with or without systemic antimicrobials.
  - **Trimethoprim-sulfamethoxazole DS** (TMP 160 mg/SMX 800 mg), 1–2 tablets twice daily. Children, dose based on TMP: 8–12 mg/kg/day in 2 doses.

TISSUE DAMAGE

Abrasion is damage to superficial layers of skin, such as with road burn or ligature marks.

Contusion occurs when friction or pressure causes damage to underlying vessels, resulting in bruising. Contusions that are bright red/purple with clear margins have occurred within 48 hours and those with receding edges or yellow-brown discoloration are older than 48 hours.

Laceration is a tear in the skin resulting from blunt force, often from falls on protuberances, such as elbows, or other blunt trauma. Lacerations may be partial to full-thickness.

Avulsion is tissue that is separated from its base and lost or without adequate base for attachment.

Treatments include:

- Local anesthetic if needed
- Low pressure, high volume irrigation with 35–50 mL syringe of open wound with normal saline, water, or non-antiseptic nonionic surfactants, and mechanical scrubbing of surrounding tissue with disinfectant
- Topical antibiotics as indicated
- Prophylactic antibiotics or antibiotic irrigation if wound contaminated
- Suturing/debridement as needed
- Hydrocolloids, Steri-Strips, and transparent dressings to stabilize flaps

Musculoskeletal Pathophysiology

IMMOBILITY

Critical care patients are often **immobile** for extended periods of time, thereby increasing their risk of skin breakdown and the development of pressure-related injuries, deep vein thrombosis, functional decline, decreased muscle mass, impaired coordination and gait, cardiovascular deconditioning, depression, and constipation. Immobility leads to impaired physical functioning in which muscle mass is lost and weakness develops. Intensive care unit acquired weakness can develop during hospitalization and is associated with an increased hospital length of stay as well as an increased mortality rate. ICU acquired weakness may last years after discharge with residual effects often affecting the patient's quality of life. Progressive mobility is defined as the gradual progression of positioning and mobility techniques and should be utilized to improve muscle strength and provide the patient a greater ability to resume activities of daily living. Patients should be assessed daily for their readiness to progress in their mobility goals in order to prevent the adverse effects of immobility.

GAIT DISORDERS

Functional movement disorders are defined as an involuntary, abnormal movement of part of the body in which pathophysiology is not fully understood. Functional tremors are the most frequent type of functional movement disorder. Dystonia, myoclonus, and Parkinsonism are other types of functional movement disorders. Functional gait disorders are another type of functional movement disorder and are common in the elderly. Gait disorders can manifest as a dragging gait, knee buckling, small slow steps or "walking on ice," swaying gait, fluctuating gait, hesitant gait, and hyperkinetic gait in which there is excessive movement of the arms, trunk, and legs when ambulating. Patients with gait disorders are at an increased risk of falling. Gait disorders are diagnosed by a thorough clinical examination (including a neurologic assessment) and health history. Treatment for functional gait disorders includes strength and balance training. Assistive devices such as walkers and canes may also be utilized.

FALLS

Falls are the most commonly occurring adverse event in the hospital setting. Confusion and agitation are factors that contribute to an increased risk for falling. In addition, impaired balance or gait, orthostatic hypotension, altered mobility, a history of falling, advanced age and the use of certain medications are additional risk factors. Approximately 30% of patient falls result in injury, some of which can significantly contribute to an increase in morbidity and mortality including fractures and subdural hematomas. Both physical and environmental factors contribute to patient falls, some of which are preventable. Fall prevention strategies include utilization of a standardized fall risk assessment to determine the patient's level of risk and subsequent care planning and interventions individualized to the patient. Fall prevention should also be balanced with progressive mobility. Many falls are related to toileting needs, and nurses often utilize scheduled rounding to address such needs.

> **Review Video: Fall Prevention**
> Visit mometrix.com/academy and enter code: 972452

CARPAL TUNNEL SYNDROME

Carpal tunnel syndrome is a type of entrapment neuropathy in which the median nerve is compressed by thickening of the flexor tendon sheath, skeletal encroachment, or mass in the soft tissue. Carpal tunnel syndrome is often associated with repetitive hand activities, arthritis, hypothyroidism, diabetes, and pregnancy. Patients complain of pain in wrist, radiating to forearm, and numbness and tingling in the first 2–3 fingers, especially during the night.

Diagnosis is based on symptoms and tests such as:

- **Positive Tinel test**: Gentle percussion over medial nerve in inner aspect of wrist elicits numbness and pain.
- **Positive Phalen test**: The backs of the hands are pressed together and the wrists sharply flexed for 1 minute to elicit pain and numbness.

Treatment includes identifying and treating the underlying cause:

- Steroid injection may relieve symptoms
- Splint during the night or during repetitive activities
- Modification of activities
- Referral for decompression surgery in recalcitrant cases or those with severe loss of sensation

INFECTIOUS ARTHRITIS

Infectious arthritis may be bacterial, viral (rubella, parvovirus, and hepatitis B), parasitic, or fungal, with bacterial arthritis causing the most rapid destruction to the joint. *Neisseria gonorrhoeae* (most common), *Staphylococcus*, *Streptococcus*, and *Escherichia coli* are the most common bacterial agents. The infection may be bloodborne or spread from an infection near the joint or from direct implantation or postoperative contamination of the wound. Usually, the infection involves just one joint.

Symptoms include acute edema, erythema, and pain in a joint. Systemic reactions, such as fever and polyarthralgia, may occur, especially with gonorrhea.

Diagnosis requires a complete history and physical examination, arthrocentesis and synovial fluid culture, and WBC.

Treatment includes:

- Antibiotics as indicated by organism
- Arthrocentesis to drain fluid accumulation in joint (may need to be repeated)
- Analgesia

BURSITIS AND TENDINITIS

Bursitis is inflammation of the bursa, fluid-filled spaces or sacs that form in tissues to reduce friction, causing thickening of the lining of the bursal walls. This can be the result of infection, trauma, crystal deposits, or chronic friction from trauma.

Tendinitis is inflammation of the long, tubular tendons and tendon sheaths adjacent to the bursa. Causes of tendinitis are similar to bursitis but tendinitis may also be caused by quinolone antibiotics. Frequently, both bursa and tendons are inflamed. Common types of bursitis include shoulder, olecranon (elbow), trochanteric (hip), and prepatellar (front of knee). Common types of tendinitis include wrist, Achilles, patellar, and rotator cuff.

Symptoms include pain with movement, edema, dysfunction, and decreased range of motion.

Diagnosis is by clinical examination, although x-rays may rule out fractures. The bursa may be aspirated diagnostically to aid in ruling out other diagnosis, like gout or infection.

Treatment for bursitis and tendinitis includes:

- Rest and immobilization
- NSAIDs
- Application of cold packs to affected area
- Steroid injections

JOINT EFFUSION AND ARTHROCENTESIS

Joint effusion is the accumulation of fluid (clear, bloody, or purulent) within a joint capsule. Joint effusion can cause pressure on the joint and severe pain. Arthrocentesis relieves the pressure and the fluid aspirated can be examined to aid in diagnosis. Arthrocentesis is usually contraindicated in the presence of overlying infection, prosthetic joint, and coagulopathy without referral to an orthopedic specialist.

Procedure:

1. Patient is **positioned** according to joint to be aspirated and encouraged to relax muscles.
2. **Overlying area** is cleansed with povidone-iodine solution, air-dried a few minutes, and cleansed of iodine with alcohol wipe.
3. **Local anesthetic** is given to the area (but not into the joint) with 25- to 30-gauge needle (lidocaine 1–2%) or a regional nerve block for severe pain.
4. The joint is **aspirated** with insertion in a straight line, using a 30–60 mL syringe (depending upon expected amount of fluid) and an 18- to 22-gauge needle or IV catheter.
5. The joint is completely **drained** of fluid.
6. Observe for **complications**: bleeding, infection, or allergic reaction.

LUMBOSACRAL PAIN

Lumbosacral (low back) pain may be related to strain, muscular weakness, osteoarthritis, spinal stenosis, herniated disks, vertebral fractures, bony metastasis, infection, or other musculoskeletal disorders. Disk herniation or other joint changes put pressure on nerves leaving the spinal cord, causing pain to radiate along the nerve. Pain may be acute or chronic (more than 3 months).

Symptoms include local or pain radiating down the leg (radiculopathy), impaired gait and reflexes, difference in leg lengths, decreased motor strength, and alteration of sensation, including numbness.

Diagnosis is by careful clinical examination and history as well as x-ray (fractures, scoliosis, dislocations), CT (identifies underlying problems), MRI (spinal pathology), and/or EMG and nerve conduction studies. Diagnostic studies may be deferred in many cases for 4–6 weeks as symptoms may resolve over time.
Treatments for nonspecific back pain include:

- Analgesia: acetaminophen, NSAIDS, opiates
- Encourage activity to tolerance but not bed rest
- Muscle relaxants: diazepam 5–10 mg every 6–8 hours
- Cold and heat compresses

STRAINS AND SPRAINS

A **strain** is an overstretching of a part of the musculature ("pulled muscle") that causes microscopic tears in the muscle, usually resulting from excess stress or overuse of the muscle. Onset of pain is usually sudden with local tenderness on use of the muscle. A **sprain** is damage to a joint, with a partial rupture of the supporting ligaments, usually caused by wrenching or twisting that may occur with a fall. The rupture can damage blood vessels, resulting in edema, tenderness at the joint, and pain on movement with pain increasing over 2–3 hours after injury. An avulsion fracture (bone fragment pulled away by a ligament) may occur with strain, so x-rays rule out fractures.

Treatment for both strains and sprains includes:

- **PRICE protocol**: protection, rest, ice, compression, and elevation
- **Ice compresses** (wet or dry) applied 20–30 minutes intermittently for 48 hours and then intermittent heat 15–20 minutes 3–4 times daily
- Monitor **neurovascular status** (especially for sprain)
- **Immobilization** as indicated for sprains for 1–3 weeks

FRACTURES
PEDIATRIC FRACTURES

Pediatric fracture types include the following:

- **Bend**: Children's flexible bones may bend up to 45° without breaking. While they will slowly straighten, they will not do so completely. Bends are most common in the ulna with fracture of the radius and in the fibula with fracture of the tibia.
- **Buckle**: When porous bone is compressed, a bulging occurs, usually near the metaphysis. Buckles are most common in younger children.
- **Complete**: The bone fragments are completely separated but may be attached on one side by a periosteal hinge.
- **Comminuted**: A comminuted fracture involves bone fragments chipping off from the broken bone and lying in the surrounding tissue. Because children's bones are more pliable than adults', comminuted fractures are rare but may occur in adolescents.
- **Greenstick**: This is an incomplete fracture on one side of a bone.
- **Spiral**: This spiraling, circular fracture goes around the bone shaft and often results from child abuse.

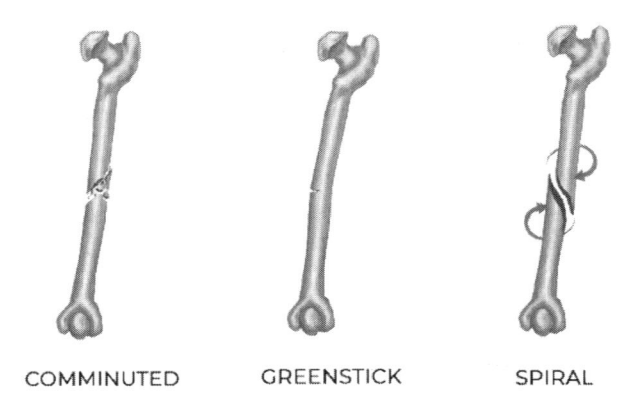

COMMINUTED   GREENSTICK   SPIRAL

DIAGNOSIS AND TREATMENT

Fractures and dislocations are commonly diagnosed by clinical examination, history, and radiographs. Careful inspection, observation of range of motion, palpation, and observation of abnormalities are important because pain may be referred. Neurovascular assessment should be done immediately to prevent vascular compromise. Radiographs should usually precede reduction of dislocations to ensure there are no fractures and follow reduction to ensure the dislocation is reduced. **Treatment** includes:

- Analgesia and sedation as indicated
- Application of cold compresses and elevation of fractured area to reduce edema
- Reduction of fracture: Steady and gradual longitudinal traction to realign bone
- Immobilization with brace, cast, sling, or splint indicated
- Reduction of dislocation: Varies according to area of dislocation
- Open fracture:
    - Wound irrigation with NS
    - Tetanus prophylaxis
    - Antibiotic prophylaxis
    - Referral to orthopedic specialist for open fractures, irreducible dislocations, and complications such as compartment syndrome or circulatory impairment

FRACTURED RIBS

Fractured ribs are usually an indication of severe injury in children because the elasticity of their ribs generally makes them resistant to fracture. Most fractures are the result of severe trauma, such as blunt force from a motor vehicle accident or physical abuse. Children presenting with rib fractures from "falls" or other vague reports of injury should be examined for signs of abuse and have a radionuclide bone scan that will show both new and old fractures. Since much force is required to fracture a child's ribs, underlying injuries should be expected according to the area of fractures.

- **Upper 4 ribs**: Injuries to trachea, bronchi, or great vessels
- **Middle ribs (5-9)**: Pneumothorax or hemothorax from penetration wounds
- **Lower ribs**: Trauma to liver, kidney, and/or spleen

Treatment is primarily supportive as rib fractures usually heal in about 6 weeks. Underlying injuries are treated according to the type and degree of injury. Supplemental oxygen is provided if indicated. Administer analgesia. Provide pulmonary physiotherapy.

FRACTURE OF THE CLAVICLE

Fracture of the clavicle is the most common pediatric fracture, with some associated with childbirth trauma and half occurring <age 7. There are three **classes**:

- **Middle third of clavicle** (80%): Usually from force on the lateral shoulder related to fall, motor vehicle accident, or sports injury. Treatment includes sling or figure-eight immobilization. Displaced fractures may be surgically repaired.
- **Lateral third** (15%): Usually from force on top of shoulder and may be nondisplaced (type I), displaced (type II), or involving the articular surface of the joint (type III). Treatment includes ice (initially) and sling. Displaced fractures usually require surgical repair.
- **Medial third** (5%): Usually from force against the anterior chest. Treatment includes ice (initially), reduction if displaced, sling, and close observation for intrathoracic injury.

Indications include pain, restricted movement of upper extremity, edema, deformity, and bruising. With compression of nerves or vasculature, circulatory compromise and numbness or weakness may be evident. In rare cases, pneumothorax may occur.

Fracture of the Wrist

A wrist fracture can occur in the distal radius (thumb side), ulna, or the wrist joint. The radius is the most commonly fractured, but both the radius and ulna may be fractured. Fracture usually occurs from falls with the weight falling on an outstretched hand, resulting in hyperextension, or direct blunt trauma. It is most common in sports such as football, soccer, hockey, skiing, and ice-skating. Pain is usually severe and deformity may be obvious. Mobility is often markedly decreased and the child has an inability to bear any weight on the wrist. Edema often begins immediately, and there may be tingling or numbness as nerves are compressed. Any bleeding should be controlled with compression and dressings applied to open wounds. The bones are aligned and wrist casted or splinted. If both bones are broken, internal fixation may be required.

Elbow Dislocation/Fracture

Dislocation or fracture of an elbow may present with similar symptoms and radiograph may be needed for diagnosis. The injury usually results from fall or blunt trauma to the elbow. The child complains of severe pain, and muscle spasms may occur. Mobility is limited and there may be obvious deformity. Usually, edema begins immediately after injury. There may be pallor and coolness of the arm and hand distal to the injury. The child may exhibit signs of shock. Immediate care includes treating for shock, monitoring pulses, and splinting the elbow. No attempt should be made to change the position of the elbow as it may increase damage to nerves and vessels. It should be splinted as found and ice applied initially. Supracondylar fractures are common in children <8 while epicondylar fractures are common in children 9-14. Growth plate fractures may arrest growth. **Treatment** depends on degree and specific site of injury and may include manipulation; immobilization in sling, cast, or splint; or surgical repair.

Fracture of the Tibia/Fibula

Fracture of the tibia or fibula, or both bones, may occur as a result of a twisting injury at any point from the proximal to the distal ends. The fibula is more protected by tissue, and fracture of this bone alone may be more difficult to detect as the tibia provides a natural splint. There may be little obvious deformity, and the child may be able to walk. Tibia fractures are more likely to result in an open fracture because of proximity to the skin surface. If both bones are fractured, there is usually pronounced deformity and edema at the site of the fractures with severe pain and marked tenderness on palpation. Immediate treatment includes stopping blood flow with compression, monitoring pulses, applying dressing to an open wound, splinting the leg with rigid splints on each side of the leg to prevent the legs from rotating, and parenteral analgesia. **Treatment** may include immobilization with cast or splint or surgical fixation, depending on site and degree of injury.

Sprain Injuries

A sprain is damage to a joint, with a partial rupture of the supporting ligaments, usually caused by wrenching or twisting that may occur with a fall. The rupture can damage blood vessels, resulting in edema, tenderness at the joint, and pain on movement with pain increasing over 2–3 hours after injury. An avulsion fracture (bone fragment pulled away by a ligament) may occur with strain, so x-rays rule out fractures. Sprains may be **classified** according to severity.

- **1st degree**: This is a relatively mild degree of injury, usually associated with good range of motion and mild pain. Swelling may vary considerably, depending upon whether vessels are disrupted by the sprain.
- **2nd degree**: This comprises a wide range of signs and symptoms, as there is further injury and partial rupture of the ligaments. Usually range of motion is limited by pain. Edema and bruising are usually present but vary in degree. The joint may be somewhat unstable.
- **3rd degree**: This involves total rupture of the ligament with immediate marked pain (although sometimes less than with 2nd degree), bruising, edema, and decreased range of motion. The joint is usually markedly unstable.

Muscle Strain

A strain is an overstretching of a part of the musculature ("pulled muscle") that causes microscopic tears in the muscle or tendon, usually resulting from excess stress or overuse of the muscle. Strains may be caused by blunt trauma to a muscle or overstretching related to sports activities, such as field events, football, and soccer. Common sites for strains include the ankle, back, and hamstrings. Neglect of warm-up routines and fatigue may increase risk of strains. Onset of pain is usually sudden with local tenderness on use of the muscle.

Strains are **classified** according to severity of injury.

- **1st degree**: This injury is relatively mild, and symptoms, such as slight discomfort and tenderness to palpation, may be delayed until the following day, as the athlete may be unaware of the injury. Range of motion remains intact.
- **2nd degree**: This injury comprises a wide range of symptoms resulting from stretching or partial tearing of the muscle or tendon. Pain is usually felt on injury with tenderness on palpation and decreased passive and active range of motion, depending upon the site of injury. There may be signs of injury, such as edema and bruising. Pain increases with passive stretching or active contraction of injured muscles.
- **3rd degree**: The muscle or tendon is completely ruptured and pain occurs with injury. A defect may be palpable. Often there is extensive edema and bruising from injury to vasculature. While loss of function in affected muscle occurs, strength and loss of range of motion varies according to site of injury.

Neurological Pathophysiology

ENCEPHALOPATHIES

HYPERTENSIVE ENCEPHALOPATHY WITH CEREBRAL EDEMA

Hypertensive encephalopathy can occur as part of a hypertensive crisis. With chronic hypertension, the brain adapts to higher pressures to regulate blood flow, but in a hypertensive crisis, autoregulation of the blood-brain barrier is overwhelmed and the capillaries leak fluid into the tissue and vasodilation takes place with resultant cerebral edema. Damage to arterioles occurs, causing increasing neurological deficits and papilledema. Hypertensive encephalopathy is relatively rare, but carries a high mortality rate and is most common in middle-aged males with long-standing hypertension. **Symptoms** usually develop over 1–2 days and include:

- Non-specific neurological deficits, such as weakness and visual abnormalities
- Alterations in mental status, including confusion
- Headache, often constant
- Nausea and vomiting
- Seizures
- Coma

TREATMENT FOR HYPERTENSIVE ENCEPHALOPATHY WITH CEREBRAL EDEMA

Hypertensive encephalopathy with cerebral edema requires prompt treatment in order to prevent neurological damage.

Treatment includes identifying and treating the underlying causes for the hypertensive crisis and taking steps to lower the blood pressure:

- **Nitroprusside sodium** is usually used initially to lower BP. However, caution must be used not to lower the blood pressure too quickly, as this can lead to cerebral ischemia. Other antihypertensive medications used include clevidipine, nicardipine, fenoldopam, and labetalol.
- **Positioning** of the patient to prevent obstruction of venous return from the head
- **Monitoring blood gas** and maintaining $PaCO_2$ at 33–37 mmHg to facilitate vasoconstriction of cerebral arteries
- **Preventing hyperthermia** with antipyretics and cooling devices
- **BP monitoring** and maintenance
- **Seizure control** with phenobarbital and/or phenytoin
- **Lidocaine** through endotracheal tube or intravenously prior to nasotracheal suctioning
- **Diuretics**, such as osmotic agents (mannitol) and loop diuretics (furosemide) to control fluid volume
- **Controlling metabolic demand** by measures to increase pain control and reduce stimulation
- **Barbiturates** (pentobarbital, thiopental) in high doses may be used if other treatments fail to decrease intracranial pressure

Hypoxic Encephalopathy

Cerebral hypoxia (hypoxic encephalopathy) occurs when the oxygen supply to the brain is decreased. If hypoxia is mild, the brain compensates by increasing cerebral blood flow, but it can only double in volume and cannot compensate for severe hypoxic conditions. Hypoxia may be the result of insufficient oxygen in the environment, inadequate exchange at the alveolar level of the lungs, or inadequate circulation to the brain. Brain cells may begin dying within 5 minutes if deprived of adequate oxygenation, so any condition or trauma that interferes with oxygenation can result in brain damage:

- Near-drowning
- Asphyxia
- Cardiac arrest
- High altitude sickness
- Carbon monoxide
- Diseases that interfere with respiration, such as myasthenia gravis and amyotrophic lateral sclerosis
- Anesthesia complications

Symptoms include increasing neurological deficits, depending upon the degree and area of damage, with changes in mentation that range from confusion to coma. Prompt identification of the cause and increase in perfusion to the brain is critical for survival.

Metabolic Encephalopathy

Metabolic encephalopathy (hepatic encephalopathy) is damage to the brain resulting from a disturbance in metabolism, primarily hepatic failure to remove toxins from the blood. There may be impairment in cerebral blood flow, cerebral edema, or increased intracranial pressure. It can occur as the result of the ingestion of drugs or toxins which can have a direct toxic effect on neurons, but it can also occur with liver disease, especially when stressed by co-morbidities, such as hemorrhage, hypoxemia, surgery, trauma, renal failure with dialysis, or electrolyte imbalances.

Symptoms may vary:

- Irritability and agitation
- Alterations in consciousness
- Dysphonia
- Lack of coordination, spasticity
- Seizures are common and may be the presenting symptom
- Disorientation progressing to coma

Prompt diagnosis is important because the condition may be reversible if underlying causes are identified and treated before permanent neuronal damage occurs.

Treatment varies according to the underlying cause.

Infectious Encephalopathy

Infectious encephalopathy is an encompassing term describing encephalopathies caused by a wide range of bacteria, viruses, or prions. Common to all infections are altered brain function that results in alterations in consciousness and personality, cognitive impairment, and lethargy. A wide range of neurological symptoms may occur: myoclonus, seizures, dysphagia, and dysphonia, neuromuscular impairment with muscle atrophy and tremors or spasticity. **Treatment** depends on the underlying cause and response to treatment. Prion infections are not treatable, but bacterial infections may respond to antibiotic therapy, and viral infections may be self-limiting. HIV-related encephalopathy results from opportunistic infections as immune responses decrease, usually indicated by CD4 counts <50. Aggressive antiretroviral treatment and treatment of the infection may reverse symptoms if permanent damage has not occurred for HIV-related encephalopathy.

Treatment for other infectious encephalopathies varies according to the type of infection and underlying causes.

CEREBRAL ANEURYSMS

Cerebral aneurysms, the weakening and dilation of a cerebral artery, are usually congenital (90%) while the remaining (10%) result from direct trauma or infection. Aneurysms are usually 2–7 mm in size and occur in the Circle of Willis at the base of the brain.

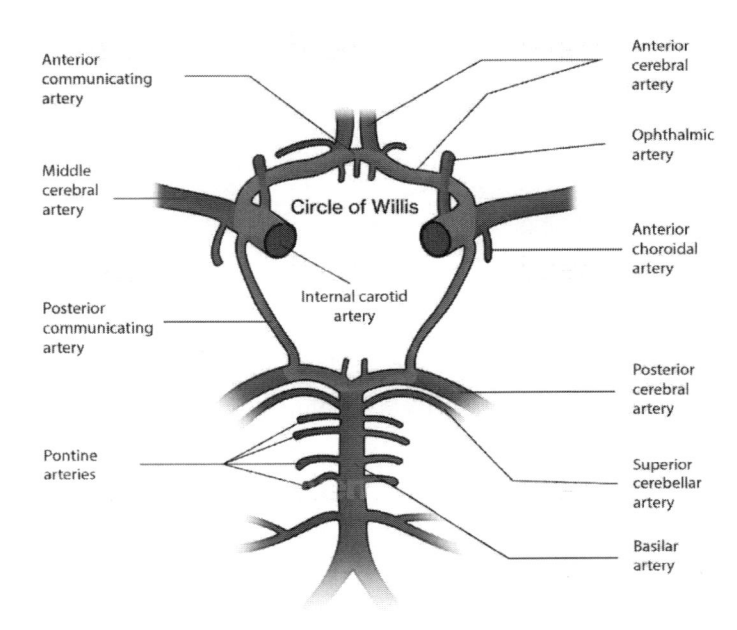

A rupturing aneurysm may decrease perfusion as well as increasing pressure on surrounding brain tissue. Cerebral aneurysms are classified as follows:

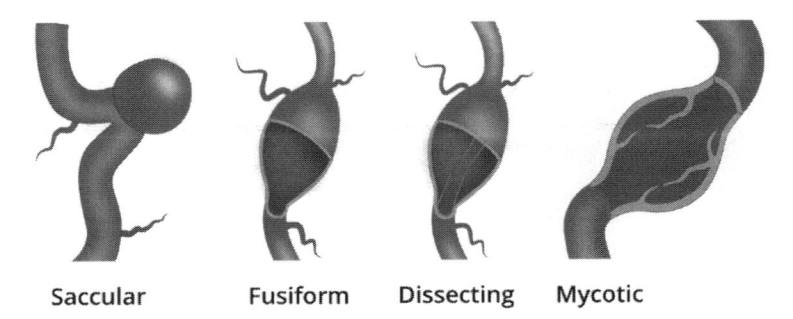

- **Berry/saccular:** The most common congenital type occurs at a bifurcation and grows from the base on a stem, usually at the Circle of Willis.
- **Fusiform**: Large and irregular (>2.5 cm) and rarely ruptures but causes increased intracranial pressure. Usually involves the internal carotid or vertebrobasilar artery.
- **Mycotic**: Rare type that occurs secondary to bacterial infection and aseptic emboli.
- **Dissecting**: Wall is torn apart and blood enters layers. This may occur during angiography or secondary to trauma or disease.
- **Traumatic Charcot-Bouchard (pseudoaneurysm):** Small lesion resulting from chronic hypertension.

ARTERIOVENOUS MALFORMATION

Arteriovenous malformation (AVM) is a congenital abnormality within the brain consisting of a tangle of dilated arteries and veins without a capillary bed. AVMs can occur anywhere in the brain and may cause no significant problems. Usually the AVM is "fed" by one or more cerebral arteries, which enlarge over time, shunting more blood through the AVM. The veins also enlarge in response to increased arterial blood flow because of the lack of a capillary bridge between the two. Because vein walls are thinner and lack the muscle layer of an artery, the veins tend to rupture as the AVM becomes larger, causing a subarachnoid hemorrhage. Chronic ischemia that may be related to the AVM can result in cerebral atrophy. Sometimes small leaks, usually accompanied by headache and nausea and vomiting, may occur before rupture. AVMs may cause a wide range of neurological symptoms, including changes in mentation, dizziness, sensory abnormalities, confusion, increasing ICP, and dementia.

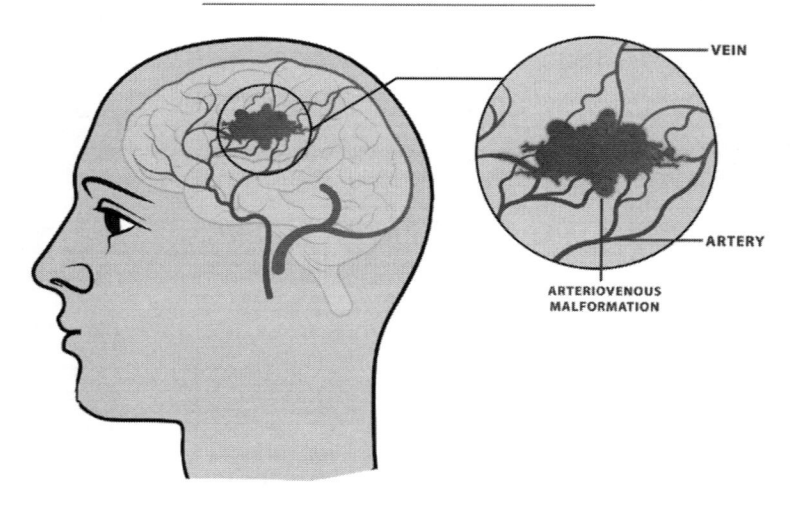

Treatment includes:

- Supportive management of symptoms
- Surgical repair or focused irradiation (definitive treatments)

HYDROCEPHALUS

COMMUNICATING AND NONCOMMUNICATING

The ventricular system produces and circulates cerebrospinal fluid (CSF). The right and left lateral ventricles open into the third ventricle at the interventricular foramen (foramen of Monro). The aqueduct of Sylvius connects the third and fourth ventricles. The fourth ventricle, anterior to the cerebellum, supplies CSF to the subarachnoid space and the spinal cord (dorsal surface). The CSF circulates and then returns to the brain and is absorbed in the arachnoid villi. **Hydrocephalus** occurs when there is an imbalance between production and absorption of cerebrospinal fluid in the ventricles, resulting from impaired absorption or obstruction, which may be congenital or acquired. There are two common types of hydrocephalus:

- **Communicating:** CSF flows (communicates) between the ventricles but is not absorbed in the subarachnoid space (arachnoid villi).
- **Noncommunicating:** CSF is obstructed (non-communicating) between the ventricles, with the obstruction most often due to stenosis of the aqueduct of Sylvius.

SYMPTOMS

Symptoms of hydrocephalus depend on the age of onset. In *early infancy*, before closure of cranial sutures, head enlargement is the most common presentation, but in adults with less elasticity in the skull, neurological symptoms usually relate to increasing pressure on structures of the brain. Hydrocephalus may occur at any age, but the type that occurs in *young/middle-aged adults* is different than that common in children or those >50. Hydrocephalus in young and middle-aged adults may result from a congenital defect, hydrocephalus of infancy with shunt failure, or trauma and is characterized by:

- Headache relieved by vomiting
- Papilledema
- Lack of bladder control
- Strabismus and other visual disorders
- Ataxia
- Irritability
- Lethargy
- Confusion and impairment of cognitive abilities

With **adult-onset normal pressure hydrocephalus** (>50) cerebrospinal fluid increases and dilates the ventricles, but frequently without increasing intracranial pressure. The cause is often unclear. Symptoms include gait disturbance, bladder control issues, and mild dementia

TREATMENT

Hydrocephalus is diagnosed through CT and MRI scans, which help to determine the cause. **Treatment** may vary somewhat depending upon the underlying disorder. For example, if obstruction is caused by a tumor, surgical excision to directly remove the obstruction is required. Generally, however, most hydrocephalus is treated with shunts:

- **Ventricular-peritoneal shunt:** This procedure is the most common and consists of placing a ventricular catheter directly into the ventricles (usually lateral) at one end with the other end in the peritoneal area to drain away excess CSF. There is a one-way valve near the proximal end that prevents backflow but opens when pressure rises to drain fluid. In some cases, the distal end drains into the right atrium.
- **Third ventriculostomy:** A small opening is made in the base of the third ventricle so CSF can bypass an obstruction. This procedure is not common and is done with a small endoscope.

NEUROLOGIC INFECTIOUS DISEASE

BACTERIAL MENINGITIS

Bacterial meningitis may be caused by a wide range of bacteria, including *Streptococcus pneumoniae* and *Neisseria meningitidis.* Bacteria can enter the CNS from distant infection, surgical wounds, invasive devices, nasal colonization, or penetrating trauma. The infective process includes inflammation, exudates, WBC accumulation, and brain tissue damage with hyperemia and edema. Purulent exudate covers the brain and invades and blocks the ventricles, obstructing CSF and leading to increased intracranial pressure. **Symptoms** include abrupt onset, fever, chills, severe headache, nuchal rigidity, and alterations of consciousness with seizures, agitation, and irritability. Antibodies specific to bacteria don't cross the blood brain barrier, so immune response is poor. Some may have photophobia, hallucinations, and/or aggressive behavior or may become stuporous and lapse into coma. Nuchal rigidity may progress to opisthotonos. Reflexes are variable but Kernig and Brudzinski signs are often positive. Signs may relate to particular bacteria, such as rashes, sore joints, or a draining ear. **Diagnosis** is usually based on lumbar puncture examination of cerebrospinal fluid and symptoms. **Treatment** includes IV antibiotics and supportive care: fluids, a dark and calm environment, measures to reduce ICP, etc.

Fungal Meningitis

Fungal meningitis is the least common cause of meningitis. It occurs when a fungal organism enters into the subarachnoid space, cerebral spinal fluid, and meninges. Immune deficient patients such as those with HIV, cancer, or immunodeficiency syndromes are most at risk for the development of fungal meningitis. The most common organisms causing fungal meningitis are candida albicans and Cryptococcus neoformans. Fungal meningitis caused by candida may occur in immunosuppressed patients, in those who have had a ventricular shunt placed, or in those that have had a lumbar puncture performed. Cryptococcus is a fungus found in soil throughout the world and does not usually affect people with a healthy immune system. Cryptococcal meningitis is most commonly seen in patients with HIV/AIDS and is one of the leading causes of death in HIV/AIDS patients in certain parts of Africa.

Signs/symptoms: Headache, fever, nausea and vomiting, stiff neck, photophobia, and mental status changes.

Diagnosis: Lumbar puncture with subsequent culture of cerebral spinal fluid. In addition, blood cultures may be obtained as well as a CT of the head.

Treatment: The treatment of fungal meningitis involves a long course of anti-fungal medications, including Amphotericin B, flucytosine, and fluconazole. Anticonvulsants may be administered for seizure control.

> **Review Video: Meningitis**
> Visit mometrix.com/academy and enter code: 277418

Viral Infections That Can Impact the Neurological System

Many different types of viral infections can impact the neurological system either by direct infection transmitted through the bloodstream or by spreading along the nerve pathways (such as rabies). Common viral infections affecting the neurological system include:

- **Viral encephalitis**: Arboviral infections are transmitted from an animal host to an arthropod (typically a mosquito or tick) to humans, who are typically dead-end hosts. Arboviral infections include western equine encephalitis, eastern equine encephalitis, St. Louis encephalitis, Powassan encephalitis, Colorado tick fever and La Crosse encephalitis. West Nile virus may also invade the CNS and cause encephalitis.
- **Viral meningitis**: Viral meningitis is usually self-limiting within 7–10 days and is less severe than bacterial meningitis.
- **Herpes virus**: Herpes simplex virus can invade the nervous system and cause herpes simplex encephalitis, which has a high mortality rate.
- **HIV**: Inflammation may affect the CNS and interfere with neuronal functions.

Neuromuscular Disorders
Multiple Sclerosis

Multiple sclerosis is an autoimmune disorder of the CNS in which the myelin sheath around the nerves is damaged and replaced by scar tissue that prevents conduction of nerve impulses.

Symptoms vary widely and can include problems with balance and coordination, tremors, slurring of speech, cognitive impairment, vision impairment, nystagmus, pain, and bladder and bowel dysfunction. Symptoms may be relapsing-remitting, progressive, or a combination. Onset is usually at 20–30 years of age, with incidence higher in females. Patient may initially present with problems walking or falling or optic neuritis (30%) causing loss of central vision. Males may complain of sexual dysfunction as an early symptom. Others have dysuria with urinary retention.

Diagnosis is based on clinical and neurological examination and MRI. **Treatment** is symptomatic and includes treatment to shorten duration of episodes and slow progress.

- **Glucocorticoids**: Methylprednisolone
- **Immunomodulator**: Interferon beta, glatiramer acetate, natalizumab
- **Immunosuppressant**: Mitoxantrone
- **Hormone**: Estriol (for females)

> **Review Video: Multiple Sclerosis (MS)**
> Visit mometrix.com/academy and enter code: 417355

ALS

Amyotrophic lateral sclerosis (ALS) is a progressive degenerative disease of the upper and lower motor neurons, resulting in progressively severe symptoms such as spasticity, hyperreflexia, muscle weakness, and paralysis that can cause dysphagia, cramping, muscular atrophy, and respiratory dysfunction. ALS may be sporadic or familial (rare). Speech may become monotone; however, cognitive functioning usually remains intact. Eventually, patients become immobile and cannot breathe independently.

Diagnosis is based on history, electromyography, nerve conduction studies, and MRI. Treatment includes riluzole to delay progression of the disease. Patients in the ED usually have been diagnosed and have developed an acute complication, such as acute respiratory failure, aspiration pneumonia, or other trauma.

Treatment includes:

- Nebulizer treatments with bronchodilators and steroids
- Antibiotics for infection
- Mechanical ventilation

If **ventilatory assistance** is needed, it is important to determine if the patient has a living will expressing the wish to be ventilated or not or has assigned power of attorney for health matters to someone to make this decision.

> **Review Video: Amyotrophic Lateral Sclerosis (ALS)**
> Visit mometrix.com/academy and enter code: 178603

PARKINSON'S DISEASE

Parkinson's disease (PD) is an extrapyramidal movement motor system disorder caused by loss of brain cells that produce dopamine. Typical symptoms include tremor of face and extremities, rigidity, bradykinesia, akinesia, poor posture, and a lack of balance and coordination causing increasing problems with mobility, talking, and swallowing. Some may suffer depression and mood changes. Tremors usually present unilaterally in an upper extremity.

Diagnosis includes:

- **Cogwheel rigidity test**: The extremity is put through passive range of motion, which causes increased muscle tone and ratchet-like movements.
- **Physical and neurological exam**
- **Complete history** to rule out drug-induced Parkinson akinesia

Treatment includes:

- Symptomatic support
- Dopaminergic therapy: Levodopa, amantadine, and carbidopa

- Anticholinergics: Trihexyphenidyl, benztropine
- For drug-induced Parkinson's, terminate drugs

Drug therapy tends to decrease in effectiveness over time, and patients may present with a marked increase in symptoms. Discontinuing the drugs for 1 week may exacerbate symptoms initially, but functioning may improve when drugs are reintroduced.

GUILLAIN-BARRÉ SYNDROME

Guillain-Barré syndrome (GBS) is an autoimmune disorder of the myelinated motor peripheral nervous system, causing ascending and descending paralysis. GBS is often triggered by a viral infection, but may be idiopathic in origin. Diagnosis is by history, clinical symptoms, and lumbar puncture, which often show increased protein with normal glucose and cell count although protein may not increase for a week or more.

> **Review Video: Guillain-Barre Syndrome**
> Visit mometrix.com/academy and enter code: 742900

Symptoms include:

- Numbness and tingling with increasing weakness of lower extremities that may become generalized, sometimes resulting in complete paralysis and inability to breathe without ventilatory support.
- Deep tendon reflexes are typically absent and some people experience facial weakness and ophthalmoplegia (paralysis of muscles controlling movement of eyes).

Treatment includes:

- Supportive: Fluids, physical therapy, and antibiotics for infections
- Patients should be hospitalized for observation and placed on ventilator support if forced vital capacity is reduced.
- While there is no definitive treatment, plasma exchange or IV immunoglobulin may shorten the duration of symptoms.

MUSCULAR DYSTROPHY

Muscular dystrophies are genetic disorders with gradual degeneration of muscle fibers and progressive weakness and atrophy of skeletal muscles and loss of mobility. **Pseudohypertrophic (Duchenne) muscular dystrophy** is the most common form and the most severe. It is an X-linked disorder in about 50% of the cases with the rest sporadic mutations, affecting males almost exclusively. Children typically have some delay in motor development with difficulty walking and have evidence of muscle weakness by about age 3. Pseudohypertrophic refers to enlargement of muscles by fatty infiltration associated with muscular atrophy, which causes contractures and deformities of joints. Abnormal bone development results in spinal and other skeletal deformities. The disease progresses rapidly, and most children are wheelchair bound by about 12 years of age. As the disease progresses, it involves the muscles of the diaphragm and other muscles needed for respiration. Mild to frank mental deficiency is common. Facial, oropharyngeal, and respiratory muscles weaken late in the disease. Cardiomegaly commonly occurs. Death most often relates to respiratory infection or cardiac failure by age 25. Treatment is supportive.

CEREBRAL PALSY

Cerebral palsy (CP) is a non-progressive motor dysfunction related to CNS damage associated with congenital, hypoxic, or traumatic injury before, during, or ≤2 years after birth. It may include visual defects, speech impairment, seizures, and intellectual disability. There are four **types of motor dysfunction:**

- **Spastic**: Damage to the cerebral cortex or pyramidal tract. Constant hypertonia and rigidity lead to contractures and curvature of the spine.
- **Dyskinetic**: Damage to the extrapyramidal, basal ganglia. Tremors and twisting with exaggerated posturing and impairment of voluntary muscle control.
- **Ataxic**: Damage to the extrapyramidal cerebellum. Atonic muscles in infancy with lack of balance, instability of muscles, and poor gait.
- **Mixed**: Combinations of all three types with multiple areas of damage.

Characteristics of CP include:

- Hypotonia or hypertonia with rigidity and spasticity
- Athetosis (constant writhing motions)
- Ataxia
- Hemiplegia (one-sided involvement, more severe in upper extremities)
- Diplegia (all extremities involved, but more severe in lower extremities)
- Quadriplegia (all extremities involved with arms flexed and legs extended)

MYASTHENIA GRAVIS

Myasthenia gravis is an autoimmune disorder that results in sporadic, progressive weakness of striated (skeletal) muscles because of impaired transmission of nerve impulses. Myasthenia gravis usually affects muscles controlled by the cranial nerves although any muscle group may be affected. Many patients also have thymomas.

Signs/symptoms include weakness and fatigue that worsens throughout the day. Patients often exhibit ptosis and diplopia. They may have trouble chewing and swallowing and often appear to have masklike facies. If respiratory muscles are involved, patients may exhibit signs of respiratory failure. Myasthenic crisis occurs when patients can no longer breathe independently.

Diagnosis includes electromyography and the Tensilon test (an IV injection of edrophonium or neostigmine, which improves function if the patient has myasthenia gravis, but does not improve function if the symptoms are from a different cause). CT or MRI to diagnose thymoma.

Treatment includes anticholinesterase drugs (neostigmine, pyridostigmine) to relieve some muscle weakness, but these drugs lose effectiveness as the disease progresses. Corticosteroids may be used. Thymectomy is performed if thymoma is present. Tracheotomy and mechanical ventilation may be needed for myasthenic crisis.

> **Review Video: Myasthenia Gravis**
> Visit mometrix.com/academy and enter code: 162510

SEIZURE DISORDERS
PARTIAL SEIZURES
Partial seizures are caused by electrical discharges to a localized area of the cerebral cortex, such as the frontals, temporal, or parietal lobes with seizure characteristics related to the area of involvement. They may begin in a focal area and become generalized, often preceded by an aura.

- **Simple partial:** Unilateral motor symptoms including somatosensory, psychic, and autonomic
    - Aversive: Eyes and head turned away from focal side
    - Sylvan (usually during sleep): Tonic-clonic movements of the face, salivation, and arrested speech
- **Special sensory:** Various sensations (numbness, tingling, prickling, or pain) spreading from one area. May include visual sensations, posturing or hypertonia.
- **Complex (psychomotor):** No loss of consciousness, but altered consciousness and non-responsive with amnesia. May involve complex sensorium with bad tastes, auditory or visual hallucinations, feeling of déjà vu, strong fear. May carry out repetitive activities, such as walking, running, smacking lips, chewing, or drawling. Rarely aggressive. Seizure usually followed by prolonged drowsiness and confusion. Most common ages 3 through adolescence.

GENERALIZED SEIZURES
Generalized seizures lack a focal onset and appear to involve both hemispheres, usually presenting with loss of consciousness and no preceding aura.

- **Tonic-clonic (Grand Mal):** Occurs without warning
    - Tonic period (10–30 seconds): Eyes roll upward with loss of consciousness, arms flexed; stiffen in symmetric tonic contraction of body, apneic with cyanosis and salivating
    - Clonic period (10 seconds to 30 minutes, but usually 30 seconds). Violent rhythmic jerking with contraction and relaxation. May be incontinent of urine and feces. Contractions slow and then stop.

Following seizures, there may be confusion, disorientation, and impairment of motor activity, speech, and vision for several hours. Headache, nausea, and vomiting may occur. Person often falls asleep and awakens more lucid.

- **Absence (Petit Mal):** Onset is at ages 4–12 and usually ends in puberty. Onset is abrupt with brief loss of consciousness for 5–10 seconds and slight loss of muscle tone but often appears to be daydreaming. Lip smacking or eye twitching may occur.

EPILEPSY
Epilepsy is diagnosed based on a history of seizure activity as well as supporting EEG findings. Treatment is individualized. First line treatments include antiepileptic medications for partial and generalized tonic-clonic seizures. Usually, treatment is started with one medication, but this may need to be changed, adjusted, or an additional medication added until the seizures are under control or to avoid adverse effects, which include allergic reactions, especially skin irritations and acute or chronic toxicity. Milder reactions often subside with time or adjustment in doses. Toxic reactions may vary considerably, depending upon the medication and duration of use, so close monitoring is essential. Severe rash and hepatotoxicity are common toxic reactions that occur with many of the antiepileptic drugs. Dosages of drugs may need to be adjusted to avoid breakthrough seizures during times of stress, such as during illness or surgery. Alcohol/drug abuse and sleep deprivation may also cause breakthrough seizures. Most anticonvulsant drugs are teratogenic.

STATUS EPILEPTICUS

Status epilepticus (SE) is usually generalized tonic-clonic seizures that are characterized by a series of seizures with intervening time too short for regaining of consciousness. The constant assault and periods of apnea can lead to exhaustion, respiratory failure with hypoxemia and hypercapnia, cardiac failure, and death.

Causes: Uncontrolled epilepsy or non-compliance with anticonvulsants, infections such as encephalitis, encephalopathy or stroke, drug toxicity (isoniazid), brain trauma, neoplasms, and metabolic disorders.

Treatment includes:

- Anticonvulsants usually beginning with a fast-acting benzodiazepine (lorazepam), often in steps, with administration of medication every 5 minutes until seizures subside.
- If cause is undetermined, acyclovir and ceftriaxone may be administered.
- If there is no response to the first 2 doses of anticonvulsants (refractory SE), rapid sequence intubation (RSI), which involves sedation and paralytic anesthesia, may be done while therapy continues. Combining phenobarbital and benzodiazepine can cause apnea, so intubation may be necessary.
- Antiepileptic medications are added.

> **Review Video: Seizures**
> Visit mometrix.com/academy and enter code: 977061

BRAIN TUMORS

Any type of brain tumor can occur in adults. Brain tumors may be primary, arising within the brain, or secondary as a result of metastasis:

- **Astrocytoma**: This arises from astrocytes, which are glial cells. It is the most common type of tumor, occurring throughout the brain. There are many types of astrocytomas, and most are slow growing. Some are operable while others are not. Radiation may be given after removal. Astrocytomas include glioblastomas, aggressively malignant tumors occurring most often in adults 45–70.
- **Glioblastoma**: This is the most common and most malignant adult brain tumor/astrocytoma. Treatment includes surgery, radiation, and chemotherapy, but survival rates are very low.
- **Brain stem glioma**: This may be fast or slow growing but is generally not operable because of location, although it may be treated with radiation or chemotherapy.
- **Craniopharyngioma**: This is a congenital, slow-growing, recurrent (especially if >5 cm) and benign cystic tumor that is difficult to resect and is treated with surgery and radiation.
- **Meningioma**: Slow growing recurrent tumors are usually benign and most often occur in women, ages 40–70; however, they can cause severe impairment/death, depending on size and location. Meningiomas are surgically removed if causing symptoms.
- **Ganglioglioma**: This can occur anywhere in the brain and is usually slow growing and benign.
- **Medulloblastoma**: There are many types of medulloblastoma, most arising in the cerebellum, malignant, and fast growing. Surgical excision is often followed by radiation and chemotherapy although recent studies show using just chemotherapy controls recurrence with less neurological damage.
- **Oligodendroglioma**: This tumor most often occurs in the cerebrum, primarily the frontal or temporal lobes, involving the myelin sheath of the neurons. It is slow growing and most common in those age 40–60.
- **Optical nerve glioma**: This slow growing tumor of the optic nerve is usually a form of astrocytoma. Optic nerve glioma is often associated with neurofibromatosis type I (NF1), occurring in 15–40% of patients with NF1. Despite surgical, chemotherapy, or radiotherapy treatment, it is usually fatal.

STROKES

HEMORRHAGIC STROKES

Hemorrhagic strokes account for about 20% of all strokes and result from a ruptured cerebral artery, causing not only a lack of oxygen and nutrients but also edema that causes widespread pressure and damage:

- **Intracerebral** is bleeding into the substance of the brain from an artery in the central lobes, basal ganglia, pons, or cerebellum. Intracerebral hemorrhage usually results from atherosclerotic degenerative changes, hypertension, brain tumors, anticoagulation therapy, or use of illicit drugs, such as cocaine.
- **Intracranial aneurysm** occurs with ballooning cerebral artery ruptures, most commonly at the Circle of Willis.
- **Arteriovenous malformation**. Rupture of AVMs can cause brain attack in young adults.
- **Subarachnoid hemorrhage** is bleeding in the space between the meninges and brain, resulting from aneurysm, AVM, or trauma. This type of hemorrhage compresses brain tissue.

Treatment includes: The patient may need airway protection/artificial ventilation if neurologic compromise is severe. Blood pressure is lowered to control rate of bleeding but with caution to avoid hypotension and resulting cerebral ischemia (Goal – CPP >70). Sedation can lower ICP and blood pressure, and seizure prophylaxis will be indicated as blood irritates the cerebral cells. An intraventricular catheter may be used in ICP management; correct any clotting disorders if identified.

ISCHEMIA STROKES

Strokes (brain attacks, cerebrovascular accidents) result when there is interruption of the blood flow to an area of the brain. The two basic types are ischemic and hemorrhagic. About 80% are **ischemic**, resulting from blockage of an artery supplying the brain:

- **Thrombosis** in a large artery, usually resulting from atherosclerosis, may block circulation to a large area of the brain. It is most common in the elderly and may occur suddenly or after episodes of transient ischemic attacks.
- **Lacunar infarct** (a penetrating thrombosis in a small artery) is most common in those with diabetes mellitus and/or hypertension.
- **Embolism** travels through the arterial system and lodges in the brain, most commonly in the left middle cerebral artery. An embolism may be cardiogenic, resulting from cardiac arrhythmia or surgery. An embolism usually occurs rapidly with no warning signs.
- **Cryptogenic** has no identifiable cause.

Medical management of ischemic strokes with tissue plasminogen activator (tPA) or tenecteplase, the primary treatment, should be initiated within 3 hours (or up to 4.5 hours if inclusion criteria are met):

- **Thrombolytic,** such as tPA or tenecteplase, which is produced by recombinant DNA and is used to dissolve fibrin clots. It is given intravenously (0.9 mg/kg up to 90 mg) with 10% injected as an initial bolus and the rest over the next hour.
- **Antihypertensives** if MAP >130 mmHg or systolic BP >220
- **Cooling** to reduce hyperthermia
- **Osmotic diuretics** (mannitol), hypertonic saline, loop diuretics (Lasix), and/or corticosteroids (dexamethasone) to decrease cerebral edema and intracranial pressure
- **Aspirin/anticoagulation** may be used with embolism
- Monitor and treat hyperglycemia
- **Surgical Intervention:** Used when other treatment fails, may go in through artery and manually remove the clot

Symptoms of Brain Attacks in Relation to Area of Brain Affected

Brain attacks most commonly occur in the right or left hemisphere, but the exact location and the extent of brain damage from a brain attack affects the type of presenting symptoms. If the frontal area of either side is involved, there tends to be memory and learning deficits. Some symptoms are common to specific areas and help to identify the area involved:

- **Right hemisphere**: This results in left paralysis or paresis and a left visual field deficit that may cause spatial and perceptual disturbances, so people may have difficulty judging distance. Fine motor skills may be impacted, resulting in trouble dressing or handling tools. People may become impulsive and exhibit poor judgment, often denying impairment. Left-sided neglect (lack of perception of things on the left side) may occur. Difficulty following directions, short-term memory loss, and depression are also common. Language skills usually remain intact.
- **Left hemisphere**: Results in right paralysis or paresis and a right visual field defect. Depression is common and people often exhibit slow, cautious behavior, requiring repeated instruction and reinforcement for simple tasks. Short-term memory loss and difficulty learning new material or understanding generalizations is common. Difficulty with mathematics, reading, writing, and reasoning may occur. Aphasia (expressive, receptive, or global) is common.
- **Brain stem**: Because the brain stem controls respiration and cardiac function, a brain attack in the brain stem frequently causes death, but those who survive may have a number of problems, including respiratory and cardiac abnormalities. Strokes may involve motor or sensory impairment or both.
- **Cerebellum**: This area controls balance and coordination. Brain attacks in the cerebellum are rare but may result in ataxia, nausea and vomiting, and headaches and dizziness or vertigo.

TIA

Transient ischemic attacks (TIAs) from small clots cause similar but short-lived (minutes to hours) symptoms. Emergent treatment includes placing patient in semi-Fowlers or Fowler's position and administering oxygen. The patient may require oral suctioning if secretions pool. The patient's circulation, airway, and breathing should be assessed and IV access line placed. Thrombolytic therapy to dissolve blood clots should be administered within 1–3 hours. While a patient can recover fully from a TIA, they should be educated, because having a TIA increases an individual's risk for a stroke.

> **Review Video: Overview of Strokes**
> Visit mometrix.com/academy and enter code: 310572

Delirium

Delirium is an acute, sudden, and fluctuating change in consciousness. Delirium occurs in 10–40% of hospitalized older adults and about 80% of patients who are terminally ill. Delirium may result from drugs, infections, hypoxia, trauma, dementia, depression, vision and hearing loss, surgery, alcoholism, untreated pain, fluid/electrolyte imbalance, and malnutrition. If left untreated, delirium greatly increases the risk of morbidity and death.

Signs/symptoms: Reduced ability to focus/sustain attention, language and memory disturbances, disorientation, confusion, audiovisual hallucinations, sleep disturbance, and psychomotor activity disorder.

Diagnosis: Patient interview, history/chart/medication review, and possible blood tests to identify electrolyte imbalance/abnormalities.

Treatment includes:

- **Medications**: Trazodone, lorazepam, haloperidol—though these may make confusion worse in elderly patients
- **Procedures**: Provide a sitter to ensure safety, decreasing dosage of hypnotics and psychotropics, correct underlying cause

Prevention: Reorient patient frequently, ensure adequate rest/nutrition, monitor response to medications, and treat infections and dehydration/malnutrition early.

AGITATION

Agitation is a common occurrence in the critically ill patient. Factors contributing to the development of agitation include drug or alcohol withdrawal, sleep deprivation, hypoxemia, electrolyte or metabolic imbalance, anxiety, pain, and adverse drug reactions. Delirium may also include agitation as a manifestation.

Diagnosis: The physiologic effects of agitation may include increases in heart rate, respiratory rate, blood pressure, intracranial pressure, and oxygen consumption. In addition, agitation can contribute to the self-removal of lines or tubes and combative behavior that may result in patient harm.

Treatment: Treatment of agitation involves the identification and correction of causative factors. The use of pharmacologic agents to manage pain, anxiety, and agitation are often utilized. Non-pharmacologic interventions including verbal de-escalation (when possible). The promotion of normal sleep patterns and relaxation techniques may also be effective. Early identification of signs and symptoms is also critical in the successful management of agitation.

DEMENTIA

Dementia is a chronic condition in which there is progressive and irreversible loss of memory and function. There are many types of dementia a nurse may encounter:

- **Creutzfeldt-Jakob disease**: Rapidly progressive dementia with impaired memory, behavioral changes, and incoordination
- **Dementia with Lewy Bodies**: Similar to Alzheimer's, but symptoms may fluctuate frequently; may also include visual hallucinations, muscle rigidity, and tremors
- **Frontotemporal dementia**: Causes marked changes in personality and behavior; characterized by difficulty using and understanding language
- **Mixed dementia**: Combination of different types of dementia
- **Normal pressure hydrocephalus**: Characterized by ataxia, memory loss, and urinary incontinence
- **Parkinson dementia**: Involves impaired decision making and difficulty concentrating, learning new material, understanding complex language, and sequencing
- **Vascular dementia**: Memory loss less pronounced than that common to Alzheimer's, but symptoms are similar

Nursing considerations: Distraction is usually the best course of action to deter the patient with dementia. Reorient frequently, but do not argue with the patient. Avoid restraints or sedatives, which worsen confusion.

INCREASED INTRACRANIAL PRESSURE

Increased intracranial pressure is a pressure build up inside the cranium that results in altered neurological function. Causes can include intracranial bleeding, tumors, cerebrospinal fluid (CSF) build up, or edema. These alterations can be caused by head trauma, hydrocephalus, meningitis, encephalitis, brain tumors, intracerebral hemorrhage, or Guillain-Barre syndrome. The brain has mechanisms to deal with rising intracranial volume; when the rising volume is too much for these mechanisms, less blood will be able to get to the brain, leading to increased edema which further raises the ICP. This cycle will continue until no blood reaches the brain and the brain dies. If the brain stem is pushed downwards and herniates, the body's vital functions cease to operate.

MONITORING OF INTRACRANIAL PRESSURE

Monitoring of intracranial pressure in pediatric patients is of special importance because of the danger of herniation with increased pressure. Studies indicate that intracranial pressure requires treatment if ≥20 mmHg, although some authorities believe that infants and young children may need treatment at lower pressures. **Monitoring** of intracranial pressure can be done in a number of ways:

- Intraventricular catheter attached to a transducer to record pressure (most accurate)
- Subarachnoid bolt
- Epidural or subdural catheter
- Fiber-optic transducer-tipped catheter placed in the ventricular or subdural space
- External anterior fontanel monitor

CSF may be drained continuously or intermittently and must be monitored hourly for amount, color, and character. For ICP measurement, the patient's head must be elevated to 30–45° and the transducer leveled to the outer canthus of the eye. Normal ICP values (manometer):

- Infant: 1.5–6.0 mmHg
- Young child: 3–7 mmHg
- Older child: 2–7 mmHg
- 18 years: 0–15 mmHg

MONRO-KELLIE HYPOTHESIS AND SYMPTOMS OF INCREASED ICP

The Monro-Kellie hypothesis states that to maintain a normal intracranial pressure (ICP), a change in volume in one compartment must be compensated by a reciprocal change in volume in another compartment. The three brain compartments are brain tissue, CSF, and blood. The CSF and blood can change more easily to accommodate changes in pressure than tissue, so medical intervention focuses on cerebral blood flow and drainage. **Symptoms** include:

- **Infants**: Bulging fontanels without normal pulsations, distention of scalp veins, and increased head circumference. Infants may be irritable with high-pitched cries and poor feeding.
- **Children**: Headache, vomiting without associated nausea, double and blurred vision, and seizures. Behavioral and personality changes may occur, increased lethargy, memory loss, and inability to follow directions.
- **Late signs**: Decreased level of consciousness, motor response, and response to painful stimuli. Pupil size and reactivity change, decerebrate or decorticate posturing, respiratory depression with Cheyne-Stokes and papilledema. Cushing's triad:
  - Increased systolic pressure with widened pulse pressure
  - Bradycardia in response to increased pressure
  - Decreased respirations

As the pressure becomes severe, the child will become lethargic which may progress to coma, be unable to move on command, react more violently to pain stimuli, have decreased pupil size and reactivity, display decerebrate (the arms and legs will extend and turn inward) or decorticate (the arms are flexed toward the body, hands clenched on chest, with legs extended) posturing, have swelling of the optic nerve at the back of the eye, and/or have abnormal respirations.

Diagnosis and Care

ICP is measured by various means. CT or MRI is used to find the cause of the increased ICP. The child should be monitored for changes in vital signs, LOC, activity, behavior, and pupils. Various tools to measure ICP can be used: intraventricular catheter, subarachnoid screw, fiber-optic sensor, or fiber-optic transducer-tipped catheter. Medications include diuretics, anticonvulsants, and corticosteroids. The head and neck should be kept in a neutral, well-aligned position to prevent compression. Suctioning and respiratory PT may increase ICP and should be avoided. Maintain good respiratory status and O_2 saturation. Keep fluids balanced. Monitor I&Os. Raise the head of bed to 15–30°. Prevent constipation and straining by using laxatives and diet control. Provide a nutritious diet to prevent weight loss. Watch for skin breakdown. Watch for signs of diabetes insipidus (low BP, high HR, weight loss, thirst, apathy or depression, excess urination, constipation, dilute urine, low blood volume and high blood sodium) and syndrome of inappropriate antidiuretic hormone (weight gain, high BP, seizures, coma, vomiting, concentrated low volume urine output, increased blood volume, and low blood sodium).

Hydrocephalus in Pediatric Patients

Symptoms of hydrocephalus depend on the age of onset. In early infancy, before closure of cranial sutures, head enlargement is the most common presentation, but in older children with less elasticity in the skull, neurological symptoms usually relate to increasing pressure on structures of the brain:

- **Early infancy**: Bulging, non-pulsating fontanels (usually anterior) usually with increasing head circumference, dilated scalp veins, separating sutures, and positive Macewen sign (resonance on tapping near the frontal-temporal-parietal juncture)
- **Later signs**: Enlargement of frontal area with depressed eyes, setting sun sign (sclera evident above iris), and pupils sluggish and unequally reactive
- **Throughout infancy**: Increased irritability, lethargy, high-pitched crying, delayed responses, change in level of consciousness, opisthotonos, spasticity, difficulty feeding, and cardiopulmonary compromise
- **Childhood** (related to increased intracranial pressure): Headache relieved by vomiting, papilledema, strabismus, ataxia, irritability, lethargy, confusion, and difficulty communicating

Treatment

Hydrocephalus is diagnosed through CT and MRI, which help to determine the cause. Treatment may vary somewhat depending upon the underlying disorder, which may require treatment. For example, if obstruction is caused by a tumor, surgical excision to directly remove the obstruction is required. Generally, however, most hydrocephalus is **treated** with shunts:

- **Ventricular-peritoneal shunt**: This procedure is the most common and consists of placement of a ventricular catheter directly into the ventricles (usually lateral) at one end with the other end in the peritoneal area to drain away excess CSF. There is a one-way valve near the proximal end that prevents backflow but opens when pressure rises to drain fluid. In some cases, the distal end drains into the right atrium.
- **Endoscopic third ventriculostomy (ETV)**: A small opening is made in the base of the third ventricle so CSF can bypass an obstruction. This procedure is not universally effective and is done with a small endoscope.

MIGRAINE AND TENSION HEADACHES

Headaches are common in children and usually benign. About 3% of children develop migraine headaches before age 7 and up to 23% by age 11 or older, and many experience tension headaches. Sudden onset of headache or persistent or severe headache may indicate a pathological condition, such as increased intracranial pressure or tumor, so headaches should be evaluated carefully.

Type	Symptoms	Treatment
Migraine	Unilateral or bilateral, moderate to severe throbbing pain persisting ≤72 hours and sometimes preceded by visual or motor aura. Co-morbidities include nausea, vomiting, photophobia, or phonophobia. Young children may exhibit head banging, irritability, general malaise, and head holding.	NSAIDs, acetaminophen. Relaxation techniques. Biofeedback. Adolescents: Sumatriptan nasal spray. Identifying and eliminating triggers, such as caffeine, foods, or additives
Tension	Dull, aching, mild to moderate bilateral constricting pain about head, neck, and sometimes shoulders persisting hours or days. Pain unrelated to physical activity.	NSAIDs, acetaminophen. Ice pack. Rest. Relaxation techniques

REBOUND AND SINUS- OR DENTAL-RELATED HEADACHES

Type	Symptoms	Treatment
Rebound (from excess medication use)	Vary but may be bilateral or unilateral in frontal area with frequency increasing with increased medication use. Tend to occur at least 5 times weekly or 15 times per month.	Withdrawal of medications (NSAIDs, acetaminophen, other drugs). Substitution with other drugs if headaches persist. Clonidine for withdrawal symptoms if necessary.
Sinus- or dental-related	Dull constant pain and pressure over affected areas of sinus or dental abscess. Fever. Changing head position may vary pain.	NSAIDs, acetaminophen. Antibiotics. Application of cold or heat. Surgical drainage of sinus may be indicated for severe infection. Dental treatment as needed.

SPINA BIFIDA AND MYELOMENINGOCELE

The terms spina bifida and myelomeningocele are often used interchangeably, but there is a distinction. Spina bifida is a neural tube defect with an incomplete spinal cord and often missing vertebrae that allow the meninges and spinal cord to protrude through the opening. There are five basic types:

- **Spina bifida**: Defect in which the vertebral column is not closed, with varying degrees of herniation through the opening
- **Spina bifida occulta**: Failure of the vertebral column to close, but no herniation through the opening so the defect may not be obvious
- **Spina bifida cystica**: Defect in closure with external sac-like protrusion with varying degrees of nerve involvement
- **Meningocele**: Spina bifida cystica with meningeal sac filled with spinal fluid
- **Myelomeningocele**: Spina bifida cystica with meningeal sac containing spinal fluid and part of the spinal cord and nerves

Physical Manifestations and Management Related to Myelomeningocele

Myelomeningocele, which involves spina bifida cystica with a meningeal sac containing spinal fluid and part of the spinal cord and nerves, comprises about 75% of the total cases of spina bifida. There are numerous physical manifestations:

- **Exposed sac** poses the danger of infection and cerebrospinal fluid leakage; so surgical repair is usually done within the first 48 hours although it may be delayed for a few days, especially if the sac is intact.
- **Chiari type II malformation** comprises hypoplasia of the cerebellum and displacement of the lower brainstem into the upper cervical area, which impairs circulation of spinal fluid. It may result in symptoms of cranial nerve dysfunction (dysphonia, dysphagia) and weakness and lack of coordination of upper extremities.
- **Neurogenic bladder** is common and may require credé massage for infants and later intermittent clean catheterization.
- **Fecal incontinence** is common and may be controlled, as the child gets older, with diet and bowel training.
- **Musculoskeletal abnormalities** depend upon the level of the myelomeningocele and the degree of impairment but often involve the muscle and joints of the lower extremities and sometimes the upper. Dysfunction often increases with the number of shunts. Scoliosis and lumbar lordosis are common. Hip contractures may cause dislocations.
- **Paralysis/paresis** may vary considerably and be spastic or flaccid. Many children require wheelchairs for mobility although some are fitted with braces for assisted ambulation.
- **Seizures** occur in about a quarter of those affected, sometimes related to shunt malfunction.
- **Hydrocephalus** is present in about 25-35% of infants at birth and 60-70% after surgical repair with ventriculoperitoneal shunt. Untreated, the ventricles will dilate and brain damage can occur.
- **Tethered spinal cord** occurs when the distal end of the spinal cord becomes attached to the bone or site of surgical repair and does not move superiorly with growth, causing increased pain, spasticity, and disability and requiring surgical repair.

Respiratory Pathophysiology

ACUTE PULMONARY EMBOLISM

Acute pulmonary embolism occurs when a pulmonary artery or arteriole is blocked, cutting off blood supply to the pulmonary vessels and subsequent oxygenation of the blood. While most pulmonary emboli are from thrombus formation, they can also be caused by air, fat, or septic embolus (from bacterial invasion of a thrombus). Common originating sites for thrombus formation are the deep veins in the legs, the pelvic veins, and the right atrium. Causes include stasis related to damage to endothelial wall and changes in blood coagulation factors. Atrial fibrillation poses a serious risk because blood pools in the right atrium, forming clots that travel directly through the right ventricle to the lungs. The obstruction of the artery/arteriole causes an increase in alveolar dead space in which there is ventilation but impairment of gas exchange because of the ventilation/perfusion mismatching or intrapulmonary shunting. This results in hypoxia, hypercapnia, and the release of mediators that cause bronchoconstriction. If more than 50% of the vascular bed becomes excluded, pulmonary hypertension occurs.

SYMPTOMS AND DIAGNOSIS

Clinical manifestations of acute pulmonary embolism (PE) vary according to the size of the embolus and the area of occlusion.

Symptoms include:

- Dyspnea with tachypnea
- Cyanosis; may turn grey or blue from nipple line up (massive PE)
- Anxiety and restlessness, feeling of doom
- Chest pain, tachycardia, may progress to arrhythmias (PEA)
- Fever
- Rales
- Cough (sometimes with hemoptysis)
- Hemodynamic instability

Diagnostic tests are as follows:

- ABG analysis may show hypoxemia (decreased PaO_2), hypocarbia (decreased $PaCO_2$) and respiratory alkalosis (increased pH).
- D-dimer will show elevation with PE but is not definitively diagnostic without a CT scan.
- ECG may show sinus tachycardia or other abnormalities.
- Echocardiogram can show emboli in the central arteries and can assess the hemodynamic status of the right side of the heart.
- Spiral CT may provide definitive diagnosis.
- V/Q scintigraphy can confirm diagnosis.
- Pulmonary angiograms also can confirm diagnosis.

MEDICAL MANAGEMENT

Medical management of pulmonary embolism starts with preventive measures for those at risk, including leg exercises, elastic compression stockings, and anticoagulation therapy. Most pulmonary emboli present as medical emergencies, so the immediate task is to stabilize the patient. **Medical management** may include:

- **Oxygen** to relieve hypoxemia
- **Intravenous infusions:** Dobutamine (Dobutrex) or dopamine (Intropin) to relieve hypotension
- **Cardiac monitoring** for dysrhythmias and issues due to right sided heart failure
- **Medications** as indicated: digitalis glycosides, diuretic, and antiarrhythmics
- Intubation and mechanical ventilation may be required

- **Analgesics** (such as morphine sulfate) or sedation to relieve anxiety
- **Anticoagulants** to prevent recurrence (although it will not dissolve clots already present), including heparin and warfarin (Coumadin)
- **Placement of percutaneous venous filter** (Greenfield) in the inferior vena cava to prevent further emboli from entering the lungs, if anticoagulation therapy is contraindicated
- **Thrombolytic therapy,** recombinant tissue-type plasminogen activator (rt-PA) or streptokinase, for those severely compromised, but these treatments have limited success and pose the danger of bleeding

TRAUMATIC ASPHYXIA

Asphyxia may relate to a number of different injuries:

- **Traumatic asphyxia** most commonly involves a crush injury of the thorax and possibly traumatic injuries to multiple organs. Crush injuries are characterized by petechiae in the area of compression although tight-fitting clothing, such as a woman's bra, may prevent petechiae from forming.
- **Manual strangulation** may involve crush injuries to the throat, such as hyoid fracture. Often the face appears cyanotic while the rest of the body does not. Petechiae may be present on the face as well. Bruising may be noted about the throat.
- **Ligature strangulation** is similar to manual although throat markings are different, with an indented area surrounding the neck.
- **Hanging** produces a V-shaped marking on the throat and does not encircle the neck.
- **Choking** obstructs the airway. (May require bronchoscopy to remove foreign object).

In all cases, immediate establishment of airway, breathing, and circulation (ABCs) takes precedence. Surgical intervention may be needed for traumatic crush injuries.

SUBMERSION ASPHYXIA

Submersion (near-drowning) asphyxiation can cause profound damage to the central nervous system, pulmonary dysfunction related to aspiration, cardiac hypoxia with life-threatening arrhythmias, fluid and electrolyte imbalances, and multi-organ damage, so treatment can be complex. Hypothermia related to near drowning has some protective affect because blood is shunted to the brain and heart. **Treatment** includes:

- Immediate establishment of airway, breathing and circulation (ABCs)
- NG tube and gastric decompression to reduce risk of aspiration
- Neurological evaluation
- Pulmonary management includes monitoring for ≥72 hours for respiratory deterioration. Ventilation may need positive-end expiratory pressure (PEEP), but this poses danger to cardiac output and can cause barotrauma, so use should be limited.
- In patients that are symptomatic but do not yet need intubation, use supplemental oxygen to keep $SpO_2 > 94\%$
- Monitoring of cardiac output and function
- Neurological care to reduce cerebral edema and increased intracranial pressure and prevent secondary injury
- Rewarming if necessary (0.5–1.0 °C/hr)

PNEUMONIA

Pneumonia is inflammation of the lung parenchyma, filling the alveoli with exudate. It is common throughout childhood and adulthood. Pneumonia may be a primary disease or may occur secondary to another infection or disease, such as lung cancer. Pneumonia may be caused by bacteria, viruses, parasites, or fungi. Common causes for community-acquired pneumonia (CAP) include:

- *Streptococcus pneumoniae*
- *Legionella* species
- *Haemophilus influenzae*
- *Staphylococcus aureus*
- *Mycoplasma pneumoniae*
- Viruses

Pneumonia may also be caused by chemical damage. Pneumonia is characterized by **location**:

- **Lobar** involves one or more lobes of the lungs. If lobes in both lungs are affected, it is referred to as bilateral or double pneumonia.
- **Bronchial/lobular** involves the terminal bronchioles, and exudate can involve the adjacent lobules. Usually, the pneumonia occurs in scattered patches throughout the lungs.
- **Interstitial** involves primarily the interstitium and alveoli where white blood cells and plasma fill the alveoli, generating inflammation and creating fibrotic tissue as the alveoli are destroyed.

> **Review Video: Pneumonia**
> Visit mometrix.com/academy and enter code: 628264

HOSPITAL-ACQUIRED PNEUMONIA

Hospital-acquired pneumonia (HAP) is defined as pneumonia that did not appear to be present on admission that occurs at least 48 hours after admission to a hospital. **Healthcare-associated pneumonia (HCAP)** is defined as pneumonia that occurs in a patient within 90 days of being hospitalized for 2 or more days at an acute care hospital or LTAC. **Ventilator-associated pneumonia (VAP)** is one type of hospital acquired pneumonia that a patient acquires more than 48 hours after having an ETT placed. The most common way that the patient is infected is via aspiration of bacteria that is colonized in the upper respiratory tract Critically ill individuals are highly susceptible to colonization with multidrug resistant bacteria within 48 hours of entering an ICU. Aspiration occurs at a higher rate in those patients with HAP, HCAP, and VAP. The frequency of patients developing these types of pneumonia is increasing, with those at highest risk being those with immunosuppression, septic shock, currently hospitalized for more than five days, and those who have had antibiotics for another infection within the previous three months. These types of pneumonia should be considered if a patient already hospitalized has purulent sputum or a change in respiratory status such as deoxygenating, in combination with a worsening or new chest x-ray infiltrate.

Treatment includes:

- Antibiotic therapy
- Using appropriate isolation and precautions with infected patients
- Preventive measures including maintaining ventilated patients in 30° upright positions, frequent oral care for vent patients, and changing ventilator circuits as per protocol

Antibiotic treatment options for HAP, HCAP, and VAP should take into account many factors, including culture data (when available), patient's comorbidities, flora in the unit, any recent antibiotics by the patient, and whether the patient is at high risk for having multidrug resistant bacteria. As most critical care patients are at high risk, due to factors such as being in an ICU setting, ventilators, and comorbidities, antibiotic recommendations to follow are for coverage for patients with risk factors for multidrug resistant bacteria.

Only one of the following:

- Ceftazidime 2 g every 8 hours IV
- Cefepime 2 g every 8 hours IV
- Imipenem 500 mg every 6 hours IV
- Piperacillin-tazobactam 4.5 g every 6 hours IV

If the patient has a positive MRSA swab or risk of MRSA, add **only one** of the following:

- Vancomycin 15–20 mg/kg every 8–12 hours IV
- Linezolid 600 mg every 12 hours IV

Aspiration Pneumonitis/Pneumonia

Aspiration pneumonitis/pneumonia may occur as the result of any type of aspiration, including foreign objects. The aspirated material creates an inflammatory response, with the irritated mucous membrane at high risk for bacterial infection secondary to the aspiration, causing pneumonia. Gastric contents and oropharyngeal bacteria are commonly aspirated. Gastric contents can cause a severe chemical pneumonitis with hypoxemia, especially if the pH is <2.5. Acidic food particles can cause severe reactions. With acidic damage, bronchospasm and atelectasis occur rapidly with tracheal irritation, bronchitis, and alveolar damage with interstitial edema and hemorrhage. Intrapulmonary shunting and V/Q mismatch may occur. Pulmonary artery pressure increases. Non-acidic liquids and food particles are less damaging, and symptoms may clear within 4 hours of liquid aspiration or granuloma may form about food particles in 1–5 days. Depending upon the type of aspiration, pneumonitis may clear within a week, ARDS or pneumonia may develop, or progressive acute respiratory failure may lead to death.

There are a number of risk factors that can lead to **aspiration pneumonitis/pneumonia:**

- Altered level of consciousness related to illness or sedation
- Depression of gag, swallowing reflex
- Intubation or feeding tubes
- Ileus or gastric distention
- Gastrointestinal disorders, such as gastroesophageal reflux disorders (GERD)

Diagnosis is based on clinical findings, ABGs showing hypoxemia, infiltrates observed on x-ray, and elevated WBC if infection is present.

Symptoms: Similar to other pneumonias:

- Cough often with copious sputum
- Respiratory distress, dyspnea
- Cyanosis
- Tachycardia
- Hypotension

Treatment includes:

- Suctioning as needed to clear upper airway
- Supplemental oxygen
- Antibiotic therapy as indicated after 48 hours if symptoms not resolving
- Symptomatic respiratory support

FOREIGN BODY ASPIRATION

Foreign body aspiration can cause obstruction of the pharynx, larynx, or trachea, leading to acute dyspnea or asphyxiation, and the object may also be drawn distally into the bronchial tree. With adults, most foreign bodies migrate more readily down the right bronchus. Food is the most frequently aspirated, but other small objects, such as coins or needles, may also be aspirated. Sometimes the object causes swelling, ulceration, and general inflammation that hampers removal.

Symptoms include:

- **Initial**: Severe coughing, gagging, sternal retraction, wheezing. Objects in the larynx may cause inability to breathe or speak and lead to respiratory arrest. Objects in the bronchus cause cough, dyspnea, and wheezing.
- **Delayed**: Hours, days, or weeks later, an undetected aspirant may cause an infection distal to the aspirated material. Symptoms depend on the area and extent of the infection.

Treatment includes:

- Removal with laryngoscopy or bronchoscopy (rigid is often better than flexible)
- Antibiotic therapy for secondary infection
- Surgical bronchotomy (rarely required)
- Symptomatic support

CHRONIC BRONCHITIS

Chronic bronchitis is a pulmonary airway disease characterized by severe cough with sputum production for at least 3 months a year for at least 2 consecutive years. Irritation of the airways (often from smoke or pollutants) causes an inflammatory response, increasing the number of mucus-secreting glands and goblet cells while ciliary function decreases so that the extra mucus plugs the airways. Additionally, the bronchial walls thicken, alveoli near the inflamed bronchioles become fibrotic, and alveolar macrophages cannot function properly, increasing susceptibility to infections. Chronic bronchitis is most common in those >45 years old and occurs twice as frequently in females as males.

Symptoms include:

- Persistent cough with increasing sputum
- Dyspnea
- Frequent respiratory infections

Treatment includes:

- Bronchodilators
- Long term continuous oxygen therapy or supplemental oxygen during exercise
- Pulmonary rehabilitation to improve exercise and breathing
- Antibiotics during infections
- Corticosteroids for acute episodes

EMPHYSEMA

Emphysema, the primary component of COPD, is characterized by abnormal distention of air spaces at the ends of the terminal bronchioles, with destruction of alveolar walls so that there is less and less gaseous exchange and increasing dead space with resultant hypoxemia, hypercapnia, and respiratory acidosis. The capillary bed is damaged as well, altering pulmonary blood flow and raising pressure in the right atrium (cor pulmonale) and pulmonary artery, leading to cardiac failure. Complications include respiratory insufficiency and failure. There are two primary types of emphysema (and both forms may be present):

- **Centrilobular** (the most common form) involves the central portion of the respiratory lobule, sparing distal alveoli, and usually affects the upper lobes. Typical symptoms include abnormal ventilation-perfusion ratios, hypoxemia, hypercapnia, and polycythemia with right-sided heart failure.
- **Panlobular** involves enlargement of all air spaces, including the bronchiole, alveolar duct, and alveoli, but there is minimal inflammatory disease. Typical symptoms include hyperextended rigid barrel chest, marked dyspnea, weight loss, and active expiration.

COPD

STAGES

Functional dyspnea, body mass index (BMI), and spirometry are used to assess the **stages of chronic obstructive pulmonary disease (COPD)**. Spirometry measures used are the ratio of forced expiratory volume in the first second of expiration (FEV_1) after full inhalation to total forced vital capacity (FVC). Normal lung function decreases after age 35; so normal values are adjusted for height, weight, gender, and age:

- **Stage 1** (mild): Minimal dyspnea with or without cough and sputum. FEV_1 is ≥80% of predicted rate and FEV_1:FVC <70%.
- **Stage 2** (moderate): Moderate to severe chronic exertional dyspnea with or without cough and sputum. FEV_1 is 50–80% of predicted rate and FEV_1:FVC <70%.
- **Stage 3** (severe): Same as stage 2 but with repeated episodes with increased exertional dyspnea and condition impacting quality of life. FEV_1 is 30–50% of predicted rate and FEV_1:FVC <70%.
- **Stage 4** (very severe): Severe dyspnea and life-threatening episodes that severely impact quality of life. FEV_1 is 30% of predicted rate or <50% with chronic respiratory failure and FEV_1:FVC <70%.

MANAGEMENT

COPD is not reversible, so management aims at slowing its progression, relieving symptoms, and improving quality of life:

- Smoking cessation is the primary means to slow progression and may require smoking cessation support in the form of classes or medications, such as bupropion, nicotine patches or gum, clonidine, or nortriptyline.
- Bronchodilators, such as albuterol and salmeterol, relieve bronchospasm and airway obstruction.
- Corticosteroids, both inhaled (budesonide, beclomethasone) and oral (prednisone) may improve symptoms but are used mostly for associated asthma.
- Oxygen therapy may be long term continuous or used during exertion.
- Bullectomy (for bullous emphysema) to remove bullae (enlarged airspaces that do not ventilate).
- Lung volume reduction surgery may be done if involvement in the lung is limited; however, mortality rates are high.
- Lung transplantation is a definitive high-risk option.
- Pulmonary rehabilitation includes breathing exercises, muscle training, activity pacing, and modification of activities.

> **Review Video: Respiratory Diseases**
> Visit mometrix.com/academy and enter code: 973392

CHRONIC VENTILATORY FAILURE

Chronic ventilatory failure occurs when alveolar ventilation fails to increase in response to increasing levels of carbon dioxide, usually associated with chronic pulmonary diseases, such as asthma and COPD, drug overdoses, or diseases that impair respiratory effort, such as Guillain-Barré and myasthenia gravis. Normally, the ventilatory system is able to maintain PCO_2 and pH levels within narrow limits, even though PO_2 levels may be more variable, but with ventilatory failure, the body is not able to compensate for the resultant hypercapnia and pH falls, resulting in respiratory acidosis. Symptoms include increasing dyspnea with tachypnea, gasping respirations, and use of accessory muscles. Patients may become confused as hypercapnia causes increased intracranial pressure. If pH is <7.2, cardiac arrhythmias, hyperkalemia, and hypotension can occur as pulmonary arteries constrict and the peripheral vascular system dilates. Diagnosis is per symptoms, ABGs consistent with respiratory acidosis (PCO_2 >50 and pH <7.35), pulse oximetry, and chest x-ray. Treatment can include non-invasive PPV (BiPAP), endotracheal mechanical ventilation, corticosteroids, and bronchodilators.

CHRONIC ASTHMA

The three primary symptoms of chronic asthma are cough, wheezing, and dyspnea. In cough-variant asthma, a severe cough may be the only symptom, at least initially. Chronic asthma is characterized by recurring bronchospasm and inflammation of the airways resulting in airway obstruction. Asthma affects the bronchi and not the alveoli. While no longer considered part of COPD because airway obstruction is not constant and is responsive to treatment, over time fibrotic changes in the airways can result in permanent obstruction, especially if asthma is not treated adequately. **Symptoms** of chronic asthma include nighttime coughing, exertional dyspnea, tightness in the chest, and cough. Acute exacerbations may occur, sometimes related to triggers, such as allergies, resulting in increased dyspnea, wheezing, cough, tachycardia, bronchospasm, and rhonchi. **Treatment** of chronic asthma includes chest hygiene, identification and avoidance of triggers, prompt treatment of infections, bronchodilators, long-acting β-2 agonists, and inhaled glucocorticoids.

STATUS ASTHMATICUS

PATHOPHYSIOLOGY

Status asthmaticus is a severe acute attack of asthma that does not respond to conventional therapy. An acute attack of asthma is precipitated by some stimulus, such as an antigen that triggers an allergic response, resulting in an inflammatory cascade that causes edema of the mucous membranes (swollen airway), contraction of smooth muscles (bronchospasm), increased mucus production (cough and obstruction), and hyperinflation of airways (decreased ventilation and shunting). Mast cells and T lymphocytes produce cytokines, which continue the inflammatory response through increased blood flow coupled with vasoconstriction and bronchoconstriction, resulting in fluid leakage from the vasculature. Epithelial cells and cilia are destroyed, exposing nerves and causing hypersensitivity. Sympathetic nervous system receptors in the bronchi stimulate bronchodilation.

CLINICAL SYMPTOMS

The person with status asthmaticus will often present in acute distress, non-responsive to inhaled bronchodilators. **Symptoms** include:

- Signs of airway obstruction
- Sternal and intercostal retractions
- Tachypnea and dyspnea with increasing cyanosis
- Forced prolonged expirations
- Cardiac decompensation with increased left ventricular afterload and increased pulmonary edema resulting from alveolar-capillary permeability. Hypoxia may trigger an increase in pulmonary vascular resistance with increased right ventricular afterload.
- Pulsus paradoxus (decreased pulse on inspiration and increased on expiration) with extra beats on inspiration detected through auscultation but not detected radially. Blood pressure normally decreases slightly during inspiration, but this response is exaggerated. Pulsus paradoxus indicates increasing severity of asthma.
- Hypoxemia (with impending respiratory failure)
- Hypocapnia followed by hypercapnia (with impending respiratory failure)
- Metabolic acidosis

INDICATIONS FOR MECHANICAL VENTILATION FOR STATUS ASTHMATICUS

Mechanical ventilation (MV) for status asthmaticus should be avoided, if possible, because of the danger of increased bronchospasm as well as barotrauma and decreased circulation. However, there are some absolute indications for the use of intubation and ventilation and a number of other indications that are evaluated on an individual basis.

The following are **absolute indications for MV**:

- Cardiac and/or pulmonary arrest
- Markedly depressed mental status (obtundation)
- Severe hypoxia and/or apnea

The following are **relative indications for MV**:

- Exhaustion/muscle fatigue from exertion of breathing
- Sharply diminished breath sounds and no audible wheezing
- Pulse paradoxus >20–40 mmHg; absent = imminent respiratory arrest
- PaO_2 <70 mmHg on 100% oxygen
- Dysphonia
- Central cyanosis
- Increased hypercapnia
- Metabolic/respiratory acidosis: pH <7.20

In this patient population, ventilator goal is to minimize airway pressures while oxygenating the patient. Vent settings include: low tidal volume (6–8 mL/kg), low respiratory rate (10–14 respirations/minute), and high inspiratory flow rate (80–100 L/min).

> **Review Video: Mechanical Ventilation**
> Visit mometrix.com/academy and enter code: 679637

AIR LEAK SYNDROMES

Air leak syndromes may result in significant respiratory distress. Leaks may occur spontaneously or secondary to some type of trauma (accidental, mechanical, iatrogenic) or disease. As pressure increases inside the alveoli, the alveolar wall pulls away from the perivascular sheath and subsequent alveolar rupture allows air to follow the perivascular planes and flow into adjacent areas. There are two categories:

- **Pneumothorax:**
    - Air in the pleural space causes a lung to collapse.
- **Barotrauma/volutrauma** with air in the interstitial space (usually resolve over time):
    - Pneumoperitoneum is air in the peritoneal area, including the abdomen and occasionally the scrotal sac of male infants.
    - Pneumomediastinum is air in the mediastinal area between the lungs.
    - Pneumopericardium is air in the pericardial sac that surrounds the heart.
    - Subcutaneous emphysema is air in the subcutaneous tissue planes of the chest wall.
    - Pulmonary interstitial emphysema (PIE) is air trapped in the interstitium between the alveoli.

PNEUMOTHORAX

Pneumothorax occurs when there is a leak of air into the pleural space, resulting in complete or partial collapse of a lung.

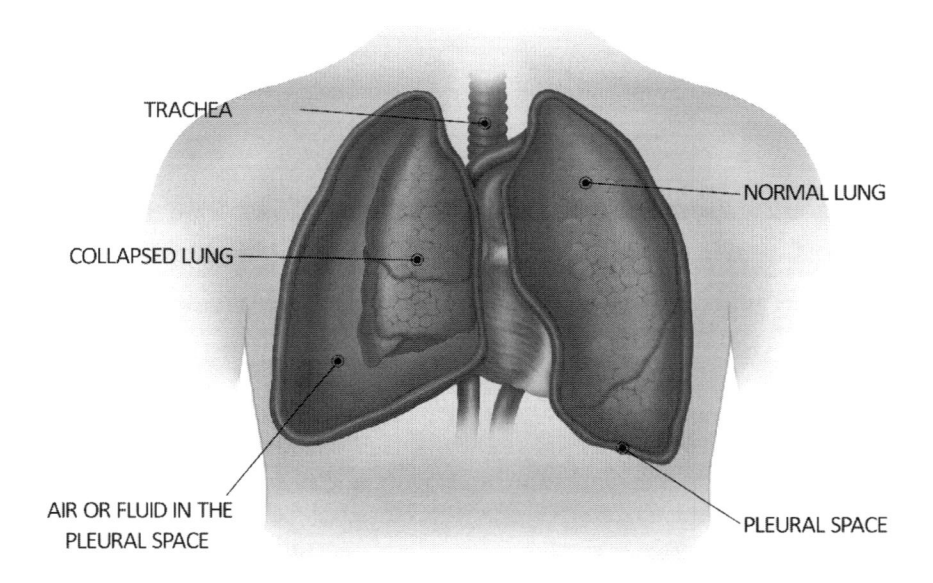

PNEUMOTHORAX

Symptoms: Vary widely depending on the cause and degree of the pneumothorax and whether or not there is an underlying disease. Symptoms include acute pleuritic pain (95%), usually on the affected side, and decreased breath sounds. In a *tension pneumothorax,* symptoms include tracheal deviation and hemodynamic compromise.

Diagnosis: Clinical findings; radiograph: 6-foot upright posterior-anterior; ultrasound may detect traumatic pneumothorax.

Treatment: Chest-tube thoracostomy with underwater seal drainage is the most common treatment for all types of pneumothorax.

- Tension pneumothorax: Immediate needle decompression and chest tube thoracostomy
- Small pneumothorax, patient stable: Oxygen administration and observation for 3–6 hours. If no increase is shown on repeat x-ray, patient may be discharged with another x-ray in 24 hours.
- Primary spontaneous pneumothorax: Catheter aspiration or chest tube thoracostomy

> **Review Video: Pneumothorax**
> Visit mometrix.com/academy and enter code: 186841

CLINICAL INDICATIONS OF ACUTE RESPIRATORY INFECTIONS
FEVER, LYMPH NODES, AND MENINGEAL IRRITATION

Children with acute respiratory infections may manifest a wide range of symptoms:

- **Fever** is usually absent in neonates but is highest in those from 6 months to 3 years of age, and may reach 103–105 °F. Sudden temperature rises to 104 °F may result in seizures in children <4 years of age. Fever may result in some children being listless and others hyperactive.
- **Cervical lymph nodes** may be tender and enlarged.
- **Meningeal irritation** occurs in some children without meningitis in the presence of an abrupt increase in fever and may manifest with headaches, nuchal rigidity and pain, as well as positive Kernig and Brudzinski signs.
    - Kernig sign: Flex each hip and then try to straighten the knee while the hip is flexed. Spasm of the hamstrings makes this painful and difficult.
    - Brudzinski sign: With the child lying supine, flex the neck by pulling head toward chest. The neck stiffness causes the hips and knees to pull up into a flexed position.

NASAL AND RESPIRATORY SYMPTOMS

Nasal and respiratory symptoms are indicative of acute respiratory infection:

- **Nasal symptoms** may include swelling of nasal passages, causing obstruction that can interfere with feeding in small infants. Exudate may be thin and watery or thick and purulent, depending on the type of infection. Irritation about the nares and upper lip related to exudate is common in infants and small children.
- **Sore throat** is usually a complaint of older children. Small infants and children may have an inflamed throat but appear to suffer less discomfort.
- **Cough** is a common symptom that may occur only during the acute phase of the respiratory infection or may persist for months after initial infection.
- **Change in respiratory sounds** may include wheezing and hoarseness in addition to cough. On auscultation, abnormal sounds may occur, such as hyperresonance, fine to coarse rales, wheezing, or absence of breath sounds in areas of the lungs.

GASTROINTESTINAL SYMPTOMS

Children with respiratory infections may initially manifest with gastrointestinal symptoms:

- **Poor appetite** or poor feeding is often the initial symptom and may persist throughout the febrile and convalescent period. This is a common symptom of acute infection in children.
- **Nausea and vomiting** may occur before other symptoms by several hours and usually subsides fairly quickly although it may persist with some children. It is most common in small children.
- **Diarrhea** is common with respiratory infections, especially those of viral origin. In most children it is mild and short lasting, but in others it may be severe and increase dehydration.
- **Abdominal pain** may be related to muscle spasms from vomiting or lymphadenitis of mesentery, especially if the child is very tense. The type of pain may be similar to or indistinguishable from pain associated with appendicitis.

BRONCHIOLITIS

Bronchiolitis is inflammation of the bronchiolar level and is usually caused by the **respiratory syncytial virus (RSV)** although rhinovirus, adenoviruses, parainfluenza, coronavirus, and *M. pneumoniae* have also been implicated. It is most common in very small children between the ages of 2 months and 2 years and rarely occurs after that age. Most children who require hospitalization are infants under 6 months of age. The infection is usually seasonal and mild although it can result in severe respiratory complications, so children should be observed carefully. Symptoms include dyspnea, a paroxysmal cough that is non-productive, tachypnea, and wheezing. The infection is usually self-limiting and runs its course in 8–15 days but is highly contagious.

Treatment is aimed at symptom management and depends on severity. Fever management, fluid status, and oxygen status are of primary importance. Hospitalization is required if the child is appearing lethargic or is presenting with apnea, hypoxemia, poor feeding, or respiratory distress. Common treatment includes:

- **Antipyretics**, such as acetaminophen
- **Oxygen therapy** with CPAP or BiPAP is often effective, but intubation and mechanical ventilation may be required in the presence of severe disease and respiratory compromise

BACTERIAL PHARYNGITIS AND BACTERIAL TONSILLITIS

Bacterial pharyngitis and bacterial tonsillitis are caused by group A beta-hemolytic *streptococci*.

Bacterial pharyngitis presents as a sore throat, lethargy, high fever, headache, stomachache and possibly trouble swallowing. The throat is red, the tonsils are enlarged, red, and may have a white discharge, and the soft palate may have petechiae on it.

Bacterial tonsillitis presents with headache, sudden high fever, vomiting, and aches. A throat culture is needed to determine a bacterial infection. Antibiotics (penicillin) are used for 10 days. Follow care guidelines for upper respiratory infection. Tonsillectomy may be indicated if there are recurrent infections, abscess or chronic enlargement of tonsils. Pre-op care involves teaching the family and child about what to expect post-surgery. Post-op care includes watching for increased bleeding, taking vital signs, watching for signs of respiratory distress and cyanosis, and encouraging fluids. Administer pain meds as indicated, discourage coughing (prevent bleeding), and apply ice as directed.

SPREAD AND SYMPTOMS OF TONSILLITIS AND INDICATIONS FOR TONSILLECTOMY

Tonsillitis is a contagious disease that is typically caused by a virus or infection with group A *Streptococcus* bacterium. Tonsillitis is treated with antibiotics if the cause of the condition is a bacterial infection; a viral infection is typically treated with rest and fluids. Recommendations vary among physicians, but children who get this condition more than five times in a year may be candidates for a tonsillectomy.

POST-TONSILLECTOMY COMPLICATIONS

A tonsillectomy, often combined with adenoidectomy, may be performed by a variety of different methods, with some posting more risk of postoperative bleeding than others. Hemorrhage may occur in the initial 24-hour postoperative period (primary) or after 7–10 days (secondary) when the scar begins to slough. Indications of bleeding include evidence of bright red blood in the mouth, spitting up of blood, or excessive swallowing as blood runs down the back of the child's throat. The first indication the child has been swallowing blood may be hematemesis. Bleeding may occur from either the tonsillectomy or adenoidectomy site. Other indications include pallor, restlessness, thirst, hypotension, and tachycardia (>100 bpm). Initial treatment includes starting IV-line, blood sample for type and crossmatch, and gentle suctioning of large clots. Small bleeding sites or those slowly oozing may be cauterized. The child should sit upright with an ice collar. Uncontrollable bleeding requires immediate surgical intervention with rapid sequence induction. Blood transfusions may be necessary with severe bleeding.

ACUTE LTB AND SPASMODIC CROUP

Acute laryngotracheobronchitis (LTB) is a narrowing of the throat and trachea, with inflammation, and is caused by a virus. It starts after a URI moves down the respiratory tract into the trachea. The symptoms come on gradually and include a hoarse voice, stridor, fever, crankiness, retractions, wheezing, crackles, rales and diminished breath sounds in some areas of the lungs, cyanosis and severe respiratory distress.

Spasmodic croup is not viral, but may have genetic or allergic origins. It begins suddenly in the middle of the night when the child wakes with a barking cough and difficulty breathing. Assess the child for signs of respiratory distress and treat with oxygen, humidity, and medications (bronchodilator, anti-inflammatory). The parents should be taught, when the child wakes up with a barking cough, to take the child into the bathroom, close the door, and run a hot shower to create warm humidity. This will help open the child's airway.

TREATMENT FOR CROUP

Croup occurs when the structures of the upper airway become inflamed; it is typically caused by a viral infection. The most common symptom of croup is a barky cough, although a child also develops a hoarse voice, congestion, and fever. Untreated, the condition may worsen and lead to respiratory distress and cyanosis. Parents monitoring a child with mild croup from home should be educated on signs/symptoms of deterioration (stridor, bluing of the lips, drooling, or worsening of symptoms) The most common form of treatment is providing a steroid (dexamethasone) and nebulized epinephrine for moderate to severe cases. Humidified air, which eases breathing, can also be used in mild cases. Children may sit with their parents in a steam-filled area, such as a bathroom while running a hot shower. A steam tent is also used for treatment. More severe cases may require additional respiratory support such as high flow nasal cannula or other non-invasive measures, Heliox (a combination of helium and oxygen), or—when these measures fail—intubation and mechanical ventilation.

ACUTE EPIGLOTTITIS

Acute epiglottitis (supraglottitis) occurs in children primarily from 1–8 years of age although it can occur at any age. It requires immediate medical attention as it can rapidly become obstructive. The onset is usually very sudden and often occurs during the night. The child may awaken suddenly with a fever but usually does not have a cough. The **symptoms** include:

- **Tripod position**: Child sits upright, leaning forward with chin out, mouth open, and tongue protruding.
- **Agitation**: The child appears restless, tense, and agitated.
- **Drooling**: Excess secretions combined with pain or dysphagia and mouth open position cause drooling.
- **Voice**: The child is not hoarse, but their voice sounds thick and "froglike."
- **Cyanosis**: Color is usually pale and sallow initially but may progress to frank cyanosis.
- **Throat**: On examination, the epiglottis appears bright red and swollen.
  NOTE: the child's throat should not be examined with a tongue blade unless intubation and tracheostomy equipment are immediately available as the examination can trigger obstruction.

BRONCHOPULMONARY DYSPLASIA

Bronchopulmonary dysplasia (**BPD**) is a chronic lung disease characterized by alveolar damage resulting from abnormal development with inflammation and development of scar tissue. Risk factors include:

- Prematurity of >10 weeks prior to due date
- Birthweight <2.5 lb or 1000 g
- Hyaline membrane disease or respiratory distress syndrome (RDS) at birth
- Long-term ventilatory support/oxygen

Most of the infants with BPD have immature lungs with inadequate surfactant to allow the lungs to expand properly, so they cannot breathe without assistance. **Symptoms** include severe respiratory distress and cyanosis. Their lungs often have fewer but enlarged alveoli with inadequate blood supply. BPD is usually diagnosed if respiratory symptoms do not improve after 28 days.

Supportive **treatment** provides oxygenation, protects vital organs, and allows the lungs to mature. Treatment may include any of the following:

- Surfactant
- Nasal continuous positive airway pressure (NCPAP)
- Mechanical ventilation or high-frequency jet ventilation (HFJV)
- Supplemental oxygen
- Bronchodilators (albuterol) to open airways (only for infants with acute deterioration due to an overreactive airway)
- Diuretics (chlorothiazide, hydrochlorothiazide, or furosemide) to reduce pulmonary edema or a fluid restriction
- Gastric/enteral feedings or total parenteral nutrition (TPN)

Complications: Most infants are hospitalized for about 4 months but may need treatment for months or years at home. Most will eventually develop nearly normal lung function as new lung tissue grows and takes over the function of the scarred tissue. Some long-term complications may occur:

- Increased risk of bacterial and viral infections, such as RSV and pneumonia
- Chronic or recurrent pulmonary edema
- Pulmonary hypertension
- Side effects related to long-term use of diuretics, such as hearing deficits, renal calculi, and electrolyte imbalances
- Slow growth patterns

CONGENITAL DIAPHRAGMATIC HERNIA

Congenital diaphragmatic hernia (**CDH**) may cause severe respiratory distress. The primary CDHs that affect children are posterolateral (Bochdalek):

- Left sided (85%) includes herniation of the large and small intestine and intraabdominal organs into the thoracic cavity.
- Right sided (13%) may be asymptomatic. It usually involves just liver herniation or part of the large intestine.

Symptoms	Treatment
- Neonates with left CDH may exhibit severe respiratory distress and cyanosis. The lungs may be underdeveloped because of pressure exerted from displaced organs during fetal development. - There may be a left hemothorax with a mediastinal shift and the heart pressing on the right lung, which may be hypoplastic. - Bowel sounds are heard over the chest area. - Pulmonary hypertension and cardiopulmonary failure may occur.	- Surgical repair once the patient is stabilized - Intubation and mechanical ventilation as soon as the diagnosis is made - Extracorporeal membrane oxygenation (ECMO) for cardiopulmonary dysfunction - Despite treatment, mortality rates are 50%, and children who survive may have emphysema, with larger volume but inadequate numbers of alveoli

PULMONARY HYPOPLASIA

Pulmonary hypoplasia occurs when the lungs and component parts are present but severely underdeveloped with less volume, decreased alveoli, fewer airway generations, and decreased pulmonary arteries. Pulmonary hypoplasia may result from congenital diaphragmatic hernia or embryologic defect that may include various other anomalies, such as prune-belly or Potter syndrome. Fetal urine in the amniotic fluid is necessary for development of fetal lungs, so renal agenesis or obstruction results in pulmonary hypoplasia. Hypoplasia is usually a secondary rather than primary disorder. If the hypoplasia is the result of compression caused by a diaphragmatic hernia, then after surgical repair, the lung will partially recover. Mortality rates range from 70-95%, depending upon severity and other anomalies. Preventive methods include providing amnioinfusions for preterm ruptured membranes <32 weeks to reduce hypoplasia. After birth, **treatment** includes:

- Respiratory support: supplemental oxygen or ventilation (HFOV and EMCO)
- Surfactants to improve ventilation and oxygenation
- Surgical repair as indicated
- Vasodilators and/or bronchodilators as indicated

CHOANAL ATRESIA

If the nurse is unable to pass a suctioning tube through the nares of the newborn, the infant may have choanal atresia, a rare condition that occurs in approximately 1 in 10,000 live births. It occurs in females twice as often as males. The choana are the two openings in the posterior nares that connect the nasal passages with the nasopharynx. Newborns are obligate nasal breathers. Successful nose breathing requires air to pass through the choana, so if these openings fail to form during fetal development, the infant must become a mouth breather. If atresia occurs only on one side (unilaterally), the infant may have no symptoms at birth. The infant with bilateral choanal atresia has periods of respiratory distress and cyanosis that are alleviated by crying. Bilateral choanal atresia often becomes a medical emergency requiring intubation, but definitive treatment requires surgical perforation of the atresia to create an opening, sometimes with insertion of a stent.

ESOPHAGEAL ATRESIA

Esophageal atresia often occurs with **tracheoesophageal fistula (TEF)**. In esophageal atresia, the esophagus has a blind pouch and does not completely pass to the stomach. In TEF, an abnormal connection is present between the trachea and the esophagus. A congenital tracheoesophageal fistula (TEF) may be associated with genetic anomalies, such as trisomy 13, 18, or 21 and various other anomalies. TEF is often associated with polyhydramnios, as esophageal atresia prevents the fetus from swallowing amniotic fluid. Acquired TEF may be secondary to intubation trauma or neoplasms.

Symptoms	Treatment
- Fine, white, frothy bubbles of mucous in the mouth and nose - Copious secretions, despite suctioning - Episodes of coughing, choking, and cyanosis, which worsen with feeding	- Surgery to separate the trachea and esophagus (for TEF) - Enteral feedings or gastrostomy feedings - Mechanical ventilation and a cuffed endotracheal tube (preventing reflux until the child stabilizes enough for surgical repair) - Maintaining cuff pressures <25 mmHg (helps prevent traumatic TEF)

CHILDHOOD ASTHMA

Asthma is a chronic reversible or partially reversible inflammation of the airway (especially the lower airways) that results in obstruction associated with genetic predisposition, environmental exposures, viral illnesses, and allergens. Children usually experience their first asthma attack between ages 3 and 8. In some cases, children may complain of a prodromal itch in the neck or upper part of the back prior to an episode. Childhood asthma is characterized by increased airway reactivity with obstruction related to inflammation and edema of mucous membranes, accumulation of secretions, and spasms of the smooth muscles of the bronchi and bronchioles. This bronchial constriction increases airway resistance that results in forced expiration through the constricted lumens. Symptoms may include dyspnea, inspiratory and expiratory high-pitched wheezing, cough, prolonged expiration, anxiety, sweating, and cyanosis. Wheezing and crackles may be heard throughout lung fields. Older children often sit upright with shoulders hunched over. Initial cough is usually hacking and nonproductive but then becomes productive of frothy gelatinous sputum. The three primary symptoms of asthma are cough, wheezing, and dyspnea.

GUIDELINES FOR DIAGNOSIS AND TREATMENT

The National Institutes of Health (NIH) and National Heart Blood and Lung Institute (NHBLI) have developed guidelines for the diagnosis and treatment of asthma. Component 1 of these guidelines addresses the assessment and monitoring of asthma.

The severity of the disease (including degree of impairment and risks), the degree of control, and the responsiveness to therapy must be assessed. Assessment is emphasized for initial diagnosis and monitoring for continued care. **Diagnosis** is based on:

- **History**: Cough, wheeze, triggers (precipitating factors or co-morbid conditions), and time of day variations.
- **Physical exam**: Hyperexpansion of thorax, wheezing, increased nasal secretions, polyps, swelling, and allergic skin conditions.
- **Spirometry** (for those 5 and older): Episodic symptoms of airflow obstruction that are at least partially reversible and not caused by other conditions. Responsiveness to therapy is demonstrated by FEV1 increase ≥12% from baseline or ≥10% of predicted FEV1 after inhalation of a short-acting bronchodilator. Additional pulmonary function studies, bronchoprovocation, chest x-ray, allergy testing, and biomarkers for inflammation may be assessed.

EXERCISE-INDUCED ASTHMA

Exercise-induced asthma (bronchospasm) is especially a risk for those with pre-existing asthma or allergies, especially with high pollen counts, high levels of smog, and cold dry weather. Children usually begin to cough, wheeze, and complain of shortness of breath and chest tightness after about 5 minutes of exercise. The symptoms may increase 5 to 10 minutes after exercise ceases, but symptoms usually recede by 30 minutes. Children should be cautioned to regularly take all prescribed preventive medications and warm up for 5 to 10 minutes before doing strenuous exercise. Additionally, they should breathe through their noses to warm the air and learn to monitor their own breathing. Immediate care includes stopping activity, positioning the person in an upright position, and having them use an inhaled bronchodilator. If symptoms are severe and do not begin to subside after ceasing activity and using bronchodilator, the child may require emergent treatment.

ASSESSMENT CRITERIA BASED ON SEVERITY OF ASTHMA ATTACKS

Assessment criteria for the severity of asthma attacks is as follows:

Mild	Moderate	Severe
- Peak expiratory flow rate (PEFR) 70–90% of normal - Respiratory rate ≤30% above average - Remains alert and no cyanosis or pallor - Dyspnea: Mild or absent with no or mild intercostal retractions - Pulsus paradoxus <10 mmHg - Oxygen saturation >95% and PCO_2 <35 - End expiratory wheeze only on auscultation	- PEFR 50–70% of normal - Respiratory rate 30–50% above average - Remains alert but pale - Moderate dyspnea but can speak in phrases - Moderate intercostal retractions with tracheosternal retractions and use of accessory muscles - Pulsus paradoxus 10–20 mmHg - Oxygen saturation 90–95% and PCO_2 <40 - Inspiratory and expiratory wheeze on auscultation	- PEFR <50% of normal - Respiratory rate >50% above average - Less alert and may be cyanotic - Severe dyspnea with difficulty speaking and severe retractions with nasal flaring and hyperinflation of chest - Pulsus paradoxus 20–40 mmHg - Oxygen saturation <90% and PCO_2 <40 - Breath sounds increasingly inaudible

GINA Treatment Recommendations Children Ages 12+ with Asthma

The **Global Initiative for Asthma (GINA)** updated their recommendations for asthma treatment and management in 2019 after compiling evidence of the ineffectiveness of a short-acting bronchodilator alone (SABA) approach to asthma management. Years of research supported their recommendation that low dose inhaled corticosteroids (ICS) significantly reduce asthma exacerbations in individuals (age 12 and older) with moderate to severe asthma, but it was also recommended for mild asthma. Guidelines were further updated in 2024, recommending that initial treatment for asthma in adolescents and adults be low-dose ICS-formoterol only when needed. Daily low-dose ICS is recommended only if asthma symptoms continue daily despite the as-needed use of ICS. This is referred to as MART (maintenance and reliever therapy). The SABA recommendation only remains for those with exacerbations twice a month or less with no risk factors for asthma exacerbations. GINA acknowledged that the likelihood of patient adherence to a daily ICS may be a barrier to improved outcomes in the population with mild asthma, but maintained this recommendation regardless. GINA breaks their recommendations down into two tracks: Track 1 (preferred) and Track 2 as an alternate. Track 1 is broken into 5 steps:

- Steps 1 and 2 (Less than two exacerbations a month): As needed low-dose ICS-formoterol.
- Step 3 (Moderate asthma; two or more exacerbations despite low dose ICS-formoterol as needed): Daily low dose maintenance ICS-formoterol.
- Step 4 (Severe asthma not controlled by low dose ICS-formoterol): Medium dose daily ICS-formoterol.
- Step 5 (Severe asthma not controlled by medium dose ICS-formoterol): Long-acting muscarinic antagonist (LAMA) and high dose daily ICS-formoterol with a referral for phenotypic assessment and potential add-on therapies.

Tracheal Stenosis

Tracheal stenosis is a marked narrowing of the trachea caused by a congenital malformation or trauma, such as from long-term intubation. Congenital tracheal stenosis may not be evident at birth, but may appear later as the child develops a respiratory infection, which further impinges on the airway, and exhibits signs of respiratory distress, such as cough, wheezing, and biphasic stridor. Children with tracheal stenosis often hyperextend the neck because this helps to open the airway. Diagnosis is per bronchoscopy although CT or MRI may also be used if severe stenosis precludes bronchoscopy. Treatment for mild stenosis includes a series of tracheal dilations with dilators or rigid bronchoscopy in increasing sizes. Complications of dilation include perforation and airway obstruction (blood, edema). Medications to reduce edema obstruction include epinephrine and corticosteroids. With severe stenosis, tracheostomy, tracheal reconstruction with stents, or tracheal resection may be necessary.

Tracheomalacia

Congenital tracheomalacia is a condition in which the tracheal cartilage is not fully developed at birth so that the trachea is not stable. The degree of respiratory impairment depends on the extent of the abnormality. In most cases, the cartilage develops adequately by 2 years, and surgical repair, which can include tracheostomy, stent placement, and repair of underlying cause, is rarely necessary. **Diagnosis** is per laryngoscopy.

Symptoms (may be mild to severe)	Treatment (conservative measures)
- Noisy, audible breathing sounds, especially when the patient's position is changed - Dyspnea, respiratory distress - High-pitched or rattling breathing sounds	- Providing humidified air - Elevating the child's head and upper body for feeding to prevent aspiration - Feeding slowly - Providing chest physiotherapy - Controlling infections with antibiotics as indicated

Multisystem Pathophysiology

ANAPHYLACTIC SHOCK

Anaphylactic reaction or anaphylactic shock, another form of distributive shock, may present with a few symptoms or a wide range of potentially lethal effects.

Symptoms may recur after the initial treatment (biphasic anaphylaxis), so careful monitoring is essential:

- Sudden onset of weakness, dizziness, confusion
- Severe generalized edema and angioedema; lips and tongue may swell
- Urticaria
- Increased permeability of vascular system and loss of vascular tone leading to severe hypotension and shock
- Laryngospasm/bronchospasm with obstruction of airway causing dyspnea and wheezing
- Nausea, vomiting, and diarrhea
- Seizures, coma, and death

Treatments:

- Establish patent airway and intubate if necessary, for ventilation
- Provide oxygen at 100% high flow
- Monitor VS
- Administer epinephrine (Epi-pen or solution)
- Albuterol per nebulizer for bronchospasm
- Intravenous fluids to provide bolus of fluids for hypotension
- Diphenhydramine if shock persists
- Methylprednisolone if no response to other drugs

HEAT-RELATED ILLNESS

Children and the elderly are particularly vulnerable to heat-related illness, especially when heat is combined with humidity. Heat-related illnesses occur when heat accumulation in the body outpaces dissipation, resulting in increased temperature and dehydration, which can then lead to thermoregulatory failure and multiple organ dysfunction syndromes. Each year in the United States, about 29 children die from heat stroke after being left in automobiles. At temperatures of 72–96 °F, the temperature in a car rises 3.2 °F every 5 minutes, with 80% of rise within 30 minutes. Temperatures can reach 117 °F even on cool days. There are three **types of heat-related illness**:

- **Heat stress**: Increased temperature causes dehydration. Patient may develop swelling of hands and feet, itching of skin, sunburn, heat syncope (pale moist skin, hypotension), heat cramps, and heat tetany (respiratory alkalosis). Treatment includes removing from heat, cooling, hydrating, and replacing sodium.
- **Heat exhaustion**: Involves water or sodium depletion, with sodium depletion common in patients who are not acclimated to heat. Heat exhaustion can result in flu-like aching, nausea and vomiting, headaches, dizziness, and hypotension with cold, clammy skin and diaphoresis. Temperature may be normal or elevated to less than 106 °F. Treatment to cool the body and replace sodium and fluids must be prompt in order to prevent heat stroke. Careful monitoring is important and reactions may be delayed.
- **Heat stroke**: Involves failure of the thermoregulatory system with temperatures that may be more than 106 °F and can result in seizures, neurological damage, multiple organ failures, and death. Exertional heat stroke often occurs in young athletes who engage in strenuous activities in high heat. Young children are susceptible to nonexertional heat stroke from exposure to high heat. Treatment includes evaporative cooling, rehydration, and supportive treatment according to organ involvement.

Hypothermia

Hypothermia occurs with exposure to low temperatures that cause the core body temperature to fall below 95 °F (35 °C). Hypothermia may be associated with immersion in cold water, exposure to cold temperature, metabolic disorders (hypothyroidism, hypoglycemia, hypoadrenalism), or CNS abnormalities (head trauma, Wernicke disease). Many patients with hypothermia are intoxicated with alcohol or drugs.

Symptoms of hypothermia include pallor, cold skin, drowsiness, alterations in mental status, confusion, and severe shivering. The patient can progress to shock, coma, dysrhythmias (T-wave inversion and prolongation of PR, QRS, and QT) including atrial fibrillation and AV block, and cardiac arrest.

Diagnosis requires low-reading thermometers to verify temperature.

Treatment includes:

- Passive rewarming if cardiac status stable
- Active rewarming (external) with immersion in warm water or heating blankets at 40 °C, radiant heat
- Active rewarming (internal) with warm humidified oxygen or air inhalation, heated IV fluids, and internal (bladder, peritoneal pleural, GI) lavage
- Warming with extracorporeal circuit, such as arteriovenous or venovenous shunt that warms the blood
- Supportive treatment as indicated

Localized Cold Injuries

Frostnip is a superficial freeze injury that is reversible. Frostbite is damage to tissue caused by exposure to freezing temperatures, most often affecting the nose, ears, and distal extremities. As frostbite develops, the affected part feels numb and aches or throbs, becoming hard and insensate as the tissue freezes, resulting in circulatory impairment, necrosis of tissue, and gangrene. There are **three zones of injury:**

- **Coagulation** (usually distal): severe, irreversible cellular damage
- **Hyperemia** (usually proximal): minimal cellular damage
- **Stasis** (between other 2 zones): severe but sometimes reversible damage

Symptoms vary according to the degree of freezing:

- **Partial freezing** with erythema and mild edema, stinging, burning, throbbing pain
- **Full-thickness freezing** with increased edema in 3–4 hours, edema and clear blisters in 6–24 hours, desquamation with eschar formation, numbness, and then aching and throbbing pain
- Prognosis is very good for **first-degree** and good for **second-degree** frostbite
- Full-thickness and into **subdermal tissue** freezing with cyanosis, hemorrhagic blisters, skin necrosis, and "wooden" feeling, severe burning, throbbing, and shooting pains
- Freezing extends into **subcutaneous tissue**, including muscles, tendons, and bones with mottled appearance, non-blanching cyanosis, and eventual deep black eschar

Prognosis is poor for **third-degree** and **fourth-degree** freeze injuries. Determining the degree of injury can be difficult because some degree of thawing may have occurred prior to admission to the hospital.

Treatment includes:

- Rapid rewarming with warm water bath (40–42 °C [104–107.6 °F]) 10–30 minutes or until the frostbitten area is erythematous and pliable
- Treatment for generalized hypothermia

Treatment **after warming**:

- Debridement of clear blisters but not hemorrhagic blisters
- Aloe vera cream every 6 hours to blistered areas
- Dressings, separating digits
- Tetanus prophylaxis
- Ibuprofen 12 mg/kg daily in divided doses
- Antibiotic prophylaxis if indicated (penicillin G 500,000 units IV every 6 hours for 24–72 hours)

TOXIC EXPOSURES
CARBON MONOXIDE POISONING

Carbon monoxide (CO) poisoning occurs with inhalation of fossil fuel exhausts from engines, emission of gas or coal heaters, indoor use of charcoal, and smoke and fumes. The CO binds with hemoglobin, preventing oxygen carriage and impairing oxygen delivery to tissue.

Diagnosis includes history, on-site oximetry reports, neurological examination, and CO neuropsychological screening battery (CONSB) done with patient breathing room air, CBC, electrolytes, ABGs, ECG, chest radiograph (for dyspnea); *pulse oximetry is not accurate in these patients.*

Symptoms:

- Cardiac: chest pain, palpitations, decreased capillary refill, hypotension, and cardiac arrest
- CNS: malaise, nausea, vomiting, lethargy, stroke, coma, and seizure
- Secondary injuries: Rhabdomyolysis, AKI, non-cardiogenic pulmonary edema, multiple organ failure (MOF), DIC, and encephalopathy

Treatment includes:

- Immediate support of airway, breathing, and circulation
- Non-barometric oxygen (100%) by non-breathing mask with reservoir or ETT if necessary
- Mild: Continue oxygen for 4 hours with reassessment
- Severe: hyperbaric oxygen therapy (usually 3 treatments) to improve oxygen delivery

CYANIDE POISONING

Cyanide poisoning, from hydrogen cyanide (HCN) or cyanide salts, can result from sodium nitroprusside infusions, inhalation of burning plastics, intentional or accidental ingestion or dermal exposure, occupation exposure, ingestion of some plant products, and the manufacture of PCP. Inhalation of HCN causes immediate symptoms, and the ingestion of cyanide salts causes symptoms within minutes.

Diagnosis is by history, clinical examination, normal PaO_2 and metabolic acidosis.

Symptoms: Increase in severity and alter with the amount of exposure: tachycardia, hypertension, leading to bradycardia, hypotension, and cardiac arrest. Pink or cherry-colored skin because of oxygen remaining in the blood. Other symptoms include headaches, lethargy, seizures, coma, dyspnea, tachypnea, and respiratory arrest.

Treatment includes:

- Supportive care as indicated
- Removal of contaminated clothes
- Gastric decontamination
- Copious irrigation for topical exposure
- Antidotes:
    - Amyl nitrate ampule cracked and inhaled 30 seconds
    - Sodium nitrite (3%) 10 mL IV
    - Sodium thiosulfate (25%) 50 mL IV

CAUSTIC INGESTIONS

Caustic ingestions of acids (pH <7) such as sulfuric, acetic, hydrochloric, and hydrofluoric found in many cleaning agents and alkalis (pH >7) such as sodium hydroxide, potassium hydroxide, sodium tripolyphosphate (in detergents) and sodium hypochlorite (bleach) can result in severe injury and death. Acids cause coagulation necrosis in the esophagus and stomach and may result in metabolic acidosis, hemolysis, and renal failure if systemically absorbed. Alkali injuries cause liquefaction necrosis, resulting in deeper ulcerations, often of the esophagus, but may involve perforation and abdominal necrosis with multi-organ damage.

Diagnosis is by detailed history, airway examination (oral intubation if possible), arterial blood gas, electrolytes, CBC, hepatic and coagulation tests, radiograph, and CT for perforations.

Symptoms may vary but can include pain, dyspnea, oral burns, dysphonia, and vomiting.

Treatment includes:

- Supportive and symptomatic therapy
- NO ipecac, charcoal, neutralization, or dilution
- NG tube for acids only to aspirate residual
- Endoscopy in first few hours to evaluate injury/perforations
- Sodium bicarbonate for pH <7.10
- Prednisolone (alkali injuries)

ALLERGIC REACTIONS

Exposure to certain toxins, medications, illegal substances, and allergens can cause life threatening effects in some patients. The physiologic response of the patient is dependent on the agent and the degree of exposure. Tissue hypoperfusion and lactic acidosis often occur as a result of the exposure. This can lead to metabolic acidosis, shock, organ failure, and death.

Signs/symptoms: In allergic type reactions, urticaria, pruritus, chest, back or abdominal pain, facial flushing, shortness of breath, wheezing and stridor may occur. Beta- and alpha-adrenergic responses may occur with exposure to amphetamines, cocaine, ephedrine, and pseudoephedrine. This response is manifested by diaphoresis, hypertension, tachycardia, and mydriasis. Diarrhea, nausea, and vomiting can occur with exposure to certain toxins.

Diagnosis: Physical assessment and testing to discover the toxin, drug, or allergen the patient was exposed to. Labs—blood gases, BMP, complete blood count, toxicology screen, urinalysis, and allergy testing.

Treatment: Priority is to eliminate exposure to the drug/toxin/allergen. Antidotes (if available) may be administered in the case of toxin exposure. Activated charcoal may be administered in the case of medication/drug overdose. For allergic reactions, antihistamines and corticosteroids may be administered. Severe allergic reactions may need to be treated with epinephrine. Dialysis may be indicated in some patients.

Sodium bicarbonate may be administered for the treatment of metabolic acidosis caused by many toxic reactions.

ACETAMINOPHEN TOXICITY

Acetaminophen toxicity from accidental or intentional overdose has high rates of morbidity and mortality unless promptly treated. **Diagnosis** is by history and acetaminophen level, which should be completed within 8 hours of ingestion if possible. Toxicity occurs with dosage >140 mg/kg in one dose or >7.5g in 24 hours.

Symptoms occur in stages:

- (Initial) Minor gastrointestinal upset
- (Days 2–3) Hepatotoxicity with RUQ pain and increased AST, ALT, and bilirubin
- (Days 3–4) Hepatic failure with metabolic acidosis, coagulopathy, renal failure, encephalopathy, nausea, vomiting, and possible death
- (Days 5–12) Recovery period for survivors

Treatment includes:

- GI decontamination with activated charcoal (orally or NG); this is most effective when administered within 4 hours of ingestion
- Toxicity is plotted on the Rumack-Matthew nomogram with serum levels >150 requiring antidote. The antidote is most effective ≤8 hours of ingestion but decreases hepatotoxicity even >24 hours.
- Antidote: 72-hour N-acetylcysteine (NAC) protocol includes 140 mg/kg initially and 70 mg/kg every 4 hours for 17 more doses (orally or IV)
- Supportive therapy: Continuous dialysis, fluids, blood pressure medications

AMPHETAMINE AND COCAINE TOXICITY

Amphetamine toxicity may be caused by IV, inhalation, or insufflation of various substances that include methamphetamine (MDA or "ecstasy"), methylphenidate (Ritalin), methylenedioxymethamphetamine (MDMA), and ephedrine and phenylpropanolamine. Cocaine may be ingested orally, IV or by insufflation while crack cocaine may be smoked. Amphetamines and cocaine are CNS stimulants that can cause multi-system abnormalities.

Symptoms may include chest pain, dysrhythmias, myocardial ischemia, MI, seizures, intracranial infarctions, hypertension, dystonia, repetitive movements, unilateral blindness, lethargy, rhabdomyolysis with acute kidney failure, perforated nasal septum (cocaine), and paranoid psychosis (amphetamines). Crack cocaine may cause pulmonary hemorrhage, asthma, pulmonary edema, barotrauma, and pneumothorax. Swallowing packs of cocaine can cause intestinal ischemia, colitis, necrosis, and perforation. **Diagnosis** includes clinical findings, CBC, chemistry panel, toxicology screening, ECG, and radiography.

Treatment includes:

- Gastric emptying (<1 hour). Charcoal administration
- IV access. Supplemental oxygen
- Sedation for seizures: Lorazepam 2 mg, diazepam 5 mg IV titrated in repeated doses
- Agitation: Haloperidol
- Hypertension: Nitroprusside/nicardipine, phentolamine IV
- Cocaine quinidine-like effects: Sodium bicarbonate

Salicylate Toxicity

Salicylate toxicity may be acute or chronic and is caused by ingestion of OTC drugs containing salicylates, such as ASA, Pepto-Bismol, and products used in hot inhalers.

Diagnosis is by ferric chloride or Ames Phenistix tests. Symptoms vary according to age and amount of ingestion. Co-ingestion of sedatives may alter symptoms.

Symptoms include:

- <150 mg/kg: Nausea and vomiting
- 150–300 mg/kg: Vomiting, hyperpnea, diaphoresis, tinnitus, and alterations in acid-base balance
- >300 mg/kg (usually intentional overdose): Nausea, vomiting, diaphoresis, tinnitus, hyperventilation, respiratory alkalosis, and metabolic acidosis
- Chronic toxicity results in hyperventilation, tremor, and papilledema, alterations in mental status, pulmonary edema, seizures, and coma

Treatment includes:

- Gastric decontamination with lavage (≤1 hour) and charcoal
- Volume replacement (D5W)
- Sodium bicarbonate 1–2 mEq/kg
- Monitoring of salicylate concentration, acid-base, and electrolytes every hour
- Whole-bowel irrigation (sustained release tablets)

Benzodiazepine Toxicity

Benzodiazepine toxicity may result from accidental or intentional overdose with such drugs as Xanax, Librium, Valium, Ativan, Serax, Versed, and Restoril. Mortality is usually the result of co-ingestion of other drugs.

Diagnosis is based on history and clinical exam, as benzodiazepine level does not correlate well with toxicity.

Symptoms: Non-specific neurological changes: Lethargy, dizziness, alterations in consciousness, and ataxia. Respiratory depression and hypotension are rare complications. Coma and severe central nervous depression are usually caused by co-ingestions.

Treatment includes:

- Gastric emptying (<1 hour)
- Charcoal
- Concentrated dextrose, thiamine, and naloxone if co-ingestions suspected, especially with altered mental status
- Monitoring for CNS/respiratory depression
- Supportive care
- Flumazenil (antagonist) 0.2 mg each minute to total 3 mg may be used in some cases but not routinely advised because of complications related to benzodiazepine dependency or co-ingestion of cyclic antidepressants. Flumazenil is contraindicated in patients with increased ICP.

Ethanol Overdose

Ethanol overdose affects the central nervous system as well as other organs in the body. Alcohol is an inhibitory neurotransmitter that depresses the central nervous system. In most states, the legal intoxication blood alcohol level is defined as 100 mg/dL. Blood alcohol levels of **500 mg/dL or greater** are associated with a high mortality rate. The central nervous system depressant effect is further enhanced when alcohol is mixed with other agents.

Ethanol is absorbed through the mucosa of the mouth, stomach, and intestines, with concentrations peaking about 30–60 minutes after ingestion. If people are easily aroused, they can usually safely sleep off the effects of ingesting too much alcohol, but if the person is semi-conscious or unconscious, emergency medical treatment should be initiated.

Symptoms include:

- Altered mental status with slurred speech and stupor
- Nausea and vomiting
- Hypotension
- Bradycardia with arrhythmias
- Respiratory depression and hypoxia
- Cold, clammy skin or flushed skin (from vasodilation)
- Acute pancreatitis with abdominal pain
- Lack of consciousness
- Circulatory collapse

Treatment includes:

- Careful monitoring of arterial blood gases and oxygen saturation
- Ensure patent airway with intubation and ventilation if necessary
- Intravenous fluids
- Dextrose to correct hypoglycemia if indicated
- Maintain body temperature (warming blanket)
- Dialysis may be necessary in severe cases

GASTRIC EMPTYING FOR TOXIC SUBSTANCE INGESTION

Gastric emptying for toxic substance ingestion should be done ≤60 minutes of ingestion for large life-threatening amounts of poison. The patient requires IV access, oximetry, and cardiac monitoring. Sedation (1–2 mg IV midazolam) or rapid sequence induction and endotracheal intubation may be necessary. Patients should be positioned in left lateral decubitus position with head down at 20° to prevent passage of stomach contents into duodenum, although intubated patients may be lavaged in the supine position. With a bite block in place, an orogastric Y-tube (36–40 Fr. for adults) should be inserted after estimating length. Placement should be confirmed with injection of 50 mL of air confirmed under auscultation and aspiration of gastric contents, as well as abdominal x-ray (pH may not be reliable depending on substance ingested). Irrigation is done by gravity instillation of about 200–300 mL warmed (45 °C) tap water or NS. The instillation side is clamped and drainage side opened. This is repeated until fluid returns clear. A slurry of charcoal is then instilled, and the tube is clamped and removed when procedures completed.

LEAD TOXICITY

Children at risk for lead toxicity include those who live in older homes that may have lead-based paint or plumbing. Lead can also be found in soil, batteries, items made from pewter, and the paint of some toys. Children can develop lead toxicity if they ingest any materials, dust, or water that has been exposed to lead. Lead toxicity causes complications associated with memory and learning, decreased attention span, and chronic problems with nerves, muscles, and kidneys.

Lead levels can be checked via blood or urine test. Normal values are as follows:

- Whole blood: <10 µg/dL
- Urine: <80 µg/dL

LEAD POISONING

Lead poisoning occurs with serum levels >10 µg/dL although some children may experience cognitive impairment at lower levels. Lead poisoning is especially dangerous for developing children ages <7 because it interferes with normal cell function, especially in the nervous system, blood cells, and kidneys. **Treatment** involves removing the source of lead and providing chelation therapy for levels >25 µg/dL. Agents used for chelation include calcium disodium ethylenediamine tetraacetate (CaNa$_2$EDTA), dimercaprol (BAL), d-penicillamine, or succimer (DMSA), usually for 5–7 days and then repeated. Classification of lead exposure and poisoning is as follows:

Class	Serum Level	Signs and Symptoms
Class I	<9 µg/dL	Usually asymptomatic or slight neurological deficits
Class II A	10–14 µg/dL	Anemia; mild cognitive, growth, and fine motor impairment
Class II B	15–19 µg/dL	Same as Class II A
Class III	20–44 µg/dL	Anemia, fatigue, difficulty concentrating, headache, motor impairment, tremors, paresis, paralysis, abdominal pain, nausea, vomiting, constipation, weight loss
Class IV	45–69 µg/dL	Anorexia, vomiting, severe intermittent abdominal cramping, hyperirritability, increased lethargy, blue-black lead line on gums
Class V	>70 µg/dL	Encephalopathy, ataxia, seizures, coma, death

ANIMAL BITES

Animal bites, including human, are frequent causes of traumatic injury. There is not a single preferred topical therapy for traumatic wounds because they vary so widely in the type and degree of injury.

General treatment includes:

- **Cleanse** wound by flushing with 10–35 cc syringe with 18-gauge Angiocath to remove debris and bacteria using normal saline or diluted Betadine solution.
- Hand, puncture, and infected wounds or those more than 12 hours old may be closed by **secondary intention**.
- **Moisture-retentive dressings** are used as indicated by the size and extent of the wound left open. Dry dressings may be applied to injuries with closure by primary intention.
- **Topical antibiotics** may be indicated, although systemic antibiotics are commonly prescribed for animal bites.
- **Tetanus toxoid** or **immune globulin** is routinely administered.

SPIDER BITES

Spider bites are frequently a misdiagnosis of a *Staphylococcus aureus* or MRSA infection, so unless the spider was observed, the wound should be cultured and antibiotics started. If the wound responds to the antibiotic, then it probably was not a spider bite. There are two main types of venomous spider bites:

- Those producing **neurological symptoms** (black widow).
- Those producing **local necrosis** (brown recluse, yellow sac, and hobo spiders).

General treatment includes:

- Cleanse wound, apply cool compress, and elevate body part if possible.

Treatment for black widow bites:

- Narcotic analgesics.
- Nitroprusside to relieve hypertension.
- Calcium gluconate 10% solution IV for abdominal cramps.
- Antivenin *Latrodectus mactans* for those with severe reaction.

Treatment for necrotic/ulcerated bites (e.g., brown recluse):

- There is no consensus on the best treatment, as ulceration caused by the venom may be extensive and **surgical repair** with grafts may be needed.
- Necrotic ulcers should be treated **moisture-retentive dressings** as indicated, and monitored for complications.
- **Hyperbaric oxygen therapy** (HBOT) has been used in some cases.

SNAKE BITES

About 45,000 snake bites occur in the United States each year, with about 8,000 from poisonous snakes. In the United States, about 25 species of snakes are venomous. There are two types of snakes that can cause serious injury, classified according to the type of fangs and venom.

CORAL SNAKES

Coral snakes have short fixed permanent fangs in the upper jaw and venom that is primarily neurotoxic, but may also have hemotoxic and cardiotoxic properties:

- Wounds show no fang marks but there may be scratches or semi-circular markings from the teeth.
- There may be little local reaction, but neurological symptoms may range from mild to acute respiratory and cardiovascular failure.

Treatment includes the following:

- Cleanse the wound thoroughly of dirt and debris and either leave it open to air or cover it with a dry dressing.
- Administer antivenin immediately even without symptoms, which may be delayed.
- Administer tetanus toxoid or immune globulin.
- Antibiotics are not usually indicated.

PIT VIPERS

A second type of snake that can cause serious injury is the pit viper. Pit vipers (**rattlesnakes, copperheads, and cottonmouths**) have erectile fangs that fold until they are aroused, and venom is primarily hemotoxic and cytotoxic but may also have neurotoxic properties:

- Wounds usually show one or two fang marks.
- Edema may begin immediately or may be delayed up to six hours.
- Pain may be severe.
- There may be a wide range of symptoms, including hypotension and coagulopathy with defibrination that can lead to excessive blood loss, depending upon the type and amount of venom.
- There may be local infection and necrosis.

Treatment includes the following:

- Cleanse the wound thoroughly and apply dressings as indicated.
- Administer tetanus toxoid or immune globulin.
- Administer analgesics, such as morphine sulphate, as needed.
- Avoid NSAIDs and aspirin because of anticoagulation properties.
- Mark edema every 15 minutes.
- Administer antivenin therapy if indicated. Observe for serum sickness if horse serum used.
- Administer prophylactic antibiotics for severe tissue necrosis.
- Administer platelets, plasma, or packed RBCs for coagulopathy.

SHARK BITES

Even small shark bites can crush bones. Hit and run attacks may cause small lacerations or minimal damage, but other types of attacks can result in loss of limbs or large chunks of flesh, with loss of muscle and bone. Internal organs may be exposed and damaged. Extensive soft tissue trauma and damage to arteries and veins may occur, as well as crushing internal injuries. The wounds are often contaminated with sand, algae, fragments of shark teeth, and other materials and pathogens, such as *Mycobacterium marinum* and *Vibrio spp.* Life-threatening injuries need to be addressed first, including control of hemorrhage:

- Administer IV fluids and blood products.
- Administer tetanus toxoid or tetanus immune globulin.
- Wounds must be flushed with copious amounts of normal saline and debris removed.
- Treat for hypothermia if needed.
- X-rays are ordered to identify fractures or debris in wound.
- Fixation of fractures.
- Administer prophylactic antibiotics:
    - Ciprofloxacin
    - Trimethoprim-sulfamethoxazole
    - Doxycycline
- Surgical repair, debridement, and/or skin grafting if indicated.

ALLIGATOR BITES

Alligators are found in ten coastal states in the southeastern United States with the largest population in Florida, where most injuries are reported. Animals between four and eight feet often bite once and release, but larger animals may bite repeatedly, engaging in typical biting and feeding activities, which result in severe injury, amputations, or death. Most wounds involve the limbs, with the hands and arms the most frequently bitten.

Treatment includes:

- Treat for shock and blood loss.
- Apply pressure to wound.
- Retrieve amputated limbs if possible.
- Flush wound(s) with copious amounts of normal saline to reduce contamination.
- Collect wound cultures.
- Administer prophylactic broad-spectrum antibiotics for gram-negative organisms, such as *Aeromonas hydrophila* and *Clostridium.*
- Observe for signs of infection, such as erythema, cellulitis, exudate, and necrosis.
- Administer tetanus toxoid or immune globulin.
- Repair fractures.
- Surgical repair and debridement as indicated, with wounds usually healing by secondary intention or delayed primary closure.

STINGRAY STINGS

Stingrays can induce injury when their tail is thrust forward, driving serrated spines into the victim, resulting in a jagged laceration. The spines of the stingray tail contain a venom that is injected upon impact, causing severe pain. The resulting wounds often become infected.

Symptoms include:

- Intense, excruciating pain with envenomation lasting two to three days.
- Bleeding.
- Systemic symptoms: Dizziness, GI upset, seizures, hypotension.

Treatment includes the following:

- **Rinse** the wound with fresh water or saline and remove visible pieces of spine with forceps or tweezers.
- **Heat immersion**: Deactivate the venom and relieve pain by immersing the wound in hot water for 30–90 minutes at 110–115 °F (45 °C). May repeat up to 2 hours.
- **Radiographs** may be necessary to locate the spine or fragment.
- Administer tetanus toxoid or tetanus immune globulin.
- Inject the wound with a **local anesthetic**, such as lidocaine or bupivacaine, to relieve severe pain.
- Administer **opiates** for pain.
- **Open wounds** are usually allowed to heal without primary closure or with loose primary closure.
- **Prophylactic antibiotics** may be given for five days to prevent infections.

INSECT STINGS AND BITES
BEE STINGS

Bees and wasps sting by puncturing the skin with a hollow stinger and injecting venom. Wasps and bumblebees can sting more than once but honeybees have barbs on their stingers, and the barbs embed the stinger into the skin. **Local reactions** to bee sting include the following:

- Raised white **wheal** with central red spot of about 10 mm appearing within a few minutes and lasting 20 minutes (honeybees).
- **Edema and erythema**, which may last several days (vespid wasps).
- Pain, swelling, and redness confined to sting site.
- Swelling may extend **beyond the sting site** and may, for example, involve swelling of an entire limb.

Some people may develop an anaphylactic reaction, including a **biphasic reaction**, in which the symptoms recede and then return two to three hours later. About 50% of deaths occur within 30 minutes of the sting, and 75% within four hours.

Symptoms of an allergic reaction/anaphylaxis may become increasingly severe with generalized urticaria, edema, hypotension, and respiratory distress.

Treatment of bee stings initially includes the following:

- Wash the site with soap and water.
- Remove stinger using 4×4-inch gauze wiped over the area or by scraping a sharp instrument over the area.
- NEVER squeeze the stinger or use tweezers, as this will cause more venom to go into the skin.
- Apply ice to reduce the swelling (10–20 minutes on, 10–20 minutes off, for 24 hours).
- Antihistamines may be prescribed.
- A paste of baking soda and water or meat tenderizer and water may reduce itching.
- Topical corticosteroids may relieve itching.
- Administer tetanus toxoid or tetanus immune globulin as needed.

Allergic responses/anaphylaxis requires immediate, aggressive medical intervention:

- Administer epinephrine.
- Administer antihistamines.
- Administer corticosteroids.
- Administer IV fluids as needed.
- Provide oxygen and other supportive treatments.

People with extensive local or anaphylactic reactions should be advised to carry an epinephrine autoinjector for emergency use if stung.

SCORPION STINGS

Symptoms

- Note: Children <6 are most at risk of death from severe reactions. Symptoms vary widely depending on individual reaction and amount of venom.
- **Local (most common):** Neurotoxic effects include itching, redness, edema, and ascending hyperesthesia. Tap test: Paresthesia worsens if area tapped.
- **Cytotoxic effects** include development of macule or papule within an hour. Purpuric plaque becomes necrotic and ulcerates and venom spreads through the lymph system.
- **Nonlethal response** includes pain, induration, redness, and wheal.
- **Neurologic:** Severe wide-ranging symptoms include strokes, altered consciousness, muscle rigidity, paralysis, and seizures.
- **Multiple organ:** Can include hypertension, tachycardia, respiratory distress, generalized allergic response, dysphagia, hepatitis, priapism, acute tubular necrosis, DIC, hyperglycemia, lactic acidosis.

Treatment

- Note: Meperidine and morphine may potentiate symptoms.
- Hospital admission for 24 hours unless symptoms very mild.
- Cool compresses, acetaminophen, topical anesthetics for pain.
- Tetanus toxoid or tetanus immune globulin as needed.
- Antivenom (available only for Centruroides).
- Complex supportive care may include intubation and ventilation.

FIRE ANT BITES
Symptoms

- Note: Multiple bites, sometimes hundreds, are common. Deaths are rare but do occur if children have a severe systemic reaction or bites about the head and neck.
- **Local reaction:** A severely itching wheal develops and subsides in 30–60 minutes, followed by a blister within 4 hours. The blister fills with milky dead tissue in 8–24 hours with redness at base and severe itching and burning. The blister ruptures and crusts over within 72 hours but redness pain and itching may persist for days.
- **Systemic reaction:** Edema, urticaria, nausea, vomiting, bronchospasm, dyspnea, slurred speech, anaphylaxis.

Treatment

- **Local reaction:** Cold compresses, weak bleach solution (within 15 minutes of bites), or topical anesthetic for pain. Cleanse with soap and water without breaking blisters. NSAIDS for pain. Topical corticosteroids for itching. Antihistamines. Tetanus toxoid or tetanus immune globulin as needed.
- **Systemic reaction:** As for anaphylaxis, depending on degree of symptoms, including epinephrine.

HUMAN BITES

Human "bites" occur when the teeth of one person injure another. This is not uncommon in contact sports. Intentional biting is common among children but usually presents mild injury. Human bites may also be the result of altercations and are referred to as "fist-bites." There are 3 common **types** of fist-bites:

- Closed fist bite resulting in small wound on the metacarpophalangeal joint of the middle finger. Bacteria enter the wound when the person extends the fingers, carrying bacteria to the extensor tendons, which can result in infection.
- Finger bite in which a finger may be partially or completely severed
- Puncture bite, usually on the face, from contact with another person's tooth

Immediate treatment of bites includes applying pressure to stop bleeding and then thoroughly flushing the wound with dilute Betadine, dilute peroxide, or normal saline solution. Protective dressings should be applied. Large wounds or those with skin flaps or signs of more serious tissue injury may require surgical repair.

Acid Base Imbalances

INVASIVE BLOOD GAS MONITORING

Invasive blood gas monitoring options include the following:

- **Arterial blood gas (ABG)** is the most informative measurement of blood gas status. If an arterial catheter is in place, it is easily obtained by aspirating 1–2 mL of blood.
- **Venous blood gas (VBG)** is easier to obtain if an arterial catheter is not in place. In order to compare the values in the VBG with an ABG, make the following calculations:
  - Add 0.05 to the pH of the VBG.
  - Subtract 5–10 mmHg from the PCO_2 of the VBG.
- **Capillary blood gas (CBG)** can be obtained with a heel stick, without a venous or arterial line, but the values obtained in a CBG are the least accurate and are rarely useful. This is used most often in neonates.

COMPONENTS OF A BLOOD GAS READING

The following are components of a blood gas reading:

- **pH** measures the circulating acid and base levels. Neutral pH for humans is 7.4. A value below 7.35 indicates acidosis and a value greater than 7.45 indicates alkalosis.
- **pCO$_2$** is the partial pressure of carbon dioxide and it determines the respiratory component of pH. An elevated pCO_2 lowers the pH. A low pCO_2 raises the pH. The pCO_2 value is dependent on adequate pulmonary ventilation and respiration. Changes in respiratory status quickly alter this value. Normal value range for pCO_2 is 35–45 mmHg.
- **pO$_2$** is the partial pressure of oxygen, which indicates how well the individual is transporting oxygen from the lungs into the bloodstream. Normal value is 75–100 mmHg.
- **HCO$_3^-$** is bicarbonate, the metabolic component of pH. This value may slowly change in response to abnormal pH, or a disease process may cause an elevation or depression. Low values decrease the pH and high values raise the pH. Normal value for bicarbonate is 22–26 mEq/L.

> **Review Video: Acid-Base Balance & Blood Gas Interpretation**
> Visit mometrix.com/academy and enter code: 611909

Metabolic and Respiratory Acidosis

Pathophysiology
- Metabolic acidosis
  - Increase in fixed acid and inability to excrete acid, or loss of base, with compensatory increase of CO_2 excretion by lungs
- Respiratory acidosis
  - Hypoventilation and CO_2 retention with renal compensatory retention of bicarbonate (HCO_3) and increased excretion of hydrogen

Laboratory
- Metabolic acidosis
  - Decreased serum pH (<7.35) and PCO_2 normal if uncompensated and decreased if compensated
  - Decreased HCO_3
- Respiratory acidosis
  - Decreased serum pH (< 7.35) and increased PCO_2
  - Increased HCO_3 if compensated and normal if uncompensated

Causes
- Metabolic acidosis
  - DKA, lactic acidosis, diarrhea, starvation, renal failure, shock, renal tubular acidosis, starvation
- Respiratory acidosis
  - COPD, overdose of sedative or barbiturate (leading to hypoventilation), obesity, severe pneumonia/atelectasis, muscle weakness (Guillain-Barré), mechanical hypoventilation

Symptoms
- Metabolic acidosis
  - Neuro/muscular: Drowsiness, confusion, headache, coma
  - Cardiac: Decreased BP, arrhythmias, flushed skin
  - GI: Nausea, vomiting, abdominal pain, diarrhea
  - Respiratory: Deep inspired tachypnea
- Respiratory acidosis
  - Neuro/muscular: Drowsiness, dizziness, headache, coma, disorientation, seizures
  - Cardiac: Flushed skin, VF, ↓BP
  - GI: Absent
  - Respiratory: Hypoventilation with hypoxia

Metabolic and Respiratory Alkalosis

Pathophysiology
- Metabolic alkalosis
  - Decreased strong acid or increased base with possible compensatory CO_2 retention by lungs
- Respiratory alkalosis
  - Hyperventilation and increased excretion of CO_2 with compensatory HCO_3 excretion by kidneys

Laboratory
- Metabolic alkalosis
  - Increased serum pH (>7.45)
  - PCO_2 normal if uncompensated and increased if compensated
  - Increased HCO_3
- Respiratory alkalosis
  - Increased serum pH (>7.45)
  - Decreased PCO_2
  - HCO_3 normal if uncompensated and decreased if compensated

Causes
- Metabolic alkalosis
  - Excessive vomiting, gastric suctioning, diuretics, potassium deficit, excessive mineralocorticoids and $NaHCO_3$ intake
- Respiratory alkalosis
  - Hyperventilation associated with hypoxia, pulmonary embolus, exercise, anxiety, pain, and fever
  - Encephalopathy, septicemia, brain injury, salicylate overdose, and mechanical hyperventilation

Symptoms
- Metabolic alkalosis
  - Neuromuscular: Dizziness, confusion, nervousness, anxiety, tremors, muscle cramping, tetany, tingling, seizures
  - Cardiac: Tachycardia and arrhythmias
  - GI: Nausea, vomiting, anorexia
  - Respiratory: Compensatory hypoventilation
- Respiratory alkalosis
  - Neuro/muscular: Light-headedness, confusion, lethargy
  - Cardiac: Tachycardia and arrhythmias
  - GI: Epigastric pain, nausea, and vomiting
  - Respiratory: Hyperventilation

Fluid and Electrolyte Imbalances

SODIUM IMBALANCE

Sodium (**Na**) regulates fluid volume, osmolality, acid-base balance, and activity in the muscles, nerves, and myocardium. It is the primary **cation** (positive ion) in extracellular fluid (ECF), necessary to maintain ECF levels that are needed for tissue perfusion:

- Normal range: 135–145 mEq/L
- Hyponatremia: <135 mEq/L
- Hypernatremia: >145 mEq/L

Hyponatremia may result from inadequate sodium intake, excess sodium loss through diarrhea, vomiting, or NG suctioning, or illness, such as severe burns, fever, SIADH, and ketoacidosis.

- **Symptoms**: Irritability to lethargy and alterations in consciousness, cerebral edema with seizures and coma, dyspnea to respiratory failure.
- **Treatment**: Identify and treat the underlying cause and provide Na replacement.

Hypernatremia may result from renal disease, diabetes insipidus, and fluid depletion.

- **Symptoms**: Irritability to lethargy to confusion to coma; seizures; flushing; muscle weakness and spasms; thirst.
- **Treatment**: Identify and treat the underlying cause, monitor Na levels carefully, and give IV fluid replacement.

POTASSIUM IMBALANCE

Potassium (**K**) is the primary **electrolyte** in intracellular fluid (ICF), with about 98% inside cells and only 2% in ECF, although this small amount is important for neuromuscular activity. Potassium influences activity of the skeletal and cardiac muscles. Its level is dependent upon adequate renal functioning because 80% is excreted through the kidneys and 20% through the bowels and sweat:

- Normal range: 3.5–5.5 mEq/L
- Hypokalemia: <3.5 mEq/L. Critical value: <2.5 mEq/L
- Hyperkalemia: >5.5 mEq/L. Critical value: >6.5 mEq/L

A healthy NPO patient will need about 40 mEq of K per day to maintain serum K levels. Expect alterations in renal disease and other disease processes.

Hypokalemia is caused by alkalosis, decreased intake associated with starvation, nephritis, and loss of potassium through diarrhea, vomiting, gastric suction, and diuresis.

- **Symptoms**: Lethargy and weakness; nausea and vomiting; paresthesia and tetany; muscle cramps with hyporeflexia; hypotension; dysrhythmias with EKG changes: PVCs or flattened T-waves.
- **Treatment**: Treatment involves identifying and treating the underlying cause and replacing K. When possible, oral replacement is preferable to IV, as it allows slower adjustment of K levels. When given IV, K should be given no faster than 20 mEq/hour via central line if possible. If given peripherally, 10 mEq/hour is preferable for patient comfort.

Hyperkalemia is caused by renal disease, adrenal insufficiency, metabolic acidosis, severe dehydration, burns, hemolysis, and trauma. It rarely occurs without renal disease but may be induced by treatment (such as NSAIDs and potassium-sparing diuretics). Untreated renal failure results in reduced excretion. Those with Addison disease and deficient adrenal hormones suffer sodium loss that results in potassium retention.

- **Symptoms**: The primary symptoms relate to the effect on the cardiac muscle: ventricular arrhythmias with increasing changes in EKG lead to cardiac and respiratory arrest, weakness with ascending paralysis and hyperreflexia, diarrhea, and increasing confusion.
- **Treatment**: Treatment includes identifying the underlying cause and discontinuing sources of increased K. Calcium gluconate to decrease cardiac effects. Sodium bicarbonate, insulin, and hypertonic dextrose shift K into the cells temporarily. Cation exchange resin (Kayexalate) to decrease K. Peritoneal dialysis or hemodialysis to remove excess K.

Note: When a tourniquet is on, a patient opening and closing their hand can lead to falsely elevated K levels.

CALCIUM IMBALANCE

More than 99% of calcium (**Ca**) is in the skeletal system with 1% in serum, but it is important for transmitting nerve impulses and regulating muscle contraction and relaxation, including the myocardium. Calcium activates enzymes that stimulate chemical reactions and has a role in the coagulation of blood:

- Normal range: 8.2–10.2 mg/dL
- Hypocalcemia: <8.2. Critical value: <7 mg/dL
- Hypercalcemia: >10.2 mg/dL. Critical value: >12 mg/dL

Hypercalcemia may be caused by acidosis, kidney disease, hyperparathyroidism, prolonged immobilization, and malignancies. Crisis carries a 50% mortality rate.

- **Symptoms**: Increasing muscle weakness with hypotonicity; anorexia; nausea and vomiting; constipation; bradycardia and cardiac arrest.
- **Treatment**: Identify and treat underlying cause, loop diuretics, IV fluids, phosphate.

Hypocalcemia may be caused by damage to the parathyroid resulting in hypoparathyroidism (directly decreasing calcium production), vitamin D resistance or inadequacy, or liver/kidney disease.

- **Symptoms**: Muscle cramping or spasms; seizures; numbness or tingling of the feet, hands, or lips; tetany if severe.
- **Treatment**: Identify and treat underlying cause, replace calcium by administering IV calcium gluconate in acute circumstances or increasing oral Vitamin D and calcium in chronic cases.

PHOSPHORUS IMBALANCE

Phosphorus, or phosphate, (**PO$_4$**) is necessary for neuromuscular and red blood cell function, the maintenance of acid-base balance, and provides structure for teeth and bones. About 85% is in the bones, 14% in soft tissue, and <1% in ECF.

- Normal range: 2.4–4.5 mEq/L
- Hypophosphatemia: <2.4mEq/L
- Hyperphosphatemia: >4.5 mEq/L

Hypophosphatemia occurs with severe protein-calorie malnutrition, hyperventilation, severe burns, diabetic ketoacidosis, and excess antacids with magnesium, calcium, or aluminum.

- **Symptoms**: Irritability, tremors, seizures to coma; hemolytic anemia; decreased myocardial function; respiratory failure.
- **Treatment**: Identify and treat underlying cause and replace phosphorus.

Hyperphosphatemia occurs with renal failure, hypoparathyroidism, excessive intake, neoplastic disease, diabetic ketoacidosis, muscle necrosis, and chemotherapy.

- **Symptoms**: Tachycardia; muscle cramping; hyperreflexia and tetany; nausea and diarrhea.
- **Treatment**: Identify and treat underlying cause, correct hypocalcemia, and provide antacids and dialysis.

MAGNESIUM IMBALANCE

Magnesium (**Mg**) is the second most common intracellular electrolyte (after potassium) and activates many intracellular enzyme systems. Mg is important for carbohydrate and protein metabolism, neuromuscular function, and cardiovascular function, producing vasodilation and directly affecting the peripheral arterial system:

- Normal range: 1.7–2.2 mg/dL
- Hypomagnesemia critical value: <1.2 mg/dL
- Hypermagnesemia critical value: >4.9 mg/dL

Hypomagnesemia occurs with chronic diarrhea, chronic renal disease, chronic pancreatitis, excess diuretic or laxative use, hyperthyroidism, hypoparathyroidism, severe burns, and diaphoresis.

- **Symptoms**: Neuromuscular excitability or tetany; confusion, headaches, dizziness; seizure and coma; tachycardia with ventricular arrhythmias; respiratory depression.
- **Treatment**: Identify and treat underlying cause, provide magnesium replacement. IV magnesium is a vasodilator, 2 g over 60 mins.

Hypermagnesemia occurs with renal failure or inadequate renal function, diabetic ketoacidosis, hypothyroidism, and Addison disease.

- **Symptoms**: Muscle weakness, seizures, and dysphagia with decreased gag reflex; tachycardia with hypotension.
- **Treatment**: Identify and treat underlying cause, IV hydration with calcium, and dialysis.

> **Review Video: Fluid and Electrolyte Balance**
> Visit mometrix.com/academy and enter code: 384389

FLUID BALANCE IN INFANTS AND CHILDREN

Body fluid is primarily **intracellular fluid (ICF)** or **extracellular space (ECF)**. Infants and children have proportionately more extracellular fluid (ECF) than adults. At birth, more than half of the child's weight is ECF, but by 3 years of age, the child's balance is more like adults:

- ECF: 20-30% (interstitial fluid, plasma, transcellular fluid)
- ICF: 40-50% (fluid within the cells)

The fluid compartments are separated by semipermeable membranes that allow fluid and solutes (electrolytes and other substances) to move by osmosis. Fluid also moves through diffusion, filtration, and active transport. In fluid volume deficit, fluid is out of balance and ECF is depleted; an overload occurs with increased concentration of sodium and retention of fluid. Signs of **fluid deficit** include:

- Thirsty, restless to lethargic
- Increasing pulse rate, tachycardia
- Fontanels depressed (infants)
- Decreased urinary output
- Normal BP progressing to hypotension
- Dry mucous membranes
- 3-10% decrease in body weight

NORMAL VALUES FOR ELECTROLYTES IN THE PEDIATRIC POPULATION

Electrolyte	Normal Range(s)
Potassium	Infant: 4.1-5.3 mEq/L Child: 3.4-4.7 mEq/L
Calcium	11 days to 2 years: 9-11 mg/dL 3-12 years: 8.8-10.8 mg/dL 13-18 years: 8.4-10.2 mg/dL
Phosphate	1-3 years: 3.9-6.5 mg/dL 4-6 years: 4.0-5.4 mg/dL 7-11 years: 3.7-5.6 mg/dL 12-13 years: 3.3-5.4 mg/dL 14-15 years: 2.9-5.4 mg/dL 16-19 years: 2.8-4.6 mg/dL
Magnesium	1.7-2.1 mEq/L

Infectious Diseases

VIRAL INFECTIONS

HERPES SIMPLEX VIRUS INFECTIONS

There are 2 types of the herpes simplex virus (HSV), human herpesvirus 1 and 2. **HSV-1** usually causes a **gingivostomatitis** (often referred to as "cold sores" or "fever blisters") and is transmitted through **close contact**. **HSV-2** usually causes painful **genital lesions** through **sexual contact**. Either may be found in other areas of the body.

- **Incubation** period is around 2–12 days.
- The primary infection is usually more severe (causes systemic **symptoms**) than the reactivated infection, but it may be asymptomatic. After the primary infection, the virus remains dormant in the nerve ganglia, and can be reactivated especially during times of stress, illness, immunosuppression, or sun exposure. While patients are most contagious during times of active lesions, the disease may be spread while asymptomatic. The frequency of the outbreaks usually decreases over time.
- HSV **lesions** are grouped vesicles with an erythematous base. They are usually painful, and a prodrome of tingling, pain, or burning sensations may be felt hours to a couple days before the eruption. Lesions last for approximately 2–3 weeks in primary infection (up to 4 weeks with genital HSV), and 1–2 weeks in recurrent infections.
- HSV is **diagnosed** clinically and confirmed with a + culture, PCR test, or HSV antibody tests (HSV-1 or HSV-2: IgM= active or recent infection; IgG= previous infection).
- Symptomatic **treatment**, proper wound care, and antivirals (acyclovir, valacyclovir, or famciclovir) may be given.
- **Complications** include perinatal infection, keratitis, herpetic whitlow, herpes gladiatorum, secondary infections, and encephalitis.

EPSTEIN-BARR INFECTION

Epstein-Barr virus (EBV) is a **herpesvirus** (human herpesvirus 4) and is responsible for causing **infectious mononucleosis**. After the initial infection, it remains latent in B cells and epithelial cells. It has been linked to certain epithelial and lymphatic neoplasms (e.g., nasopharyngeal carcinoma, Burkitt lymphoma, Hodgkin lymphoma).

- EBV is **transmitted** through **body fluids** like saliva, so it is sometimes referred to as the kissing disease. It is most common in teenagers and college-age young adults
- **Incubation** period is typically 30–50 days.
- **Symptoms** of EBV infection range from being asymptomatic to swollen painful lymph nodes, pharyngitis (can mimic strep pharyngitis), extreme fatigue, fever, and possibly hepatosplenomegaly. The WBC count is elevated (~10,000–20,000 cells/mL) with 10–30% atypical lymphocytes in the differential.
- Confirm **diagnosis** with a Mono Spot test or EBV antibody serology tests.
- **Treatment** is supportive, and antibiotics are not helpful in treating this viral infection. Therefore, avoid unnecessary antibiotics in those with EBV, especially since administration of ampicillin or amoxicillin is often associated with a pruritic, maculopapular rash. Analgesics, warm salt water gargles, increased fluid intake, and rest will help to relieve some of the symptoms. Symptoms may last for several weeks and fatigue may last even longer. Patients should avoid contact sports for up to 2 months.
- **Complications** include hepatitis, cytopenias (e.g., thrombocytopenia), Guillain Barré syndrome, and splenic rupture.

MEASLES, MUMPS, AND RUBELLA

Measles (rubeola) virus is highly contagious, is spread through **respiratory secretions** (incubation is 7–14 days), and peaks in late winter to spring. It causes a prodrome of high fever (4–7 days), cough, congestion, conjunctivitis; then Koplik spots (pathognomonic), and finally a maculopapular rash (spreads cephalocaudally). Report suspected cases immediately to the health dept. **Diagnose** with a + IgM antibody test (collected after 3 days of rash), viral culture, or PCR. **Treatment** is supportive.

Mumps (parotitis) is a viral infection that is spread via **saliva** (incubation is 12–24 days), and often occurs during winter and spring. It causes painful swelling of the salivary glands (parotid). Report to health dept. Supportive **treatment**. Complications include orchitis (infertility), pancreatitis, and meningitis.

Rubella (German measles) is a virus that spreads via **respiratory droplets** (incubation is 2–3 weeks), and peaks in the spring. There is a mild prodrome (fever, aches, sore throat, conjunctivitis, swollen nodes [esp. suboccipital, postauricular, & posterior cervical]), then a maculopapular rash (face first, then down). Report to health dept. Confirm with rubella antibodies IgM or IgG. Symptomatic care.

INFLUENZA

Influenza is a highly contagious viral infection that affects the entire **respiratory system** from the nose to the lungs. There are 3 types of **influenza virus**: **A** (causes epidemics), **B** (only in humans), and **C**. Types A and B are seen most often and are the strains that the annual flu vaccine is most effective against; and type C is not as common and much less severe.

- Prevention is key and annual, age-appropriate influenza **vaccines** should be given to those ≥6 months; 2 vaccines are required in first-time vaccine patients if 6 mo. through 8-year-olds (separated by 28 days).
- **Incubation** period is 1–4 days and it is spread via respiratory droplets.
- Though **symptoms** can be very similar, the flu and the common cold differ in that the flu has a very sudden onset. Symptoms of influenza include a high fever (may last up to 5 days), headache, myalgias, dry cough, rhinorrhea, and fatigue. There may also be vomiting and diarrhea, although children are more prone to this.
- Clinical judgment, community patterns, and rapid influenza tests (high specificity, but lower sensitivity) aid in **diagnosis**, but RT-PCR or viral culture definitively confirm the diagnosis; pulse oximetry and CXR as needed for pulmonary issues.
- Antibiotic **treatment** is not effective unless there is a secondary bacterial infection (e.g., pneumonia). Look for signs of secondary infections (e.g., dyspnea, cyanosis, fever that goes away and returns, confusion/lethargy). Supportive treatment with rest, fluids, and analgesics. Antivirals should be considered in those who are at high risk (<5 years old, elderly, pregnant, chronic conditions). These are most effective if initiated within 24–48 hours of symptom onset. The neuraminidase inhibitors (oseltamivir, zanamivir) treat type A, type B, and avian H5N1. There is extensive resistance to the adamantanes (amantadine, rimantadine) so they are rarely used.
- **Complications** include pneumonia, ARDS, and death.

CORONAVIRUS

A coronavirus is a common virus that causes cold-like symptoms, including a cough, runny nose, sore throat, and congestion. Most cases of coronavirus are not dangerous and are often given little attention or go entirely unnoticed. However, specific coronavirus strains have led to two worldwide pandemics. The first, **severe acute respiratory syndrome (SARS)**, appeared in China in 2002 and quickly spread worldwide. Presenting symptoms of SARS were fever, cough, dyspnea, and general malaise. It was extremely virulent, spreading easily from person to person through close contact by way of contaminated droplets produced by coughing or sneezing. SARS was also very deadly, with a case fatality rate of nearly 10%. High rates of infection occurred in health care workers and others in contact with infected patients, so prompt diagnosis and proper isolation were essential. By 2004, there were no longer any documented active cases of SARS.

The most recent coronavirus outbreak was the **COVID-19** strain, which first appeared in China in 2019 and quickly became a global pandemic. Presentation of COVID-19 was similar to that of SARS, with the notable additional symptom of acute loss of taste/smell as a unique identifier.

Precautions to take when treating patients with COVID-19 include the following:

- Contact and droplet precautions, including eye protection and appropriate personal protection equipment.
- Airborne precautions (recommended by the CDC), especially with aerosol-producing procedures (ventilators, nebulizers, intubation).
- Activity restrictions of exposed health care workers planned in coordination with public health officials.

CYTOMEGALOVIRUS

Cytomegalovirus (CMV) is a herpes virus, occurring in most people by the time they are adults.

- **Transmission** can occur through secretions during personal contact and from mother to baby before, during or after birth.
- Most cases have no **symptoms**, although a few infants will have fetal damage, such as jaundice, hepatitis, brain damage, or growth retardation.
- **Treatment** for those with severe infections is with ganciclovir, an antiviral drug.

RESPIRATORY SYNCYTIAL VIRUS

Respiratory syncytial virus (RSV) is a virus that infects the respiratory tract, causing symptoms of nasal congestion, cough, sore throat, and headache. Severe cases can lead to high fever, breathing difficulties, severe cough, and cyanosis.

- Respiratory syncytial virus may **manifest** as a cold in adults and older children; however, there are some children who are more at risk of developing complications.
- **Transmission** is through contact with droplets from an infected person's nose or throat, generally through coughing and sneezing.
- Infants born prematurely, children with chronic lung disease, children with cystic fibrosis, and children who are in an immunocompromised state because of surgery or illness are at **high risk** of breathing difficulties, poor oxygenation, and even death from RSV.

Vaccination for RSV is now recommended for at-risk populations, including pregnant women, infants who are less than 8 months old and entering into season of high RSV spread (fall to spring), adults ages 60–74 with increased risk for complications, and all adults ages 75 and older. Vaccination may not prevent the disease, but will lessen its severity.

FIFTH DISEASE

Fifth disease, or **erythema infectiosum**, is a viral illness caused by parvovirus B19. It is most prevalent in the spring, with outbreaks in preschools, daycares, and elementary schools.

- The **incubation** period is 4-20 days, and it may be communicable for several days before the rash appears.
- **Transmission** occurs through oral and nasal secretions and possibly blood.
- **Symptoms** are possible fever, headache, nasal congestion, general unwell feeling, and rash starting on the cheeks (slapped cheek appearance). The rash typically spreads to the rest of the body as a lacy red rash that may come and go for up to a month.

- Use over-the-counter fever medications as needed and provide **supportive care**.
- The virus can cause fetal death if contracted during pregnancy. There is no vaccine for fifth disease, and because it is a viral infection, it is not treated with antibiotics.

CHICKENPOX

Chickenpox (Varicella) is a viral infection, most prevalent in the late winter and early spring in children under 10 years of age.

- It has an **incubation** period of 10-21 days and is communicable from 1-2 days before the rash appears to after all lesions have dried up.
- **Transmission** is through direct contact and contact with respiratory droplets.
- **Symptoms** are low fever and feeling unwell, followed by the itchy rash (raised red bumps that develop vesicles which then ooze and crust over).
- The patient should be isolated until all lesions are dry. Aveeno baths and Benadryl help with the itching. Ibuprofen or acetaminophen can be used for the fever, and acyclovir is indicated in some cases. Encourage the patient not to scratch the lesions to prevent secondary infections. Provide supportive care as indicated.

ROSEOLA

Roseola is a viral illness, most prevalent in children 6-24 months of age.

- The **incubation** period is about 9 days.
- **Transmission** may be through oral and nasal.
- The illness begins with a high fever for 3-5 days; the patient appears well otherwise. The fever drops and then the rash appears. The rash is a light pink maculopapular rash which lasts 1-2 days.
- Parents should **treat the fever** as needed with anti-inflammatory medications.

POLIOMYELITIS

Poliomyelitis (commonly referred to as **polio**) is caused by an enterovirus and occurs most often in babies and young children.

- The **incubation** period is 3-14 days, and transmission occurs through direct contact with respiratory secretions and the oral-fecal route.
- The **symptoms** are slight fever, sore throat, general malaise, nausea and vomiting, headache, stomach ache, and constipation, but there can be severe pain, muscular weakness, and then paralysis.
- There are no drug therapies for polio. Observe for respiratory distress, provide general support measures, and provide for physical therapy.

ROTAVIRUS

Rotavirus is a viral illness that causes diarrhea, fever, and vomiting in children.

- It can be extremely **contagious** within groups where large numbers of children are present, such as in daycare centers, preschools, pediatric offices, clinics, and children's units in hospitals.
- Rotavirus can be prevented through **immunization** with a vaccine, as recommended by the American Academy of Pediatrics. Immunization can prevent up to 98% of severe cases of the illness.
- Children should wash their hands before eating and after using the bathroom to avoid spreading the disease. Caregivers should wash their hands before preparing food, after changing diapers, and after using the bathroom; they should avoid letting small children place toys or other items in their mouths and should disinfect surfaces after use.

BACTERIAL INFECTIONS
DIPHTHERIA
Diphtheria, caused by **Corynebacterium diphtheriae**, is most prevalent in fall and winter.

- The **incubation** period is 2–7 days, possibly longer, and transmission is through direct contact with nasal, eye, and oral secretions.
- The **symptoms** are slight fever, nasal discharge, sore throat, feeling unwell, poor appetite, and swelling of the airway.
- If the disease is severe, death can result. The patient requires isolation, bed rest, fluids, antibiotics, medication for fever, and an antitoxin. The patient may also require oxygen therapy and tracheostomy if the airway is obstructed.

TETANUS
Tetanus, caused by **Clostridium tetani**, occurs all over the world. The spores formed by the bacillus are present in soil, dust, and the GI tracts of animals and humans.

- The **incubation** period is 3–21 days.
- **Symptoms** start with headache, irritability, jaw muscle spasms, and inability to open the mouth. This is followed by severe back muscle spasms, seizures, incontinence, and fever.
- **Treatment** requires human tetanus immune globulin, penicillin G, Valium, and placement on a ventilator. The environment should be kept quiet because the spasms are initiated by stimuli.

SCARLET FEVER
Scarlet fever, caused by **group A beta-hemolytic streptococci**, is most prevalent in school-age children during the fall, winter, and spring.

- The **incubation** period is 1-7 days, and transmission occurs through direct or indirect contact with oral and nasal secretions.
- The illness begins with a high fever, very sore throat, headache, malaise, chills and possibly vomiting and stomach pain. A rash appears in about 12 hours as sandpapery red pinpoints in creases of the skin, flushed face and then a strawberry tongue.
- Antibiotics will be prescribed, but patients should be isolated until taking the antibiotic for 24 hours. Analgesics are needed to bring down the fever and the patient should be encouraged to drink plenty of fluids.

WHOOPING COUGH
Whooping cough, caused by **Bordetella pertussis bacillus**, is most prevalent in infants and children who were not immunized.

- The **incubation** period is 6-20 days, and transmission occurs through direct contact with oral and nasal secretions.
- The **symptoms** are cold symptoms for 1-2 weeks, when the cough will worsen and progress to a whoop sound, usually occurring at night. Vomiting will usually follow an episode of intense coughing. As the patient recovers, the coughing will subside. In babies, a mucus plug or apnea can result in death by respiratory arrest. Hospitalization is usually required for infants less than 6 months of age and those with a severe case of pertussis.
- The patient needs isolation and bed rest, with a calm, quiet environment to limit coughing spells. Fluid intake needs to be monitored and humidified air will help.
- Watch for signs of respiratory distress and give antibiotic and pertussis immune globulin as prescribed.

IMPETIGO

Impetigo is a skin infection that is most commonly seen in preschool children or those in young childhood.

- Impetigo causes blister-like sores on skin areas that may already be compromised, such as under the nose, on the hands or neck, or in the diaper area. It is caused by a bacterial infection, most commonly *Staphylococcus aureus* or group A *Streptococcus*. The sores may itch or the patient may already have irritation at the site, such as a diaper rash.
- To **prevent the spread of infection**, children and caregivers should wash their hands frequently and avoid scratching the sores and then touching items. Isolation by staying home from school or daycare may be necessary until the sores have crusted over. Treating skin irritations, such as poison ivy or eczema, can also prevent infection from spreading to impetigo.

FUNGAL INFECTIONS

CRYPTOCOCCOSIS

Cryptococcosis is an infection resulting from inhaling the **fungus** *Cryptococcus neoformans,* which is found worldwide in soil (can be associated with bird droppings), or *Cryptococcus gattii,* which is associated with certain trees in the Northwest.

- Cryptococcosis is most often due to *C. neoformans*. It is often found among those with compromised immune systems and is an **AIDS-defining opportunistic infection**.
- Healthy patients may be asymptomatic and the only finding may be pulmonary lesions on CXR that resolve spontaneously. The fungus can disseminate and cause meningitis, encephalitis, cutaneous lesions, and affect long bones and other tissues. **Symptoms** are based on the area of involvement. Patients may experience cough, pleuritic chest pain, weight loss, and fever if there is pulmonary involvement; headache, double vision, light sensitivity, N/V, and confusion if CNS involvement; cutaneous lesions (papules, pustules, nodules, ulcers) if the skin is involved.
- **Diagnosis** includes microscopic analysis, culture (gold standard), or an antigen test (highly sensitive; good for detecting early infection) for *Cryptococcus* using CSF, tissue, sputum, blood, or urine. Check CSF by India ink (limited sensitivity) or culture so meningitis can be ruled out. Confirm that no mass lesion is present by CT or MRI before LP is performed.
- Mild cases may only require monitoring to ensure that the infection does not spread. In more advanced cases, the infection is treated with different antifungal medications (e.g., fluconazole for pulmonary infections, amphotericin B ± flucytosine for meningitis). The patient should also be monitored for CNS infection and medication side effects. AIDS patients may need lifelong antifungals.
- **Complications** include cryptococcal meningitis, neural deficits, optic nerve damage, and hydrocephalus.

HISTOPLASMOSIS

Histoplasmosis is an infection caused by inhalation of **spores** from the fungus *Histoplasma capsulatum* that is found in soil and is associated with bird and bat droppings (e.g., chicken coops, caves).

- Healthy patients are usually asymptomatic and those with symptoms are typically immunocompromised or those who've had a heavy exposure to spores. The primary **pulmonary infection** occurs 3–17 days after exposure and can present with flu-like symptoms. It is typically self-limited but may become chronic. Histoplasmosis can also spread through the **blood** and can cause progressive disseminated disease in the immunocompromised (high mortality rate); this is an **AIDS-defining illness**.
- **Diagnose** through antigen tests (urine, serum), histopathology, or cultures; order a CXR. Mild and even moderate acute pulmonary histoplasmosis may resolve on its own.
- If needed, **treat** mild to moderate infections with itraconazole and severe illness with amphotericin B.

PNEUMOCYSTIS

Pneumocystis jiroveci is a **fungus** (previously known as *Pneumocystis* carinii) that causes **pneumonia** (PJP, previously PCP) in the immunocompromised. Most people have been exposed to this by the age of 3 or 4.

- **Symptoms** of PJP include a dry nonproductive cough, fever, dyspnea, and weight loss.
- CXR may show diffuse bilateral infiltrates or it may be normal; and pulse oximetry may be low, especially on exertion. **Diagnosis** is confirmed with sputum histopathology using sputum induction or bronchoalveolar lavage.
- **Treat** immediately with TMP-SMX (trimethoprim/sulfamethoxazole) for 21 days if HIV + and for 14 days in other cases. Steroids may be added for HIV patients with severe PJP. HIV/AIDS patients with CD4 counts <200/µL should receive PJP prophylaxis with TMP-SMX. Dapsone and pentamidine are alternatives.
- **Complications** include ARDS and death.

CANDIDAL INFECTIONS

Candida is a type of yeast that may cause a variety of infections:

- **Oral thrush** is commonly seen in diabetic patients and those who are immunosuppressed (HIV or underlying neoplasm). Patients often complain of burning on the tongue or in the mouth, associated with "curd-like" white patches that can be scraped away leaving reddish tissue underneath. Diagnosis is with KOH prep. Treatment is with oral or topical antifungals, including nystatin (swish and swallow or troches).
- **Candida esophagitis** also occurs in the immunosuppressed population, and patients may complain of dysphasia, odynophagia, and chest pain. This is diagnosed on EGD and may be treated with oral or IV antifungals (ketoconazole).
- **Candidal intertrigo**, or diaper rash, presents with beefy-red lesions at skin fold areas as well as satellite lesions. Treatment is with topical antifungals.
- **Candidemia** is diagnosed with fungal blood cultures and may lead to osteomyelitis, endocarditis, and other complications. Treatment is with IV antifungals.

RINGWORM

Ringworm is caused by an infection from the ***Tinea* fungus**, which produces patches on the skin that have normal centers, giving the appearance of a ring.

- The fungus can cause hair loss and patches of scaly skin that may develop blisters that ooze or crust.
- It is **transmitted** by touching the affected skin or through objects that have touched the affected skin.
- Ringworm may be **diagnosed** by viewing the skin section under a Wood's lamp. Skin cultures may also be taken for examination to identify the fungus. A potassium hydroxide (KOH) exam involves scraping the affected skin and placing the skin sample in KOH to test for the presence of the fungus.

VECTOR-BORNE AND PARASITIC INFECTIONS
MALARIA

Malaria is a **blood-borne disease** caused by a **parasite** from the genus *Plasmodium and* found in tropical areas. There are 4 known to cause disease in humans (*P. malariae, P. vivax, P. ovale*, and *P. falciparum*). These protozoa are transmitted by the **female *Anopheles* mosquito**. They travel to the **liver** where they multiply, are released, and then infect the RBCs, where they continue to multiply. Incubation time can be as little as 9 days or as much as multiple years depending on the species of the infecting parasite.

- **Signs/symptoms** include headache, high fever with shaking chills and sweating (rigors; occurs when merozoites, an immature form of the parasite, are released from RBCs), jaundice, anemia, and hepatosplenomegaly. Take a thorough history including recent travel.
- **Diagnose** with 3 thin and thick blood smears (gold standard) stained with Giemsa (preferred) and obtained 12–24 hours apart. Labs typically show elevated LDH, thrombocytopenia, and atypical lymphocytes. Rapid antigen tests are also available as well as PCR.
- **Treat** with chloroquine. If travelling, chemoprophylaxis depends on the area of travel due to species and resistance patterns, and may include chloroquine, primaquine, mefloquine, Malarone, or doxycycline. Report infections to your local or state health department.
- **Complications** include severe anemia and hemolysis, organ failure (liver, spleen, kidneys), cerebral malaria, ARDS, and death.

LYME DISEASE

Lyme disease occurs from a bite from a **deer tick** (blacklegged tick) infected with the **spirochete bacterium** *Borrelia burgdorferi*. It is the most common tick-borne disease in the U.S. and is more prevalent in heavily wooded areas. Adult ticks are more active during colder times whereas the nymphs (<2 mm in size) are more active in the warm, spring or summer months. Once the tick bites, it stays attached; however, it takes about 36–48 hours for nymphs and about 48–72 hours for adult ticks before the spirochete is transmitted to the person. **Incubation** period is 3–30 days. There are 3 stages to this disease: early localized, early disseminated, and chronic disseminated.

- At **Stage 1**, 75% have the characteristic expanding red rash (erythema migrans; can be large, ~30cm) which can progress to have central clearing (bull's eye), headache, fever, chills, myalgias, and fatigue.
- **Stage 2** occurs weeks to months after initial infection and involves systemic symptoms (flu-like), neck stiffness, headaches, migrating pain in muscles and joints, rashes, paresthesias, Bell's palsy, confusion, fatigue, myocarditis, and heart palpitations.
- **Stage 3** occurs months to years after initial infection and involves neurologic (e.g., encephalitis) and rheumatologic issues, especially arthritis of large joints (e.g., knee).

> **Review Video: Lyme Disease**
> Visit mometrix.com/academy and enter code: 505529

DIAGNOSIS AND TREATMENT OF LYME DISEASE

Diagnose Lyme disease using 2-tiered testing: antibodies (IgM, IgG), then Western blot. Antibiotic treatment for localized Lyme disease involves 2–3 weeks of doxycycline, amoxicillin, or cefuroxime axetil is started immediately after diagnosis. IV antibiotics may be needed for severe disease (e.g., IV ceftriaxone). Prevention is key by wearing clothes covering the skin, using tick repellents, showering soon after being outdoors in tick-prone areas, and thoroughly checking for ticks (especially in hard to see areas by using a mirror). The Lyme vaccine is no longer available and previous vaccine recipients are still at risk of contracting the disease as protection decreases over time. Complications are prevalent with untreated Lyme disease and include chronic arthritis, fatigue, chronic musculoskeletal issues, acrodermatitis chronica atrophicans, and memory and concentration issues. Report cases to the local health dept.

ROCKY MOUNTAIN SPOTTED FEVER

Rocky Mountain spotted fever is a tick-borne illness caused by **Rickettsia rickettsii**. It tends to occur in spring and summer throughout the United States.

- **Incubation** period is about one week.
- **Symptoms** include headache, fever, nausea, vomiting, loss of appetite, muscle pain, and rash on the ankles and wrists.
- **Treatment** requires an antibiotic, usually doxycycline.

ZIKA VIRUS IN PREGNANT WOMEN

Zika virus is a **flavivirus** that is transmitted by the *Aedes* mosquito and through sexual contact. This virus can be passed on to an unborn baby causing severe congenital defects while causing mild or no disease in the mother. It is advised that all pregnant women avoid traveling to areas with the Zika virus (e.g., Central and South America, Mexico, Caribbean, Africa).

- **Incubation** period is 3–14 days and symptoms may last 4–7 days. The virus has been found to remain longer in semen than in other body fluids.
- If **symptoms** are present, they may include fever, headache, myalgias, arthralgias, a maculopapular rash, and conjunctivitis. Congenital defects include severe microcephaly, severe brain abnormalities, macular scarring, hearing loss, motor disabilities (e.g., hypertonia), and contractures. Women should be screened for Zika exposure at each prenatal visit.
- **Diagnostic** testing is recommended for all asymptomatic pregnant women who have continued exposure to Zika and for all symptomatic pregnant women who have possibly been exposed to the Zika virus. Testing includes RNA NAT testing on serum and urine, and serum IgM Zika antibody testing. Prenatal ultrasound helps determine if the effects of Zika are present. Report cases to the state health department; and the CDC can be consulted.
- There is **no treatment** or cure for the Zika virus.

HELMINTH INFESTATIONS

Helminth infestations (worms) include **roundworms** [nematodes: *Ascaris*, hookworms (cause anemia), **filariae** (cause elephantiasis)] and **flatworms** [tapeworms (cause weight loss); **flukes** (intestinal or liver)]. **Pinworms** are a type of roundworm that cause enterobiasis and is the most common helminth infestation. Pinworms are more prevalent in warmer areas of the country and infestations occur more frequently in children. The worms lay eggs within the digestive tract and then travel to the anal area where they are usually found. Pinworms are highly contagious. As a patient itches the anal area where the eggs are located, the eggs cling to the fingers and can easily be transmitted to other people either directly or through food or surfaces. The eggs can survive for 2–3 weeks on inanimate objects.

- Patients may be asymptomatic or have intense anal itching that is usually worse at night and can cause insomnia. Abdominal pain, nausea, and vomiting can also occur.
- **Diagnose** with the "tape test" which involves pressing cellophane tape over the perianal area to pick up eggs or worms and examine under the microscope. Most other helminth infestations can be diagnosed with a stool sample for ova and parasites; filariasis requires a blood smear or antigen test.
- Anthelmintic medications are given in a single dose and repeated in 2 weeks to kill the pinworms and their larvae (mebendazole, albendazole, or pyrantel pamoate). The entire family and close contacts should be treated simultaneously since pinworms are so contagious.

GIARDIA LAMBLIA

Giardia lamblia is a **protozoan** that infects water supplies and spreads to children through the fecal-oral route. It is the most common cause of non-bacterial diarrhea in the United States, causing about 20,000 cases of infection each year in all ages.

- Children often become infected after swallowing recreational waters (pools, lakes) while swimming or putting contaminated items into the mouth. *Giardia* live and multiply within the small intestine where cysts develop.
- **Symptoms** occur 7–14 days after ingestion of 1 or more cysts and include diarrhea with greasy floating stools (rarely bloody), stomach cramps, nausea, and flatulence, lasting 2–6 weeks. A chronic infection may develop that can last for months or years.
- **Treatment** includes furazolidone 5–8 mg/kg/day in 4 doses for 7–10 days or metronidazole 40 mg/kg/day in 3 doses for 7–10 days. Chronic infections are often very resistant to treatment.

TOXOPLASMOSIS

Toxoplasmosis is an infection caused by the **parasite *Toxoplasma gondii***, which is commonly found in soil. It is widespread and transmitted through cat feces; however, it also may be contracted by eating undercooked meat (especially pork, lamb, or venison) or poorly washed vegetables. Toxoplasmosis can cause serious disease and can affect various organs; and immunocompromised and pregnant women and their unborn babies are especially likely to have side effects of the disease (the "T" in congenital TORCH infections).

- Healthy patients are usually asymptomatic; however, once infected the parasite can remain latent until the patient becomes immunocompromised and the parasite is reactivated causing **symptoms**. The disease can cause a flu-like illness with fever, myalgias, and lymphadenopathy. More serious effects include retinochoroiditis, brain lesions, and encephalitis. Congenital toxoplasmosis may cause retinochoroiditis, microcephaly, hydrocephalus, intellectual disability, and possibly miscarriage or stillbirth.
- **Diagnose** with serology for *Toxoplasma* antibodies IgM and IgG. Also, PCR may be used to test amniotic fluid, CSF, or tissue.
- **Treat** with pyrimethamine (preferred) plus folinic acid or sulfadiazine plus folinic acid. Pregnant women should avoid high-risk practices like changing the cat litter and should avoid sand boxes.

HEALTHCARE ASSOCIATED CONDITIONS
CLABSI

Intensive care patients routinely have central venous catheters placed for the administration of fluids, medications, parenteral nutrition, and other supportive therapies. **Central line blood stream infections (CLABSI)** occur when a confirmed (by laboratory analysis) bloodstream infection occurs in a patient with a central line in place for greater than 2 calendar days on the date of the confirmed infection. Central line blood stream infections contribute to an increase in hospital length of stay, a marked increase in healthcare costs, and a higher mortality rate for those patients that acquire them. CLABSI is often a preventable occurrence and many evidence-based practices have been identified in their prevention. Strategies aimed at prevention of CLABSI include hand hygiene, strict aseptic technique in accessing and maintaining the catheter, thorough assessment of the catheter insertion site daily, and appropriate site care.

- **Signs and symptoms**: Fever, chills, hypotension, tachycardia, erythema, edema and/or drainage at the catheter site, and pain/tenderness at the catheter site
- **Diagnosis**: CBC, blood cultures, and culture of the catheter tip
- **Treatment**: Once the causative organism is identified, antimicrobial treatment will be initiated. The central venous catheter may also be removed.

CAUTI

Urinary tract infections that occur in the hospitalized patient are most often associated with the use of a urinary catheter. **Catheter associated urinary tract infections (CAUTIs)** occur when a urinary tract infection develops in a patient with an indwelling urinary catheter in place during the 48 hour period before the development of the infection. CAUTI is the most common healthcare associated infection. Like other health care associated infections, catheter associated urinary tract infections contribute to increased healthcare costs, increased length of stay and higher morbidity and mortality rates. Evidence based strategies aimed at prevention of CAUTIs include using urinary catheters only when appropriately indicated, discontinuation of the urinary catheter as soon as possible, utilization of aseptic technique and sterile equipment during insertion, hand hygiene, utilization of a closed drainage system and securement of the urinary catheter.

- **Signs and symptoms**: Fever, urinary urgency, urinary frequency, dysuria, pressure or pain in lower abdomen or back, flank pain, fatigue, nausea and vomiting, and mental status changes
- **Diagnosis**: Physical assessment, urinalysis, and urine culture
- **Treatment**: Treatment of a catheter associated urinary treatment infection includes removal of the catheter, antibiotics, and administration of fluids.

VENTILATOR ASSOCIATED EVENTS

Ventilator associated events (VAE) include a broad range of complications that may occur in the ventilated patient. Aspiration is a potential complication of intubation and greatly increases the risk of developing ventilator associated pneumonia in the critical care patient. **Ventilator associated pneumonia (VAP)** is a healthcare associated infection that develops in a patient with an endotracheal tube or tracheostomy that has been mechanically ventilated for at least 48 hours when the infection is identified. Risk factors for the development of VAP include advanced age, immobility, post-operative status, and immunocompromised immune system.

- **Signs and symptoms**: Fever, purulent drainage/sputum, cough, hypoxemia
- **Diagnosis**: Perform physical assessment and chest x-ray to confirm the presence of infiltrates. Samples of respiratory secretions may also be obtained and sampled
- **Treatment**: Once the organism causing the pneumonia has been identified, treatment will include the administration of the appropriate antibiotic. Prevention includes keeping the HOB raised 30°, frequent mouth care (usually every 2 hours), routine changing of in-line suction and tubing, and early mobility

RESISTANT INFECTIOUS DISEASES
MRSA

Methicillin resistant staphylococcus aureus (MRSA) is a drug resistant form of staph aureus that accounts for 10-50% of all staph infections. It is associated with an increased risk of morbidity and mortality and can manifest as a skin infection, bloodstream infection, urinary tract, respiratory infection, or wound infection. Risk factors for the development of MRSA are recent antibiotic therapy, recent or current hospitalization (risk increases with longer hospitalizations), and immunosuppression.

- **Signs and symptoms**: Depending on the site of infection, symptoms may include fever, chills, headache, fatigue, malaise, rash, shortness of breath, cough, and delayed healing. Skin infection symptoms may include erythema, edema, and drainage.
- **Diagnosis**: The diagnosis of MRSA is made through a laboratory culture of the suspected site (i.e., wound, sputum, urine, blood).
- **Treatment**: MRSA is treated by antibiotic therapy. Laboratory cultures can assist in determining the sensitivity of the organism to antibiotics. Skin infections may require an irrigation and debridement.

MULTIDRUG RESISTANT VRE

Enterococcus bacteria may cause infections of the urinary tract, blood stream, endocardium and meninges. **Vancomycin resistant enterococcus (VRE)** is a drug resistant organism that is most likely to develop in hospitalized or immunosuppressed patients. Post-operative patients, patients who have been on long term antibiotic therapy and those with an indwelling intravenous or urinary catheter are also at an increased risk of developing VRE.

- **Signs and symptoms**: Dependent on the site of infection—fever, chills, fatigue and malaise. Urinary tract infection symptoms may include back pain, urinary frequency and urgency and painful urination. Wound infection symptoms include erythema, edema, pain and drainage.
- **Diagnosis**: The diagnosis of VRE is made through a laboratory culture of the suspected area.
- **Treatment**: VRE is treated with antibiotic therapy. Laboratory cultures can assist in determining the sensitivity of the organism to antibiotics. These patients are placed in strict contact precautions.

CARBAPENEM RESISTANT ENTEROBACTERIACEAE

Carbapenem resistant Enterobacteriaceae (CRE) are a family of resistant organisms that were formerly susceptible to the antibiotic class carbapenems. The majority of CRE infections are caused by the *Klebsiella pneumonia* organism. CRE infections are associated with an increased mortality rate and are more likely to occur in hospitalized patients who are mechanically ventilated, have an indwelling intravenous or urinary catheter or have received a long-term course of antibiotic therapy.

- **Signs and symptoms**: Dependent on the site of infection—fever, chills, malaise and delayed wound healing. CRE infections may manifest as wound, urinary, respiratory, or bloodstream infections.
- **Diagnosis**: The diagnosis of CRE is made through a laboratory culture of the suspected area.
- **Treatment**: CRE is treated with antibiotic therapy. Laboratory cultures can assist in determining the sensitivity of the organism to antibiotics. Hand hygiene, meticulous cleaning/sterilization of patient equipment and supplies and limited use of antibiotic therapy may be effective in decreasing the risk of healthcare acquired CRE infections. These patients are placed in strict contact precautions.

PEDIATRIC INFECTIOUS DISEASE RISKS

TODDLERS AND PRESCHOOLERS

These children will still put toys in their mouths, which can transmit infections. Toilet training is still in the early stages, and their hand washing may need more practice, leading to transmitting fecal-oral germs. Toddlers and preschoolers are at risk for infections from animal scratches and bites, such as ringworm of the body. Daycare centers can be breeding grounds for germs, and these children are very susceptible to any infections in their environment. Day care workers should wear gloves and clean diaper changing areas with a disinfectant each time a diaper is changed. Children should be assisted in hand washing (after toileting, before and after eating, and after coughing or sneezing) and should be educated in these areas.

SCHOOL AGE CHILDREN

School environments are similar to daycare centers. Children may not always use good hand washing after toileting and before meals. They tend to share personal objects, which can lead to the spread of lice, scabies, tinea corporis, tinea capitis, and pinworms. Children with respiratory illnesses who don't cover their mouth and nose when coughing or sneezing and don't wash their hands afterwards can spread common illnesses. Pneumonia in this age group is usually caused by Mycoplasma pneumoniae and is very contagious. Fifth's disease is also common, very contagious, and causes a lacy rash that can come and go for up to a month. The child is contagious before the rash appears.

ADOLESCENTS

Adolescents are normally fairly healthy individuals and so aren't often seen at the doctor's office. This puts them at risk of skipping any needed immunizations or boosters. Without the boosters, they will be susceptible to measles, mumps, rubella, hepatitis B, and chickenpox. The MMR vaccine should not be given to females who may be pregnant. Sexually active teens are at risk for sexually transmitted infections and HIV. Adolescents tend to believe they won't get infections from their partners and that they won't get pregnant. Teens using crack cocaine are at higher risk for becoming infected with STIs and HIV. Teens should be given a private room, away from parents, when visiting the doctor so that an accurate portrayal of the teen's knowledge of STIs and sexual behaviors can be gleaned.

Geriatric Pathophysiology

GERIATRIC SYNDROMES

Geriatric syndromes represent a category of illnesses that is comprised of the most common non-disease conditions that are seen amongst the geriatric community. It is the responsibility of the nurse to be competent in these critical areas:

- **Falls**: As individuals age, their senses dull, leaving them vulnerable to falls due to a combination of sensory decline and chronic disease. Patients and caregivers should be provided with recommendations for fall prevention, and health care providers should create safe inpatient environments with proper fall prevention protocols.
- **Frailty**: A syndrome characterized by decreased stamina, strength, weight, and speed. This combination of issues results from the natural decline of aging and presents specific risks (falls, confusion, and depression) that must be assessed amongst the geriatric population.
- **Incontinence**: Urinary incontinence is an especially common ailment amongst the elderly population due to neurological conditions, physical limitations, and cognitive decline. This particular ailment is not only physically limiting and introduces risks for skin breakdown and infection, but it is socially limiting and can lead to psychological issues as well.
- **Delirium**: Confusion is the most common manifestation of any physical ailment amongst the elderly, along with the prevalence of dementia amongst the elderly. Delirium should never be cast aside in an elderly individual. Though common, it may be an indication of other more serious issues.
- **Functional Decline**: Functional decline is the diminished ability of an individual to carry out the activities of daily living to sustain independence and perform self-care. With this, comes the consideration for additional support, be it live-in care, nursing homes, or assisted living communities.

ADDITIONAL HEALTH ISSUES FOR THE ELDERLY

The following are additional health issues for the elderly:

- **Antibodies and Immunity**: An elderly patient can react to an infection with antibodies that have been created by the body before, but if the infection is new, it is more difficult for the body to respond appropriately. Cells in the immune system cannot proliferate as easily in an older patient as in a younger one. The number of T-cells is stable, but they do not work as well and can have less cytotoxicity. Additionally, there is not as much thymus-gained immunity because the thymus gland is smaller. This also means it is harder for an older patient to make antibodies.
- **Allergies**: Identify the type of allergic response the patient has and to what allergens, especially when getting the patient history. Determine if the response is actually an allergy to a medication or an adverse effect of it.
- **Driving**: An elderly patient senses change with age. A decreased ability to hear does not mean a patient cannot drive, but sight is very important, including binocular sight, ability to see color, and ability to see in the dark.
- **REM**: Rapid eye movement starts approximately 120 minutes after going to sleep, and happens again in 3–4 evenly spread out increments that last 10–15 minutes. It is linked to skeletal muscle atonia, rapid eye movements, and dreaming. REM sleep occurs less frequently as one gets older. With aging, the patient is more likely to wake up, which affects their sleep quality.

Urinary Incontinence

Urinary incontinence (UI) is the involuntary loss of urine. Incidence increases with age and is more common in women. There are several **types of urinary incontinence**:

- **Transient**: Adverse medication reaction, urinary tract infection, severe constipation, immobility, mental disorders.
- **Urge or Reflex**: Detrusor muscle spasms cause an urgent desire to urinate because of neurological impairment in Parkinson's, stroke, Alzheimer's, and sitting. Can be triggered by drinking, or hearing or seeing running water.
- **Stress (SUI)**: Increased intra-abdominal pressure from sneezing, coughing, laughing, pregnancy, childbirth damage to the detrusor muscle and pelvic floor fascia, and menopausal hormone changes. Twice as common in women as men.
- **Enuresis**: Bedwetting while asleep.

Decreased bladder strength, diminished ability to concentrate urine, and decreased urethral closing pressure following menopause are common causes of incontinence in the elderly. Incontinence is also influenced by depression, less mobility, decreased vision, and less awareness of feeling a full bladder. Voiding routines are helpful in managing incontinence among the elderly. The typical voiding routine for a fully-grown adult patient is as follows: The initial urge to go to the bathroom happens at the point of the bladder having 200-300 mL in it. Grown patients generally void 4-6 times daily, and most will not need to go during the night except when there is a condition that makes it so or if the patient is using diuretic medication. The sensation of the bladder beginning to fill up begins at 90-150 mL, and the need to go starts at 200-300 mL. Usually, an hour or two will elapse between the first feeling of needing to go and the bladder being at full capacity. Full, easy capacity is around 300-600 mL. There should not be any leaking if going to the bathroom has to be postponed.

Age-Related Changes in Respiratory System

As a patient ages, the respiratory system changes in the following ways:

- **Rib cage becomes more rigid.** There will be more width measured across the anteroposterior chest. When a patient gets old, the number of alveoli decreases. They get inflexible and can no longer draw back. This means that the patient cannot breathe out as well, leading to more residual volume. There is less basilar inflation and the patient cannot get foreign bodies out as well. This condition also happens to someone who has kyphosis.
- **Decreased ability for the chest wall to work** so that it is harder to take a deep inhalation.
- **Trachea and bronchi increase in measurement** so that there is more unused area and lessened air volume that gets to the alveoli. Small airway shutting means there is less vital capacity and more residual volume.
- **Lung parenchyma is not as elastic** so that the alveoli do not function as effectively.
- **Breaths are not as deep and coughs are not as forceful** because the muscles are not as strong.

CHRONIC DIARRHEA

Chronic diarrhea is more than three bowel movements per day, with watery stools lasting more than two weeks. It is more common and potentially more serious for the elderly population. The most common cause is infectious, but **chronic diarrhea** in the elderly population can also be caused by inflammatory bowel disease, diverticulitis, colon cancer, medication side effects, and irritable bowel syndrome. Take a careful history, including a list of travel destinations. Look for these signs and **symptoms of dehydration** in the physical exam:

- Flushed, dry skin
- Dark, scanty urine
- Fast pulse and respiration
- Fever
- Vomiting or nausea
- Head rushes
- Thirst
- Dry mouth
- Anorexia
- Chills
- Tingling
- Cramps
- Exhaustion
- Confusion
- Seizures
- Unconsciousness

Send stools to the lab for culture, ova and parasites, occult blood, fecal leukocytes, and *C. difficile* toxin, especially if the patient was recently hospitalized. Collect blood for a CBC and electrolytes. Order an abdominal x-ray, and follow up with a barium enema or colonoscopy, if indicated. Treat the underlying cause. Significantly dehydrated patients require hospital admission for IV therapy.

FRACTURES

Fractures are a common cause of disability in the elderly population. The elderly population is at higher risk for sustaining **fractures** due to decreased bone mass and strength, and increased risk for falls due to poor vision and balance. The most common locations for fractures in the elderly are the distal radius, proximal humerus, proximal femur and tibia, vertebrae, hip, and pubic ramus. Most fractures are the result of minor trauma. Fractures are slightly more common in women. Make the diagnosis based on the history, physical exam, and x-ray results. Immobilize the fracture above and below the break. Administer analgesics. Refer the patient to a physiotherapist, an orthopedic surgeon, and a PSW. The goal of treatment is as rapid a return to normal activity as is possible. The elderly population is more vulnerable to complications, such as permanent functional impairment, bedsores, and pulmonary embolism. The aide, nurse, or caregiver must turn the patient every two hours to minimize complications.

AGE-RELATED CATARACTS

The lens is the clear part of the eye behind the pupil that focuses light on the retina. **Cataracts** are categorized by gradual clouding or opacification of the lens. One or both eyes can be affected, and cataracts can be congenital. Incidence increases with age and affects 70% of people over the age of 75. Risk factors include trauma, radiation, diabetes, family history, smoking, alcoholism, sun exposure, steroid use, and previous eye surgery. Signs and symptoms for cataracts include gradual lens clouding; blurry vision; decreased night vision; brown tint or color fading; halo or glare around lights; diplopia (double vision); trouble distinguishing blue and purple. An ophthalmologist makes the diagnosis by slit lamp exam and retinal exam. Cataracts are followed until they cause significant visual loss and then are treated by surgical removal of the clouded lens and replacement with a permanent intraocular or removable external lens.

> **Review Video: Glaucoma vs. Cataracts**
> Visit mometrix.com/academy and enter code: 279024

HEARING LOSS

Approximately 25% of adults over the age of 65 have varying degrees of hearing loss. Risk factors for hearing loss include:

- A positive family history
- Chronic exposure to loud noises, especially if hearing protection was not worn
- Use of ototoxic drugs, like Gentamicin, NSAIDs, loop diuretics, or cancer chemotherapy

Hearing loss can be either peripheral or central. **Peripheral hearing loss** results when the ear canal is obstructed by impacted wax, a foreign object, or damage to the middle or inner ear. **Central hearing loss** is the result of damage to the portions of the brain that are needed for hearing: Vestibulocochlear nerve, brain stem, contralateral inferior colliculus, superior olivary nucleus, inferior colliculi, ipsilateral medial geniculate nucleus of the thalamus, and primary auditory cortex below the superior temporal gyrus in the temporal lobe.

Psychosocial Pathophysiology

DEVELOPMENTAL DELAYS AND INTELLECTUAL DISABILITY

Developmental delays occur when a patient does not progress mentally at the same rate as the general population. Intellectual disability is a condition in which individuals may have difficulty adapting to changing environments, need guidance in decision-making, and have self-care or communication deficits. Behaviors range from shy and passive to hyperactive and aggressive. Intellectual disability may be inherited (Tay-Sachs), toxin-related (maternal alcohol consumption), perinatal (hypoxia), environmental (lack of stimulation/neglect), or acquired (encephalitis, brain injury). **Diagnosis** involves performance results from standardized tests with behavior analysis. Intellectual disability classifications are based on IQ:

- **55–69 (mild, 85% of cases):** Educable to about 6th grade level. May not be diagnosed until adolescence. Usually able to learn skills and be self-supporting but may need assistance and supervision.
- **40–54 (moderate, 10% of cases):** Trainable and may be able to work and live in sheltered environments or with supervision.
- **25–39 (severe, 3–4% of cases):** Language usually delayed and can learn only basic academic skills and perform simple tasks.
- **≤25 (profound, 1–2% of cases):** Usually associated with neurological disorder with sensorimotor dysfunction. Require constant care and supervision.

Nursing considerations: Always treat patients according to their developmental level, not their physical age. This is especially important when considering education and consent. People with developmental delays are at increased risk for injury and abuse.

PERSONALITY DISORDER

A personality disorder is a fixed and enduring set pattern or traits of behavior that **deviate from expected behaviors within a culture**. These disorders inhibit the individual's ability to have meaningful interpersonal relationships, to be fulfilled, or to enjoy life. Onset usually occurs during adolescence or early adulthood. A personality disorder is an attitude directed toward the whole world including one's own self. This attitude is expressed through thoughts, feelings, and behaviors. Many times, the behaviors will become less extreme as the person gets older.

DSM CLASSIFICATION GROUPINGS

The DSM-5-TR lists 10 personality disorders grouped into three clusters: A, B, and C.

- **Cluster A** includes disorders that are characterized by odd or eccentric behaviors and a tendency for social awkwardness and withdrawal.
- **Cluster B** includes disorders that are characterized by erratic, highly emotional, dramatic, or impulsive behaviors.
- **Cluster C** includes disorders that are characterized predominantly by fearful or anxious symptoms.

SPECIFIC DIAGNOSES INCLUDED IN CLUSTER A FOR PERSONALITY DISORDERS

Cluster A: The classification of Cluster A for personality disorders includes the diagnoses of paranoid, schizoid, and schizotypal personality disorders.

- The **paranoid** individual is very distrustful and suspicious of others. They believe that other people are up to no good, are keeping secrets, and may intend to harm them. There is usually no basis or evidence to support this belief.
- The **schizoid** individual exhibits a consistent social detachment. Many of their behaviors indicate a restricted emotional response and can include appearing cold and indifferent, having no desire for close personal relationships, having no desire for intimacy, choosing solidarity over socializing, and usually having no close friends or relatives.
- Like the schizoid individual, the **schizotypal** individual tends to lack intimate relationships, but this is due to social ineptitude and fear rather than a lack of interest in relationship. They also experience cognitive and perceptual distortions, seeing or hearing things that are not there, and hold odd or superstitious beliefs.

SPECIFIC DIAGNOSES INCLUDED IN CLUSTER B FOR PERSONALITY DISORDERS

Cluster B: The classification of Cluster B for personality disorders includes the diagnoses of antisocial, borderline, histrionic, and narcissistic personality disorders.

- The **antisocial** individual exhibits a blatant disregard for other people. They frequently lie, manipulate, exploit, and commit illegal acts.
- The **borderline** individual has a markedly unstable self-image. They are very impulsive, self-destructive, have unstable and intense interpersonal relationships, mood instability, inappropriate and intense anger, and may have recurrent suicidal or self-mutilating behaviors.
- The **histrionic** individual is extremely emotional and desires to be the center of attention. They often perform attention-seeking behaviors and have frequent, intense, and short-lived relationships.
- The **narcissistic** individual has a great sense of self-importance and is often arrogant. They lack empathy for others and can be exploitative and manipulative, and they tend to react violently if they perceive disrespect or opposition.

SPECIFIC DIAGNOSES INCLUDED IN CLUSTER C FOR PERSONALITY DISORDERS

Cluster C: The classification of Cluster C for personality disorders includes the diagnoses of avoidant, dependent, and obsessive-compulsive personality disorders.

- The **avoidant** individual is socially inhibited and consequently avoids interaction with others. They are very sensitive to criticism or rejection and often have feelings of inadequacy.
- The **dependent** individual has very low self-esteem and will be submissive and dependent in behaviors and relationships, making them susceptible to being taken advantage of. If they lose their primary supportive relationship, they will quickly seek to establish another one.
- The **obsessive-compulsive** individual will have an extreme preoccupation with minute details, and will possess an inflexible perfectionism and desire for control. They also exhibit cold, unfeeling, and superior attitudes towards others.

BIPOLAR DISORDER

Bipolar disorder causes severe mood swings between hyperactive states and depression, accompanied by impaired judgment because of distorted thoughts. The hypomanic stage may allow for creativity and good functioning in some people, but it can develop into more severe mania, which may be associated with psychosis and hallucinations with rapid speech and bizarre behavior, and then into periods of profound depression. While most cases are diagnosed in late adolescence, there is increasing evidence that some children present with symptoms earlier; especially at risk are children with a bipolar parent. Bipolar disorder is associated with high rates of suicide, so early diagnosis and treatment is critical.

Symptoms may be relatively mild or involve severe rapid cycling between mania and depression.

Treatment includes both medications (usually given continually) to prevent cycling and control depression and psychosocial therapy, such as cognitive therapy, to help control disordered thought patterns and behavior. Psychiatric referral should be made.

OBSESSIVE-COMPULSIVE DISORDER

Anxiety disorders also include the diagnosis of obsessive-compulsive disorder (OCD). OCD involves either **obsessions** or **compulsions** that are persistent impulses or thoughts that are uncontrollable by the person. These thoughts lead to an **abnormally elevated anxiety response**. Some examples of obsessions can include fear of dirt, germs, robbery, contracting a medical disease, unintentional discarding of important information, having images of a sexual nature, or things not being symmetrical or completed. Compulsions are when the individual is driven to perform certain repetitive behaviors in ritualistic order with the outcome being resolution of the anxiety caused by the obsession.

Some examples of **compulsive repetitive behaviors** can include hand washing, checking locks, counting objects found routinely within their normal day, hoarding, ordering or arranging items, or saying words silently.

> **Review Video: Obsessive-Compulsive Disorder (OCD)**
> Visit mometrix.com/academy and enter code: 499790

COMORBIDITIES

When an individual has two or more disorders occurring at the same time, these disorders are considered to share **comorbidity**. Obsessive-compulsive disorder (OCD) is often found sharing comorbidity with other psychological disorders. Many times, individuals with OCD also have Tourette's syndrome, depression, panic attacks, mood disorders, social and specific phobias, eating disorders, or personality disorders. It has been found that Tourette's syndrome and OCD actually cause similar brain dysfunctions. Depression is commonly seen in patient's suffering from OCD due to the isolating effects it can have upon their lifestyle. It is also common for these individuals to have substance abuse problems due to trying to self-medicate to solve their struggles with OCD.

DEPRESSION

Depression is a mood disorder characterized by profound feelings of sadness and withdrawal. It may be acute (such as after a death) or chronic with recurring episodes over a lifetime. The cause appears to be a combination of genetic, biological, and environmental factors. A major depressive episode is a depressed mood, profound and constant sense of hopelessness and despair, or loss of interest in all or almost all activities for a period of at least two weeks. Some drugs may precipitate depression: diuretics, Parkinson's drugs, estrogen, corticosteroids, cimetidine, hydralazine, propranolol, digitalis, and indomethacin. Depression is associated with neurotransmitter dysregulation, especially serotonin and norepinephrine. Major depression can be mild, moderate, or severe.

Symptoms include changes in mood, sadness, loss of interest in usual activities, increased fatigue, changes in appetite and fluctuations in weight, anxiety, and sleep disturbance.

Treatment includes tricyclic antidepressants (TCAS) and SSRIs, but SSRIs have fewer side effects and are less likely to cause death with an overdose. Counseling, undergoing cognitive behavioral therapy, treating underlying cause, and instituting an exercise program may help reduce depression.

> **Review Video: Major Depression**
> Visit mometrix.com/academy and enter code: 632694

ANXIETY AND DEPRESSION DUE TO INTENSIVE CARE STAYS

Anxiety and depression affect over half of patients who are treated in intensive care not only during the stay but also after discharge, especially if care is long-term or if their needs for moderate or high care continue. Additionally, studies have shown that those who suffer depression during and after ICU stays have increased risk of mortality over the next two years. Patients with anxiety may appear restless (thrashing about the bed), have difficulty concentrating, exhibit tachycardia and tachypnea, experience insomnia and feelings of dread, and complain of various ailments, such as stomach ache and headache. Symptoms of depression may overlap (and patients may have both anxiety and depression) and may also include fatigue, insomnia, withdrawal, appetite change, irritability, pessimistic outlooks, feelings of worthlessness, sadness, and suicidal ideation. Brief screening tools for anxiety and depression should be used with all ICU patients and interventions per psychological referral made as needed.

ANXIETY DISORDERS

Anxiety is a human emotion and experience that everyone has at some point during their life. Feelings of uncertainty, helplessness, isolation, alienation, and insecurity can all be experienced during an **anxiety response**. Many times, anxiety occurs without a specific known object or source. It can occur because of the unknown. Anxiety occurs throughout the life cycle, and therefore anxiety disorders can affect people of all ages. Populations that are most commonly affected include women, smokers, people under the age of 45, individuals that are separated or divorced, victims of abuse, and people in the lower socioeconomic groups. An individual can have one single anxiety disorder, experience more than one anxiety disorder, or have other mental health disorders all occurring at the same time.

> **Review Video: Different Types of Anxiety Disorders**
> Visit mometrix.com/academy and enter code: 366760

GENERALIZED ANXIETY DISORDER

Generalized anxiety disorder can be very insidious and occurs when an individual consistently experiences **excessive anxiety and worry**. This anxiety and worry will be present almost every day and lasts for a period of at least six months. The worry and anxiety will be uncontrollable, intrusive, and not related to any medical disease process. It will pertain to real-life events, situations, or circumstances and may occur along with mild depression symptoms. The individual will also experience three or more of the following symptoms: fatigue, inability to concentrate, irritability, insomnia, restlessness, loosing thought processes or going blank, and muscle tension. The continued anxiety and worry will eventually affect daily functioning and cause social and occupational disturbances.

COMORBIDITIES

Individuals with generalized anxiety disorder (GAD) will often have **other mental health disorders**. When a person has more than one psychological disorder occurring at the same time, these disorders are considered to be **comorbid**. Most patients suffering from GAD will have at least one more psychiatric diagnosis. The most common comorbid disorders can include major depressive disorder, social or specific phobias, panic disorder, and dysthymic disorder. It is also common for these individuals to have substance abuse problems, and they may look to alcohol or barbiturates to help control their symptoms of anxiety.

Levels of Anxiety

There are four main levels of anxiety that were named by Peplau. They are as follows:

- **Mild anxiety** is associated with normal tensions of everyday life. It can increase awareness and motivate learning and creativity.
- **Moderate anxiety** occurs when the individual narrows their field of perception and focuses on the immediate problem. This level decreases the perceptual field; however, the person can tend to other tasks if directed.
- **Severe anxiety** leads to a markedly reduced field of perception and the person focuses only on the details of the problem. All energy is directed at relieving the anxiety and the person can only perform other tasks under significant persuasion.
- **Panic** is the most extreme level of anxiety and associated with feelings of dread and terror. The individual is unable to perform any other tasks no matter how strongly they are persuaded to do so. This level can be life-threatening with complete disorganization of thought occurring.

Stress

Relationship Between Stress and Disease

Stress causes a number of physical and psychological changes within the body:

- Cortisol levels increase
- Digestion is hindered and the colon stimulated
- Heart rate increases
- Perspiration increases
- Anxiety and depression occur and can result in insomnia, anorexia or weight gain, and suicide
- Immune response decreases, making the person more vulnerable to infections
- Autoimmune reaction may increase, leading to autoimmune diseases

The body's **compensatory mechanisms** try to restore homeostasis. When these mechanisms are overwhelmed, pathophysiological injury to the cells of the body result. When this injury begins to interfere with the function of the organs or systems in the body, symptoms of dysfunction will occur. If the conditions are not corrected, the body changes the structure or function of the affected organs or systems.

Adaptation of Cells to Stress

The most common stressors to cells include the lack of oxygen, presence of toxins or chemicals, and infection. **Cells react to stress** by making the following changes:

- **Hypertrophy**: Cells swell, leading to an overall increase in the size of the affected organ.
- **Atrophy**: Cells shrivel and the overall organ size decreases in size.
- **Hyperplasia**: The cells divide and overgrowth and thickening of the tissue results.
- **Dysplasia**: The cells are changed in appearance as a result of irritation over an extended period of time, sometimes leading to malignancy.
- **Metaplasia**: Cells change type as a result of stress.

If the stress that caused the cells to change continues, the cells become injured and die. When enough cells die, organ and systemic failure occur.

Psychological Response to Stress

When stress is encountered, a person **responds** according to the threat perceived to compensate. The threat is evaluated as to the amount of harm or loss that has occurred or is possible. If the stress is benign (such as with marriage), then a challenge is present that demands change. Once the threat or challenge is defined, the person can gather information, resources, and support to make the changes needed to resolve the stress to the greatest degree possible. Immediate psychological response to stress may include shock, anger, fear, or excitement. Over time, people may develop chronic anxiety, depression, flashbacks, thought disturbances, and sleep disturbances. Changes may occur in emotions and thinking, in behavior, or in the person's environment. People may be more able to adapt to stress if they have many varied experiences, a good self-esteem, and a support network to help as needed. A healthy lifestyle and philosophical beliefs, including religion, may give a person more reserve to cope with stress.

Impact of Different Kinds of Stress

Everyone encounters **stress** in life and it **impacts** each person differently. There are the small daily "hassles," major traumatic events, and the periodic stressful events of marriage, birth, divorce, and death. Compounded stress experienced on a daily basis can impact health status over time. Stressors that occur suddenly are the hardest to overcome and result in the greatest tension. The length of time that a stressor is present affects the impact with long-term, relentless stress, such as that generated by poverty or disability, resulting in disease more often. If there is **ineffective coping**, a person will suffer greater changes resulting in even more stress. The nurse can help patients to recognize those things that induce stress in their lives, find ways to reduce stress when possible, and teach effective coping skills and problem-management.

Substance Abuse

Substance abuse is the abuse of drugs, medicines, or alcohol that causes mental and physical problems for the abuser and family. Abusers use substances out of boredom, to hide negative self-esteem, to dampen emotional pain, and to cope with daily stress. As the abuse continues, abusers become unable to take care of daily needs and duties. They lack effective coping mechanisms and the ability to make healthy choices. They can't identify and prioritize stress or choose positive behavior to resolve the stress in a healthy way. Some family members may act as codependents because of their desire to feel needed by the abuser, to control the person, and to stay with him or her. The nurse can help the family to confront an individual with their concerns about the person and their proposals for treatment. Family members can enforce consequences if treatment is not sought. Family members may also need counseling to learn new behaviors to stop enabling the abuser to continue substance abuse.

Pathophysiology of Addiction

Genetic, social, and personality factors may all play a role in the development of **addictive tendencies**. However, the main factor of the development of substance addiction is the pharmacological activation of the **reward system** located in the central nervous system (CNS). This reward systems pathway involves **dopaminergic neurons**. Dopamine is found in the CNS and is one of many neurotransmitters that play a role in an individual's mood. The mesolimbic pathway seems to play a primary role in the reward and motivational process involved with addiction. This pathway begins in the ventral tegmental area of the brain (VTA) and then moves forward into the nucleus accumbens located in the middle forebrain bundle (MFB). Some drugs enhance mesolimbic dopamine activity, therefore producing very potent effects on mood and behavior.

INDICATORS OF SUBSTANCE ABUSE

Many people with substance abuse (alcohol or drugs) are reluctant to disclose this information, but there are a number of **indicators** that are suggestive of substance abuse:

Physical signs include:

- Burns on fingers or lips
- Pupils abnormally dilated or constricted, eyes watery
- Slurring of speech, slow speech
- Lack of coordination, instability of gait, tremors
- Sniffing repeatedly, nasal irritation, persistent cough
- Weight loss
- Dysrhythmias
- Pallor, puffiness of face
- Needle tracks on arms or legs
- Odor of alcohol/marijuana on clothing or breath

Behavioral signs include:

- Labile emotions, including mood swings, agitation, and anger
- Inappropriate, impulsive, or risky behavior
- Lying
- Missing appointments
- Difficulty concentrating, short term memory loss, blackouts
- Insomnia or excessive sleeping; disoriented, confused
- Lack of personal hygiene

ALCOHOL WITHDRAWAL

Chronic abuse of ethanol (alcoholism) can lead to physical dependency. Sudden cessation of drinking, which often happens in the inpatient setting, is associated with **alcohol withdrawal syndrome.** It may be precipitated by trauma or infection and has a high mortality rate, 5–15% with treatment and 35% without treatment.

Signs/symptoms: Anxiety, tachycardia, headache, diaphoresis, progressing to severe agitation, hallucinations, auditory/tactile disturbances, and psychotic behavior (delirium tremens).

Diagnosis: Physical assessment, blood alcohol levels (on admission).

Treatment includes:

- Medication: IV benzodiazepines to manage symptoms; electrolyte and nutritional replacement, especially magnesium and thiamine.
- Use the CIWA scale to measure symptoms of withdrawal; treat as indicated.
- Provide an environment with minimal sensory stimulus (lower lights, close blinds) & implement fall and seizure precautions.
- Prevention: Screen all patients for alcohol/substance abuse, using CAGE or other assessment tool. Remember to express support and comfort to patient; wait until withdrawal symptoms are subsiding to educate about alcohol use and moderation.

EATING DISORDERS
ANOREXIA NERVOSA

Eating disorders are a profound health risk and can lead to death, especially for adolescent girls, although boys also have eating disorders, often presenting as excessive exercise. Anorexia nervosa is characterized by profound fear of weight gain and severe restriction of food intake, often accompanied by abuse of diuretics and laxatives, which can cause electrolyte imbalances, kidney and bowel disorders, and delay or cessation of menses.

- **Symptoms** include growth retardation, amenorrhea (missing 3 consecutive periods), unexplained and sometimes precipitous weight loss (at least 15% below normal weight), dehydration, loss of appetite, hypoglycemia, hypercholesterolemia, or carotenemia with yellowing of skin, emaciated appearance, osteoporosis, bradycardia, and food obsessions and rituals.
- **Diagnosis** includes complete history, physical, and psychological exam with CBC and chemical panels to rule out other disorders.
- **Treatment** includes volume and electrolyte replacement initially with referral to psychiatric care for long-term management of the disorder and nutritional plans.

BULIMIA NERVOSA

Bulimia nervosa includes binge eating followed by vomiting (at least 2 times monthly for at least 3 months), often along with diuretics, enemas, and laxatives. Some may engage in periods of fasting or excessive exercise rather than vomiting to offset the effects of binging. Gastric acids from purging can damage the throat and teeth. While bulimics may maintain a normal weight, they are at risk for severe electrolyte imbalances that can be life-threatening. Binge eating affects 2–5% of females and includes grossly overeating, often resulting in obesity, depression, and shame. Symptoms include hypokalemia, metabolic acidosis, fluctuations of weight, dental caries and loss of enamel, knuckle scars (from contact with teeth while inducing vomiting), parotid and submandibular gland enlargement, and insulin-dependent diabetes. Diagnosis includes complete history, physical, and psychological exam with CBC and chemical panels to rule out other disorders. Treatment includes volume and electrolyte replacement initially with referral to psychiatric care for long-term management of the disorder and nutritional plans, as well as SSRIs, naltrexone, and ondansetron.

INTELLECTUAL DISABILITY

Intellectual disability is usually diagnosed <18. Individuals may have difficulty adapting to changing environments, need guidance in decision-making, and have self-care or communication deficits. Behaviors range from shy and passive to hyperactive or aggressive. Those with associated physical characteristics (Down syndrome) or problems are often diagnosed early. Intellectual disability may be inherited (Tay-Sachs), toxin-related (maternal alcohol consumption), perinatal (hypoxia), environmental (lack of stimulation/neglect), or acquired (encephalitis, brain injury). Diagnosis involves performance results from standardized tests along with behavior analysis. **Intellectual disability classifications** are divided into mild, moderate, severe, and profound with criteria broken down across three domains: conceptual, social, and practical.

- **Mild (85% of cases)**: Educable to about 6th grade level. May not be diagnosed until adolescence. Usually able to learn skills and be self-supporting but may need assistance and supervision.
- **Moderate (10% of cases)**: Trainable and may be able to work and live in sheltered environments or with supervision.
- **Severe (3-4% of cases)**: Language usually delayed and can learn only basic academic skills and perform simple tasks.
- **Profound (1-2% of cases)**: Usually associated with neurological disorder with sensorimotor dysfunction. Require constant care and supervision.

ATTENTION-DEFICIT HYPERACTIVITY DISORDER

A child with attention-deficit hyperactivity disorder (ADHD) may display some or all of the following symptoms:

- Inattention (short attention span, distractible)
- Hyperactivity (can't sit still, moves constantly)
- Impulsivity (impatience, acts before thinking)

Inattention and hyperactivity/impulsivity can be present separately or in combination. A diagnosis of ADHD is based on several criteria. The most important criteria are that symptoms of impulsivity/hyperactivity and/or inattention be present for at least 6 months and that some symptoms were present before the age of 12.

TREATMENT

Treatment for ADHD is aimed at controlling the behavior (pharmacotherapy and behavior management), controlling the environment (educational interventions) and educating the family. Medications used include stimulants (Ritalin, Dexedrine, and Adderall), antihypertensives (Catapres, Tenex), antidepressants (Wellbutrin), or Strattera, a nonstimulant. Stimulants are addictive and the side effects include weight loss, insomnia, headache, palpitations, and high blood pressure. Behavior therapy involves using positive reinforcement to help the child follow rules, stay on task, and have more self-control. ADHD is a developmental disorder, meaning that the school system must provide accommodations for these children in mainstreamed classrooms if at all possible. Families should be educated as to the nature of ADHD and coping skills. Some controversial treatments are used, although they are part of the standard of care. These can include vitamins, mineral and herbal supplements, biofeedback, dietary changes, and chiropractic care.

AUTISM SPECTRUM DISORDERS

Autism spectrum disorders (ASD) affect approximately 3.4 per 1000 children in the United States and present with a wide range of symptoms, including impairment in thinking and expressions of emotion, using language, and communicating and relating with others. Some children are profoundly impaired and are diagnosed early, but more high functioning children, such as those with Asperger's, may go undiagnosed. All exhibit some degree of impairment in 3 areas:

- Social interaction
- Communication (verbal and nonverbal)
- Repetitive behavior

Because they may lack social skills, children with ASD are often isolated and bullied. They may do well in school or have some degree of intellectual disability. About 25% suffer from seizure disorders as well. ASD may be identified through developmental screening, and/or specific screening instruments for autism. Intervention includes referrals to special education programs, including early intervention programs for children under the age of 3 and may include behavioral and speech therapy. Early diagnosis helps maximize the child's potential and may allow the child to live independently as an adult.

EARLY INDICATORS OF AUTISM

Although there is no specific test that defines a diagnosis of autism, there are many indications that can point to autistic development that caregivers should be aware of. Further testing may be indicated with a child who does not make sounds such as babbling or giggling; fails to show positive facial expressions or mimic smiles or laughter; lacks the ability to repeat activities, words, or sounds when another person initiates these; fails to utter speech sounds at all by 16 months of age; fails to initiate gestures, such as waving, pointing to objects, or reaching for items; and appears to turn backwards in development, such as a sudden loss of speech, words, or social skills.

Rett's Syndrome

Rett's syndrome is a pervasive developmental disorder in females, characterized by normal prenatal development, normal motor development in the first five months of life and a normal head circumference. However, between 5-48 months of age, head growth decelerates and the loss of purposeful use of the hands, along with gait abnormalities, seizures, and intellectual disability appears.

- **I (Early onset)** 6-18 months: The infant begins to exhibit less eye contact, diminished interest in playing, and delays in motor skill development (crawling and sitting).
- **II (Rapid destruction)** 1-4 years: Previously gained skills, such as use of hands and speech, are lost. Purposeless hand movements such as wringing, grasping or finger wriggling begin while the child is awake, but disappear when the child is asleep. Deceleration of head growth is usually evident.
- **III (Pseudo-stationary)** 2-10 years: Apraxia and seizures are prominent. A child may show more interest in her surroundings than she did during Stage II, and her alertness, attention span, and communication skills may improve. Many girls remain in this stage for most of their lives.
- **IV (Motor deterioration)** ≥10 years: Characterized by reduced mobility, muscle weakness, and rigidity spasticity. Dystonia and scoliosis are common features. Girls who were previously able to walk may stop walking. Generally, there is no decline in cognition, communication, or hand skills. Repetitive hand movements may decrease, and eye gaze usually improves.

Mood Disorders

Mood disorders can be broken down into two types: **bipolar** (depression alternating with mania) and **depressive** (chronic or episodic). The major symptom of mood disorders is depression, usually lasting 7–9 months. Other symptoms to watch for are disinterest in activities the child used to enjoy, changes in eating or sleeping patterns, agitation or anxiety, low self-esteem, being more tired than usual, problems with concentration, and suicidal thoughts. They may also exhibit physical complaints, such as stomach aches, diarrhea, and headaches.

Bipolar Disorder

In children with bipolar disorder, the hallmark symptom is intense rage. They may experience rage episodes lasting for 2–3 hours. Many parents do not seek treatment for younger children for several years until the child becomes older and the behavior becomes more disruptive. For many younger children, the first symptom exhibited is depression. Symptoms in children under the age of nine usually include labile emotions and irritability rather than more classic manic symptoms. However, as the child becomes older and enters adolescence, the symptoms become more classic-like and include abnormally elevated mood and delusions of grandeur. They may exhibit racing thoughts and pressured speech. Bipolar disease may occur with ADHD, depression, reactive attachment disorder, conduct disorder, and oppositional defiant disorder, so diagnosis and treatment may be complicated. Children often experience academic and behavioral problems as well as suicidal ideation. Initial treatment is monotherapy with a mood stabilizer, such as lithium, carbamazepine, divalproex, or atypical antipsychotics.

Depression

Depression is increasingly recognized as a risk factor for children, manifesting in young children as feigning illness or refusal to go to school and in older children as behavioral problems, negativity, and difficulties at school rather than the more common withdrawal and overt depression of some adults. However, children may feel persistent anxiety and sadness, and they often have profound fears that something will happen to a parent. Usually changes in behavior become apparent. One study showed that 29% of children with depression had suicidal thoughts, making early diagnosis and intervention very important. While there is some concern about antidepressants and children, suicide is a leading cause of death in teenagers, so medications with careful monitoring along with psychotherapy, such as cognitive behavioral therapy, seem to provide the best form of treatment, providing >70% with clinical improvement.

ANXIETY DISORDERS IN CHILDREN

Some anxiety is normal and assists the child in adjusting to new situations. Overwhelming anxiety to unspecific events can produce psychological and physical symptoms. Classifications of anxiety disorders in children include the following:

- **Social anxiety disorder** occurs when the child feels embarrassed, judged, or humiliated in the social environment.
- **Specific phobia** involves extreme fear/anxiety when exposed to a specific object/scenario, which may present as crying/screaming or freezing in the child.
- **Separation anxiety disorder** occurs when the child becomes stressed upon being separated from familiar surroundings or people.
- **Generalized anxiety disorder** presents as excessive worry over future events or day-to-day situations. Symptoms of anxiety may include stomachaches, nausea, vomiting, headaches, dizziness, palpitations, slight fever, tiredness, crying, irritability, and sleeping and eating difficulties.

TREATMENT AND NURSING MANAGEMENT

Treatment for anxiety disorders focuses on relieving symptoms and normalizing the child's daily activities. Education of the child and family, cognitive behavioral, family, and individual therapy, and medication are some treatment modalities. School teachers should be involved in the plan of care. To return the child to school, cognitive therapies such as desensitization and conditioning can be used. Medication is used in combination with therapy; antidepressants or anti-anxiety drugs are commonly used.

Assess for physical symptoms of anxiety (stomachaches or headaches that go away later in the day) and excessive absences from school. Diagnoses can include fear of separation, fear of interacting with others outside the home, and poor coping skills. A good outcome might include being able to be away from home for extended periods of time with little anxiety, attending school with little anxiety, good coping skills, and good social skills. The family should be included in the implementation of therapy. They can be taught signs of anxiety and ways to help the child gain independence and increase self-confidence.

PHYSIOLOGICAL EFFECTS OF CHRONIC STRESS ON A CHILD'S BODY

Children experience and struggle with stress, even at a very young age. Stressful situations can cause potential harm when a child lives in a chronic state of stress. Physiologically, a child who experiences continuous life stress may secrete increased levels of cortisol from the adrenal glands. This can contribute to a decreased immune response, resulting in increased illnesses and diminished protection from diseases. Increased levels of cortisol also damage the part of the brain that promotes memory and learning, which can lead to learning disabilities and difficulties in school. **Chronic stress** can alter brain growth, and when begun at a very early age, it can result in a smaller brain. Finally, continuous levels of stress may make a child less likely to tolerate stressful situations in life, leading to a decreased threshold for tolerating demanding activities.

SUICIDAL IDEATION/SUICIDE ATTEMPTS

Suicide is the third leading cause of death among adolescents, with about 1 million attempting suicide in the US each year. Additionally, antidepressants and atypical antipsychotics may increase suicidal ideation and depression.

Suicidal Ideation Indications	High Risk for Repeated Suicide Attempt
<ul><li>Depression or dysphoria</li><li>Hostility to others</li><li>Problems with peer relationships, and lack of close friends</li><li>Post-crisis stress (divorce, death in family, graduation, college)</li><li>Withdrawn personality</li><li>Quiet, lonely appearance, behavior</li><li>Change in behavior (drop in grades, wearing black clothes, unkempt appearance, sleeping excessively, or not sleeping)</li><li>Co-morbid psychiatric problems (bipolar, schizophrenia)</li><li>Drug abuse</li></ul>	Children who actually attempt suicide should be hospitalized and assessed for repeated suicide risk after initial treatment:<ul><li>Violent suicide attempt (knives, gunshots)</li><li>Suicide attempt with low chance of rescue</li><li>Ongoing psychosis or disordered thinking</li><li>Ongoing severe depression and feeling of helplessness</li><li>History of previous suicide attempts</li><li>Lack of social support system</li></ul>

HOMICIDAL IDEATION/ATTEMPTS

Homicidal ideation or attempts are rare in young children but can occur during adolescence for a variety of reasons.

- **Sociopathy/psychopathy**: These children usually appear quite normal and may even seem charming, but they can be very dangerous because they lack empathy for others. Some are involved in gangs in which violent behavior is expected and valued.
- **Psychosis**: Uncontrolled schizophrenia and paranoia may result in a child behaving in a homicidal manner.
- **Medications**: Medications such as antidepressants, SSRIs, and antipsychotics as well as interferon have been associated with homicidal ideation in some patients. Children on multiple medications may experience involuntary intoxication that results in rage reactions and sometimes even the death of others.

Children who express homicidal ideation or who have attempted homicide require immediate psychiatric referral and may require restraint. The nurse should conduct a complete review of medications and notify security personnel if the child poses a danger.

BEHAVIORAL AND ENVIRONMENTAL CAUSES OF FAILURE TO THRIVE

Failure to thrive (FTT) is a descriptive term for children who exhibit inadequate growth and development, usually measured by the child's being below the 5th percentile for weight (and sometimes height). FTT may relate to physical causes (such as renal disease or congenital heart disease), psychosocial factors (such as poverty, neglect) or idiopathic factors (unexplained). However, many issues may be involved other than just the parent-child relationship:

- **Income**: Inability to buy sufficient or nutritional food.
- **Health beliefs**: Child subjected to extreme or fad diets (Vegan, low fat) without ensuring proper nutrition.
- **Lack of education**: Inadequate knowledge of proper nutritional requirements for children.
- **Stress**: Illness, single-family home, divorce, lack of employment, incarceration.
- **Psychosocial issues**: Postpartum depression, other mental illnesses, or Munchausen syndrome by proxy.
- **Resistance to feeding**: History of NG feedings, cleft lip/palate, or esophageal atresia,
- **Inadequate supply of milk**: Poor breastfeeding technique or poor milk supply.

DIAGNOSIS AND MANAGEMENT

FTT is diagnosed first by identifying children at risk by evidence of growth failure.

Diagnostic Measures

- Weight/height percentile (5th percentile for weight indicative of FTT)
- Dietary intake history: Previous 24 hours and 3- to 5-day period.
- Evaluation of genetic factors:
  - Family history, including heights/weights of parents
  - Identification of food allergies and food restrictions
  - Evaluation of meal behaviors and practices.
  - Lab tests as indicated to check for conditions such as anemia, parasites, and lead poisoning.
- Observation of family interactions and situation

Management

- Nutritional program to reverse evidence of malnutrition:

$$\text{kcal per day} = \text{recommended daily allowance} \times \frac{\text{ideal weight}}{\text{actual weight}}$$

- Vitamin and mineral supplements: For infants (young), provide supplements to formula. Kcal per ounce of formula should not exceed 24. For toddlers, provide high-caloric milk drink (PediaSure).
- Provide referrals to social workers, welfare, and child protective services as indicated.
- Behavior modification related to meal times and eating habits interfering with nutrition. Family therapy as indicated.
- Family education. Structured supportive environment for feeding, Persistence in feeding and elimination of distractions.
- Slow introduction of new foods.

Diagnostic Testing

SOURCES AND PROCEDURES FOR OBTAINING DIAGNOSTIC STUDIES AND TEST RESULTS

The advent of the electronic health record has somewhat simplified the procedures for obtaining diagnostic studies and test results.

- **Laboratory systems** are typically stand-alone systems that must be interfaced with the electronic health record. The laboratory component of the electronic health record often is utilized as a means to coordinate laboratory orders, laboratory results, and administrative details.
- **Radiology information systems** are typically utilized to enable unification of patient data such as orders, results, and actual images. Radiology information can be accessed using a picture archive and communication system (PACS). PACS can be used to obtain diagnostic medical scans from a variety of imaging devices.

ANALYZING NORMAL AND ABNORMAL TEST RESULTS AND DIAGNOSTIC STUDIES

Knowledge of normal and abnormal values for test results and for diagnostic studies is a vital component of the nursing assessment. Nurses should have a basic knowledge of the purpose and procedures for typical laboratory tests, such as a blood test for complete blood count (CBC), and diagnostic practices, such as x-rays for bone fractures, as well as the specialized tests and studies relevant to their field of expertise. In addition, they should understand accepted standards or **norms**, and how normal values are defined by the facility where they are employed. These norms offer general guidelines for assessing any individual test results or diagnostic studies. Interpreting abnormal test results requires knowing what potential problems may be responsible and what mitigating factors in the patient's history, such as current medications or timing of the last meal, might be influencing these results. Often nurses are the first to review/receive critically abnormal lab results and must be sure to notify the physician immediately in case emergency interventions (such as electrolyte replacement or blood transfusions) must be ordered.

MEDICAL REASONING, DIAGNOSTIC REASONING, THERAPEUTIC REASONING, AND THERAPEUTIC UNCERTAINTY

Medical reasoning refers to the process by which clinicians gather data and information about a patient, and then use those data to arrive at a diagnosis and treatment plan. Diagnostic reasoning and therapeutic reasoning are subsets of medical reasoning. **Diagnostic reasoning** is the process that is used to determine the most likely diagnosis, while **therapeutic reasoning** is the process used to determine what the best treatment is for that particular patient suffering from that particular disease. While the patient is undergoing treatment, it is necessary for the clinician to evaluate the patient's response to treatment on a regular basis. If it is not clear whether the patient is improving, or whether another treatment might be more beneficial, a degree of **therapeutic uncertainty** is introduced. There is also therapeutic uncertainty when the clinician is trying to decide which treatment option to use if the first treatment fails.

IMPORTANCE OF DATA GATHERING TO DIAGNOSTIC REASONING

The gathering and recording of data are of utmost importance to the diagnostic evaluation process. The history and physical section of the patient chart contains a wealth of information (ideally) and should always be taken into consideration when developing a care plan for the patient. Because any number of clinicians can add information to the patient chart (and because all of these clinicians will be reading this information), it is important to record all information clearly and in an organized manner. This can be a daunting task when considering all of the different sources of information, including the patient interview, family member interviews, previous charts, and lab results. By keeping this information clear and concise, errors are minimized, and the differential diagnosis is comprehensive.

SENSITIVITY AND SPECIFICITY IN RELATION TO DIAGNOSTIC TESTING

Some degree of error is inherent in almost all diagnostic testing. When ordering a diagnostic test for a patient, how confident should the practitioner be that the result will be accurate? The terms **sensitivity and specificity** are used to illustrate the accuracy of diagnostic tests.

- The **sensitivity** of a diagnostic test refers to its ability to correctly identify patients who *do have the disease*. If a test is administered to 1000 patients with diabetes, and all 1000 patients test positive, the test is considered to have a sensitivity of 100%. If only 850 test positive, however, that means that the test has a false-negative rate of 15%, and a sensitivity of 85%.
- The **specificity** of a diagnostic test refers to its ability to identify patients who *do not have the disease*. If 1000 nondiabetic patients are tested for diabetes, and 200 of them test positive, the test has a false-positive rate of 20% and a specificity of 80%.

DIFFERENTIAL DIAGNOSIS PROCESS

The differential diagnosis is an important tool that allows the clinician to familiarize him or herself with the patient's condition, understand the condition, create an effective treatment plan, and follow the progress of the patient. To start, thoroughly examine the patient's chart, making a list of all of the abnormal test results and laboratory values. Add to this list all of the patient's complaints. Once this list is complete, organize the test results, labs, and complaints by anatomic location or organ system. After breaking the list down by organ site, look for any relationships between symptoms and/or results. Create another list of those data that seem to be related, and list all of the diseases or conditions that explain the findings, eliminating any that do not fit.

ANALYTICAL DECISION-MAKING

An **analytical decision** is one that is made after a systematic review and analysis of all factors involved in the decision. Concentration and awareness are important in the analytical decision-making process. In contrast with an intuitive decision, an analytical decision takes longer to make, because it is not automatic. The analysis involves an in-depth look at all factors and is based on scientific evidence (i.e., based on the outcomes of previous similar situations). Because an analytical decision is based on scientific evidence and facts, the outcome of the decision has a high predictive value; this means that by looking at previous outcomes, it is possible to predict the current outcome. Because the clinician has so carefully reviewed all factors, he or she will most likely not experience the emotional anxiety associated with an intuitive decision.

INTUITIVE DECISION-MAKING

When a clinician makes an **intuitive decision**, he or she is making a decision not necessarily based on fact, but more so because it feels like the right decision. Of course, in most cases, one would not want a doctor making decisions this way, although in certain cases (say, a choice between 2 different types of treatment, each of which has the same general risks, or when all other options have been exhausted), it may be necessary. Although these decisions are not based on an analysis of the facts, there is something to be said about the so-called "gut instinct," which years of training and experience can hone. These decisions are made without spending a lot of time on the process of decision-making; though they are based on experience, the clinician may suffer some degree of anxiety about the decision and its outcome.

INFLUENTIAL FACTORS IN CLINICAL DECISION-MAKING PROCESS

Although one would like to think that there isn't much variation in the clinical decision-making process, this simply is not true. The process, of course, will differ depending on the patient, the differential diagnosis, and the clinician. The first variable to consider is the clinician. The way that the clinician conducts the clinical decision-making process is influenced by the knowledge base of the clinician, as well as the level of his experience, the ability he possesses to think both critically and creatively, and the confidence that he has in his ability to make educated decisions. The acuity level of the patient is also a factor in the clinical decision-making process, as is the length of the differential. A time stressor is placed on the clinician when the condition of the patient is critical, and when there are more diseases that must be eliminated from the differential. An element of stress may also exist if the clinician has a high number of patients, especially if he has multiple high-acuity patients.

QUESTIONS TO CONSIDER WHEN DEALING WITH DIAGNOSTIC AND THERAPEUTIC UNCERTAINTY

Diagnosis and subsequent treatment are not easily arrived at for every patient because every patient is different. The clinical presentation of a heart attack, for example, may include severe chest pain, sweating, and nausea for one patient, and may have very mild, almost unnoticeable symptoms in another. **Diagnostic uncertainty** is especially prominent when dealing with diseases that have nonspecific symptoms; in these cases, it is important that the clinician recognize which of the possible diagnoses are life-threatening, and which are not. Ruling out the life-threatening possibilities should be higher on the clinician's list of priorities than the nonlife-threatening ones. Diagnostic testing, and subsequent treatment options, should also be evaluated according to the risks and benefits to the patient.

DEGREE OF CLINICAL UNCERTAINTY

Although the degree of uncertainty is somewhat dependent on the patient, the clinical setting can have an influence on the degree of uncertainty that the clinician is likely to encounter. For example, a clinic, such as a dermatology clinic, is a setting in which the degree of uncertainty is likely to be low; this is because the clinic is nonemergent, and because the clinic treats a specific, limited group of diseases with which the clinicians are very familiar. An urgent care clinic would fall somewhere in the middle because, although there is a wider range of diagnostic possibility, life-threatening emergencies are rarely encountered. An emergency room or a trauma center, on the other hand, sees a high degree of uncertainty because the clinicians see a wide range of diagnostic possibilities, and are expected to work at a fast pace.

PREDICTIVE VALUES IN RELATION TO DISEASE PROBABILITY

Sensitivity and specificity are useful in evaluating the efficacy of a diagnostic test, but the predictive value of a test is more immediately relevant to individual patients. The **positive predictive value (PPV)** of a test is the likelihood that a patient who has *tested positive* truly has the condition that is being tested for. Similarly, the **negative predictive value (NPV)** of a test is the likelihood that a patient who has *tested negative* truly does not have the condition being tested for.

For a given controlled trial, PPV is calculated by dividing the number of true positive results by the number of total positive results (true and false positives). NPV is calculated by dividing the number of true negative results by the number of total negative results. Calculating the PPV and NPV is straightforward, but in order for these values to be applied to an individual patient, the assumption has to be made that the patient's pre-test likelihood of having the tested condition matches that of the trial's population.

Cardiovascular Diagnostics

CARDIAC ENZYMES

While creatine kinase (CK) and CK-MB levels used to be the mainstay for diagnosing acute myocardial infarction, they are no longer commonly used in the United States. CK is a reflection of muscular infarction, but is not specific to the heart muscle. CK-MB adds slightly more specificity to the heart but not as much as the gold standard, which is **troponin**. Troponin, which is found in cardiac and skeletal muscle, is a type of protein. Both troponin I and T (isolates of troponin) are found in the myocardium, but troponin T is also found in skeletal muscle, so it is less specific than troponin I. Troponin I, therefore, may be used to detect a myocardial infarction after non-cardiac surgery and to detect acute coronary syndrome. Troponin is released into the bloodstream when injury to the tissue (such as the myocardium) occurs and causes damage to the cell membranes, as occurs with myocardial injury.

- **Troponin I** (<0.05 ng/mL): Appears in 2–6 hours, peaks at 15–20 hours and returns to normal in 5–7 days. Exhibits a second but lower peak at 60–80 hours (biphasic).
- **Troponin T** (<0.2 ng/mL): Increases 2–6 hours after MI and stays elevated. Returns to normal in 7 days. (Less specific than troponin I)

ECHOCARDIOGRAPHY

Echocardiography is a non-invasive ultrasound technology that is very useful for assessing and diagnosing anatomic heart abnormalities, blood flow, and valvular lesions:

- The **standard "2D Echo"** is used best for basic structural imaging, such as valvular lesions and assessment of pericardial disorders.
- The **transesophageal (TEE)** probe is an improved version of echocardiography, which allows better visualization of the left atrium and more precise evaluation of the valvular structure. TEE is also the best modality for evaluation of the thoracic aorta in the setting of suspected aortic dissection or aneurysm.
- **Doppler imaging** is used to measure blood flow, often in the context of velocity across a valve and a pressure gradient.
- **Bubble study** (which is done by injecting saline contrast that has been agitated to include bubbles) is an addition to echocardiography allowing the study to determine if there is right to left blood flow through a patent foramen ovale or a more distal intrapulmonary shunt of blood.

STRESS ECHOCARDIOGRAPHY

Basic **cardiac stress testing** consists of exercise EKG testing (EET) and exercise imaging testing. The exercise imaging testing may be broken down into exercise, or "stress" echocardiography, and exercise myocardial perfusion imaging.

Exercise imaging testing is usually performed with echocardiography. Stress echocardiography is performed similarly to **exercise EKG testing** and also requires that the patient meet at least 85% maximum heart rate in order to attain optimum sensitivity and specificity. (The maximum heart rate formula is 220 minus the person's age.) Of note, chemicals may substitute for exercise during the "stress" portion of the test. This may be performed with dobutamine (beta-1-agonist: cannot be used after beta-blocker administration) or adenosine (causes diffuse coronary dilatation, leading to decreased perfusion pressure and unmasking of defects, and cannot be used with asthma). Stress imaging allows the study to determine the actual area of ischemia and whether or not this is a reversible defect. Additional information obtained during echocardiography is cardiac output and measurement of viability.

Endocrine Diagnostics

GLUCOSE LABORATORY TEST

Glucose is manufactured by the liver from ingested carbohydrates and is stored as glycogen for use by the cells. If intake is inadequate, glucose can be produced from muscle and fat tissue, leading to increased wasting. High levels of glucose are indicative of diabetes mellitus, which predisposes people to skin injuries, slow healing, and infection. **Fasting blood glucose levels** are used to diagnose and monitor this condition:

- Normal values: 70–99 mg/dL
- Impaired: 100–125 mg/dL
- Diabetes: ≥126 mg/dL

There are a number of different conditions that can increase glucose levels, including stress, renal failure, Cushing syndrome, hyperthyroidism, and pancreatic disorders. Medications, such as steroids, estrogens, lithium, phenytoin, diuretics, tricyclic antidepressants, may increase glucose levels. Other conditions, such as adrenal insufficiency, liver disease, hypothyroidism, and starvation can decrease glucose levels.

HEMOGLOBIN A1C LABORATORY TEST

Hemoglobin A1c comprises hemoglobin A with a glucose molecule because hemoglobin holds onto excess blood glucose, so it shows the average blood glucose levels over a 3-month period and is used primarily to monitor long-term diabetic therapy:

- Normal value: <6%

BASIC THYROID FUNCTION TESTING AND ANTIBODY TESTING

Thyroid stimulating hormone (TSH) is produced by the pituitary as a result of thyrotropin releasing hormone (TRH) from the hypothalamus. TSH stimulates the thyroid to produce T4 (mostly) and T3. T4 is deiodinated to T3 (active hormone), and the free hormone is active while the majority is bound to albumin and thyroxine-binding globulin. The best testing of thyroid function is the free T4 (unbound). Free T4 and TSH testing allows appropriate screening for thyroid disease.

Additionally, certain antibodies are used to screen for thyroid disease. Thyroglobulin antibodies are found in 50% of patients with Graves' disease and about 90% of those with Hashimoto's thyroiditis. Thyroid peroxidase antibodies are detected in >90% of those with Hashimoto's thyroiditis. TSH receptor antibodies (TSHR) may be either thyroid stimulating immunoglobulin (TSI) which stimulate the receptor to produce thyroid hormone (found in Graves' disease), or TSHR-blocking antibodies, which may inhibit production of thyroid hormone.

Lab values to consider include:

- **Thyroid stimulating hormone (TSH)** (0.4–6.15 mIU/L). Increase in TSH indicates hypothyroidism and decrease indicates hyperthyroidism.
- **Free thyroxine**: (FT4) (0.9–2.4 ng/dL). FT4 is used to confirm TSH abnormalities. Serum T3 (80–180 ng/dL) and T4 (4.5–11.5 mcg/dL) usually increase together, but T3 more accurately diagnoses hyperthyroidism. T3 resin uptake (25–35%) increases with hyperthyroidism and decreases with hypothyroidism.

ADDITIONAL ENDOCRINE FUNCTION STUDIES

There is a wide range of endocrine function studies:

- **Pituitary:** Serum levels of pituitary hormones and hormones of target organs, dependent on stimulation by pituitary hormones, are measured to determine abnormalities.
- **Parathyroid:** Parathyroid hormone (PTH) level (10–65 ng/L) and serum calcium levels (8.5–10.2 mg/dL) both increase with hyperparathyroidism. Calcium levels decrease with hypoparathyroidism, and phosphate levels (2.5–4.5 mg/dL) increase.
- **Adrenal**: Catecholamine (urine and serum) levels: Epinephrine (<75 ng/L) and norepinephrine (<100–550 ng/mL) elevate with pheochromocytoma. Electrolyte and glucose levels.
- **ACTH** and **serum cortisol levels** and **ACTH stimulation test** to evaluate for Addison. Dexamethasone suppression test for Cushing's disease.

Gastrointestinal Diagnostics

LIVER FUNCTION STUDIES

Liver function studies are described below:

- **Bilirubin:** Determines the ability of the liver to conjugate and excrete bilirubin, direct 0.0–0.3 mg/dL, total 0.0–0.9 mg/dL, and urine bilirubin, which should be 0
- **Total protein:** Normal: 6.0–8.0 g/dL (Albumin: 4.0–5.5 g/dL, Globulin: 1.7–3.3 g/dL); normal albumin/globulin (A/G) ratio: 1.5:1 to 2.5:1, measured by serum protein electrophoresis
- **Prothrombin time (PT):** 100% or clot detection in 10–14 seconds; PT increases with liver disease
   - International normalized ratio (PT result/normal average): <2 for those not receiving anticoagulation, 2–3 for those receiving anticoagulation, critical value >3 in patients receiving anticoagulation therapy
- **Alkaline phosphatase:** 36–93 units/L in adults (normal values vary with method); indicates biliary tract obstruction if no bone disease
- **AST (SGOT):** 10–40 units (increases with liver cell damage)
- **ALT (SGPT):** 5–35 units (increases with liver cell damage)
- **GGT, GGTP:** 5–55 µ/L females, 5–85 µ/L males (increases with alcohol abuse)
- **LDH:** 100–200 units (increases with alcohol abuse)
- **Serum ammonia:** 150–250 mg/dL (increases with liver failure)
- **Cholesterol:** Increases with bile duct obstruction and decrease with parenchymal disease

NUTRITIONAL LAB MONITORING

TOTAL PROTEIN AND ALBUMIN

Total protein levels can be influenced by many factors, including stress and infection, but it may be monitored as part of an overall nutritional assessment. Protein is critical for general health and wound healing, and because metabolic rate increases in response to a wound, protein needs increase:

- Normal values: 6–8 g/dL
- Diet requirements for wound healing: 1.25–1.5 g/kg/day

Albumin is a protein that is produced by the liver and is a necessary component for cells and tissues. Levels decrease with renal disease, malnutrition, and severe burns. Albumin levels are the most common screening to determine protein levels. Albumin has a half-life of 18–20 days, so it is sensitive to long-term protein deficiencies more than short-term.

- Normal values: 3.5–5.5 g/dL
- Mild deficiency: 3.0–3.5 g/dL
- Moderate deficiency: 2.5–3.0 g/dL
- Severe deficiency: <2.5 g/dL

Levels below 3.2 correlate with increased morbidity and death. Dehydration (poor intake, diarrhea, or vomiting) elevates levels, so adequate hydration is important to ensure meaningful results.

Prealbumin

Prealbumin (transthyretin) is most commonly monitored for acute changes in nutritional status because it has a half-life of only 2–3 days. Prealbumin is a protein produced in the liver, so it is often decreased with liver disease. Oral contraceptives and estrogen can also decrease levels. Levels may rise with Hodgkin's disease or the use of steroids or NSAIDS. Prealbumin is necessary for transportation of both thyroxine and vitamin A throughout the body, so if **prealbumin levels** fall, both thyroxine and vitamin A utilization are also affected:

- Normal values: 16–40 mg/dL
- Mild deficiency: 10–15 mg/dL
- Moderate deficiency: 5–9 mg/dL
- Severe deficiency: <5 mg/dL

Prealbumin is a good measurement because it quickly decreases when nutrition is inadequate and rises quickly in response to increased protein intake. Protein intake must be adequate to maintain levels of prealbumin. Death rates increase with any decrease in prealbumin levels.

Transferrin

Transferrin, which transports about one-third of the body's iron, is a protein produced by the liver. It transports **iron** from the intestines to the bone marrow where it is used to produce **hemoglobin**. The half-life of transferrin is about 8–10 days. It is sometimes used as a measure of nutritional status; however, transferrin levels are sensitive to many factors. Levels rapidly decrease with protein malnutrition. Liver disease and anemia can also depress levels, but a decrease in iron, commonly found with inadequate protein, stimulates the liver to produce more transferrin, which increases transferrin levels but also decreases production of albumin and prealbumin. Transferrin levels may also increase with pregnancy, use of oral contraceptives, and polycythemia. Thus, **transferrin levels** alone are not always reliable measurements of nutritional status:

- Normal values: 200–400 mg/dL
- Mild deficiency: 150–200 mg/dL
- Moderate deficiency: 100–150 mg/dL
- Severe deficiency: <100 mg/dL

> **Review Video: Transferrin**
> Visit mometrix.com/academy and enter code: 267479

EGD

Esophagogastroduodenoscopy (EGD) with a flexible fiberscope equipped with a lighted fiberoptic lens allows direct inspection of the mucosa of the esophagus, stomach, and duodenum. The scope has a still or video camera attached to a monitor for viewing during the procedure. The scope may be used for biopsies or therapeutically to dilate strictures or treat gastric or esophageal bleeding. The patient is positioned on the left side (head supported) to allow saliva drainage. Conscious sedation (midazolam, propofol) is commonly used along with a topical anesthetic spray or gargle to facilitate placing the lubricated tube through the mouth into the esophagus. Atropine reduces secretions. A bite guard in the mouth prevents the patient from biting the scope. The airway must be carefully monitored through the procedure (which usually takes about 30 minutes), including oximeter to measure oxygen saturation. While perforation, bleeding, or infection may occur, most complications are cardiopulmonary in nature and relate to drugs (conscious sedation) used during the procedure, so reversal agents (flumazenil, naloxone) should be available.

> **Review Video: Diagnostic Procedures of the GI System**
> Visit mometrix.com/academy and enter code: 645436

Genitourinary Diagnostics

RENAL FUNCTION STUDIES

Renal function studies are described below:

- **Osmolality (urine):** Normal: 350–900 mOsm/kg/day. Shows early changes when the kidney has difficulty concentrating urine.
- **Osmolality (serum):** Normal: 275–295 mOsm/kg. Gives a picture of the amount of solute in the blood.
- **Uric acid:** Normal: 3.0–7.2 mg/dL. Increases with renal failure.
- **Creatinine clearance (24-hour):** Normal: 75–125 mL/min. Evaluates the amount of blood cleared of creatinine in 1 minute. Approximates the GFR.
- **Serum creatinine:** Normal: 0.6–1.2 mg/dL. Increase with decreased renal function, urinary tract obstruction, and nephritis.
- **Urine creatinine:** Normal: 11–26 mg/kg/day. Product of muscle breakdown. Increase with decreased renal function.
- **Blood urea nitrogen (BUN):** Normal: 7–8 mg/dL (8–20 mg/dL if age >60). An increase indicates impaired renal function, as urea is the end product of protein metabolism.
- **BUN/creatinine ratio:** Normal: 10:1. Increases with hypovolemia. With intrinsic kidney disease, the ratio is increased.
- **Urinalysis:** Tests various qualities of a urine sample that are reflective of kidney function and other disease processes.

URINALYSIS

Urinalysis components and normal findings are described below:

- **Color:** Pale yellow/amber and darkens when urine is concentrated or other substances (such as blood or bile) are present.
- **Appearance:** Clear but may be slightly cloudy.
- **Odor:** Slight. Bacteria may give urine a foul smell, depending upon the organism. Some foods, such as asparagus, change the odor.
- **Specific gravity:** Normal: 1.005–1.025. May increase if protein levels increase or if there is fever, vomiting, or dehydration.
- **pH:** Usually ranges from 4.5–8 with an average of 5–6.
- **Sediment:** Red cell casts from acute infections, broad casts from kidney disorders, and white cell casts from pyelonephritis. Leukocytes >10 per mL^3 are present with urinary tract infections.
- **Glucose, ketones, protein, blood, bilirubin, and nitrate:** Negative. Urine glucose may increase with infection (with normal blood glucose). Frank blood may be caused by some parasites and diseases but also by drugs, smoking, excessive exercise, and menstrual fluids. Increased red blood cells may result from lower urinary tract infections.
- **Urobilinogen:** 0.1–1.0 units.

IVP AND RADIONUCLEOTIDE RENAL SCAN

Intravenous pyelogram (IVP) is done to identify structural defects and tumors and to observe urinary structures. The patient is administered an IV contrast medium and may be administered antihistamine or corticosteroid before the test to minimize allergic response. Serum creatinine and BUN are done prior to the IVP to ensure that the contrast medium can be excreted. During the procedure, radiographs are taken once every minute for five minutes and then again after 15 minutes (giving the contrast medium time to pass into the bladder). A post-voiding radiograph shows how efficiently the bladder is able to empty. Fluid intake should be increased post-procedure to flush contrast.

Radionucleotide renal scan with dimercaptosuccinic acid (DMSA) requires IV administration of a radioactive element followed by a series of CT scans taken over 20 minutes to 4 hours. The scan is used to assess function and perfusion of the kidney and can detect lesions, atrophy, and scars and differentiate among different causes for hydronephrosis. The patient must be well-hydrated and may need to be catheterized to measure the output of urine.

RENAL BIOPSY

Renal biopsy to remove a small segment of cortical tissue helps to identify the extent of **kidney disease** with acute renal failure, transplant rejection, glomerulopathies, and persistent hematuria or proteinuria. Preoperative coagulation studies determine the risk of bleeding. The biopsy is done percutaneously per needle biopsy (guided by fluoroscopy or ultrasound) or surgically through a small flank incision. A urine specimen must be obtained so it can be compared with a post-procedure specimen. **Post-procedure**:

- Maintain the patient in a supine position immediately after the procedure for 4–6 hours and on bed rest overnight.
- Monitor urine for hematuria and compare it with the preop specimen.
- Monitor VS every 5–15 minutes for the first hour and then less frequently. To minimize bleeding, maintain blood pressure <140/90.
- Note anorexia, vomiting, and abdominal discomfort that may suggest bleeding.
- Note pain: Severe colicky pain may indicate a clot in the ureter.
- Monitor urinalysis and CBC post-procedure.
- Maintain fluid intake at 3,000 mL/day in absence of renal insufficiency.
- Provide blood component therapy and surgical repair if bleeding occurs.

RENAL ULTRASOUND

Renal ultrasound is a non-invasive method of viewing the **urinary structures**. Most patients that present with kidney disease of unknown origin should undergo a renal ultrasound to assess for possible obstruction. An ultrasound uses ultrasonic sound waves transmitted by a transducer, which picks up reflected sound waves that a computer converts to electronic images. An ultrasound can show fluid accumulation, the movement of blood through the kidney, masses, malformations (congenital abnormalities), changes in size of the kidney or other structures, and obstructions, such as renal calculi. An ultrasound is usually done before a renal biopsy, and may be done with a needle biopsy to guide the placement of the needle. Patient preparation includes drinking two 8-ounce glasses of water one hour before the examination to ensure that the bladder is full. The patient should be reminded not to urinate before the ultrasound. The patient usually remains in a supine position throughout the procedure but may be asked to turn to the side. No special precautions are necessary post-procedure.

Hematologic Diagnostics

RED BLOOD CELLS

Red blood cells (RBCs or erythrocytes) are biconcave disks that contain **hemoglobin** (95% of mass), which carries oxygen throughout the body. The heme portion of the cell contains **iron**, which binds to the oxygen. RBCs live about 120 days, after which they are destroyed and their hemoglobin is recycled or excreted. Normal values of **red blood cell count** vary by gender:

- Males >18 years: 4.7–6.1 million per mm^3
- Females >18 years: 4.2–5.4 million per mm^3

The most common **disorders of RBCs** are those that interfere with production, leading to various types of **anemia**:

- Blood loss
- Hemolysis
- Bone marrow failure

The **morphology** of RBCs may vary depending upon the type of anemia:

- Size: Normocytes, microcytes, macrocytes
- Shape: Spherocytes (round), poikilocytes (irregular), drepanocytes (sickled)
- Color (reflecting concentration of hemoglobin): Normochromic, hypochromic

LABORATORY TESTS

A number of different tests are used to evaluate the condition and production of red blood cells in addition to the red blood cell count.

Hemoglobin: Carries oxygen and is decreased in anemia and increased in polycythemia. Normal values:

- Males >18 years: 14.0–17.46 g/dL
- Females >18 years: 12.0–16.0 g/dL

Hematocrit: Indicates the proportion of RBCs in a liter of blood (usually about 3 times the hemoglobin number). Normal values:

- Males >18 years: 40–50%
- Females >18 years: 35–45%

Mean corpuscular volume (MCV): Indicates the size of RBCs and can differentiate types of anemia. For adults, <80 is microcytic and >100 is macrocytic. Normal values:

- Males >18 years: 84–96 μm^3
- Females >18 years: 76–96 μm^3

Reticulocyte count: Measures marrow production and should rise with anemia. Normal values: 0.5–1.5% of total RBCs.

WBC Count and Differential

White blood cell (leukocyte) count is used as an indicator of bacterial and viral infection. WBC count is reported as the total number of all white blood cells.

- Normal WBC for adults: 4,800–10,000
- Acute infection: 10,000+; 30,000 indicates a severe infection
- Viral infection: 4,000 and below

The **differential** provides the percentage of each different type of leukocyte. An increase in the white blood cell count is usually related to an increase in one type, and often an increase in immature neutrophils (bands), referred to as a "shift to the left," is an indication of an infectious process:

- Normal immature neutrophils (bands): 1–3%, increases with infection
- Normal segmented neutrophils (segs) for adults: 50–62%, increases with acute, localized, or systemic bacterial infections
- Normal eosinophils: 0–3%, decreases with stress and acute infection
- Normal basophils: 0–1%, decreases during acute stage of infection
- Normal lymphocytes: 25–40%, increases in some viral and bacterial infections
- Normal monocytes: 3–7%, increases during recovery stage of acute infection

C-Reactive Protein and Erythrocyte Sedimentation Rate

C-reactive protein is an acute-phase reactant produced by the liver in response to an inflammatory response that causes neutrophils, granulocytes, and macrophages to secrete cytokines. Thus, levels of C-reactive protein rise when there is inflammation or infection. It is helpful to measure the response to treatment for pyoderma gangrenosum ulcers:

- Normal values: <0.9 mg/dL

Erythrocyte sedimentation rate (sed rate) measures the distance erythrocytes fall in a vertical tube of anticoagulated blood in one hour. Because fibrinogen, which increases in response to infection, also increases the rate of the fall, the sed rate can be used as a non-specific test for inflammation when infection is suspected. The sed rate is sensitive to osteomyelitis and may be used to monitor treatment response. Values vary according to gender and age:

- <50: Males 0–15 mm/hr; females 0–20 mm/hr
- >50: Males 0–20 mm/hr; females 0–30 mm/hr

ELEMENTS OF THE COAGULATION PROFILE

The coagulation profile measures clotting mechanisms, identifies clotting disorders, screens preoperative patients, and diagnoses excessive bruising and bleeding. Values vary depending on lab:

- **Prothrombin time (PT)**: 10–14 seconds
    - Increases with anticoagulation therapy, vitamin K deficiency, decreased prothrombin, DIC, liver disease, and malignant neoplasm. Some drugs may shorten PT.
- **Partial thromboplastin time (PTT)**: 25–35 seconds
    - Increases with hemophilia A and B, von Willebrand disease, vitamin deficiency, lupus, DIC, and liver disease.
- **Activated partial thromboplastin time (aPTT)**: 21–35 seconds
    - Similar to PTT, but decreases in extensive cancer, early DIC, and after acute hemorrhage. Used to monitor heparin dosage.
- **Thrombin clotting time (TCT) or Thrombin time (TT)**: 7–12 seconds
    - Used most often to determine the dosage of heparin. Prolonged with multiple myeloma, abnormal fibrinogen, uremia, and liver disease.
- **Bleeding time**: 2.0–9.5 minutes
    - (Using the IVY method on the forearm) Increases with DIC, leukemia, renal failure, aplastic anemia, von Willebrand disease, some drugs, and alcohol.
- **Platelet count**: 150,000–400,000 per µL
    - Increased bleeding <50,000 (transfusion required) and increased clotting >750,000.

> **Review Video: The Coagulation Profile**
> Visit mometrix.com/academy and enter code: 423595

Neurological Diagnostics

Lumbar Puncture

The lumbar puncture (spinal tap) is done between the 3rd and 4th or between the 4th and 5th lumbar vertebrae. The patient is in the lateral recumbent position with knees drawn toward the chest during the procedure. A local anesthetic is applied to prevent pain when the needle is inserted into the subarachnoid space to withdraw CSF and measure CSF pressure, which should be 70–200 mmH$_2$O.

Queckenstedt's test: Compress jugular veins on each side of the neck during the procedure. Note pressure and then release the veins and note pressure in 10-second intervals. Pressure should rise quickly with compression and fall quickly with release. Slower or no response indicates blockage of subarachnoid pathways.

Normal values (CSF analysis):

- Clear and colorless
- Protein: 15–45 mg/dL
- Glucose: 60–80 mg/dL
- Lactic acid: <25.2 mg/dL
- Culture: Negative
- RBCs: 0
- WBCs: 0.5/mL

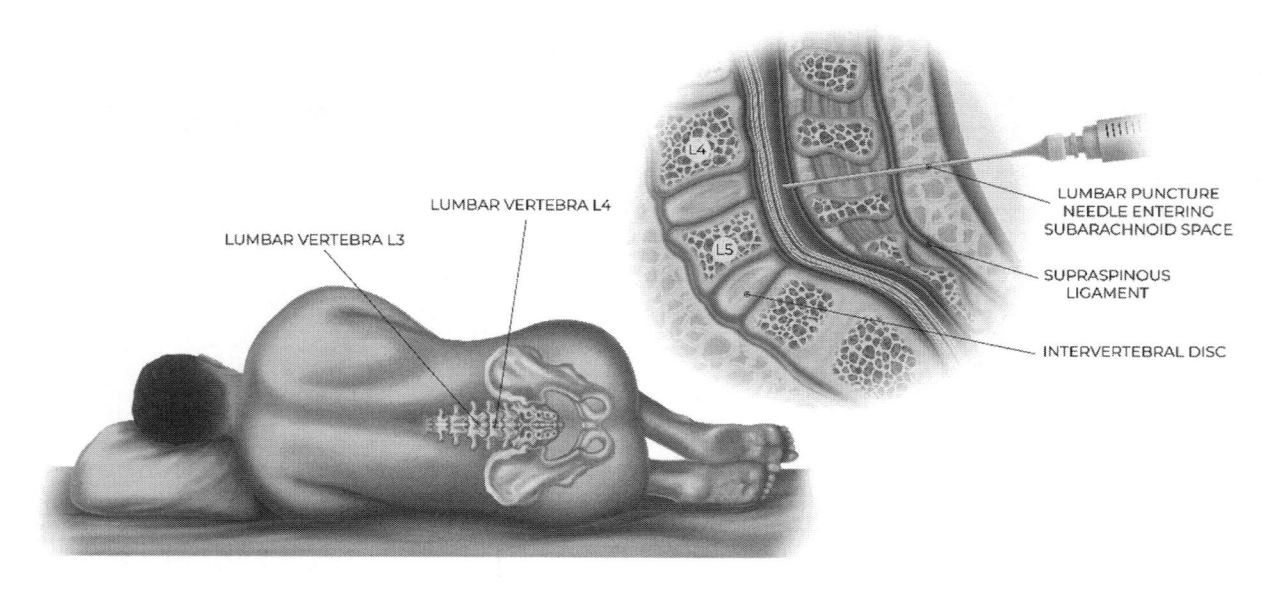

Avoiding Complications After Lumbar Puncture and Use of Epidural Blood Patch

After a lumbar puncture, the patient should remain in the prone position for at least 3 hours to ensure that the needle puncture sites through the dural and arachnoid areas remain separate in order to reduce the chance of CSF leakage. If >20 mL of CSF is removed, then the patient should remain prone for 2 hours, side-lying (flat) for 2–3 hours, and supine or prone for 6 additional hours. Relieving intracranial pressure by withdrawing CSF may cause herniation of the brain, so lumbar puncture should be done with care in the presence of increased ICP. The most common complaint is of spinal headache, which may occur within a few hours or several days of the procedure. Increased fluid intake may reduce risk of headache. If headache occurs, it may be treated with analgesics, fluids, and bed rest; however, if the headache is severe or persistent, an **epidural blood patch** may be done, with venous blood withdrawn and then injected into the epidural space at the site of the puncture to seal the leaking opening.

Planning

Nursing Care Planning

PLANNING OF NURSING CARE FOR PATIENTS

The patient's needs as defined by the **nursing diagnoses** are first prioritized with the help of the patient and family:

- **Critical needs** are met immediately and then other needs are ranked according to the patient's priorities and Maslow's Hierarchy of Needs.
- When diagnoses are prioritized, **desirable outcomes** for each diagnosis are defined. Outcomes include desirable changes in patient behavior and are the backbone of the care plan. Outcomes are used to determine whether the nursing care has met its objectives.
- **Goals** for each nursing diagnosis are devised with patient and family input. Immediate, intermediate, and long-term goals that combine to meet the desired outcome are defined along with a timetable. Intermediate and long-term goals usually pertain to the prevention of complications and patient and family teaching concerning self-care and rehabilitation needs.

Each goal is then completed by a list of specific **actions** needed to achieve the goal. These actions include nursing interventions and may also include coordination of actions by other healthcare personnel.

> **Review Video: Plan of Care**
> Visit mometrix.com/academy and enter code: 300570

RESOURCES FOR CARE PLANNING

Various resources provide lists of nursing diagnoses, interventions, and expected outcomes to help guide the nurse care planning process:

- The **North American Nursing Diagnosis Association (NANDA)** compiles a list of the most commonly used nursing diagnoses and refines them so that they are acceptable for study and nursing research. This list is updated biannually and is useful when developing care plans.
- **Nursing-Sensitive Outcomes Classification (NOC)** lists nursing outcomes for specific needs. Each outcome has an associated scale of achievement and can be used to evaluate patient progress in achieving the outcome desired.
- **Nursing Interventions Classification (NIC)** consists of interventions appropriate for specific nursing needs. These interventions can be individualized for each patient's needs.

NANDA, NIC, and NOC utilize the **Taxonomy of Nursing Practice** to classify nursing diagnoses, outcomes, and interventions. The Taxonomy of Nursing Practice divides patient problems into four domains:

- **The functional domain** includes classes consisting of patient movement, relief of symptoms, developmental status, nutrition, ADLs, sexuality, belief systems, and sleep.
- **The physiological domain** consists of bodily needs for proper functioning divided into classes concerning the cardiovascular, respiratory, gastrointestinal, genitourinary, neurological, metabolic, immune, reproductive, musculoskeletal, and integumentary systems. The effects of medications and other substances on system functioning are included.
- **The psychosocial domain** contains classes concerning emotional health (coping mechanisms, mental state, self-image, and self-esteem), mental health (knowledge and behaviors), and social status (communication with others, relationships, and support network).
- **The environmental domain** is concerned with patient populations, public and individual health and safety in the environment, healthcare delivery, and management of risks.

By using the taxonomy, all three tools describe the same problems in the same way in language that is specific and refined, yet universal.

UTILIZING CLINICAL PATHWAYS IN CARE PLANNING

Clinical pathways are written tools that direct the treatment of a specific group of patients according to diagnosis. They provide a way to standardize medical and nursing care according to evidence-based practice guidelines, predict the cost of the care, and ensure quality, timeliness, and cost-effectiveness of care. Each plan consists of the DRG or group that it addresses, time segments with specific activities, and desired outcomes for each time segment. They include a place to record activities that deviate from the pathway. Nursing care is charted according to the pathway, which serves as the patient's plan of care. Nurses are responsible for helping to formulate and change clinical pathways. They initiate the pathways when the patient presents for treatment and ensure that the care is given for each time segment. They also use the pathways to monitor patients as case managers for hospitals or insurance companies. The patient may receive a copy that the nurse then discusses to make the patient aware of the treatment course and desired goals.

INCORPORATING PATIENT AND FAMILY RIGHTS INTO PLAN OF CARE

In order for patient and family rights to be incorporated into the plan of care, the care plan needs to be designed as a **collaborative effort** that encourages participation of patients and family members. There are a number of different programs that can be useful, such as including patients and families on advisory committees. Additionally, assessment tools, such as surveys for patients and families, can be utilized to gain insight in the issues that are important to them. While infants and small children and sometimes the elderly cannot speak for themselves, the "patient" is generally understood to include not only the immediate family but also other groups or communities who have an interest in the care of the individual. Because many hospital stays are now short-term, programs that include follow-up interviews and assessments are especially valuable in determining if the needs of the patient were addressed in the care plan.

Psychosocial Factors That Affect Care Planning

There are many psychosocial factors that affect patient care. A patient's **psychological state** influences how that patient interacts with others, including nurses and hospital staff, and can also affect compliance and positive health outcomes. For instance, anxiety or depression can make a patient incapable of performing the instructions necessary for completing a full recovery; the psychological problem would need to be addressed in the patient's care plan.

Social and culture factors also shape a patient's **perception** of health and disease, communication style, and decision-making methods. It is important to understand that differences in ethnicity, race, sex, gender, religion, age, socioeconomic status, family dynamics, sexual orientation, and life experiences mean that patients experience illness and healing differently. Being sensitive to these differences can lead to more effective patient care across the spectrum.

Consideration of Comorbidities in Care Planning

Comorbidity, also known as multimorbidity, refers to the coexistence of multiple chronic or acute medical diseases within one patient. Comorbid conditions are associated with poorer outcomes, the need for more complex medical or surgical management, and elevated healthcare costs. It is now the norm, as opposed to the exception, that patients have multiple comorbid medical conditions. Some examples would be an obese patient with concomitant diabetes, heart disease, and osteoarthritis; a multi-system trauma patient with diabetes, chronic obstructive pulmonary disease, and cardiovascular disease; or a cancer patient with anxiety, depression, and multiple pulmonary emboli.

Implementation of a Nursing Plan

The patient's nursing care plan is implemented as soon as the patient has been stabilized. During stabilization, nursing care is guided by standards of practice and logarithms that define care for life-threatening situations. Once the patient is stabilized, **interventions** are guided by the patient's individualized plan of care:

- The nurse has the responsibility of performing the planned nursing interventions and of delegating and coordinating care given by others to meet the patient's needs.
- All care is documented along with patient response.
- Additional patient information, changes in condition, patient priorities, and needs guide the nurse in continuously modifying the care plan.
- Orders are analyzed, clarified, and questioned as needed to meet collaborative patient needs.
- Patient input is necessary to the evaluation of nursing care and revision of the care plan as needed. Patient response to interventions, treatments, and procedures is assessed and care is given accordingly.
- The results of labs and tests are also used to determine actions according to the care plan.

Adult Age/Disease-Related Factors that Influence Findings

LABORATORY TESTS WITH AGE-AFFECTED REFERENCE RANGES

There are times when certain conditions associated with increasing age can influence lab values. Some examples of these situations include use of several different types of medications, physiological changes in the body associated with aging, fluctuating fluid and electrolyte levels, and the presence of chronic diseases and autoimmune disorders.

The normal results of laboratory values that are reported in reference ranges may be different for older adults than for young, healthy individuals. Some laboratories use geriatric reference ranges to recognize the changes associated with aging, providing a normal set of values for adults over a certain age. This process reduces the incidence of unnecessary critical values that may only appear out of range because of age-related changes. Some examples of lab tests that may have different reference ranges for older adults include serum iron, hematocrit, hemoglobin, white blood cells, erythrocyte sedimentation rate, and platelets.

FACTORS THAT MIGHT AFFECT RESULTS OF GLUCOSE TESTS FOR OLDER ADULTS

Older adults with diabetes must regulate their blood sugar levels to avoid both hypo- and hyperglycemia. Many older adults with diabetes are accustomed to the factors that may alter their blood glucose levels; however, nurses are in a position to educate all adult patients about those elements that may cause a drop or rapid spike in blood glucose. Some factors that may be more common among older adults are prescription medications such as acetazolamide, bicalutamide (Casodex), or chlorothiazide (Diuril). Low levels of activity, increased carbohydrate intake, stress, missing medication doses, and poor skin condition at insulin injection sites may all also affect blood glucose levels in older adults.

ELEVATED PSA LEVELS

A **prostate-specific antigen (PSA)** test identifies the protein produced by the prostate, which may increase among adult men, often in cases of prostate cancer. However, there may be other reasons why an older man has an elevated PSA level that is not indicative of cancer. Benign prostatic hyperplasia (BPH), or an enlarged prostate, may cause elevated PSA levels. Inflammation of the prostate, a digital rectal exam, or a prostate biopsy may also cause elevated levels of PSA. Finally, recent pressure on the prostate, such as riding a bicycle or sexual intercourse may also cause temporarily elevated levels of PSA in the older adult male.

EFFECTS OF DEHYDRATION ON COGNITIVE LEVELS

Dehydration, or loss of fluid levels in the body, can impact an older adult's mood and cognitive levels. Mild dehydration can cause fatigue, difficulties with concentration, memory loss, and anxiety. Significant dehydration can cause confusion, difficulties with balance, dizziness, headaches, organ failure, and death. Because elderly patients may be at higher risk of dehydration because of decreased fluid intake, taking some medications that can affect fluid and electrolyte levels, or the dependence on caregivers to provide enough fluids, nurses should be alert for signs of dehydration that can affect cognitive assessment.

FACTORS THAT MAY AFFECT RESULTS OF CHOLESTEROL TESTS

There are some activities that may have an effect on **cholesterol levels**, thereby producing inaccurate results. Before performing a cholesterol check on an older adult, a nurse should provide information about what factors impact test results, so the patient can refrain from these activities. Excess alcohol consumption can cause elevated triglyceride levels, while increased intake of fat and calories over a period of time can cause elevated levels of total cholesterol. Adults who perform exercise just before the test may have lower results that are not entirely accurate. There are also some health conditions that may cause high cholesterol in previously healthy patients. Examples of these illnesses include hypothyroidism and diabetes.

Impact of Increased Age on Immune System

Advancing age can have negative effects on the **immune system**, leaving an older adult prone to increased risk of infections and illness. The thymus gland, which is responsible for secreting cells that fight off foreign invaders in the body, decreases in size, thereby producing fewer cells. The smaller size of the thymus also diminishes the body's ability to convert white blood cells into T cells, which work to provide protection. As a person ages, he or she may also be more susceptible to autoimmune disorders, as the body may produce autoantibodies that signal it to attack itself. Because of this, older adults are more prone to developing infections due to a decreased immune response, as well as autoimmune conditions that can cause negative symptoms and poor health.

Inaccurate Results from Urine Samples

Urinalysis results may have a higher risk of inaccuracy due to the method required to obtain the urine sample. Nurses should consider how the process of obtaining the urine sample was performed if the results are grossly inaccurate. For patients who must provide clean-catch urine samples, failure to adequately cleanse the area before voiding or contamination of the container may produce inaccurate results, such as bacteria from the external genitalia being present in the urine that would falsely indicate infection. Older adults who have urinary catheters typically need the nurse to obtain the urine sample. Depending on the type of test, this may need to be a sterile procedure. Any deviation from the standard procedure for collection from a catheter, such as breaking sterile technique, can cause inaccurate results in a urine test.

Improper Use of Equipment During Assessment

Nurses use many different types of **equipment** to care for older adults, whether it is to monitor vital signs, administer fluids, or measure laboratory values. Proper use of equipment is essential in order to obtain accurate results. When equipment has not been calibrated, has been placed improperly, or has not been maintained, it may not be able to fulfill its intended purpose and may even harm the client. For example, a nurse who uses a large blood pressure cuff on a client who has a small build and thin arms may achieve low blood pressure readings, believing the patient has hypotension. Failure to inspect or use equipment properly can result in mechanical failures, which could deliver the wrong amounts of medication, oxygen, fluids, or food to some patients.

Pediatric Response to Illness

INFANT RESPONSE TO ILLNESS AND HOSPITALIZATION

Infants respond to illness and pain with crying, grimacing, and withdrawal from the stimulus. Infants up to 4 months tolerate hospitalization fairly well, if their needs are met. They may exhibit separation anxiety from 4 months on, when their parents are not close by.

Nursing Interventions: Let parents participate in the care of the infant as much as possible. Keep the infant's schedule the same as the home schedule. Meet basic needs quickly and gently. Provide age-appropriate toys. Interact often with the infant (holding, talking to her). The key is to make the hospital environment match the home environment as closely as possible. This will encourage the infant to continue to trust her environment and the people in it.

TODDLER RESPONSE TO ILLNESS AND HOSPITALIZATION

Toddlers tend to experience a great deal of stress when dealing with an invasive procedure. Pain produces crying, pulling away, and resistance if they've experienced painful procedures before. Toddlers regress when hospitalized. Their usual control of their environment is lost and they will exhibit separation anxiety if their caregiver is absent.

Nursing Interventions: Encourage the parents to stay in the room. Ask them to bring items from home that remind the child of the parents. Discourage the parents from leaving the room while the child is sleeping. Keep routines the same as at home. Use terms that the child is used to. Provide age-appropriate toys and activities. Allow the child to do as much as he can for himself. Allow him some control over his environment and schedule.

PRESCHOOLER RESPONSE TO ILLNESS AND HOSPITALIZATION

Preschoolers think illness is caused by something they can see or experience and may blame their illness on something totally unrelated. They may also think the illness or hospitalization is a punishment. They fear body mutilation, and will therefore be very afraid of any invasive procedure. An IV can bring on a fear of body contents leaking out. Preschoolers, like toddlers, will exhibit regression as a defense mechanism. They experience a loss of control over their environment and fear their parents do not love them if they are separated from them.

Nursing Interventions: Keep invasive procedures to a minimum. Use dolls/puppets to show how procedures will be done. Use band-aids after giving injections. Use terms understood by the child. Give rewards. Stay with the child for procedures. Keep the routine as close to the home routine as possible. Encourage parents to stay. Provide appropriate toys and activities. Assure the child that she did not cause the illness.

SCHOOL AGE CHILDREN RESPONSE TO ILLNESS AND HOSPITALIZATION

The school age child fears being mutilated, being held down, and having to take clothes off for exams. They have a basic understanding of the severity of different illnesses and think illness is caused by something outside themselves. These children take a brave stance when they are truly scared (reaction formation). They become depressed and withdrawn when separated from family. School age children are stressed by the loss of control experienced in the hospital and by their fear of pain, injury, and death.

Nursing Interventions: Allow parents to stay. Allow the child to do things for himself. Encourage him to talk about what is happening. Let him know it's ok to be scared and cry. Be honest and use models to explain procedures. Provide appropriate play activities. Keep the routine as normal as possible, allowing the child to read, play games, and do homework. Let the child assist in his care by letting him help with charting and keeping track of procedures and medication times.

Adolescent Response to Illness and Hospitalization

Adolescents who are hospitalized experience stress due to changes in body image, loss of peer interaction, dependence on others, and fear that illness is a punishment. They use denial to deal with these feelings and tend to become angry and withdraw. Their world often revolves around peer interactions, so losing control over this part of their lives can result in many negative behaviors.

Nursing Interventions: Allow her to have as much control over her environment as possible (wear own clothes, decorate room, have telephone, have privacy). Set limits and provide appropriate activities as diversions. Allow a routine that she is comfortable with, including schoolwork, peer interactions, and self-care. Involve her in the management of her care, along with the parents.

Impact of Pediatric Chronic Illness on the Family

FEELINGS AND RESPONSE OF CHILDREN TO CHRONIC ILLNESS

The most stressful aspect of having a **chronic illness** is how much the symptoms and treatment tend to embarrass children and make them feel different. Young children tend to focus on pain, while school age children are concerned with aspects of their illness that interfere with their activities. School age children are more apt to refuse treatments because they have a limited understanding of why those treatments are necessary. As the school age child matures, he takes more responsibility for the care of his illness. In adolescence, difficulties arise when the youth seeks independence and control over his environment, which is difficult to do with a chronic illness. He may either become very controlling and preoccupied with his illness or rebel against treatments, resorting to risky behaviors. Near the end of adolescence, maturity brings a more responsible outlook on his disease, when he will want to work with his illness to fit it in around his life.

IMPACT OF CHRONIC ILLNESS ON THE CHILD

Chronic illnesses/disorders may interfere with the normal development of the child. Adjustments need to be made, as much as possible, to facilitate normal development. For example, allowing a wheelchair-bound adolescent to participate in sports designed for handicapped individuals. Schools are required by law to provide a free education for all children, regardless of handicaps. This includes any modifications that need to be made to the school environment. Most children are able to be mainstreamed into regular classrooms. Dealing with the general public's reactions to a child who looks different is difficult for most kids. The nurse and caregivers can role-play with the child to practice what to say to people who stare or make comments. School nurses should educate classmates about the child's illness and assure them that she is just like them on the inside. Most school age children adjust well to a classmate's disorder and become protective of her.

ASSISTING CHILDREN IN DEALING POSITIVELY WITH ILLNESS

Children generally want to be defined by who they are on the inside, not by the illness that changes their appearance and affects their daily life. They need help in creating a sense of normalcy in their life. Treatments may need to be modified for their situation, and they should have control over how much information is told to family and peers. A thorough assessment using open-ended questions to elicit as much information as possible on what the child wants and needs is essential. All treatment plans should involve the child's input. Assessment should include the coping strategies being used, such as social support from family, peers, and school and health officials, problem solving techniques, managing emotions (using humor, relaxation, talk therapy, distraction), and spiritual help (prayer, time with church family). If coping strategies are not working, different ones can be suggested, including support groups. Negative coping strategies might include using risky behaviors, regression, withdrawal, blaming, and antisocial behaviors.

REACTIONS OF FAMILY TO CHILD'S ILLNESS OR HOSPITALIZATION

Families may not have the coping skills in place to deal with a serious illness, increasing their levels of fear and anxiety, which in turn makes it hard for the family to help the child cope with his illness. They may regress to helplessness and display many signs of stress, such as physical ailments, guilt, anger, depression, and denial.

The nurse needs to assess the family's coping skills, support system, parenting style, present stressors, cultural and religious beliefs, education and how each parent was raised by their own parents. Identify areas that need support and allow the parents to ask questions, bring in support systems from outside and participate in support groups. Provide information on the child's treatment, progress and anticipated needs. The outcomes identified should focus on strengthening the parents and enabling them to assist the child in coping.

CHALLENGES FACED BY PARENTS OF CHRONICALLY ILL CHILDREN

Families with chronically ill children experience stress, lack of social contacts, and worry about the other family member's psychosocial health. They may cope in the following ways: educating themselves, making sure they are experts at their child's care, gaining social support, including church contacts, being positive, and recognizing that there are other's whose illnesses are worse. Parents do tend to become overwhelmed at times. They may work through the grieving process several times during their child's life, especially at milestones. Families attempt to normalize their lives as much as possible, incorporating family rituals and activities that the whole family participates in. The more the family works together and remains cohesive, the better their coping strategies will work to decrease everyone's stress and the healthier the ill child will remain. The family will be strengthened by working together and networking with other caregivers.

Parents first need to work through the emotions that come with the diagnosis of a chronic illness. Then they need to learn how to operate any equipment, troubleshoot any problems, anticipate any changes in the child's health, and recognize dangerous conditions. The caregivers need support, encouragement and assistance in setting short term goals during this time. Eventually they take over as CEO of the illness and treatments. Over time the parent will gradually give control over the disease to the child. When this will happen depends on the developmental level and readiness of the child. The **nurse plays a vital role** in this transition as a teacher and coach. Time management is another challenge, especially finding time to spend with the parent's other children and spouse. Other caregiver stressors include lack of sleep, managing conflict in the family, and roles of other family members. Nurses can help by arranging respite care for short- or long-term periods.

STRESSORS FACED BY SIBLINGS OF CHRONICALLY ILL CHILDREN

Siblings are exposed to the emotions and stress of the caretakers. They usually receive less attention and take on more responsibilities earlier. They respond better when taught about the condition and the need for treatments. Efforts need to be made for the siblings to have their own activities. They also need role-playing to learn to deal with peers' reactions to the ill child, which may transfer to themselves. They would like to be involved in the ill child's care, but need their own time also. The parents and nurse need to be aware that they do worry about what will happen to their ill sibling, as well as about their own future if they should ever be expected to take on his or her care.

NURSING MANAGEMENT OF FAMILY OF CHILD WITH CHRONIC ILLNESS

Educate the family about the condition, its expected progression, and the available treatments. Teach the family to care for the child and any equipment needed. Provide education about psychosocial aspects of caring for a chronically ill child, including normal feelings of grief, denial, anger, etc. Encourage parents to talk to siblings about the illness and to take time for them. Refer them to support groups for siblings. Make sure the family meets with the healthcare team on a regular basis and that the parent's and child's wants and needs take primary consideration. Refer them to support groups. Talk with school officials about any needed modifications and continuing education when the child cannot be at school. Encourage participation in school and community activities. Teach school personnel about any equipment to be used. Arrange any home health care that is needed.

Pediatric Evidence-Based Practices

SPECIFIC EVIDENCE-BASED INTERVENTIONS IN PEDIATRICS

KANGAROO CARE

Kangaroo care involves holding an infant with skin-to-skin contact to promote warmth and bonding between a mother and child. Ideally, kangaroo care occurs naturally, with a mother carrying her infant in this position as often as possible. However, in the neonatal intensive care unit, many infants are connected to tubing and wires and may be too medically unstable to be held in this manner. Instead, parents may perform kangaroo care during times when the infant is hemodynamically stable and for short intervals to promote bonding and breastfeeding. In this method, the infant is undressed down to a diaper and held against the mother or father's bare chest.

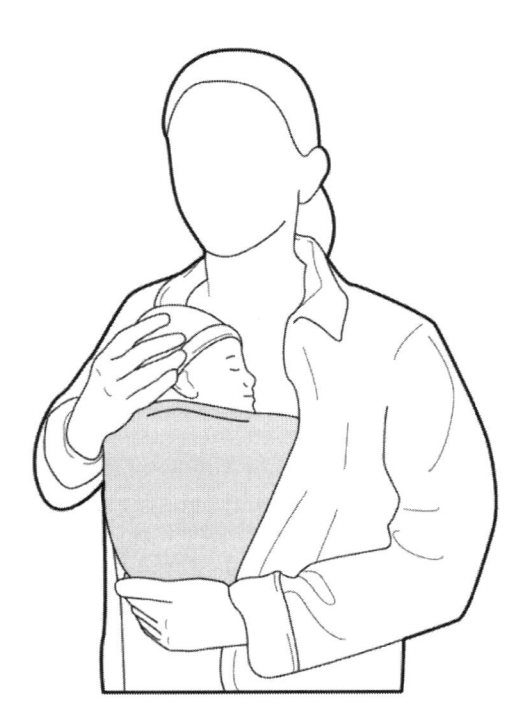

SUCTIONING A HIGH-RISK NEWBORN AND A CHILD WITH A TRACHEOSTOMY

Suctioning should not be considered a routine procedure. It is only performed when necessary, as determined by lung sounds, oximeter reading, or restlessness. Suctioning can cause bradycardia, bronchospasm, hypoxia, and increased ICP (may lead to IVH). Always use aseptic technique. The suction catheter is premeasured so that it is not inserted past the end of the endotracheal tube. The catheter should be inserted quickly and withdrawn using intermittent suction; a suctioning episode should last no more than 5 seconds. A pulse oximeter should be used before, during, and after suctioning to ascertain oxygen status, and the results should be documented. An in-line suction device can be used for very ill infants. This will ensure an adequate oxygen supply during suctioning and is more aseptic. The infant should be placed supine with the head in the sniffing position or on the side with the head in alignment. When suctioning a tracheostomy, make sure the catheter's diameter is half that of the tracheostomy tube.

Chlorhexidine (CHG) Baths and Oral Sucrose

Chlorhexidine (CHG) baths and oral sucrose are evidence-based interventions on the pediatric unit:

- **Chlorhexidine (CHG) baths**: Chlorhexidine gluconate has been used to prevent hospital acquired infections across hospital units for decades. From CHG baths, to CHG soaked dressings and skin preparation solutions, this method of infection prevention has proven effective, particularly on units with patients who are ventilated or have central lines. For that reason, many pediatric inpatient units implement daily CHG baths as part of the HAI prevention protocol.
- **Oral sucrose**: Oral sucrose, a simple sugar solution, is used as a non-pharmacologic pain reliever for infants less than 28 days old during short procedures that may induce pain or distress. The sucrose is administered orally to the infant's tongue, and its analgesic effect lasts for about five to eight minutes. This is most commonly used prior to the following procedures: heel pricks, circumcision, IV-line insertion, injections, eye examination, lumbar puncture, amongst other brief pain-inducing procedures.

ADHD Interventions

Because of research studies, interventions, surveys, and collaboration with parents and teachers, health care workers have access to evidence-based practice information about how to help children diagnosed with **attention-deficit/hyperactivity disorder (ADHD)**. Continued work with children with this condition and follow-up with practice guidelines can be successful because evidence through previous outcomes is available. Nurses can use evidence-based practices to treat as well as educate parents about their child with ADHD by performing interventions to help with decreased impulse control, short attention spans, hyperactivity, decreased concentration, and memory problems. These interventions can be implemented in any situation in which the child is having difficulty, such as at home, in the classroom, with peers, or in other group settings.

Prevention of Hospital-Acquired Infections

Hospital-acquired infections can occur in several ways among children in health care facilities, such as after surgery or invasive procedures and after exposure to infectious organisms from other patients in the hospital or from central lines or endotracheal tubes. Nurses can perform research to determine the effectiveness of interventions aimed at preventing infections. Because of the large number of studies related to infection control, many evidence-based practices are well recognized and accepted in the health care environment. Some interventions that may be used to prevent hospital-based infections include regular and appropriate hand washing between patients, use of waterless hand sanitizer, sterile technique when performing invasive procedures, proper cleaning and disinfection of reusable equipment, reducing the number of breaks in central lines, and using isolation precautions for infectious patients.

Cases of Child Abuse or Neglect

Evidence-based practices are in use for health care workers and social service workers who treat **victims of child abuse**. Evidence-based practices can be used to find case studies about treatment protocols, long-term effects of child abuse, and policies related to reporting incidents. Evidence-based practices can be used to change practices for reporting cases and prosecuting offenders; to train practitioners to recognize child abuse and methods by which to collect evidence; and to educate families about domestic violence, anger management, respite opportunities, and the negative outcomes of child abuse.

Positive Behavior Analysis

Positive behavior analysis is a treatment method that involves using certain types of techniques to affirm positive behaviors with the hope of the child repeating the positive behavior. For example, positive behavior analysis might involve giving a child a sticker when he makes a positive choice. The child may be more likely to make the same choice in a future situation if he or she remembers a positive outcome from the last time. Applied behavioral analysis, when used with children with autism, may teach them social skills and more positive interactions. This is done by setting up a situation that will teach the children something new and then help them to succeed at learning so that they associate positive outcomes with change.

Grief and Loss

GRIEF

Grief is an emotional response to a **loss** that begins at the time a loss is anticipated and continues on an individual timetable. While there are identifiable stages or tasks, it is not an orderly and predictable process. It involves overcoming anger, disbelief, guilt, and a myriad of related emotions. The grieving individual may move back and forth between stages or experience several emotions at any given time. Each person's grief response is unique to their own coping patterns, stress levels, age, gender, belief system, and previous experiences with loss.

KUBLER-ROSS'S FIVE STAGES OF GRIEF

Kubler-Ross taught the medical community that the dying patient and family welcomes open, honest discussion of the dying process and felt that there were certain **stages** that patients and family go through. The stages may not occur in order, but may vary or some may be skipped. Stages include:

- **Denial**: The person denies the diagnosis and tries to pretend it isn't true. During this time, the person may seek a second opinion or alternative therapies. They may use denial until they are better able to emotionally cope with the reality of the disease or changes that need to be made. Patients may also wish to save family and friends from pain and worry. Both patients and family may use denial as a coping mechanism when they feel overwhelmed by the reality of the disease and threatened losses.
- **Anger**: The person is angry about the situation and may focus that rage on anyone.
- **Bargaining**: The person attempts to make deals with a higher power to secure a better outcome to their situation.
- **Depression**: The person anticipates the loss and the changes it will bring with a sense of sadness and grief.
- **Acceptance**: The person accepts the impending death and is ready to face it as it approaches. The patient may begin to withdraw from interests and family.

> **Review Video: The Five Stages of Grief**
> Visit mometrix.com/academy and enter code: 648794

ANTICIPATORY GRIEF

Anticipatory grief is the mental, social, and somatic reactions of an individual as they prepare themselves for a **perceived future loss**. The individual experiences a process of intellectual, emotional, and behavioral responses in order to modify their self-concept, based on their perception of what the potential loss will mean in their life. This process often takes place ahead of the actual loss, from the time the loss is first perceived until it is resolved as a reality for the individual. This process can also blend with past loss experiences. It is associated with the individual's perception of how life will be affected by the particular diagnosis as well as the impending death. Acknowledging this anticipatory grief allows family members to begin looking toward a changed future. Suppressing this anticipatory process may inhibit relationships with the ill individual and contribute to a more difficult grieving process at a later time. However, appropriate anticipatory grieving does not take the place of grief during the actual time of death.

DISENFRANCHISED GRIEF

Disenfranchised grief occurs when the loss being experienced cannot be openly acknowledged, publicly mourned, or socially supported. Society and culture are partly responsible for an individual's response to a loss. There is a **social context** to grief; if a person incurring the loss will be putting himself or herself at risk if grief is expressed, disenfranchised grief occurs. The risk for disenfranchised grief is greatest among those whose relationship with the individual they lost was not known or regarded as significant. This is also the situation found among bereaved persons who are not recognized by society as capable of grief, such as young children, or needing to mourn, such as an ex-spouse or secret lover.

Grief vs. Depression

Normal grief is preoccupied with self-limiting to the loss itself. Emotional responses will vary and may include open expressions of anger. The individual may experience difficulty sleeping or vivid dreams, a lack of energy, and weight loss. Crying is evident and provides some relief of extreme emotions. The individual remains socially responsive and seeks reassurance from others.

Depression is marked by extensive periods of sadness and preoccupation often extending beyond 2 months. It is not limited to the single event. There is an absence of pleasure or anger and isolation from previous social support systems. The individual can experience extreme lethargy, weight loss, insomnia, or hypersomnia, and has no recollection of dreaming. Crying is absent or persistent and provides no relief of emotions. Professional intervention is required to relieve depression.

Loss

Loss is the blanket term used to denote the absence of a valued object, position, ability, attribute, or individual. The aspect of **loss** as it is associated with the death of an animal or person is a relatively new definition. Loss is an individualized and subjective experience depending on the **perceived attachment** between the individual and the missing aspect. This can range from little or no value of attachment to significant value. Loss also can be represented by the **withdrawal of a valued relationship** one had or would have had in the future. Depending on the unique and individual responses to the perception of loss and its significance, reactions to the loss will vary. Robinson and McKenna summarize the aspects of loss in three main attributes:

- Something has been removed.
- The item removed had value to that person.
- The response is individualized.

Mourning

Mourning is a public grief response for the death of a loved one. The various aspects of the mourning process are partially determined by **personal and cultural belief systems**. Kagawa-Singer defines mourning as "the social customs and cultural practices that follow a death." Durkheim expands this to include the following: "mourning is not a natural movement of private feelings wounded by a cruel loss; it is a duty imposed by the group." Mourning involves participation in religious and culturally appropriate customs and rituals designed to publicly acknowledge the loss. These rituals signify they are adjusting to the change in their relationships created by the loss, as well as mark the beginning of the reorganization and forward movement of their lives.

Bereavement

Bereavement is the emotional and mental state associated with having suffered a **personal loss**. It is the reactions of grief and sadness initiated by the loss of a loved one. Bereavement is a normal process of feeling deprived of something of value. The word bereave comes from the root "reave" meaning to plunder, spoil, or rob. It is recognized that the lost individual had value and a defining role in the surviving individual's life. Bereavement encompasses all the acts and emotions surrounding the feeling of loss for the individual. During this grieving period, there is an increased mortality risk. A **positive bereavement experience** means being able to recognize the significance of the loss while still recognizing the resilience and value of life.

Risk Factors Complicating Bereavement

The caregiver should assess for multiple **life crises** that take energy away from the grieving process. An important factor is the grieving individual's history with past grieving experiences. Assess for other recent, unresolved, or difficult losses that may need to be addressed before the individual can move toward resolution of the current loss. Age, mental health, substance abuse, extreme anger, anxiety, or dependence on the individual facing the end of life can add additional stressors and handicap natural coping mechanisms. Income strains, community support, outside and personal responsibilities, the absence of cultural and religious beliefs, the difficulty of the disease process, and age of the loved one lost can also present additional risk factors.

COUNSELING AND PROVIDING EMOTIONAL SUPPORT REGARDING GRIEF AND LOSS TO CHILDREN

The approach to counseling and providing emotional support regarding grief and loss to children is dependent on the age of the child. When available, children and family should be provided information about **peer support groups** (especially adolescents) and **bereavement art therapy groups** as these may be especially helpful. Healthcare professionals should use appropriate words (death, died) instead of euphemisms (passed on) when talking about the deceased and should encourage the child to ask questions. Children are often reluctant to express feelings directly, so it may be beneficial to encourage them to keep a journal about their feelings or draw pictures to express them. Parents should be encouraged to share their feelings of grief with their children rather than trying to hide their emotions and should be aware that children express grief in different ways and may regress or complain of physical ailments (stomach ache, headache) in response to grief. Children should be prepared for changes in routines or living situations, such as a stay-at-home parent having to take a job, which may occur as a result of a death or serious illness.

SIGNS OF A CHILD HAVING ISSUES MANAGING GRIEF

Management of **grief** comes in stages for children as well as for adults. Grief may be complicated for a child who does not understand the significance of the situation, such as in the case of a parent's death, or for someone who does not have the necessary support systems in place, as in the case of a child who has a grieving parent who consequently becomes unavailable. **Signs that a child is not coping well with grief** include extended periods of sadness, lack of interest in regular activities, sleep disturbances, loss of appetite, statements of wishing for death or joining a person who has died, difficulties with concentration, problems taking direction at school, poor school performance, and fear of being alone.

INTERVENTIONS FOR PATIENTS AND FAMILY EXPERIENCING LOSS AND GRIEF

Loss is painful and frightening. Loss can occur through death or loss of health, self-esteem, or relationships. Loss can also occur from threats, such as fire, flood, theft, or severe weather. The severity of the loss, preparation for it, and the maturity, stability, and coping mechanisms of the person all affect the grieving process. Multiple losses and substance abuse can complicate grief and recovery. Previous life experience and cultural and religious beliefs can help in resolution of grief. Many emotions are triggered, and if the loss is not acknowledged, the person may become depressed or develop health problems. **Interventions** for those experiencing grief and loss include:

- Teach patients to recognize symptoms, such as SOB, empty feelings in the chest or abdomen, deep sighing, lethargy, and weakness as signs of grief.
- Assist the patient and family to heal themselves by accepting the loss, recognizing the pain from it, making changes to adapt to and assimilate the loss, and moving toward new relationships and activity.
- Refer to groups or counseling for more intense support if needed.

Supporting Families and Patients as They Receive Bad News

It is often best if the patient can **receive bad news** while being **supported** by family, friends, physicians, nurses, support staff, social workers, and clergy if they so desire. However, the patient may not want family members or others to be present, and this too should be respected.

- Provide privacy and ensure that there will be no interruptions.
- Provide seating for all participants.
- Do not provide too much information at once, as the opening statement may be all that the patient can comprehend at one time.
- Allow time for reactions before providing more information.
- Wait for the patient to signal the need for more information and then provide an honest answer in layman's terms. Information may not be absorbed and may need to be repeated as the patient and family are ready for it later after the initial conference.
- Use techniques of therapeutic communication. People may need others to sit and listen and provide comforting empathy many times before having a conversation about problem solving.

Spirituality

Spirituality provides a connection of the self to a higher power and a way of finding meaning in life experiences. It provides guidance for behavior and can help to clarify one's purpose in life. It can offer hope to those who are ill or facing loss and grief and can give comfort, support, and guidance. **Spirituality** is not always connected to a religion and is highly individualized. A person may lose faith and confidence in his/her spiritual beliefs during trying times:

- Ask patients about their spiritual beliefs.
- Listen attentively and do not offer opinions about their beliefs or share your own unless invited.
- Show respect for their views and offer to obtain spiritual support by calling a spiritual leader or setting up a spiritual ritual that has meaning for them.

This support can help them to regain their beliefs and endure illness by helping them to rise above their suffering and find meaning in this experience.

Palliative and Hospice Care

Palliative care attempts to make the rest of the patient's life as comfortable as possible by treating distressing symptoms to keep them controlled. It does not attempt to cure but only to control discomfort caused by the disease. Palliative care does not require terminal illness/prognosis and can be implemented for any patient with chronic disease and suffering.

Hospice care uses palliative care as it supports the patient and family through the dying process. Hospice teams support the daily needs of the patient and family and provide needed equipment, medical expertise, and medications to control symptoms. They offer spiritual, psychological, and social support to the patient and family as needed and desired. Assistance with end-of-life planning is given to help the patient and family accomplish goals important to them. Bereavement support is also given. The team consists of the attending physician, hospice physician advisor, nurses, social worker, clergy, hospice aides, and volunteers. Hospice care is given in the home when the patient has family who are willing to assume care with the assistance of the hospice team. Hospice care also occurs in hospice facilities, hospitals, and extended care facilities. To qualify for Hospice care, the patient must be deemed terminal and given a 6-month or less life expectancy by two separate physicians. Should the patient survive 6 months in hospice, they can be extended for two 90-day periods, and then an unlimited number of 60-day periods per physician order.

Principles of Pharmacology

PRINCIPLES OF PHARMACOKINETICS

Pharmacokinetics relates to the route of administration, the absorption, the dosage, the frequency of administration, the distribution, and the serum levels achieved over time.

- The **drug's rate of clearance (elimination)** and **doses needed** to ensure therapeutic benefit are considered. Most drugs are cleared through the kidneys, with water-soluble compounds excreted more readily than protein-soluble compounds.
- **Volume of distribution** (IV drug dose divided by plasma concentration) determines the rate at which the drug passes into tissue. Drug distribution depends on the degree of protein binding and ion trapping that takes place.
- **Elimination half-life** is the time needed for the concentration of a particular drug to decrease to half of its starting dose in the body. Approximately five half-lives are needed to achieve steady-state plasma concentrations if giving doses intermittently.
- **Context-sensitive half-life** is the time needed to reach 50% concentration after withdrawal of a continuously-administered drug.
- **Recovery time** is the length of time it takes for plasma levels to decrease to the point that the effect is eliminated. This is affected by plasma concentration.
- **Effect-site equilibrium** is the time between administration of a drug and clinical effect (the point at which the drug reaches the appropriate receptors) and must be considered when determining dose, time, and frequency of medications.
- The **bioavailability** of drugs may vary, depending upon the degree of metabolism that takes place before the drug reaches its site of action.

PRINCIPLES OF PHARMACODYNAMICS

Pharmacodynamics relates to biological effects (therapeutic or adverse) of drug administration over time. Drug transport, absorption, means of elimination, and half-life must all be considered when determining effects. Responses may include continuous responses, such as blood pressure variations, or dichotomous responses in which an event either occurs or does not (such as death). Information from pharmacodynamics provides feedback to modify medication dosage (pharmacokinetics). Drugs provide biological effects primarily by interacting with receptor sites (specific protein molecules) in the cell membrane. Receptors include voltage-sensitive ion channels (sodium, chloride, potassium, and calcium channels), ligand-gated ion channels, and transmembrane receptors. Agonist drugs exert effects after binding with a receptor, while antagonist drugs bind with a receptor but have no effects, so they can block agonists from binding. The total number of receptors may vary, upregulating or downregulating in response to stimuli (such as drug administration). Dose-response curves show the relationship between the amount of drug given and the resultant plasma concentration and biological effects.

FIRST PASS METABOLISM AND DRUG CLEARANCE

First pass metabolism is the phenomenon that occurs to ingested drugs that are absorbed through the gastrointestinal tract and enter the hepatic portal system. Drugs metabolized on the first pass travel to the liver, where they are broken down, some to the extent that only a small fraction of the active drug circulates to the rest of the body. This first pass through the liver greatly reduces the bioavailability of some drugs. Routes of administration that avoid first pass metabolism include intravenous, intramuscular, and sublingual.

Drug clearance refers to the ability to remove a drug from the body. The two main organs responsible for clearance are the liver and the kidneys. The liver eliminates drugs by metabolizing, or biotransforming, the substance or excreting the drug in the bile. The kidneys eliminate drugs by filtration or active excretion in the urine. Drugs use either renal or hepatic methods of clearance. Kidney and liver dysfunction inhibit the clearance of drugs that rely on that organ for removal. Toxicity results from poor clearance.

Enterohepatic Recirculation of Drugs and Renally Excreted Drugs

Enterohepatic recirculation refers to the process whereby a drug is effectively removed from circulation and then reabsorbed. The drug is secreted in bile, which is collected in the gall bladder and emptied into the small intestine, from which part of it is reabsorbed and part excreted in the feces. This reabsorption reduces the clearance of these drugs and increases their duration of action. Generally, drugs susceptible to enterohepatic recirculation are those with a molecular weight greater than 300 g/mol and those that are amphipathic (have both a lipophilic portion and a polar portion).

Renally excreted drugs are metabolized (biotransformed) by the liver to a form that can be excreted by the kidneys. Others are excreted by the kidneys unchanged. Infants with decreased renal function demonstrate decreased urine output or elevated levels of BUN and creatinine. The nurse should avoid using drugs that depend on the kidneys for clearance if the infant has renal impairment, as overdose may result.

Absorption in Relation to Routes of Medication Administration

The absorption rate of a drug depends on its transfer from its site of administration to the circulatory system. Different **routes of administration** have different absorption characteristics:

- **Oral**: Ingested medications pass from the gastrointestinal tract into the bloodstream. Most absorption occurs in the small intestine and is affected by gastric motility and emptying rate, drug solubility in gastrointestinal fluids, and food presence. Orally administered drugs are susceptible to first pass metabolism by the liver.
- **Intravenous**: Medications directly administered to the bloodstream have 100% absorption. Peak serum levels are rapidly achieved. Some drugs are not tolerated intravenously, due to vein irritation or toxicity, and others must be given as an infusion.
- **Intramuscular**: Medications injected into a muscle are absorbed fairly rapidly because muscle tissue is highly vascularized. Drugs in lipid vehicles absorb more slowly than those in aqueous vehicles.
- **Subcutaneous**: Medications injected beneath the skin absorb more slowly because the dermis is less vascularized than muscle. Hypoperfusion and edema decrease absorption further.

Effects of Pharmacokinetic Characteristics on Different Age Groups
Pediatric Age Group

Infants, in particular, have unique **absorption profiles** that can dramatically impact the use of drugs in this age group. Babies have very variable rates of absorption, which precludes the use of certain routes of administration. At birth, full-gestational infants generally have a gastric pH near neutral, but after about one day, it drops to the highly acidic range (about pH 1-3). On the other hand, premature babies cannot effectively secrete acid, have a high stomach pH, and empty their stomachs more slowly. Infants also have **immature epithelial barriers** on the skin, making the skin more permeable. Infants have a larger percentage of water weight than adults, making **water-soluble drugs** more effective. However, in turn, their low protein concentrations can depress binding and distribution. Processes involved with elimination are also not fully developed in the infant until he or she is about a year old.

GERIATRIC AGE GROUP

Pharmacokinetics involves four steps: absorption, distribution, metabolism, and elimination. All of these steps are affected by the age of the patient, as the organs involved degenerate from wear and tear:

1. **Absorption** of most drugs occurs in the small intestine. Drug absorption in older adults may be delayed or decreased due to decreased blood flow to the small intestine. This could change the blood levels of drugs achieved in the geriatric patient.
2. **Distribution** of the drug is altered due to a change in body composition. Elderly patients have decreased total body water and lean muscle mass. This relative increase in total body fat may increase the duration of action of lipid-soluble drugs.
3. Most drugs are **metabolized** by either the liver or the kidneys. Decreased function of these organs leads to delayed metabolism and elimination of certain medications.
4. **Renal function** and **elimination effectiveness** diminish with age, often decreasing the kidney's ability to remove toxins and medications from the body. For this reason, drugs may remain in the body longer, therefore requiring smaller doses among the elderly.

BLOOD DRUG LEVELS

Plasma drug levels are used for **therapeutic drug monitoring** because, although plasma is often not the site of action, plasma levels correlate well with therapeutic (effective) and toxic (dose-related adverse effects) responses to most drugs. The therapeutic range of a drug is that between the minimum effective concentration (level at which there is no therapeutic benefit) and the toxic concentration (level at which toxic effects occur). To achieve drug plateau (steady state), the drug half-life (time needed to decrease drug concentration by 50%) must be considered. Most drugs reach plateau with administration equal to four half-lives and completely eliminate a drug in 5 half-lives. Because drug levels fluctuate, peak (highest drug concentration) and trough (lowest drug concentration) levels may be monitored. Samples for trough levels are taken immediately prior to administration of another dose, while peak samples are taken at various times, depending on the average peak time of the specific drug, which may vary from 30 minutes to 2 hours or so after administration.

SIDE EFFECTS OF MEDICATIONS

All drugs can have side effects, and some are toxic at certain levels or in combination with other drugs. Some side effects will be minor and may go away after a week or two. Others can be severe or life-threatening, such as anaphylaxis. Common side effects include nausea, vomiting, diarrhea, and rashes. Side effects may vary with individuals according to age, gender, and condition and may be related to non-compliance with treatment, incorrect dosage, polypharmacy, or drug interactions. Drug compendiums will list all possible side effects according to system or incidence. Pharmacologically similar medications usually have some common side effects among the drugs in that class. Nursing actions include:

- Always question the patient about allergies or previous drug reactions before administering medication.
- Educate the patient about possible side effects of all medications.
- Watch out for drug-drug and food-drug combinations that are dangerous.

Drug Interactions

Drug interactions occur when one drug interferes with the activity of another in either the pharmacodynamics or pharmacokinetics:

- With **pharmacodynamic interaction,** both drugs may interact at receptor sites causing a change that results in an adverse effect or that interferes with a positive effect.
- With **pharmacokinetic interaction**, the ability of the drug to be absorbed and cleared is altered, so there may be delayed effects, changes in effects, or toxicity. Interactions may include problems in a number of areas:
    - **Absorption** may be increased or (more commonly) decreased, usually related to the effects within the gastrointestinal system.
    - **Distribution** of drugs may be affected, often because of changes in protein binding.
    - **Metabolism** may be altered, often causing changes in drug concentration.
    - **Biotransformation** of the drug must take place, usually in the liver and gastrointestinal system, but drug interactions can impair this process.
    - **Clearance interactions** may interfere with the body's ability to eliminate a drug, usually resulting in increased concentration of the drug.

Specific Interactions

Some drugs will either increase or inhibit the actions of other drugs. They may interfere with receptor-site binding or the way in which the drug is metabolized or excreted. Certain drugs may cause drowsiness when taken together or with alcohol. Some foods will inhibit drug action, such as the inhibition of warfarin by vitamin-K-containing foods. Other foods may cause toxic levels of a drug to accumulate. Grapefruit juice, for example, is metabolized by the same enzyme that metabolizes about 50 drugs, including digoxin and statins, and this can prevent the liver from breaking down drugs and lead to severe reactions. The nurse should always obtain a complete medication list from the patient, including prescription and over-the-counter medications, herbals, vitamins, minerals, and dietary supplements that are taken regularly and occasionally. All medications taken should be checked for **potential interactions with drugs or foods**.

Principles of Adult Medication Administration

DRUG CLASSIFICATION

The following are different ways to classify drugs:

- **Therapeutic classification**: The common uses for the drug will place it in a certain therapeutic classification.
- **Pharmacological classification**: The action of the drug determines which pharmacological category a drug will be in.

All drugs have a **chemical name** and a **generic name,** which is simpler. A company making the drug can give it a **trade or brand name**. The generic form of a drug is generally cheaper but may differ in efficacy from a brand name drug due to a difference in the amount of drug that is absorbed for use in the body. The Controlled Substances Act restricts usage of certain drugs and classifies them according to schedules that include:

- **Schedule I**: Ecstasy, LSD, marijuana, peyote, mescaline, psilocybin, heroin, and others
- **Schedule II**: Amphetamine, cocaine, codeine, fentanyl, Dilaudid, Demerol, Ritalin, morphine, opium, and others
- **Schedule III**: Anabolic steroids, barbiturates, codeine, Vicodin, and pentothal
- **Schedule IV**: Xanax, Librium, Klonopin, Valium, Ativan, Versed, phenobarbital, Restoril, Ambien
- **Schedule V**: Lomotil and others

5 RIGHTS OF MEDICATION ADMINISTRATION

The 5 rights of medication administration are used to prevent/reduce medication errors in the hospital setting. Often these 5 rights are integrated into the scanning requirements of electronic documentation. The **5 rights of medication administration** must also be incorporated into the prescriber's order:

- **Right Patient**: Confirm the patient's identity using two identifiers, often being their full name and date of birth. Scanning will also confirm the patient's identity with their bar code and electronic health record.
- **Right Drug**: Check the name of the drug with the prescriber's order. By scanning the medication, the drug name will also be checked against the order.
- **Right Dose**: Check the dose of the drug with the prescriber's order. Some medications require a second nurse confirm any dosage calculations utilized before administration. Ensure the dosage is appropriate and contact the prescriber if there are any concerns.
- **Right route**: Routes include oral (PO), subcutaneous, intradermal, IV, or IM, amongst others. The route must also be confirmed with the prescriber's order.
- **Right time/frequency**: The drug may be administered as a one-time dose, PRN (as needed), or recurring administration (twice daily, every 8 hours, etc.).

CLINICAL SITUATIONS THAT HAVE IMPLICATIONS FOR MEDICATION ADMINISTRATION

It is quite important to recognize clinical situations involving patients that may have **implications for the administration of medications**. For example, many patients have co-morbid conditions that will impact decisions about their medication administration. A patient with non-insulin-dependent diabetes and coronary artery disease who is being treated for a hip fracture would require oral hypoglycemic medications, cardiovascular medications, pain medication, and anti-coagulants. Another example would be an insulin-dependent diabetic patient with concomitant hypertension and renal failure. This patient would require insulin, anti-hypertensive medications, and dosing adjustments of medications secondary to renal failure. The nurse who is responsible for the patient must ensure that the correct dosages of each prescribed medication are administered on time. Potential negative side effects and drug-drug interactions should be avoided, and the patient should be monitored for adverse reactions to newly prescribed drugs.

ROUTES OF DRUG ADMINISTRATION

The route of administration is the manner by which a drug is introduced into the body. The most **common routes of administration** are:

- Enteral (oral, rectal, or by feeding tube)
- Topical (on the skin, in the eyes or nose, vaginal, or inhaled)
- Parenteral (IV, subcutaneous, intramuscular, intracardiac, intraosseous, intradermal, intrathecal, intraperitoneal, transdermal, transmucosal, intravitreal, and epidural)

There are many variations on these three basic routes of administration. The FDA acknowledges 111 different routes of administration. When deciding on the route of administration, the doctor and pharmacist consider:

- How fast the patient requires the drug
- How effective it will be by a given route
- The likelihood of toxicity
- The discomfort it will cause
- How likely the patient is to comply with the route
- How likely the route is to play into the patient's addictive habits

INJECTIONS

The three most common types of injections and the preferred injection sites are as follows:

- **Subcutaneous Injection**: Deliver the drug under the skin with a ½ inch, 24- or 25-gauge needle held at a 45° angle to reach the fat. Choose the upper arm, abdomen, thigh, or lower back as the site. The maximum amount of subcutaneous medication is 0.5 mL. An example is insulin for a patient with diabetes.
- **Intramuscular Injection**: Deliver the drug into the muscle at a 90° angle to reach the deep tissue. Standard needle length is 1 to 1.5 inches depending on the weight of the individual. CDC guidelines recommend the use of a 22- to 25-gauge needle for adult intramuscular injections. Recommended sites for injection on the adult include deltoid (most recommended), vastus lateralis (thigh), ventrogluteal (hip), or dorsogluteal (buttocks). The maximum recommended amount of IM medication is 3 mL. An example is Vitamin B12 for a patient with pernicious anemia.
- **Intravenous Injection**: Deliver the drug into a vein of the arm, hand, leg, foot, scalp, or neck with an Angiocath, butterfly, or Insyte Autoguard needle. Use a size from 14 gauge to 26 gauge, depending on the fluid and the patient. The nurse sets the drip rate per minute by adjusting the clamp and monitoring the drip chamber. An example of a drug requiring intravenous injection is Zoledronate, which is given yearly to prevent bone fractures for individuals with osteoporosis.

> **Review Video: Calculating IV Drip Rates**
> Visit mometrix.com/academy and enter code: 396112

Two less frequently used forms of injection are: Intradermal (into the skin) for Mantoux TB test, and intraosseous access (IO) into the bone, which is used in emergency situations when other access sites are not available.

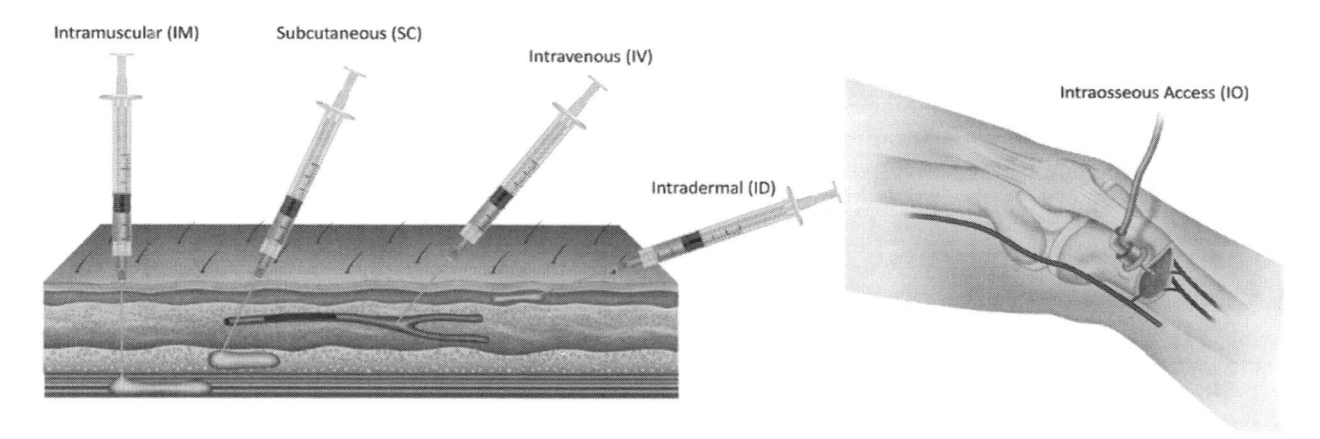

HERBAL-DRUG CONTRAINDICATIONS

Patients on certain medications should not take some herbals. Some **contraindications for common herbals** include:

- **Echinacea**: Anti-anxiety meds, antifungals, heart medications, HIV medications, anabolic steroids, methotrexate, NSAIDs
- **Gingko Biloba**: Anticoagulants, NSAIDs, aspirin, acetaminophen
- **Garlic**: Anticoagulants, oral hypoglycemics, NSAIDs
- **Licorice**: Diuretics, digoxin, antihypertensives
- **St. John's Wort**: Antidepressants, anticoagulants, Tamoxifen, oral contraceptives, HIV medications, anesthetics. Action is similar to MAO inhibitor
- **Valerian**: Sedatives, anti-seizure meds, anesthetics, alcohol, opioids
- **Feverfew**: Anticoagulants, migraine meds, NSAIDs
- **Ginger**: Anticoagulants, NSAIDs
- **Ginseng**: Anticoagulants, antihypertensives, NSAIDs, opioids. Do not take when pregnant or lactating
- **Goldenseal**: Antihypertensives, diabetic medications, meds for kidney diseases. Do not take when pregnant or lactating
- **Kava-kava**: Alcohol, anti-seizure meds, antidepressants, sedatives, anesthetics, antipsychotics, NSAIDS, opioids
- **Saw Palmetto**: Hormone therapy
- **Hawthorn**: Digoxin

Principles of Pediatric Medication Administration

LIFESPAN CONCERNS
Prescribing drugs across the lifespan requires an understanding of differences in types of medications used and dosages according to age and gender.

Dosage and administration of pediatric medications is **weight and age related**, and only pediatric medications should be prescribed if possible. Adult pills, for example, should not be cut for use for a child, as even small variations in dosage may have adverse effects. Dosage should always be checked. The Broselow tape can be used to measure the child to guide medication dosage.

PHYSIOLOGICAL AND DEVELOPMENTAL CONSIDERATIONS FOR MEDICATION ADMINISTRATION
Absorption of medications can be delayed due to delayed gastric emptying, or delayed or enhanced due to the high pH of the newborn's gastric juices or irregular peristalsis. IM medications can be affected by the small muscle mass and diminished peripheral blood flow of the young child. Topical meds are more rapidly absorbed due to their greater body surface area. The greater body fluid volume can dilute water-soluble medications, and if body fat is increased, a higher dose of a lipid-soluble drug may be needed. An immature liver and temperature fluctuations can affect drug metabolism. Immature kidney function can affect excretion of medications, causing toxicity.

Infants benefit from having the parents assist in medication administration. Toddlers benefit from simple choices, handling any equipment, a positive approach, quick administration and restraint if needed, followed by rewards for positive behavior. Preschoolers need simple explanations, to be able to play with equipment, choices, and parental assistance. School age children benefit from rewards, explanations and play therapy. Adolescents can be treated the same as adults.

SAFE ADMINISTRATION OF ORAL MEDICATIONS
Oral medications can be given by medicine spoon, oral syringe, dropper, nipple, or tube. Suspensions must be shaken. Sometimes tablets need to be crushed or capsules opened if a liquid form is unavailable. Ensure this will not interfere with the action of the drug. Drugs can sometimes be mixed with a pleasant tasting food or flavored. If using a nasogastric, gastrostomy or naso-jejunal tube, ensure proper placement of the tube, and flush the tube before and after administration of medicine.

ADMINISTERING ORAL LIQUID MEDICATIONS
Nurses may have a hard time getting children to take liquid medications and keep them down. There are, however, some methods that may help to make the process a little smoother. Liquid medications can be drawn into a syringe (without a needle) and then the medicine is inserted into the pocket of the child's cheek. Children should not be told that the medicine is candy in order to get them to take it more easily as this can be very confusing. Many medications allow for a drink afterward to wash it down. Having a glass of water on hand to drink after the medication is administered may help. If a medication is very distasteful and the children are old enough, they can drink the liquid through a straw, which may help them taste less of it.

SAFE ADMINISTRATION OF IV MEDICATIONS
IV medication administration permits better control over therapeutic blood levels and is less traumatic for the pediatric patient. The nurse should make sure the drug is given according to pharmacologic guidelines. Check for compatibility with other drugs being given. Check for a patent IV with no complications. The drug should be dissolved completely and be ready for administration prior to entering the patient's room. All ports are cleansed, lines are primed, and rates are set according to protocol. A syringe pump is used for small amounts of fluid. Larger volumes may be administered with a Buretrol or piggyback method (diluted in 50-100 cc bag of saline or dextrose water). The retrograde method can be used for a small amount of medication (injected into the IV line after clamping off close to patient, then the clamp is undone, and medication will dilute and flow with the IV fluid).

Safe Administration of IM Medications

The safe administration of IM medications is discussed below:

- Infants require a smaller needle and gauge (5/8 inch and 25-27 gauge); toddlers require 1 inch, 22- to 23-gauge needles; and school age children and older require a 1.0-1.5 inch, 22- to 23-gauge needles. Larger gauge needles are used for thicker solutions. Use the smallest gauge needle for the solution and age of the child.
- The preferred site for the infant and toddler is the vastus lateralis; if the child has been walking for at least a year the dorsogluteal muscle can be used. If the child is older than 3 years and has been walking for several years, the ventrogluteal muscle can be used. In children over age 4 or 5, the deltoid can be used.
- The skin is cleaned with alcohol and allowed to dry.
- The needle should be inserted at a 90° angle, aspirated, and then the medicine injected.
- In small infants the needle can be inserted at a 45° angle toward the knee.

Administering Intramuscular Vaccination to Infants

Many types of immunizations are given intramuscularly (IM). In infants, this process typically involves administering the drugs into the large muscles of the thighs. Children from birth until approximately 2 years of age should have IM injections in the anterolateral muscle of the thigh. After preparing the syringe and cleaning the site, the vaccination should be administered at a 90° angle through the skin and subcutaneous fat and into the muscle beneath. Before injecting the medication, aspiration is necessary to avoid giving the drug into the bloodstream. If more than one vaccination is needed, injection sites should be more than 1 inch apart but can be given in the same leg.

Proper Administration of Subcutaneous and Intradermal Medications

Subcutaneous injections are used frequently in children to administer insulin, vaccines, and allergy shots. Intradermal injections are used for tuberculin and allergy testing, and local anesthesia. Subcutaneous injections are given at a 90° angle through skin that has been pinched up to separate the fat from the muscle layer. If you are unable to pinch enough skin, administer subcutaneous injections at a 45° angle. Pain can be minimized by changing the needle to a small gauge after drawing up the medication (provides a sharper, smaller needle) and only injecting small amounts. Sites for subcutaneous injections include the abdomen, the outside of the upper arm and the front center of the thigh. Refer to protocol concerning aspiration before injection. Intradermal injections are given in the inside of the forearm.

Administration of Eye Medications

For eye medication, the child can be supine or sitting. The lower lid is pulled downward while the dominant hand rests on the forehead holding the dropper (to stabilize the dropper). The medication is placed into the conjunctival sac. Alternatively, the lower lid can be pulled down and outward to form a cup, where the medication can be placed. Wipe away excess medication after allowing the child to close his eyes gently. To prevent the medication flowing to the nasopharynx where the child can taste it, apply gentle pressure to the inside corner of the eye for one minute. In infants, place the medication in the corner of the eye with the child supine; when the infant opens their eyes, the medication will flow into the eye. Game-playing with young children may help with administration. Sometimes medication can be administered while the child is sleeping.

Rectal Administration of Medications

The rectal route is sometimes used when the child is vomiting and cannot take oral medications. Acetaminophen, aspirin, antiemetics, sedatives and analgesics are available in suppository form. The absorption of rectal medications is unpredictable due to the presence or absence of stool in the rectum. Using gloves, the suppository is lubricated and inserted into the rectum, beyond the rectal sphincter. The buttocks are held together for 5 to 10 minutes to allow the urge to defecate to pass. Altering the dose of a suppository requires cutting it, which doesn't provide an accurate dose. A retention enema is administered in the same manner.

ADMINISTRATION OF MEDICATIONS IN THE EAR AND NOSE

For the administration of ear medication, the child should be supine and turned with the ear up. Under the age of 3, the pinna is pulled downward and then straight back. Over 3 years of age, the pinna is pulled upward and straight back. Administer the medication (for cleanliness use a disposable ear speculum). Loosely placed cotton may be used to prevent the medication from flowing out of the ear canal. The child should be placed on the opposite side for a few minutes.

For nose drops, the child should be supine with the head extended. This prevents the medication flowing into the sinuses and throat where the child can taste it. Keep the child in this position for one minute after administration.

CRUSHING MEDICATIONS FOR ADMINISTRATION TO CHILDREN

Some children cannot tolerate swallowing pills and may benefit from having the pills crushed and mixed with another substance. Permission from the physician is necessary before crushing medications to ensure it will not destroy the activity of the medicine. Pills that are enteric coated, extended release, slow release, or that may irritate the gastrointestinal lining may not be crushed. Pills may be crushed between two spoons or by using a pill-crusher after verifying the correct dose. Crushed medications may be added to applesauce or pudding to assist with administration of the drugs.

GIVING MEDICATION THROUGH A GASTROSTOMY TUBE

Some children use feeding tubes for nutrition, including gastrostomy tubes, also called G-tubes. These tubes are also used for medication administration if the child cannot take medicine by mouth. Many medications are administered in liquid form through tubes; however, some may need to be crushed and diluted with water. The G-tube may have only a button at the site; if this is the case, an extension tube is attached to administer the medications. After drawing up the medicine, the tube is flushed with a small amount of water to clear the tube without adding air. Following the flush, the medication is administered into the tube using a syringe. If more than one type of medication is needed, the tube is flushed between doses with approximately 5 mL of water. Following the last medication dose, the tube is flushed with a small amount of water to ensure that the medicine clears the tube, the extension tubing is removed, and the button is closed.

PATIENT'S AND PARENT'S WILLINGNESS TO ADHERE TO MEDICATION REGIMENS

A patient's willingness to adhere to medication regimens is often critical to the medications' effectiveness. Noncompliance may result in inadequate relief of symptoms, disease complications, super infections, adverse drug effects, and even death. A patient's willingness to adhere to medication regimens depends on a number of variables. The pediatric population's adherence largely depends on parental/guardian support and understanding:

- **Knowledge base**: The patient/parents must be knowledgeable about the administration (time and dosage) of medications and should be aware of uses and adverse effects in order to understand the importance of adhering to a regimen.
- **Relief of symptoms**: Patients/parents who do not see relief of symptoms immediately may believe medications are ineffective.
- **Financial status**: Parents may not be able to afford medications.
- **Ease of administration**: Patients/parents are more likely to comply with medications that are administered orally.
- **Trust**: Patients/parents must trust healthcare providers to provide appropriate treatment.
- **Cultural values/beliefs**: A patient's and their parents' cultural attitudes may influence compliance.

Cultural Sensitivity Practice

CULTURAL CHARACTERISTICS

HISPANIC PATIENTS

Many areas of the country have large populations of Hispanics and Hispanic Americans. As always, it's important to recognize that cultural generalizations don't always apply to individuals. Recent immigrants, especially, have cultural needs that the nurse must understand:

- Many Hispanics are Catholic and may like the nurse to make arrangements for a priest to visit.
- Large extended families may come to visit to support the patient and family, so patients should receive clear explanations about how many visitors are allowed, but some flexibility may be required.
- Language barriers may exist as some may have limited or no English skills, so translation services should be available around the clock.
- Hispanic culture encourages outward expressions of emotions, so family may react strongly to news about a patient's condition, and people who are ill may expect some degree of pampering, so extra attention to the patient/family members may alleviate some of their anxiety.

Caring for Hispanic and Hispanic American patients requires understanding of cultural differences:

- Some immigrant Hispanics have very little formal education, so medical information may seem very complex and confusing, and they may not understand the implications or need for follow-up care.
- Hispanic culture perceives time with more flexibility than American culture, so if parents need to be present at a particular time, the nurse should specify the exact time (1:30 PM) and explain the reason rather than saying something more vague, such as "after lunch."
- People may appear to be unassertive or unable to make decisions when they are simply showing respect to the nurse by being deferent.
- In traditional families, the males make decisions, so a woman waits for the father or other males in the family to make decisions about treatment or care.
- Families may choose to use folk medicines instead of Western medical care or may combine the two.
- Children and young women are often sheltered and are taught to be respectful to adults, so they may not express their needs openly.

MIDDLE EASTERN PATIENTS

There are considerable cultural differences among Middle Easterners, but religious beliefs about the segregation of males and females are common. It's important to remember that segregating the female is meant to protect her virtue. Female nurses have low status in many countries because they violate this segregation by touching male bodies, so parents may not trust or show respect for the nurse who is caring for their family member. Additionally, male patients may not want to be cared for by female nurses or doctors, and families may be very upset at a female being cared for by a male nurse or physician. When possible, these cultural traditions should be accommodated:

- In Middle Eastern countries, males make decisions, so issues for discussion or decision should be directed to males, such as the father or spouse, and males may be direct in stating what they want, sometimes appearing demanding.
- If a male nurse must care for a female patient, then the family should be advised that *personal care* (such as bathing) will be done by a female while the medical treatments will be done by the male nurse.

Caring for Middle Eastern patients requires understanding of cultural differences:

- Families may practice strict dietary restrictions, such as avoiding pork and requiring that animals be killed in a ritual manner, so vegetarian or kosher meals may be required.
- People may have language difficulties requiring a translator, and same-sex translators should be used if at all possible.
- Families may be accompanied by large extended families that want to be kept informed and whom patients consult before decisions are made.
- Most medical care is provided by female relatives, so educating the family about patient care should be directed at females (with female translators if necessary).
- Outward expressions of grief are considered as showing respect for the dead.
- Middle Eastern families often offer gifts to caregivers. Small gifts (candy) that can be shared should be accepted graciously, but for other gifts, the families should be advised graciously that accepting gifts is against hospital policy.
- Middle Easterners often require less personal space and may stand very close.

ASIAN PATIENTS

There are considerable differences among different Asian populations, so cultural generalizations may not apply to all, but nurses caring for Asian patients should be aware of common cultural attitudes and behaviors:

- Nurses and doctors are viewed with respect, so traditional Asian families may expect the nurse to remain authoritative and to give directions and may not question, so the nurse should ensure that they understand by having them review material or give demonstrations and should provide explanations clearly, anticipating questions that the family might have but may not articulate.
- Disagreeing is considered impolite. "Yes" may only mean that the person is heard, not that they agree with the person. When asked if they understand, they may indicate that they do even when they clearly do not so as not to offend the nurse.
- Asians may avoid eye contact as an indication of respect. This is especially true of children in relation to adults and of younger adults in relation to elders.

Caring for Asian patients requires understanding of cultural differences:

- Patients/families may not show outward expressions of feelings/grief, sometimes appearing passive. They also avoid public displays of affection. This does not mean that they don't feel, just that they don't show their feelings.
- Families often hide illness and disabilities from others and may feel ashamed about illness.
- Terminal illness is often hidden from the patient, so families may not want patients to know they are dying or seriously ill.
- Families may use cupping, pinching, or applying pressure to injured areas, and this can leave bruises that may appear as abuse, so when bruises are found, the family should be questioned about alternative therapy before assumptions are made.
- Patients may be treated with traditional herbs.
- Families may need translators because of poor or no English skills.
- In traditional Asian families, males are authoritative and make the decisions.

Religious Objections to Treatment
Jehovah's Witnesses

Jehovah's Witnesses have traditionally shunned transfusions and blood products as part of their religious beliefs. In 2004, the *Watchtower,* a Jehovah's Witness publication, presented a guide for members. When medical care indicates the need for blood transfusion or blood products and the patient and/or family members are practicing Jehovah's Witnesses, this may present a conflict. It's important to approach the patient/family with full information and reasons for the transfusion or blood components without being judgmental, allowing them to express their feelings. In fact, studies show that while adults often refuse transfusions for themselves, they frequently allow their children to receive blood products, so one should never assume that an individual would refuse blood products based on the religion alone. Jehovah's Witnesses can receive fractionated blood cells, thus allowing hemoglobin-based blood substitutes. The following guidelines are provided to church members:

Basic **blood standards for Jehovah's Witnesses**:

- **Not acceptable**: Whole blood: red cells, white cells, platelets, plasma.
- **Acceptable**: Fractions from red cells, white cells, platelets, and plasma.

Christian Scientists

Christian Science, a religion developed by Mary Baker Eddy in 1879, promotes the belief that sickness is most effectively treated through prayer alone. While Christian Scientists do not avoid all medical interventions, their beliefs are conservative regarding medical treatment. Most notably, Christian Scientists, for the most part, do not believe in vaccinations and may only agree to such if required by law, as they do acknowledge the importance of community health. They have widely appreciated the use of exemptions from mandatory vaccines, but as these exemptions have become more limited, religious leaders have given their members the right to decide upon vaccinations.

Impact of Culture and Religion on Dietary Preferences

When performing a dietary assessment, the nurse should remember that culture and religion might dictate which foods and spices are used. The manner in which food is prepared, cooked, and served may also be specified. The utensils used at the meal as well as the persons who may eat together may be important. Mealtimes and required fasts should be determined. Holidays may be accompanied by particular foods. Alcohol (including extracts made with alcohol) and caffeine may be prohibited. The culture may also consider obesity a sign of affluence and success. The nurse should evaluate the foods that are eaten in light of the patient's medical condition. The patient may not wish to eat the usual hospital fare and may need to have a special diet prepared or food brought from home. The nurse can guide the patient and family to foods that are acceptable and within the patient's requirements for health.

Nursing Research

ELEMENTS OF RESEARCH

The following are elements of research:

- **Variable**: An entity that can be different within a population
- **Independent variable**: The variable that the researchers change to evaluate its effect
- **Dependent variable**: The variable that may be changed by alterations in the independent variable
- **Hypothesis**: The proposed explanation to describe an expected outcome in a study
- **Sample**: The selected population to be studied
- **Experimental group**: The population within the sample that undergoes the treatment or intervention
- **Control group**: The population within the sample that is not exposed to the treatment of intervention being evaluated

The nurse must be taught and must understand the process of critical analysis and know how to conduct a survey of the literature. **Basic research concepts** include:

- **Survey of valid sources**: Information from a juried journal and an anonymous website or personal website are very different sources, and evaluating what constitutes a valid source of data is critical.
- **Evaluation of internal and external validity**: Internal validity shows a cause-and-effect relationship between two variables, with the cause occurring before the effect and no intervening variable. External validity occurs when results hold true in different environments and circumstances with different populations.
- **Sample selection and sample size**: Selection and size can have a huge impact on the results, but a sample that is too small may lack both internal and external validity. Selection may be so narrowly focused that the results can't be generalized to other groups.

VALIDITY, GENERALIZABILITY, AND REPLICABILITY

Many research studies are most concerned with **internal validity** (adequate unbiased data properly collected and analyzed within the population studied), but studies that determine the efficacy of procedures or treatments, for example, should have **external validity** as well; that is, the results should be **generalizable** (true) for similar populations. **Replication** of the study under different circumstances and with different subjects and researchers should produce similar results. For various reasons, some people may be excluded from a study so that instead of randomized subjects, the subjects may be highly selected so when data is compared with another population in which there is less or more selection, results may be different. The selection of subjects, in this case, would interfere with external validity. Part of the design of a study should include considerations of whether or not it should have external validity or whether there is value for the institution based solely on internal validation.

HYPOTHESIS

A hypothesis should be generated about the probable cause of the disease/infection based on the information available in laboratory and medical records, epidemiologic study, literature review, and expert opinion. For example, a hypothesis should include the infective agent, the likely source, and the mode of transmission: "Wound infections with *Staphylococcus aureus* were caused by reuse and inadequate sterilization of single-use irrigation syringes used during wound care in the ICU."

Hypothesis testing includes data analysis, laboratory findings, and outcomes of environmental testing. It usually includes case-control studies, with 2–4 controls picked for each case of infection. They may be matched according to age, sex, or other characteristics, but they are not infected at the time they are picked for the study. Cohort studies, whose controls are picked based on having or lacking exposure, may also be instituted. If the hypothesis cannot be supported, then a new hypothesis or different testing methods may be necessary.

CRITICAL READING

There are several steps to critical reading to evaluate research:

- **Consider the source** of the material. If it is in the popular press, it may have little validity compared to something published in a peer-reviewed journal.
- **Review the author's credentials** to determine if a person is an expert in the field of study.
- **Determine the thesis**, or the central claim of the research. It should be clearly stated.
- **Examine the organization** of the article, whether it is based on a particular theory, and the type of methodology used.
- **Review the evidence** to determine how it is used to support the main points. Look for statistical evidence and sample size to determine if the findings have wide applicability.
- **Evaluate** the overall article to determine if the information seems credible and useful and should be communicated to administration and/or staff.

MAJOR STUDY TYPES UTILIZED IN STATISTICAL ANALYSIS

When conducting research, the nurse should be aware of the **types of studies** available and when each type of study is appropriate and most reliable:

- **Case-control studies** are simple. They use pre-existing cases with and without the disorder of interest. For example, case-control studies may be done with mesothelioma and exposure to possible pleural irritants. These are good for rare diseases to determine cause and effect.
- **Cross-sectional studies** utilize a cross-section of data from the population and analyze variables at one time point. They are not good for determining cause and effect, but they are useful for correlating characteristics with disorders.
- **Cohort studies** follow a cohort of a population for a period of time and attempt to make a link with diseases. As in the previous example, researchers could follow a group exposed to asbestos and study the incidence of mesothelioma.
- **Randomized controlled trial** is the gold standard, with patients assigned to the control or experimental group. This is a difficult type of test to design and implement but very useful, as the data is often well-controlled. It is the most expensive type of study.

BIAS IN RESEARCH

Selection bias occurs when the method of selecting subjects results in a cohort that is not representative of the target population because of inherent error in design. For example, if all patients who develop urinary infections are evaluated per urine culture and sensitivities for microbial resistance, but only those patients with clinically-evident infections are included, a number of patients with sub-clinical infections may be missed, skewing the results. Selection bias is only a concern when participants in studies are specifically chosen. Many surveillance studies do not involve the selection of subjects.

Information bias occurs when there are errors in classification, so an estimate of association is incorrect. Non-differential misclassification occurs when there is similar misclassification of disease or exposure among both those who are diseased/exposed and those who are not. Differential misclassification occurs when there is a differing misclassification of disease or exposure among both those who are diseased/exposed and those who are not.

QUALITATIVE AND QUANTITATIVE DATA

Both qualitative and quantitative data are used for analysis, but the focus is quite different:

- **Qualitative data**: Data are described verbally or graphically, and the results are subjective, depending upon observers to provide information. Interviews may be used as a tool to gather information, and the researcher's interpretation of data is important. Gathering this type of data can be time-intensive, and it can usually not be generalized to a larger population. This type of information gathering is often useful at the beginning of the design process for data collection.
- **Quantitative data**: Data are described in terms of numbers within a statistical format. This type of information gathering is done after the design of data collection is outlined, usually in later stages. Tools may include surveys, questionnaires, or other methods of obtaining numerical data. The researcher's role is objective.

Implementation

Legal and Ethical Implications for Healthcare

PATIENT RIGHTS AND RESPONSIBILITIES

Empowering patients and families to act as their own advocates requires that they have a clear understanding of their **rights and responsibilities.** These should be given (in print form) and/or presented (audio/video) to patients and families on admission or as soon as possible:

- **Rights** include competent, non-discriminatory medical care that respects privacy and allows participation in decisions about care and the right to refuse care. They should have clear understandable explanations of treatments, options, and conditions, including outcomes. They should be apprised of transfers, changes in care plan, and advance directives. They should have access to medical records and billing information.
- **Responsibilities** include providing honest and thorough information about health issues and medical history. They should ask for clarification if they don't understand information that is provided to them, and they should follow the plan of care that is outlined or explain why that is not possible. They should treat staff and other patients with respect.

> **Review Video: Patient Advocacy**
> Visit mometrix.com/academy and enter code: 202160

INFORMED CONSENT

The patient or their legal guardian must provide informed consent for all treatment the patient receives. This includes a thorough explanation of all procedures and treatment and associated risks. Patients/guardians should be apprised of all options and allowed to have input on the decision-making process. They should be apprised of all reasonable risks and any complications that might be life threatening or increase morbidity. The American Medical Association has established **guidelines for obtaining informed consent:**

- Explanation of the diagnosis
- Nature and reason for the treatment or procedure
- Risks and benefits of the treatment or procedure
- Alternative options (regardless of cost or insurance coverage)
- Risks and benefits of alternative options, including no treatment

Obtaining informed consent is a requirement in all states; however, a patient may waive their right to informed consent. If this is the case, the nurse should document the patient's waiving of this right and proceed with the procedure. Informed consent is not necessary for procedures performed to save life or limb in which the patient or guardian is unable to consent.

CONFIDENTIALITY

Confidentiality is the obligation that is present in a professional-patient relationship. Nurses are under an obligation to protect the information they possess concerning the patient and family. Care should be taken to safeguard that information and provide the privacy that the family deserves. This is accomplished through the use of required passwords when family calls for information about the patient and through the limitation of who is allowed to visit. There may be times when confidentiality must be broken to save the life of a patient, but those circumstances are rare. The nurse must make all efforts to safeguard patient records and identification. Computerized record keeping should be done in such a way that the screen is not visible to others, and paper records must be secured.

REGULATION OF NURSING BY STATES' NURSE PRACTICE ACT

Each state's **nurse practice act** seeks to regulate nursing within the state. It specifies the amount and type of education required to become an RN or LPN/LVN. It defines the nurse's role and responsibilities in healthcare settings. It lists actions that the nurse may take and defines advanced practice education, experience, responsibilities, and limitations. It gives nurses the authorization to perform as required. It also regulates delegation and supervision responsibilities of the nurse. Nurse practice acts are administrated by the state board of nursing, which is responsible for issuing and renewing nurse licenses as well as discipline and censure of nurses. Most state boards of nursing now have a website that provides state-specific information about licensure and nursing rights and responsibilities.

NURSE'S ACCOUNTABILITY FOR NURSING CARE

Nurses are part of an interdisciplinary team responsible for patient outcomes. Nurses have the responsibility for the outcomes of nursing care as a professional group. This responsibility is outlined in each state's nurse practice act, the American Nurses Association (ANA) practice guidelines, and the nurse's job description. Tools, such as the nursing care plan that includes standardized nursing diagnoses, interventions, and expected outcomes, enable the nurse to fulfill this responsibility. Empowerment to act as the patient advocate allows the nurse to point out factors in the patient's individual situation that can be addressed to further improve outcome. Critical thinking during decision-making and detailed documentation are also important. The nurse is held accountable for delegation as well as supervising care by others and evaluation of the outcomes of that care as well. The nurse has personal **accountability** in terms of ethical and moral conduct. Since clinical knowledge is crucial to critical thinking, the nurse must strive to increase knowledge continuously through professional development throughout his or her career.

ADVANCE DIRECTIVES

In accordance to Federal and state laws, individuals have the right to self-determination in health care, including the right to make decisions about end of life care through **advance directives** such as living wills and the right to assign a surrogate person to make decisions through a durable power of attorney. Patients should routinely be questioned about an advanced directive as they may present at a healthcare provider without the document. Patients who have indicated that they desire a do-not-resuscitate (DNR) order should not receive resuscitative treatments for terminal illness or conditions in which meaningful recovery cannot occur. Patients and families of those with terminal illnesses should be questioned as to whether the patients are Hospice patients. For those with DNR requests or those withdrawing life support, staff should provide the patient palliative rather than curative measures, such as pain control and/or oxygen, and emotional support to the patient and family. Religious traditions and beliefs about death should be treated with respect.

HIPAA

The Health Insurance Portability and Accountability Act (HIPAA) and state laws govern **who may receive healthcare information** about a person, how permission is to be obtained, how the information may be shared, and patients' rights concerning personal information. HIPAA strives to protect the **privacy** of an individual's healthcare information. Facilities must prevent this information from being accessed by unauthorized personnel. Healthcare information is required to be protected on the **administrative**, **physical**, and **technical** levels. The patient must sign a release form to allow any sharing of patient information. There are stiff penalties for violation of these laws, ranging from $100 for an unintentional violation to nearly $70,000 for a willful violation. Facilities that violate HIPAA may also be subject to corrective actions. Penalties are governed by the Department of Health and Human Services' Office for Civil Right and the state attorneys general.

APPLICATION OF HIPAA TO PRACTICE

As an integral member of the health care team, the nurse must always be aware of HIPAA regulations and apply this knowledge to practice. The nurse is responsible for the following efforts to protect and maintain patient privacy:

- The nurse must read and follow facility policies regarding the transfer of patient data.
- Communication between health care personnel about a patient should always be in a private place so that this information is not overheard by those who do not have the right to share the information.
- Access to charts must be restricted to only those health care team members involved in that patient's care.
- Patient care information for unlicensed workers cannot be posted at the bedside, but must be on a care plan or the patient chart in a protected area.
- The nurse must not give information casually to anyone (e.g., visitors or family members) unless it is confirmed that they have the right to have that information.
- Family members must not be relied upon to interpret for the patient; an interpreter must be obtained to protect patient privacy.
- Computers with patient information must have passwords and safeguards to prevent unauthorized access of patient information.
- The nurse should not leave voicemail messages containing protected healthcare information for a patient but should instead ask the patient to call back.

> **Review Video: HIPAA**
> Visit mometrix.com/academy and enter code: 412009

OSHA

The **Occupational Safety and Health Act (OSHA)** seeks to keep workers safe and healthy while on the job. OSHA mandates that employers maintain a safe environment, workers are made fully aware of any hazards, and that access to personal protective gear is made available to workers who come into contact with hazardous materials. By following these regulations, an employer keeps injury and illness of workers to an absolute minimum. This fosters productivity, since workers are not absent due to illness or injury, employee health costs are contained, and the turnover rate is decreased, saving money spent on hiring and training new employees. OSHA is concerned about healthcare employee exposure to radiation, as well as chemical and biological agents, when caring for patients. Information is available to help hospitals and other facilities write plans that comply with best practices to deal with this and other threats to employees. Cleaning procedures, decontamination, and hazardous waste disposal are all covered by OSHA and apply to everyday hospital operation as well as disaster situations.

> **Review Video: Intro to OSHA**
> Visit mometrix.com/academy and enter code: 913559

CMS

The **Centers for Medicare and Medicaid (CMS)**, part of the U.S. Department of Health and Human Service department, see to it that healthcare regulations are observed by healthcare facilities that receive federal reimbursement. They reimburse facilities for care given to Medicare, Medicaid, and the state Children's Health Insurance Program (CHIP) recipients. They also monitor adherence to HIPAA regulations concerning healthcare information portability and confidentiality. CMS examines documentation of patient care when deciding to reimburse for care given. CMS has regulations for all types of medical facilities, and these regulations have profoundly impacted nursing practice because nurses must ensure that they comply with regulations related to the quality of patient care and concerns regarding cost-containment. Each facility should provide guidelines to assist nursing staff in meeting the specific documentation requirements of CMS.

ETHICAL PRINCIPLES

Autonomy is the ethical principle that the individual has the right to make decisions about his or her own care. In the case of children or patients with dementia who cannot make autonomous decisions, parents or family members may serve as the legal decision maker. The nurse must keep the patient and/or family fully informed so that they can exercise their autonomy in informed decision-making.

Justice is the ethical principle that relates to the distribution of the limited resources of healthcare benefits to the members of society. These resources must be distributed fairly. This issue may arise if there is only one bed left and two sick patients. Justice comes into play in deciding which patient should stay and which should be transported or otherwise cared for. The decision should be made according to what is best or most just for the patients and not colored by personal bias.

Beneficence is an ethical principle that involves performing actions that are for the purpose of benefitting another person. In the care of a patient, any procedure or treatment should be done with the ultimate goal of benefitting the patient, and any actions that are not beneficial should be reconsidered. As conditions change, procedures need to be continually reevaluated to determine if they are still of benefit.

Nonmaleficence is an ethical principle that means healthcare workers should provide care in a manner that does not cause direct intentional harm to the patient:

- The actual act must be good or morally neutral.
- The intent must be only for a good effect.
- A bad effect cannot serve as the means to get to a good effect.
- A good effect must have more benefit than a bad effect has harm.

NURSING CODE OF ETHICS

There is more interest in the **ethics** involved in healthcare due to technological advances that have made the prolongation of life, organ transplants, prenatal manipulation, and saving of premature infants possible, sometimes with poor outcomes. Couple these with healthcare's limited resources, and **ethical dilemmas** abound. Ethics is the study of **morality** as the value that controls actions. The American Nurses Association Code of Ethics contains nine statements defining **principles** the nurse can use when faced with moral and ethical problems. Nurses must be knowledgeable about the many ethical issues in healthcare and about the field of ethics in general. The nurse must help a patient to reveal their values and morals to the health care team so that the patient, family, and team can resolve moral issues pertaining to the patient's care. As part of the healthcare team, the nurse has a right to express personal values and moral concerns about medical issues.

Cardiovascular Procedures and Interventions

CARDIOVERSION

Cardioversion sends a timed electrical stimulation to the heart to convert a tachydysrhythmia (such as atrial fibrillation) to a normal sinus rhythm. Usually, anticoagulation therapy is done for at least 3 weeks prior to elective cardioversion to reduce the risk of emboli, and digoxin is discontinued for at least 48 hours prior. During the procedure, the patient is usually sedated and/or anesthetized. Electrodes in the form of gel-covered paddles or pads are placed in the anteroposterior position and then connected by leads to a computerized ECG and cardiac monitor with a defibrillator. The defibrillator is synchronized with the ECG so that the electrical current is delivered during ventricular depolarization (QRS). The timing must be precise in order to prevent ventricular tachycardia or ventricular fibrillation. Sometimes, drug therapy is used in conjunction with cardioversion; for example, antiarrhythmics (Cardizem, Cordarone) may be given before the procedure to slow the heart rate.

Arrhythmia	Beginning Monophasic Shock	Beginning Biphasic Shock
Atrial Fibrillation	100 J	70 J
Atrial Flutter	50–100 J	50 J
Ventricular Tachycardia	100 J	75 J

EMERGENCY DEFIBRILLATION

Emergency defibrillation delivers a non-synchronized shock that is given to treat acute ventricular fibrillation, pulseless ventricular tachycardia, or polymorphic ventricular tachycardia with a rapid rate and decompensating hemodynamics. **Defibrillation** can be given at any point in the cardiac cycle. It causes depolarization of myocardial cells, which can then repolarize to regain a normal sinus rhythm. Defibrillation delivers an electrical discharge through pads/paddles. In an acute care setting, the preferred position to place the pads is the anteroposterior position. In this position, one pad is placed to the right of the sternum about the second to third intercostal space, and the other pad is placed between the left scapula and the spinal column. This decreases the chances of damaging implanted devices, such as pacemakers, and this positioning has also been shown to be more effective for external cardioversion (if indicated at some point during resuscitation). There are two main types of defibrillator shock waveforms: monophasic and biphasic. Biphasic defibrillators deliver a shock in one direction for half of the shock, and then in the return direction for the other half, making them more effective and able to be used at lower energy levels. Monophasic defibrillation is given at 200–360 J and biphasic defibrillation is given at 100–200 J.

CARDIOVERSION AND EMERGENCY DEFIBRILLATION DOSES FOR CHILDREN

The initial dose for cardioversion in a pediatric patient is 0.5–1.0 J/kg, doubled for subsequent doses if ineffective. The timing must be precise in order to prevent ventricular tachycardia or ventricular fibrillation. Sometimes, drug therapy is used in conjunction with cardioversion; for example, antiarrhythmics may be given before the procedure to slow the heart rate. Complications include dysrhythmias, burns, and injury to the myocardium. If ventricular fibrillation occurs, asynchronous shock is used.

The initial dose for emergency defibrillation in children is 2 J/kg, causing depolarization of myocardial cells, which can then repolarize to regain a normal sinus rhythm. Defibrillation delivers an electrical discharge usually through paddles applied to both sides of the chest. If the first shock and 2 minutes of CPR are ineffective, the dose is increased to 4 J/kg and 2 minutes of CPR and repeated if it is still ineffective.

AHA Pediatric Advanced Life Support Guidelines for Cardiac Emergencies

Cardiac Arrest

AHA Pediatric Advanced Life Support guidelines for **cardiac arrest** include:

- **Begin CPR** (30:2 for single rescuer and 15:2 for multiple) at rate of 100-120 compressions/minute and ventilate with oxygen if available. Maintain airway. Obtain IV/IO access when possible. If arrest is witnessed, obtain an AED/defibrillator immediately. If unwitnessed, begin first with compressions (CAB protocol) for 2 minutes and then obtain the AED/defibrillator and use it as soon as possible.
- **Shockable rhythm**: Defibrillate at 2 J/kg and resume CPR for 2 minutes, check rhythm, if necessary, defibrillate at 4 J/kg and continue CPR for 2 minutes. Obtain IV/IO access. Administer epinephrine 0.01 mg/kg IV/OI of a concentration of 1 g per 10,000 mL (1:10,000) every 3-5 minutes during resuscitative efforts. Continue to alternate CPR and defibrillation. The nurse may administer amiodarone 5 mg/kg up to two dosage or lidocaine 1 mg/kg.
- **Non-shockable rhythm**: Continue CPR at rate of 30 compressions:2 breaths (single rescuer) or 15:2 (multiple rescuers) and administer epinephrine 0.01 mg/kg IV/IO of 1:10,000 every 3-5 minutes.

If possible, identify the cause of the cardiac arrest and attempt treatment to reverse.

> **Review Video: Pediatric Advanced Life Support**
> Visit mometrix.com/academy and enter code: 141388

Symptomatic Tachycardia

Treatment for pediatric tachycardia depends on the type of tachycardia. The child's airway should be maintained, and respirations should be assisted with oxygen and ventilation as needed and application of cardiac monitoring, vital signs, and oxygen saturation as well as IV/IO access. A 12-lead ECG should be obtained as soon as possible although treatment should not be delayed in order to obtain the ECG:

- **Probable sinus tachycardia** (P waves normal, variable R-R, PR constant, heart rate <220 for infants and <180 for children): Identify and treat cause.
- **Probable supraventricular tachycardia** (P waves missing/abnormal, heartrate ≥220 for infants and ≥180 for children): If IV/IO is available, adenosine per rapid bolus 0.1 mg/kg (maximum 6 mg); second dose 0.2 mg/kg (maximum 12 mg). If IV/IO is unavailable or medications are ineffective, use synchronized cardioversion.
- **Possible ventricular tachycardia with cardiopulmonary compromise** (hypotension, signs of shock, altered mental status): Synchronized cardioversion is indicated. If cardiopulmonary compromise is not evident and rhythm is regular and QRS is monomorphic, then one may administer adenosine IO/IV as for probable supraventricular tachycardia.

If synchronized cardioversion carried out, it should begin with 0.5-1.0 J/kg, increasing to 2 J/kg if ineffective.

SYMPTOMATIC BRADYCARDIA

When a child presents with symptomatic bradycardia, the first step is to maintain a patent airway and assist with respirations as needed, including administration of oxygen and ventilation and application of cardiac monitoring, vital signs, and oxygen saturation as well as IV/IO access. A 12-lead ECG should be obtained as soon as possible, although treatment should not be delayed in order to obtain the ECG. Indications of cardiopulmonary compromise include hypotension, signs of shock (pallor, cool clammy skin), and altered mental status. If heart rate persists below 60 beats per minute with continued poor perfusion despite interventions, then medications should be administered:

- Epinephrine (IV/IO) 0.01 mg/kg of 1:10,000 concentration. May repeat every 3-5 minutes. Alternately, if IV/IO access is unavailable and an ET is in place, then epinephrine may be administered per the ET tube at 0.1 mg/kg of 1:1000 concentration.
- Atropine (IV/IO) 0.02 mg/kg (minimum dose 0.2 mg and maximum single dose 0.5 mg). May repeat one time. Indicated for increased vagal tone or primary atrioventricular block.

For pulseless arrest, treatment for cardiac arrest is instituted.

Gastrointestinal Procedures and Interventions

NG TUBES, SUMP TUBES, AND LEVIN TUBES

Nasogastric **(NG) tubes** are plastic or vinyl tubes inserted through the nose, down the esophagus, and into the stomach. **Sump tubes** are radiopaque with a vent lumen to prevent a vacuum from forming with high suction. **Levin tubes** have no vent lumen and are used only with low suction. NG tubes drain gastric secretions, allow sampling of secretions, or provide access to the stomach and upper GI tract. They are used for lavage after medication overdose, for decompression, and for instillation of medications or fluids. NG tubes are contraindicated with obstruction proximal to the stomach or gastric pathology, such as hemorrhage.

Tube-insertion length is estimated: earlobe to xiphoid + earlobe to nose tip + 15 cm.

The tube is inserted through the naris with the patient upright, if possible, and swallowing sips of water. Vasoconstrictors and topical anesthetic reduce gag reflex. Placement is checked with insufflation of air or aspiration of stomach contents and verified by x-ray. The NG is secured and drainage bag provided. Tubes attached to continuous low or intermittent high suction must be monitored frequently.

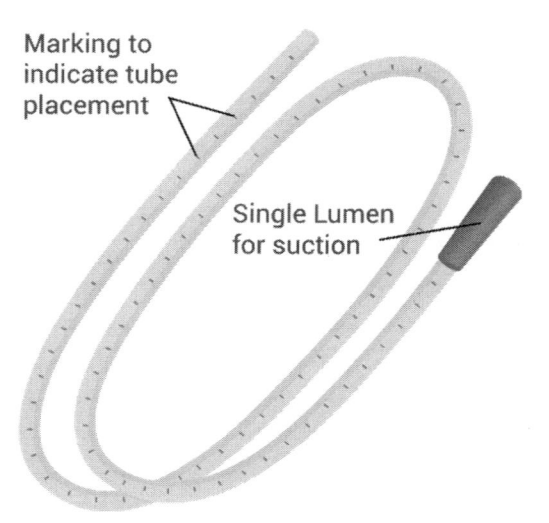

Levin Tube

PEG TUBE

Percutaneous endoscopic gastrostomy (PEG), used for tube feedings, involves intubation of the esophagus with the endoscope and insertion of a sheathed needle with a guidewire through the abdomen and stomach wall so that a catheter can be fed down the esophagus, snared, and pulled out through the opening where the needle was inserted and secured. The PEG tube should not be secured to the abdomen until the PEG is fully healed, which usually takes 2–4 weeks, because tension caused by taping the tube against the abdomen may cause the tract to change shape and direction. The tract should be straight to facilitate insertion and removal of catheters. Once the tract has healed, the original PEG tube can generally be replaced with a balloon gastrostomy tube. External stabilizing devices can be applied to the skin to hold the tube in place but should be placed 1–2 cm above the skin surface to prevent excessive tension that may result in buried bumper syndrome (BBS) in which the internal fixation device becomes lodged in the mucosal lining of the gastric wall, resulting in ulceration.

DRAINS

The following are different types of drains a patient may have, including pertinent nursing considerations:

- **Simple drains** are latex or vinyl tubes of varying sizes/lengths. They are usually placed through a stab wound near the area of involvement.
- **Penrose drains** are flat, soft rubber/latex tubes placed in surgical wounds to drain fluid by gravity and capillary action.

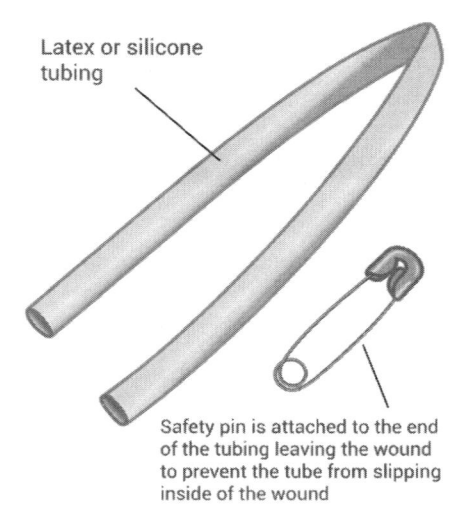

- **Sump drains** are double-lumen or tri-lumen tubes (with a third lumen for infusions). The multiple lumens produce venting when air enters the inflow lumen and forces drainage out of the large lumen.
- **A percutaneous drainage catheter** is inserted into the wound to provide continuous drainage for infection/fluid collection. Irrigation of the catheter may be required to maintain patency. Skin barriers and pouching systems may also be necessary.

SAFE PERCUTANEOUS DRAINAGE KIT

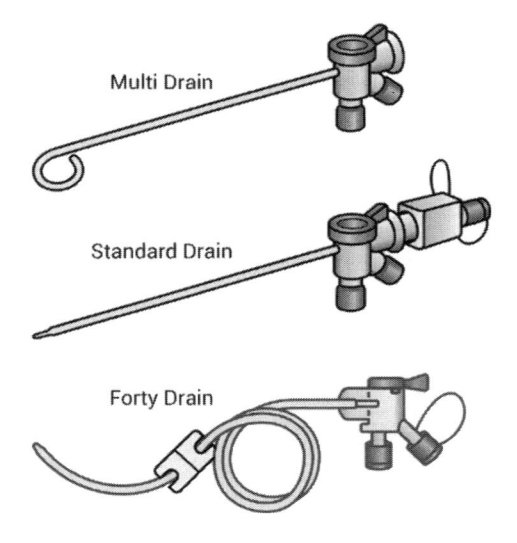

- **Closed drainage systems** use low-pressure suction to provide continuous gravity drainage of wounds. Drains are attached to collapsible suction reservoirs that provide negative pressure. The nurse must remember to always re-establish negative pressure after emptying these drains. There are two types in frequent use:
  - *Jackson-Pratt is* a bulb-type drain that is about the size of a lemon. A thin plastic drain from the wound extends to a squeeze bulb that can hold about 100 mL of drainage.

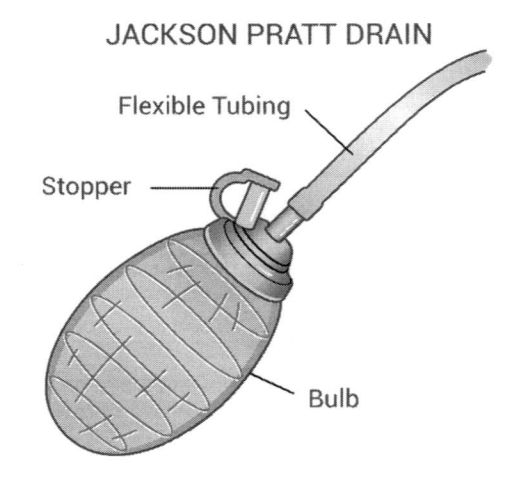

JACKSON PRATT DRAIN

Flexible Tubing

Stopper

Bulb

  - *Hemovac* is a round drain with coiled springs inside that are compressed after emptying to create suction. The device can hold up to 500 mL of drainage.

ENTERAL SUPPORT AND PARENTERAL SUPPORT

Enteral nutrition is a method of providing nutrition to a patient through a tube; the tube may be placed in either the nose (a nasogastric tube), the stomach (a percutaneous endoscopic gastrostomy [PEG] tube), or the small bowel (a percutaneous endoscopic jejunal [J] tube). When the tube has been placed, nutrition can be administered through the tube and absorbed by the patient's digestive system. Various **enteric formulas** exist, and the choice is dependent on the nutritional requirements of the patient.

Parenteral nutrition (also called total parenteral nutrition [**TPN**]) is a method of providing nutrition that completely bypasses the digestive system by administering nutrition through an intravenous line. Enteral support is the preferred method of providing nutrition, although in patients suffering from some compromise of the gastrointestinal tract, parenteral nutrition is the only option.

TROUBLE-SHOOTING PROBLEMS RELATED TO ENTERAL FEEDINGS

Feeding tubes are commonly found in the critical care setting, as many patients are intubated and unable to take oral nutrition or medication. General maintenance involves checking placement before flushing anything into the tube (prevents aspiration), flushing the tubes with at least 30 mL of water before and after use, and every 4 hours. Never crush enteric-coated medications, and keep the HOB inclined at least 30° at all times during feeding. **Complications** include:

- **Vomiting/aspiration:** Caused by incorrect placement, gastric emptying, and/or formula intolerance.
    - Treatment: Confirm placement by checking pH (preferred to air bolus); delay feeding one hour and check residual volume before resuming. Refrigerate formula, check expiration, and use only for 24 hours.
- **Diarrhea:** Caused by rapid feeding, antibiotics/medications, intolerance of formula or hypertonic formula, and/or tube migration.
    - Treatment: Reduce rate of feeding, evaluate medications, avoid hanging feedings longer than 8 hours, and add fiber or decrease sodium in the feed.
- **Displacement of tube:**
    - Treatment: For NG tube, replace using the other nostril, only if not surgically placed. For G-tube or J-tube, cover the site and notify the physician.
    - Prevention: secure all tubes with the appropriate device and mark placement to identify migration.
- **Tube occlusion:**
    - Treatment: Check for kinks and obvious problems. Aspirate fluid, instill warm water, and aspirate to loosen occlusion. The physician may order an enzyme or sodium bicarb solution.

ENTERAL FEEDINGS

Caloric and nutritional needs for **enteral feedings** are assessed according to the age of the child, size, and stress factors. Breast milk is the optimal nutrition for infants. Feedings may be adjusted because of needs associated with diseases; for example, children with HF may require fluid restriction. Formula usually contains 24–30 calories per ounce. **Caloric requirements** are based on the recommended daily allowance (RDA) and resting energy expenditure (REE), the calories needed for a child at rest.

Age	RDA (kcal/kg/day)	REE (kcal/kg/day)	Protein (g/kg/day)
6-12 months	80	55	2.0-2.5
1-3 years	80-100	50-57	1.2-3.0
4-6 years	70-90	45-48	1.1-3.0
7-10 years	60-70	40	1.0-3.0
11-13 years	45-55	28-32	1.0-2.5
14-18 years	36-45	25-27	0.8-1.2

Total energy expenditure (TEE) is calculated by multiplying the REE by stress factors:

Maintenance: 0.2
Activity: 0.1-0.25
Fever: 0.13 per degree >38 °C
Burns: 0.5-1.0

Simple trauma: 0.2
Sepsis/major trauma: 0.4-1.5
Ventilation/sedation: 1.2-1.3
Growth: 0.5

Nasogastric and Orogastric Enteral Feeding Tubes

Nasogastric/orogastric enteral feeding tubes can be inserted quickly and nonsurgically but are usually reserved for short-term (<3 months) enteral feedings. A weighted or non-weighted catheter (5-8 Fr) is used. The length of insertion can be calculated using age-related height-based measurement or measuring the distance from the nose tip to the earlobe and from the earlobe to the midpoint between the xiphoid process and the umbilicus.

1. Mark the insertion length on the tube.
2. Explain the procedure in age-appropriate terms.
3. Check nares for patency, assess gag reflex, and note any contraindications (such as basal skull fracture with NG tubes).
4. Secure the child in supine position (swaddling, holding) with head elevated to 30–45°.
5. Lubricate tube or dip in water for pre-lubricated tubes.
6. Insert the tube into the mouth or nostril, aiming posteriorly and inferiorly.
7. When the NG/OG tube is in the pharynx, instruct the child to swallow or stimulate swallowing with use of pacifier.
8. Insert to the marking on the tube and temporarily secure.
9. Verify placement with radiograph.

Gastrointestinal Feeding Tubes Placement

Feeding tubes can be placed surgically, endoscopically, or radiologically:

- **Surgical placement**: There are both open and laparoscopic surgical techniques for placing tubes to the stomach or jejunum. The three most common methods are the Janeway, the Stamm, and the Witzel techniques.
- **Endoscopic placement**: Percutaneous endoscopic gastrostomy (PEG) involves intubation of the esophagus with the endoscope and insertion of a sheathed needle with a guidewire through the abdomen and stomach wall so that a catheter can be fed down the esophagus, snared, and pulled out through the opening where the needle was inserted and secured. Similar endoscopic procedures can be done in the jejunum.
- **Radiologic placement**: Through fluoroscopy, ultrasound and/or CT, a gastrostomy tube is inserted through the epigastrium and secured with a balloon and external bumper or disk. Insertion into the jejunum is done in a similar manner through the duodenum into the jejunum. A gastrojejunostomy tube, which both drains the stomach and feeds the jejunum, is another procedure.

Preventing Displacement of Enteral Feeding Tubes

The displacement of an enteral feeding tube is usually the result of inadequate stabilization. Foley catheters must be marked where they exit the stoma to check for migration. Gastrostomy tubes with an internal balloon or mushroom tip, measured markings, and an external disk are easier to stabilize, but the internal device should be checked daily by gently pulling until resistance is felt. External stabilizing devices can be applied to the skin to hold the tube in place. The tube may also be taped to the abdomen or secured with a binder. Sometimes surgeons suture the tube in place, especially those with no balloon, such as jejunostomy tubes, which can become easily dislodged. A solid skin barrier with the tube fed through an anchored baby nipple is an inexpensive stabilizer. The position and length of the tube should be carefully documented. Balloon volume should be checked weekly to insure there are no leaks. Skin beneath disks/bumpers should be checked frequently.

PREVENTING AND TREATING OCCLUSION OF ENTERAL FEEDING TUBES

Prevention of occlusion of enteral feeding tubes involves proper administration of medications and feedings, and maintaining a regular schedule of flushing. Tubes should be flushed with 5–30 ml of water (depending on the age and size of the child) at least every 4 hours as well as before and after feedings and administration of medications. Medications should be in liquid form or crushed completely and enteric-coated or delayed release preparations should be avoided. Feeding solutions should be liquid consistency. The child should be positioned with head elevated for feedings.

Flushing of an occluded tube involves first checking for kinks or obvious problems, attaching a 20–30 mL syringe and aspirating fluid. Then, 5–10 mL of water or carbonated beverage (ginger ale, cola) can be slowly instilled (over about a minute) and aspirated a number of times to try to loosen the occlusion. After clamping for 10–15 minutes, the flushing procedure can be repeated with warm water/carbonated beverage. If the water or carbonated beverage fails, a multi-enzyme cocktail or Pancrease and sodium bicarbonate solution may succeed. If all flushing fails, the physician should be notified.

ADDITIONAL COMPLICATIONS

Additional complications of enteral feedings include:

Complication	Causes	Solutions
Vomiting/aspiration	Tube incorrectly placed Delayed gastric emptying Contaminated formula Increased residual volume	Check tube position Elevate head of bed 30-45° or have the child sit in a chair Refrigerate formula, check dates, and discard after 24 hours Delay feeding one hour and check residual volume before resuming
Diarrhea	Rapid feeding Medications (e.g., antibiotics) Contaminated formula Distal movement of tube Lactose intolerance Low-fiber/hypertonic formula	Slow rate of feeding or use continuous drip Change tubing every 24 hours and avoid hanging feedings for more than 4 hours Evaluate medications Check position of tube before feedings Change formula (add fiber, decrease sodium)
Constipation	Inadequate fluids Fecal impaction Medications Formula	Increase fluids, according to age/size Manual examination for fecal impaction Evaluate medications Consult dietitian regarding formula
Dehydration	Diarrhea/vomiting High protein formula Poor fluid intake Hyperosmotic diuresis	Treat same as for diarrhea/vomiting Consult dietitian for change in formula Increase fluids Monitor blood glucose levels

Esophagogastroduodenoscopy

Esophagogastroduodenoscopy (EGD), which is performed with a flexible fiberscope equipped with a lighted fiberoptic lens, allows direct inspection of the mucosa of the esophagus, stomach, and duodenum. The scope has a still or video camera attached to a monitor for viewing during the procedure. The scope may be used for biopsies or therapeutically to dilate strictures or treat gastric or esophageal bleeding. The child is positioned on the left side (head supported) to allow saliva drainage. Conscious sedation (midazolam, propofol) is commonly used along with a topical anesthetic spray or gargle to facilitate placing the lubricated tube through the mouth into the esophagus. Atropine reduces secretions. A bite guard in the mouth prevents the older children from biting the scope. The airway must be carefully monitored through the procedure (which usually takes about 30 minutes), including oximeter to measure oxygen saturation. While perforation, bleeding, or infection may occur, most complications are cardiopulmonary in nature and relate to drugs (conscious sedation) used during the procedure, so reversal agents (flumazenil, naloxone) should be available.

Fundoplication Surgery

Fundoplication, in which part of the fundus of the stomach (the upper portion) is wrapped either completely or partially around the distal esophagus and then sutured, is the third most common surgery for children. It is done to prevent regurgitation and strengthen the lower esophageal sphincter. When the stomach contracts, this shuts the sphincter, preventing backflow of gastric contents into the esophagus. This procedure is done for children with congenital abnormalities of the esophagus and for those with gastroesophageal reflux, if they do not respond to medical treatment. It is also a common repair after infants have had gastrostomy tubes inserted, damaging the sphincter. There are a number of different procedures, but all are basically variations of the Nissen procedure, which involves a full 360° wrap of the esophagus. In recent years, most procedures have been done with laparoscopy, allowing for small abdominal incisions and less recovery time.

Hernia Repair

Hernia repair (herniorrhaphy) is the most common surgery for infants and children and is done to repair herniation of the peritoneum and a segment of bowel through the abdominal wall. Surgery is necessary to prevent an incarcerated hernia, in which the bowel twists and blood supply is compromised. There are three main types:

- **Inguinal**: Herniation in the inguinal canal. This is common in premature or low birth-weight infants, usually males, and may occur bilaterally.
- **Femoral**: Herniation posterior to the inguinal ligament. This is more common in females.
- **Umbilical**: Herniation in the umbilical ring.

Inguinal and femoral hernias are usually repaired as soon as possible because of the danger of incarceration. Umbilical hernias pose less concern and often heal over time without surgical repair, so surgery for umbilical hernias is rarely done prior to school age. If incarceration has occurred prior to surgery, the affected segment of bowel is resected. Surgery may be done laparoscopically.

Genitourinary Procedures and Interventions

PROCEDURES FOR INSERTION AND REMOVAL OF URINARY CATHETER

Procedure for inserting and removing a urinary catheter:

1. Gather supplies (included in a urinary catheter insertion kit), perform hand hygiene, place a waterproof pad under the patient, and ensure that the light source is adequate to view the urinary meatus.
2. Place females in supine position with knees flexed and males in supine position.
3. Apply gloves and wash the perineal area with facility provided cleanser (sometimes included in the outside of the urinary catheter kit) and allow to dry.
4. Remove gloves and wash hands.
5. Using aseptic technique, place the catheter kit between the patient's legs, open the kit touching only the corners of the drape that wraps around the kit.
6. Apply sterile gloves.
7. Apply sterile drapes to the patient.
8. Following the steps provided with the kit, place the lubricant into the appropriate section of tray, remove the catheter from its plastic and place the tip into the lubricant, and pour iodine over the three cleansing swabs (if they do not come impregnated with iodine already). Attach the 10-cc syringe (filled with sterile water) to the appropriate port of the catheter.
9. Cleanse the urethral meatus with the iodine impregnated swabs.
10. Using the nondominant hand, hold the penis or open the labia to observe the urethral meatus. This hand now becomes "dirty" and cannot be used to touch the catheter.
11. Using the dominant hand, insert catheter with the drainage end attached to the collection bag. Insert until urine flows freely, advancing a little further after that point.
12. Inflate the balloon using the 10-cc sterile water syringe, and ensure the catheter is secure.
13. Secure the catheter to the patient's leg and hang the collection bag below the level of the patient. Secure any tubing to the bed and ensure no kinking is present.

Removal: Straight catheter—remove by pulling out slowly. To remove indwelling catheter, deflate the balloon using the appropriate port and gently pull the catheter out.

REDUCING INFECTION RISKS ASSOCIATED WITH URINARY CATHETERS

Strategies for reducing infection risks associated with urinary catheters include:

- Using **aseptic technique** for both the straight and indwelling catheter insertion
- **Limiting catheter use** by establishing protocols for use, duration, and removal; training staff; issuing reminders to physicians; using straight catheterizations rather than indwelling; using ultrasound to scan the bladder; and using condom catheters
- Utilizing **closed-drainage systems** for indwelling catheters
- **Avoiding irrigation** unless required for diagnosis or treatment
- Using **sampling port** for specimens rather than disconnecting catheter and tubing
- Maintaining **proper urinary flow** by proper positioning, securing of tubing and drainage bag, and keeping the drainage bag below the level of the bladder
- **Changing catheters** only when medically needed
- **Cleansing external meatal area** gently each day, manipulating the catheter as little as possible
- Avoiding placing catheterized patients adjacent to those infected or colonized with antibiotic-resistant bacteria to reduce **cross-contamination**

Renal Dialysis
Peritoneal Dialysis

Renal dialysis is used primarily for those who have progressed from renal insufficiency to uremia with end-stage renal disease (ESRD). It may also be temporarily for acute conditions. People can be maintained on dialysis, but there are many complications associated with dialysis, so many people are considered for renal transplantation. There are a number of different approaches to **peritoneal dialysis:**

- **Peritoneal dialysis:** An indwelling catheter is inserted surgically into the peritoneal cavity with a subcutaneous tunnel and a Dacron cuff to prevent infection. Sterile dialysate solution is slowly instilled through gravity, remains for a prescribed length of time, and is then drained and discarded.
- **Continuous ambulatory peritoneal dialysis:** a series of exchange cycles is repeated 24 hours a day.
- **Continuous cyclic peritoneal dialysis:** a prolonged period of retaining fluid occurs during the day with drainage at night.

Peritoneal dialysis may be used for those who want to be more independent, don't live near a dialysis center, or want fewer dietary restrictions.

> **Review Video: End-Stage Renal Disease**
> Visit mometrix.com/academy and enter code: 869617

Hemodialysis

Hemodialysis, the most common type of dialysis, is used for both short-term dialysis and long-term for those with ESRD. Treatments are usually done three times weekly for 3–4 hours or daily dialysis with treatment either during the night or in short daily periods. **Hemodialysis** is often done for those who can't manage peritoneal dialysis or who live near a dialysis center, but it does interfere with work or school attendance and requires strict dietary and fluid restrictions between treatments. Short daily dialysis allows more independence, and increased costs may be offset by lower morbidity. A vascular access device, such as a catheter, fistula, or graft, must be established for hemodialysis, and heparin is used to prevent clotting. With hemodialysis, blood is circulated outside of the body through a dialyzer (a synthetic semipermeable membrane), which filters the blood. There are many different types of dialyzers. High flux dialyzers use a highly permeable membrane that shortens the duration of treatment and decreases the need for heparin.

Dialysis Complications

There are many complications associated with dialysis, especially when used for long-term treatment:

- **Hemodialysis:** Long-term use promotes atherosclerosis and cardiovascular disease. Anemia and fatigue are common, as are infections related to access devices or contamination of equipment. Some experience hypotension and muscle cramping during treatment. Dysrhythmias may occur. Some may exhibit dialysis disequilibrium from cerebral fluid shifts, causing headaches, nausea and vomiting, and alterations of consciousness.
- **Peritoneal dialysis:** Most complications are minor, but it can lead to peritonitis, which requires removal of the catheter if antibiotic therapy is not successful in clearing the infection within 4 days. There may be leakage of the dialysate around the catheter. Bleeding may occur, especially in females who are menstruating as blood is pulled from the uterus through the fallopian tubes. Abdominal hernias may occur with long use. Some may have anorexia from the feeling of fullness or a sweet taste in the mouth from the absorption of glucose.

BLADDER TRAINING

Bladder training usually requires the person to keep a toileting diary for at least three days so patterns can be assessed. There are a number of different approaches:

- **Scheduled toileting** is toileting on a regular schedule, usually every 2-4 hours during the daytime.
- **Habit training** involves an attempt to match the scheduled toileting to a person's individual voiding habits, based on the toileting diary. This is useful for people who have a natural and fairly consistent voiding pattern. Toileting is done every 2-4 hours.
- **Prompted voiding** is often used in nursing homes and attempts to teach people to assess their own incontinence status and prompts them to ask for toileting.
- **Bladder retraining** is a behavioral modification program that teaches people to inhibit the urge to urinate and to urinate according to an established schedule, restoring normal bladder function as much as possible. Bladder training can improve incontinence in 80% of cases.

PROMPTED VOIDING

Prompted voiding is a communication protocol for people with mild to moderate **cognitive impairment**. It uses positive reinforcement for recognizing being wet or dry, staying dry, urinating, and drinking liquids.

- Ask patient **every two hours** (8 a.m. to 4-8 p.m.) whether they are wet or dry.
- Verify if they are correct and give **feedback**, "You are right, Mrs. Brown, you are dry."
- **Prompt** patient, whether wet or dry, to use the toilet or urinal. If yes, assist them, record results, and give positive reinforcement by praising and visiting for a short time. If no, repeat the request again once or twice. If they are wet, and decline toileting, change and tell them you will return in two hours and ask them to try to wait to urinate until then.
- Offer **liquids** and record amount.
- **Record** results of each attempt to urinate or wet check.

BLADDER RETRAINING

Bladder retraining teaches people to control the urge to urinate. It usually takes about three months to rehabilitate a bladder muscle weakened from frequent urination, causing a decreased urinary capacity. A short urination interval is gradually lengthened to every 2-4 hours during the daytime as the person suppresses bladder urges and stays dry.

- The patient keeps a **urination diary** for a week.
- An individual program is established with **scheduled voiding times and goals**. For example, if a patient is urinating every hour, the goal might be every 80 minutes with increased output.
- The patient is taught **techniques** to withhold urination, such as sitting on a hard seat or on a tightly rolled towel to put pressure on pelvic floor muscles, doing five squeezes of pelvic floor muscles, deep breathing, and counting backward from 50.
- When the patient consistently meets the goal, a **new goal** is established.

THE KNACK TO CONTROL URINARY INCONTINENCE

The **knack** is the use of precisely timed muscle contractions to prevent **stress incontinence**. It is "the knack" of squeezing up before bearing down. The knack is a preventive use of **Kegel exercises**. Women are taught to contract the pelvic floor muscles right before and during events that usually cause stress incontinence. For example, if a woman feels a cough or sneeze coming, she immediately contracts the pelvic floor muscles and holds until the stress event is over. This contraction augments support of the proximal urethra, reducing the amount of displacement that usually takes place with compromised muscle support, thereby preventing incontinence. It is particularly useful if used before and during stress events, such as coughing, sneezing, lifting, standing, swinging a golf club, or laughing. Studies have shown that women who are taught this technique for mild to moderate urinary incontinence and use it consistently are able to decrease incontinence by 73-98%.

Bowel Training

Bowel training for defecation includes keeping a bowel diary to chart progress:

- **Scheduled defecation** is usually daily, but for some people 3-4 times weekly, depending on individual bowel habits. Defecation should be at the same time, so work hours and activities must be considered. Defecation is scheduled for 20-30 minutes after a meal when there is increased motility.
- **Stimulation** is necessary. Drinking a cup of hot liquid may work, but initially many require rectal stimulation, inserting a gloved, lubricated finger into the anus and running it around the rim of the sphincters. Some people require rectal suppositories, such as glycerine. Stimulus suppositories, such as Dulcolax (bisacodyl), or even Fleet enemas are sometimes used, but the goal is to reduce use of medical or chemical stimulants.
- **Position** should be sitting upright with knees elevated slightly if possible and leaning forward during defecation.
- **Straining** includes attempting to tighten abdominal muscles and relax sphincters while defecating.
- **Exercise** increases the motility of the bowel by stimulating muscle contractions. **Walking** is one of the best exercises for this purpose, and the person should try to walk 1 or 2 miles a day. If the person is unable to walk, then other activities, such as chair exercises that involve the arms and legs and bending can be very effective. Those who are bed bound need to turn from side to side frequently and change position.
- **Kegel exercises** increase strength of the pelvic floor muscles. Kegel exercises for urinary incontinence and fecal incontinence are essentially the same, but the person tries to pull in the muscles around the anus, as though trying to prevent the release of stool or flatus. The person should feel the muscles tightening while holding for 2 seconds and then relaxing for 2 seconds, gradually building the holding time to 10 seconds or more. Exercises should be done 4 times a day.

Management Strategies for Constipation and Fecal Impaction

Management strategies for constipation and impaction include:

- **Enemas** and **manual removal of impaction** may be necessary initially.
- Add **fiber** with bran, fresh/dried fruits, and whole grains, to 20-35 grams per day.
- Increase **fluids** to 64 ounces each day.
- **Exercise** program should include walking if possible, and exercises on a daily basis.
- Change in **medications** causing constipation can relieve constipation. Additionally, the use of stool softeners, such as Colace (docusate), or bulk formers, such as Metamucil (psyllium), may decrease fluid absorption and move stool through the colon more quickly. Overuse of laxatives can cause constipation.
- Careful **monitoring** of diet, fluids, and medical treatment, especially for irritable bowel syndrome.
- **Pregnancy-related constipation** may be controlled through dietary and fluid modifications and regular exercise.
- **Delayed toileting** should be avoided and bowel training regimen done to promote evacuation at the same time each day. During travel, stool softeners, increased fluid, and exercise may alleviate constipation.

Purpose of Fiber in the Diet

Most constipation is caused by insufficient **fiber** in the diet, especially if people eat a lot of processed foods. An adequate amount of fiber is 20-30 grams daily. There are both soluble and insoluble forms of fiber, and both add bulk to the stool and are not absorbed into the body. Some foods have both types:

- **Soluble fiber** dissolves in liquids to form a gel-like substance, which is why liquids are so important in conjunction with fiber in the diet. Soluble fiber slows the movement of stool through the gastrointestinal system. Food sources include bananas, potatoes, dried beans, nuts, apples, oranges, and oatmeal.
- **Insoluble fiber** changes little with the digestive process and increases the speed of stool through the colon, so too much can result in diarrhea. Food sources of insoluble fiber include wheat bran, whole grains, seeds, skins of fruits, vegetables, and nuts.

Integumentary Procedures and Interventions

WOUND VACS

Wound vacuum-assisted closure (wound VAC) (i.e., negative pressure wound therapy) uses subatmospheric (negative) pressure with a suction unit and a semi-occlusion vapor-permeable dressing. The suction reduces periwound and interstitial edema, decompressing vessels, improving circulation, stimulating production of new cells, and decreasing colonization of bacteria. Wound VAC also increases the rate of granulation and re-epithelialization to hasten healing. The wound must be debrided of necrotic tissue prior to treatment. Wound VAC is used for a variety of difficult-to-heal wounds, especially those that show less than 30% healing in 4 weeks of post-debridement treatment or those with excessive exudate, including chronic stage II and IV pressure injuries, skin flaps, diabetic ulcer, acute wounds, burns, surgical wound, and those with dehiscence and nonresponsive arterial and venous ulcers. Contraindications include:

- Wound malignancy
- Untreated osteomyelitis
- Exposed blood vessels or organs
- Non-enteric, unexplored fistulas.

Nonadherent porous foam is cut to fit and cover the wound and is secured with occlusive transparent film with an opening cut to accommodate the drainage tube, which is attached to a suction canister in a closed system. The pressure should be set at 75–125 psi and the dressing changed 2–3 times weekly.

PRESSURE REDUCTION SURFACES

Pressure reduction surfaces redistribute pressure to prevent pressure injuries and reduce shear and friction. There are various types of support surfaces for beds, examining tables, operating tables, and chairs. Functions of pressure reduction surfaces include temperature control, moisture control, and friction/shear control. **General use guidelines** include:

- Pressure redistribution support surfaces should be used for patients with stage II, III, and IV pressure injuries, as well as for those that are at risk for developing pressure injuries.
- Chairs should have gel or air support surfaces to redistribute pressure for chair-bound patients, critically ill patients, or those who cannot move independently.
- Support surface material should provide at least an inch of support under areas to be protected when in use to prevent bottoming out. (Check by placing hand palm-up under the overlay below the pressure point.)
- Static support surfaces are appropriate for patients who can change position without increasing pressure to a preexisting pressure injury.
- Dynamic support surfaces are needed for those who need assistance to move or when static pressure devices provide less than an inch of support.

Negative Pressure Wound Therapy

Negative pressure wound therapy is used for slow-healing wounds with large volumes of exudate after debridement is completed, leaving the wound tissue exposed. There are a number of different electrical suction NPWT systems, such as the VAC (vacuum-assisted closure) system and the Versatile I (VI). Application steps include:

- Apply nonadherent porous foam cut to fit and completely cover the wound:
    - Polyurethane (hydrophobic, repelling moisture) is used for all wounds EXCEPT those that are painful, have tunneling or sinus tracts, deep trauma wounds, and wounds needing controlled growth of granulation.
    - Polyvinyl (hydrophilic), is used for all wounds EXCEPT deep wounds with moderate granulation, deep tissue pressure injuries and flaps.
- Secure foam occlusive transparent film.
- Cut opening to accommodate the drainage tube in the dressing and attach drainage tube.
- Attach tube to suction canister, creating closed system.
- Set pressure to 75-125 mmHg, as indicated.
- Change dressings 2-3 times weekly.
- Pediatric patients must be monitored carefully, positions changed at least every 2 hours, and adequate analgesia provided. Patients old enough to understand should be educated about the treatment and the meaning of alarms.

Incision and Drainage

Incision and drainage (I&D) is used to drain localized pockets of purulent material, such as an abscess that is causing pain and inflammation, and has not resolved with other treatment, such as antibiotics. I&D may also be used to drain a hematoma or seroma in some cases. For all I&Ds, position the patient for easy access, use sterile draping and techniques, and cleanse the abscess and 3 inches of surrounding tissue with antiseptic. Procedures:

1. **Furuncle/boil**: Apply field block about abscess (1-2% lidocaine with or without epinephrine), make the incision with #11 scalpel and express purulent material. Obtain cultures. Explore cavity with hemostat and then pack with iodoform gauze with wick protruding and cover with dressing.
2. **Paronychia**: As above. If under nail, use cautery to bore a small hole or remove part of nail to facilitate drainage.
3. **Perianal/ischiorectal abscess**: Place in lithotomy or left lateral position and explore anus/rectum with anoscope or digital exam to determine if there is a fistula present. Freeze the top of the abscess with topical anesthetic (do not use local anesthetic) and incise with a #11 scalpel. Express purulent material and irrigate with NS solution, pack with iodoform gauze with the wick protruding, and cover with dressing.

Suture Removal

Prior to suture removal, examine the suture line to determine the type of stitch. If the sutures are crusted, cleanse with a cotton-tipped applicator and hydrogen peroxide, remove hydrogen peroxide with applicator saturated with NS, and then dry with gauze. Procedure:

1. **Interrupted stitches**: Lift suture with forceps and slide scissors under the suture and clip. Grasp the knotted end with the forceps and pull suture through skin.
2. **Running stitches**: Identify the distal knotted end and lift with forceps if necessary and cut off the knot. Pull the sutures out by grasping the knot at the proximal end with the forceps and gently pulling.
3. **Closed and loop sutures or those in awkward anatomic locations**: Lift the suture with forceps and slide a #11 scalpel flat against the skin and under the suture, cutting the suture with the edge of the scalpel. Grasp the knotted end with the forceps and pull the suture through the skin.

Following suture removal, if the suture line appears weak or gaps appear, apply Steri-strips.

STAPLE REMOVAL

Staples should be removed within 7-10 days for staples in the limbs, hands, feet, and trunk, in 3-5 days for the face/neck, and 5-7 days for the ear or scalp as prolonged staple closure may result in scarring and increased risk of infection. Prior to staple removal, examine the staples and wipe with alcohol prep pad if crusted. Procedure for **complete removal**:

1. Using the staple remover, insert the prongs under the most distal staple (to avoid rubbing against other staples during removal) and depress the handle, which will cause both ends of the staple to elevate. Gently rock the remover from side to side if necessary, to loosen the staple, and lift up to remove the staple.
2. Remove all staples in the same manner.
3. Wipe incision line with an alcohol prep pad.

Procedure for **partial removal** (usually reserved for large wounds that are healing poorly or are at risk of dehiscence/evisceration):

1. Proceed as above but remove only every other staple.
2. Apply benzoin to areas where staples were removed and allow to dry until tacky and then apply Steri-strips to those areas.
3. Wipe incision line with an alcohol prep pad.

WART (VERRUCA VULGARIS) REMOVAL

Verruca vulgaris (common warts) are usually self-limiting and will disappear in time, but they can be unsightly and become easily irritated, so requests for removal are common. For all procedures, position the patient so that the lesion is easily accessible. Then cleanse the lesion and 3 inches of surrounding skin with antiseptic, don gloves, and drape the field. Possible procedures for wart removal include the following:

- **Cautery**: Inject 1% lidocaine under the lesion or use a field block for lesions over 4 mm. Use a disposable cautery pen to burn off the lesion. Wipe clean and apply antibiotic ointment and dressing.
- **Duct tape**: Cover the lesion with duct tape and leave in place for 3-6 days. Remove, soak in warm water, and use an emery board or pumice stone to reduce the wart. Wait 10 hours and reapply. Repeat the cycle until the wart disappears.
- **Salicylic acid**: Soak the lesion in warm water for 5-10 minutes, dry, use an emery board or pumice stone to smooth, apply cream to the wart, and let it dry on the skin. Do twice daily for 12 weeks or until the wart is gone.
- **Cryosurgery**: Apply gauze soaked in water to the wart for 5-10 minutes to soften, apply K-Y jelly to the lesion, use a cryoprobe with the appropriately-sized tip to freeze the lesion, and apply antibiotic ointment and dressing.

Musculoskeletal Procedures and Interventions

PELVIC STABILIZER

Pelvic stabilizers are used to prevent excessive bleeding associated with pelvic fractures, to maintain the bones in the correct position, and to prevent further damage. Maintaining pressure and reducing the fracture often reduces bleeding. Various methods of stabilizing the pelvis may be employed, including the sheet wrap method in which a sheet is folded, center under the patient, wrapped tightly about the pelvis, and secured. The pneumatic anti-shock garment (PASG) is indicated for hypovolemic shock, and hypotension associated with and for stabilization of pelvic and bilateral femur fractures. PASG is contraindicated with respiratory distress, pulmonary edema, pregnancy (after the first trimester), heart failure, myocardial infarction, stroke, evisceration, abdominal or leg impalement, head injuries, and uncontrolled bleeding above the garment. Another device is the SAM pelvic sling, which has a wide band that fits under and about the pelvis and lateral hips and a belt anteriorly that allows adjustment.

IMMOBILIZATION DEVICES

Immobilization devices include:

- **Cervical collar**: Support the head to prevent spinal cord injury with suspected injury to cervical vertebrae.
- **Cervical extrication splints**: Short board used to immobilize and protect the head and neck during extrication.
- **Backboards**: Used to immobilize the spine to prevent further injury to spinal cord. Both long and short spine boards are available in a number of different shapes and sizes.
- **Full-body splints** (such as vacuum mattress splint): Provide cushioned support to maintain body alignment.
- **Various types of splints for extremities**: Include rigid (should be padded), non-rigid (moldable), traction, and air (pneumatic devices) as well as the use of blankets, rolled towels, sheets, and pillows to maintain position. Traction splints are used for fractured femurs to keep bones in position.
- **Pneumatic anti-shock garment** (PASG): Provides pressure on lower extremities and abdomen and is used to control hemorrhage and shock to prevent pooling of blood in extremities and return blood to general circulation. Often used for pelvic fractures, but may increase risk of internal hemorrhage.

SPINAL IMMOBILIZATION

Spinal immobilization, once a standard for trauma patients, has been shown to have little effect and in some cases may cause harm. Because of these findings, spinal immobilization with backboard is now recommended only for patients with neurological complaints, such as numbness, tingling, weakness, paralysis, pain or tenderness in the spine, spinal deformity, blunt trauma associated with alterations of consciousness, and high energy injuries associated with drugs/alcohol, inability of the patient to communicate, and/or distracting injury. Cervical collars for cervical spine immobilization are to be utilized for trauma based on the NEXUS criteria or Canadian C-spine rules (CCR). According to **NEXUS criteria**, a patient who exhibits <u>all</u> of the following does <u>not</u> require a cervical collar:

- Alert and stable
- No intoxication
- No midline tenderness of the spine
- No distracting injury
- No neurological deficit

Spinal immobilization should be continued for the shortest time possible, so imaging, such as CT, should be carried out upon admission. Cervical collars are applied while the head is supported in neutral position, and the patient is logrolled onto a backboard and strapped in place.

IMMOBILIZATION OF FRACTURES AND DISLOCATIONS

Immobilization techniques for fractures and dislocations include:

- **Cast**: Plaster and fiberglass casts are applied after reduction to ensure that the bone is correctly aligned. Cast should be placed over several layers of padding that extends slightly beyond the cast ends. Cast material, such as plaster, should NOT be immersed in hot water but water slightly above room temperature (70 °F).
- **Splint**: Plaster splints use 12 or more layers of plaster measured to the correct length and then several layers of padding (longer and wider than splint should be measured and cut). The plaster splint is submerged in water to saturate, removed, laid on a flat surface, and massaged to fuse the layers. The padding is laid on top, and the splint is positioned and wrapped with gauze to hold it in place. While setting the splint, position can be maintained by holding it in place with the palm of the hand (not the fingers). After setting, the splint may be wrapped by elastic compression bandages.

TRACTION SPLINTING

Traction splints are applied for fractures of long bones, such as midshaft fractures of the femur, in order to reduce pain and prevent further damage to tissue and vasculature. Procedures may vary slightly with different types of traction splints. Two people are usually required.

1. Begin by fitting the splint to the uninjured limb so that it can be adjusted to fit properly.
2. Assess circulation including pedal pulses, toe movement, and sensation while a partner manually stabilizes the femur.
3. Apply manual traction by holding above the ankle and below the knee (only if no lower leg injury is suspected).
4. Slide the splint below the limb.
5. Secure the splint with straps, usually 2 above the knee and two below, being careful to avoid the area of fracture and attaching the ischial strap first.
6. Apply ankle strap.
7. Apply traction hook to ankle strap.
8. Adjust traction until it takes over for manual traction.
9. Reassess pain level, pedal pulses, toe movement, and sensation.

For transport, the patient is placed on a long board with the splint secured to the board.

TEACHING PATIENTS HOW TO WALK WITH CRUTCHES

Crutches should be properly fitted before a patient attempts ambulation. Correct height is one hand-width below axillae. The handgrips should be adjusted so the patient supports the body weight comfortably with elbows slightly flexed rather than locked in place. The patient should be cautioned not to bear weight under the axillae as this can cause nerve damage but to hold the crutches tightly against the side of the chest wall. The type of gait that the patient uses depends on the type of injury. Typical gaits include:

- **Two-point** in which each crutch is advanced in tandem with the opposite side leg (i.e., the left crutch is advanced at the same time as the right leg, and the right crutch is advanced at the same time as the left leg).
- **Three-point** in which the injured extremity and both crutches are advanced together and then the well leg advances to (or past) the crutches.

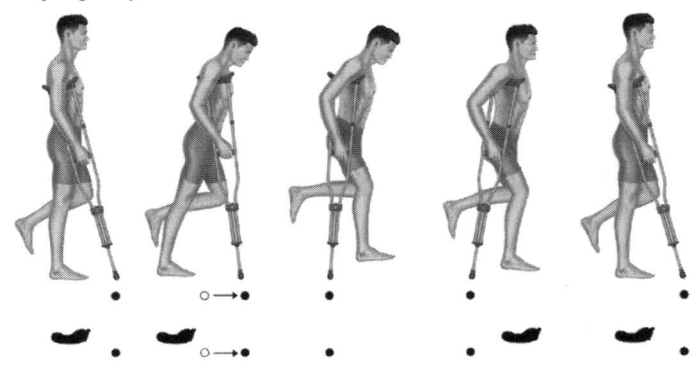

- **Four-point** in which the injured side crutch is advanced, followed by the non-injured leg, followed by the non-injured side crutch, followed by the injured leg.

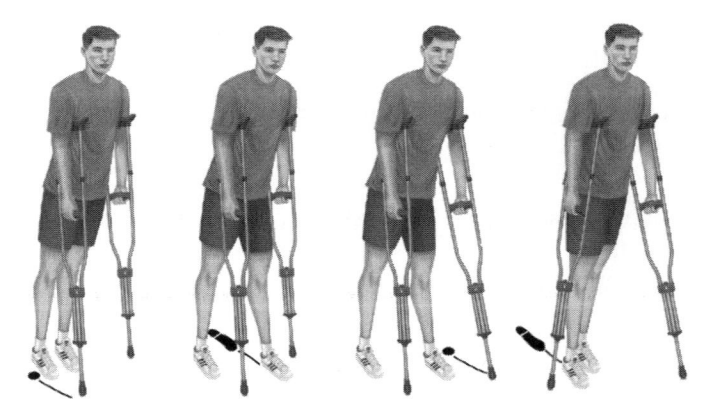

The patient should be advised whether there is partial or no weightbearing and a demonstration should be provided. Stair climbing should be practiced:

- **Ascending**: well foot goes first and then crutches and injured extremity.
- **Descending**: crutches go first and then the well foot.

REDUCTION OF NURSEMAID'S ELBOW

Nursemaid's elbow is a partial dislocation of the elbow (radial head subluxation) that typically occurs when the child is pulled suddenly, lifted by the arm, or falls on the arm. This injury is most common in children between one and four but can occur any time within the first seven years. Typically, the child has pain, will not use the affected arm, and holds it closely to the body. **Reduction procedure**:

1. Calm the child and allow the parents to hold infants and young children securely, facing the practitioner.
2. Grasp the child's forearm or wrist with one hand and the elbow and radial head with the other, placing the thumb against the radial head.
3. Extend (almost to hyperextension) the arm and turn the palm so that it is facing upward (supination) and then flex the elbow rapidly bringing the hand up to the shoulder, using the thumb to guide the radial head into place. A slight click is felt when the radial head pops back into place.
4. The child may still guard the arm for a few more minutes, so wait for 5-10 minutes to determine if the procedure needs to be repeated.

SPINAL FUSION FOR CHILDREN AND ADOLESCENTS

Spinal fusion is done to repair vertebral abnormalities, some resulting in spinal curvature of the spine with disability and deformity that can impair cardiopulmonary function and cause death. While exercises, braces, and electrical stimulation are used to treat mild conditions, **surgical correction** is often required:

- Spinal fusion usually includes spinal realignment and straightening with vertebrae fused together with **bone grafts**, usually from the child's iliac crest or a donor. The grafts may be placed posteriorly or anteriorly, often with the addition of instrumentation (hardware) in the form of rods, screws, wires, hooks, plates, and cages to stabilize and align vertebrae during fusion.
- A **posterior fusion** is done with a vertical incision along the length of the spine to be fused.
- An **anterior fusion** requires an incision to be back to front on one side of the rib cage (thoracic repair) or across the rib cage and down the abdomen (for thoracic and lumbar repair).
- **Endoscopic surgery** may be done through small incisions.

MUSCULOSKELETAL CONDITIONS THAT MAY REQUIRE SPINAL FUSION FOR CORRECTION

Spinal fusion may be needed for the following conditions:

- **Kyphosis**, a convex angulation of the thoracic spine, may be secondary, such as to arthritis or compression fractures, or may be postural, resulting from skeletal growth faster than muscular. Exercises may help postural kyphosis.
- **Lordosis**, an often-painful concave angulation of the lumbar spine, is frequently associated with obesity, flexion hip contracture, and slipped femoral capital epiphysis. Exercises may give some relief but not a permanent cure.
- **Scoliosis**, a lateral and rotational curvature of the spine, can cause alterations in the structure of the pelvis and chest. It may be nonstructural, related to some other deformity or underlying problem, or structural, with changes in the spine and vertebrae because of congenital or other disorders. It is idiopathic in 70-80% of cases.
- **Spina bifida**, a neural tube defect, results in incomplete closure of the spine with the bones over the defect underdeveloped and unfused.
- A child may have a combination, such as **scoliokyphosis**.

Psychosocial Interventions

Trauma-Informed Care

Trauma-informed care acts on the premise that many individuals have experienced some sort of trauma, and therefore every patient should be approached with sensitivity and care. Traumatic events are deeply individualized, and what may have been traumatic to one individual, may not be to the next. Withholding judgment of what qualifies as trauma is imperative for the psychiatric-mental health nurse.

The five elements of **trauma-informed care** include the following:

- **Safety**: Ensuring that the patient feels emotionally and physically safe must be the first priority in order to create a conducive environment for treatment.
- **Choice**: Treatment cannot be forced and must honor the individual's right to choose.
- **Collaboration**: The patient and the nurse must work collaboratively through shared decision-making.
- **Trustworthiness**: The patient must trust the nurse in order for treatment to be effective. Trustworthiness can be established by communicating what is happening and what will happen next to the patient.
- **Empowerment**: Empower the patient with tools to cope on their own so that their recovery extends outside the walls of treatment.

Psychiatric and Mental Health Programs

A variety of psychiatric and mental health programs are available and should be evaluated, according to the needs of the individual patient.

- **Inpatient programs** provide a secure environment and comprehensive care, often with psychologists, psychiatrists, occupational therapists, social workers, and other allied health personnel. Programs may be tailored to one specific type of patient (e.g., criminally insane, substance abusers) or to a general population. They may offer short-term or long-term care.
- **Outpatient programs** provide assessment and treatment, such as group therapy, cognitive-behavioral therapy, and family therapy. Programs may be community-based, targeting specific groups of people, such as alcoholics or the homeless.
- **Partial/day hospitalization programs** provide daily inpatient care during prescribed hours (e.g., 8 a.m. to 3 p.m.) as well as outpatient services. The stay is usually short-term (1–2 weeks) and may serve as a transition from inpatient to outpatient care.

Nonviolent Crisis Intervention and De-Escalation Techniques

Nonviolent crisis intervention and de-escalation techniques begin with self-awareness because the normal response to aggression is a stress response (freezing, fight/flight, fear). The nurse must control these responses in order to deal with the situation. The nurse should recognize signs of impending conflict (clenched fists, and sudden change in tone of voice or body stance, and change in eye contact). Steps include:

- Maintain social distance (≥12 feet) if possible and stay at the same level as the person (sitting or standing).
- Speak in a quiet calm tone of voice, limiting eye contact and avoiding changes in voice tone, facial expression, and gestures (especially avoid pointing or waving a finger at the person).
- Ask the person's name (if necessary) and use the name when addressing the person.
- Validate the person by acknowledging their issue: "I can see that you are angry about the changes in your treatment."
- Show empathy without being judgmental: "I'm sorry you are upset."
- Ignore questions that are challenging and avoid arguing.
- Practice active listening by paraphrasing and clarifying.
- Assist the person to explore options and the results of those options: "What is it that you would like to do?"

Physical Restraints

Restraints are used to restrict movement and activity when other methods of controlling patient behavior have failed and there is a risk of harm to the patient or others. There are two primary types of **physical restraints**: violent (behavioral) and non-violent (clinical). Violent restraints are more commonly used in the psychiatric unit or when individuals exhibit aggressive behavior. More commonly, non-violent restraints are used to ensure that the individual does not interfere with safe care. Non-violent restraints are commonly used in the confused elderly or intubated patient to prevent pulling out lines/removing equipment. The federal government and the Joint Commission have issued strict **guidelines** for temporary restraints or those not part of standard care (such as post-surgical restraint):

- Each facility must have a written policy and restraints are only used when ordered by a physician (usually require written/signed order every 24hrs and within 4 hours of restraint initiation).
- An assessment must be completed frequently, including circulation, toileting, and nutritional needs (generally every 1–2 hours).
- All alternative methods should be tried before applying a restraint and the least restrictive effective restraint should be used.
- A nurse must remove the restraint, assess, and document findings at least every 2 hours, every hour for violent restraints.

Key: Least restrictive option for the least amount of time.

Chemical Restraints

Chemical restraints involve the use of pharmacological sedatives to manage an individual's behavior problems. This type of restraint is indicated only when severe agitation/violence puts the patient at risk for injury to themselves or others. **Chemical restraints** inhibit the individuals' physical movements, making their behavior more manageable. It is important to realize that medication used on an ongoing basis as part of treatment is not legally considered a chemical restraint, even though the medications may be the same. There is little consensus about the use of chemical restraints, although benzodiazepines and antipsychotics are frequently used to control severe agitation (haloperidol, lorazepam, etc.). Oral medications should be tried first before injections, as oral medication is less coercive. It is important for the nurse to realize that chemical restraints are used as a last resort when other measures (such as de-escalation and environmental modification) have failed and there is an immediate risk of harm to the patient or others.

Treatments for Children and Families with Psychosocial Disorders

Treatments for children and families with psychosocial disorders includes a variety of approaches:

- **Individual therapy** involves the child and therapist working together on the psychosocial and developmental problems.
- **Family therapy** involves the whole family working with the therapist. The focus is on family relationships, communication, and assisting each family member in individual development within the family.
- **Group therapy** involves a group of children or teens working on socialization skills.
- **Play therapy** uses play to allow the child to explore and bring out his feelings. The therapist helps the child understand these emotions and use them in positive ways. The child learns to control his actions and emotions, thereby increasing his self-esteem.
- **Art therapy** uses the child's own art projects to bring out emotions and deal positively with them.

Types of Physical Restraints for Pediatric Patients

There are a number of different types of physical restraints to ensure child safety:

- **Swaddling**: Used for infants and small children for treatments and examinations of the head, neck, and throat, venipuncture, and gavage feedings to prevent movement. A papoose board with straps or a mummy wrap is used.
- **Jacket**: Used to prevent children from falling out of chairs/beds or to maintain horizontal position. A jacket is applied with ties in the back and long ties secured out of reach in the back of the wheelchair or underside of the crib.
- **Limb**: Used to prevent arm or leg movement that might cause injury or to protect IV access. Commercial restraints are sized, so they should fit properly and should be padded to prevent pressure.
- **Elbow**: This restraint is used to prevent the child from reaching the head or face, usually after surgery, or to prevent scratching. The most common restraint is a muslin wrap with pockets for tongue depressors for infants. Commercial restraints are available for older children.

Respiratory Procedures and Interventions

NON-INVASIVE VENTILATION

NASAL CANNULA

A nasal cannula can be used to deliver supplemental oxygen to a patient, but it is only useful for flow rates ≤6 L/min as higher rates are drying of the nasal passages. As it is not an airtight system, some ambient air is breathed in as well so oxygen concentration ranges from about 24–44%. The nasal cannula does not allow for control of respiratory rate, so the patient must be able to breathe independently.

NON-REBREATHER MASK

A non-rebreather mask can be used to deliver higher concentrations (60–90%) of oxygen to those patients who are able to breathe independently. The mask fits over the nose and mouth and is secured by an elastic strap. A 1.5 L reservoir bag is attached and connects to an oxygen source. The bag is inflated to about 1 liter at a rate of 8–15 L/min before the mask is applied as the patient breathes from this reservoir. A one-way exhalation valve prevents most exhaled air from being rebreathed.

NON-INVASIVE POSITIVE PRESSURE VENTILATORS

Non-invasive positive pressure ventilators provide air through a tight-fitting nasal or face mask, usually pressure cycled, avoiding the need for intubation and reducing the danger of hospital-acquired infection and mortality rates. It can be used for acute respiratory failure and pulmonary edema. There are 2 types of non-invasive positive pressure ventilators:

- **CPAP (Continuous positive airway pressure)** provides a steady stream of pressurized air throughout both inspiration and expiration. CPAP improves breathing by decreasing preload for patients with congestive heart failure. It reduces the effort required for breathing by increasing residual volume and improving gas exchange.
- **Bi-PAP (Bi-level positive airway pressure)** provides a steady stream of pressurized air as CPAP but it senses inspiratory effort and increases pressure during inspiration. Bi-PAP pressures for inspiration and expiration can be set independently. Machines can be programmed with a backup rate to ensure a set number of respirations per minute.

NEVER place a patient in wrist restraints while wearing these devices. If the patient vomits, they need to be able to remove the mask to prevent aspiration.

Face Mask

Ensuring that a face mask (Ambu bag) is the correct fit and type is important for adequate ventilation, oxygenation, and prevention of aspiration. Difficulties in management of face mask ventilation relate to risk factors: >55 years, obesity, beard, edentulous, and history of snoring. In some cases, if dentures are adhered well, they may be left in place during induction. The face mask is applied by lifting the mandible (jaw thrust) to the mask and avoiding pressure on soft tissue. Oral or nasal airways may be used, ensuring that the distal end is at the angle of the mandible. There are a number of steps to prevent mask airway leaks:

- Increasing or decreasing the amount of air to the mask to allow better seal
- Securing the mask with both hands while another person ventilates
- Accommodating a large nose by using the mask upside down
- Utilizing a laryngeal mask airway if excessive beard prevents seal

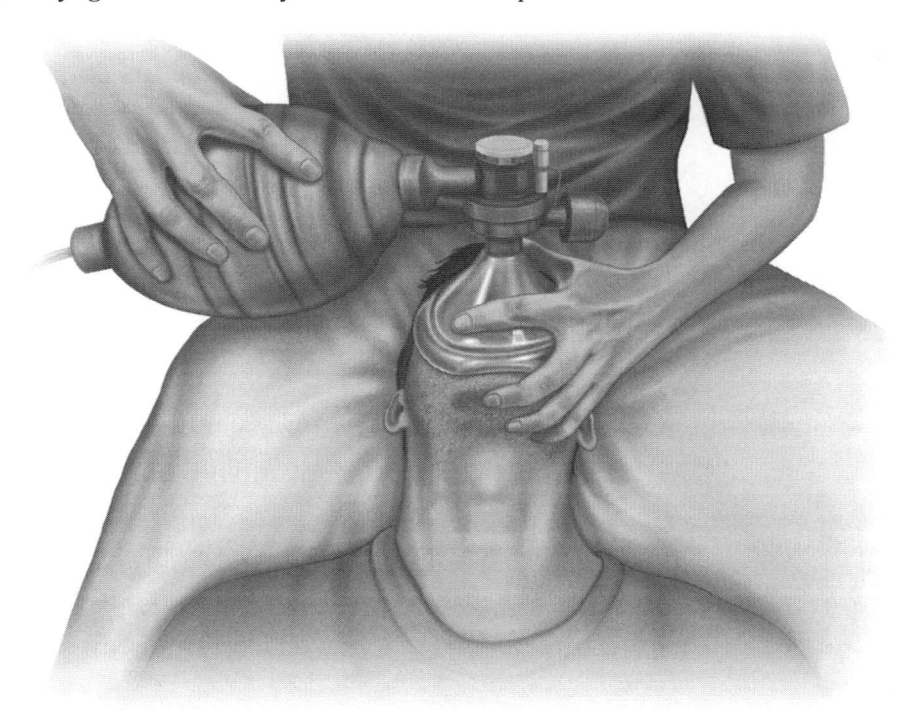

High and Low Flow Oxygen Delivery

High flow oxygen delivery devices provide oxygen at flow rates higher than the patient's inspiratory flow rate at specific medium to high FiO_2, up to 100%. However, a flow of 100% oxygen actually provides only 60–80% FiO_2 to the patient because the patient also breathes in some room air, diluting the oxygen. The actual amount of oxygen received depends on the type of interface or mask. Additionally, the flow rate is actually less than the inspiratory flow rate upon actual delivery. High flow oxygen delivery is usually not used in the sleep center. Humidification is usually required because the high flow is drying.

Low flow oxygen delivery devices provide 100% oxygen at flow rates lower than the patient's inspiratory flow rate, but the oxygen mixes with room air, so the FiO_2 varies. Humidification is usually only required if flow rate is >3L/min. Much oxygen is wasted with exhalation, so a number of different devices to conserve oxygen are available. Interfaces include transtracheal catheters and cannulae with reservoirs.

AIRWAY DEVICES
OROPHARYNGEAL, NASOPHARYNGEAL, AND TRACHEOSTOMY TUBES

Airways are used to establish a patent airway and facilitate respirations:

- **Oropharyngeal**: This plastic airway curves over the tongue and creates space between the mouth and the posterior pharynx. It is used for anesthetized or unconscious patients to keep tongue and epiglottis from blocking the airway.

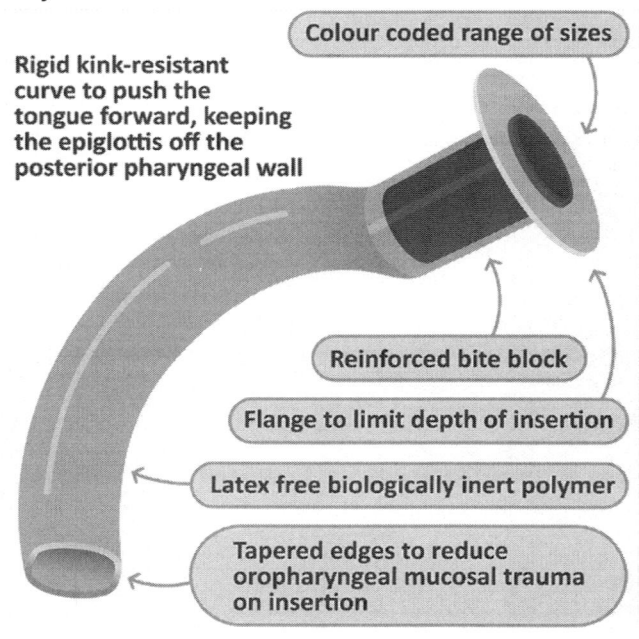

- **Nasopharyngeal** (trumpet): This smaller flexible airway is more commonly used in conscious patients and is inserted through one nostril, extending to the nasopharynx. It is commonly utilized in patients who need frequent suctioning.

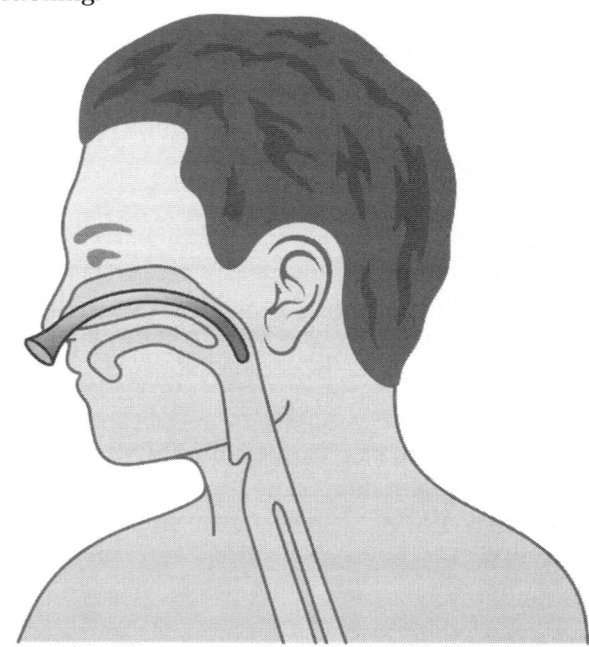

- **Tracheostomy tubes**: Tracheostomy may be utilized for mechanical ventilation. Tubes are inserted into the opening in the trachea to provide a conduit and maintain the opening. The tube is secured with ties around the neck. Because the air entering the lungs through the tracheostomy bypasses the warming and moistening effects of the upper airway, air is humidified through a room humidifier or through the delivery of humidified air through a special mask or mechanical ventilation. If the tracheostomy is going to be long-term, eventually a stoma will form at the site, and the tube can be removed.

LARYNGEAL MASK AIRWAY

The laryngeal-mask airway (LMA) is an intermediate airway allowing ventilation but not complete respiratory control. The LMA consists of an inflatable cuff (the mask) with a connecting tube. It may be used temporarily before tracheal intubation or when tracheal intubation can't be done. It can also be a conduit for later blind insertion of an endotracheal tube. The head and neck must be in neutral position for insertion of the LMA. If the patient has a gag reflex, conscious sedation or topical anesthesia (deep oropharyngeal) is required. The LMA is inserted by sliding along the hard palate, using the finger as a guide, into the pharynx, and the ring is inflated to create a seal about the opening to the larynx, allowing ventilation with mild positive-pressure. The ProSeal LMA has a modified cuff that extends onto the back of the mask to improve seal. LMA is contraindicated in morbid obesity, obstructions or abnormalities of oropharynx, and non-fasting patients, as some aspiration is possible even with the cuff seal inflated.

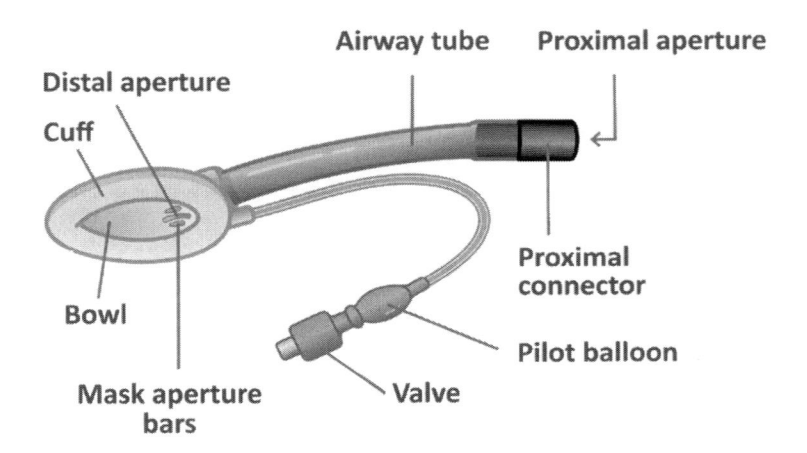

ESOPHAGEAL-TRACHEAL COMBITUBE

The esophageal tracheal Combitube (ETC) is an intermediate airway that contains two lumens and can be inserted into either the trachea or the esophagus (≤91%). The twin-lumen tube has a proximal cuff providing a seal of the oropharynx and a distal cuff providing a seal about the distal tube. Prior to insertion, the Combitube cuffs should be checked for leaks (15 mL of air into distal and 85 mL of air into proximal). The patient should be non-responsive and with absent gag reflex with head in neutral position. The tube is passed along the tongue and into the pharynx, utilizing markings on the tube (black guidelines) to determine depth by aligning the ETC with the upper incisors or alveolar ridge. Once in place the distal cuff is inflated (10–15 mL) and then placement in the trachea or esophagus should be determined, so the proper lumen for ventilation can be used. The proximal cuff is inflated (usually to 50–75 mL) and ventilation begun. A capnogram should be used to confirm ventilation.

THORACENTESIS

A thoracentesis (aspiration of fluid or air from pleural space) is done to make a diagnosis, relieve pressure on the lung caused by pleural effusion, or instill medications. A chest x-ray is done prior to the procedure. A sedative may be given. The patient is in a sitting position, leaning onto a padded bedside stand, straddling a chair with head supported on the back of the chair, or lying on the opposite side with the head of the bed elevated 30–45° to ensure that fluid remains at the base. The patient should avoid coughing or moving during the procedure. The chest x-ray or ultrasound determines needle placement. After a local anesthetic is administered, a needle (with an attached 20-mL syringe and 3-way stopcock with tubing and a receptacle) is advanced intercostally into the pleural space. Fluid is drained, collected, examined, and measured. The needle is removed and a pressure dressing applied. A chest x-ray is done to ensure there is no pneumothorax. The patient is monitored for cough, dyspnea, and hypoxemia.

> **Review Video: Thoracentesis**
> Visit mometrix.com/academy and enter code: 321111

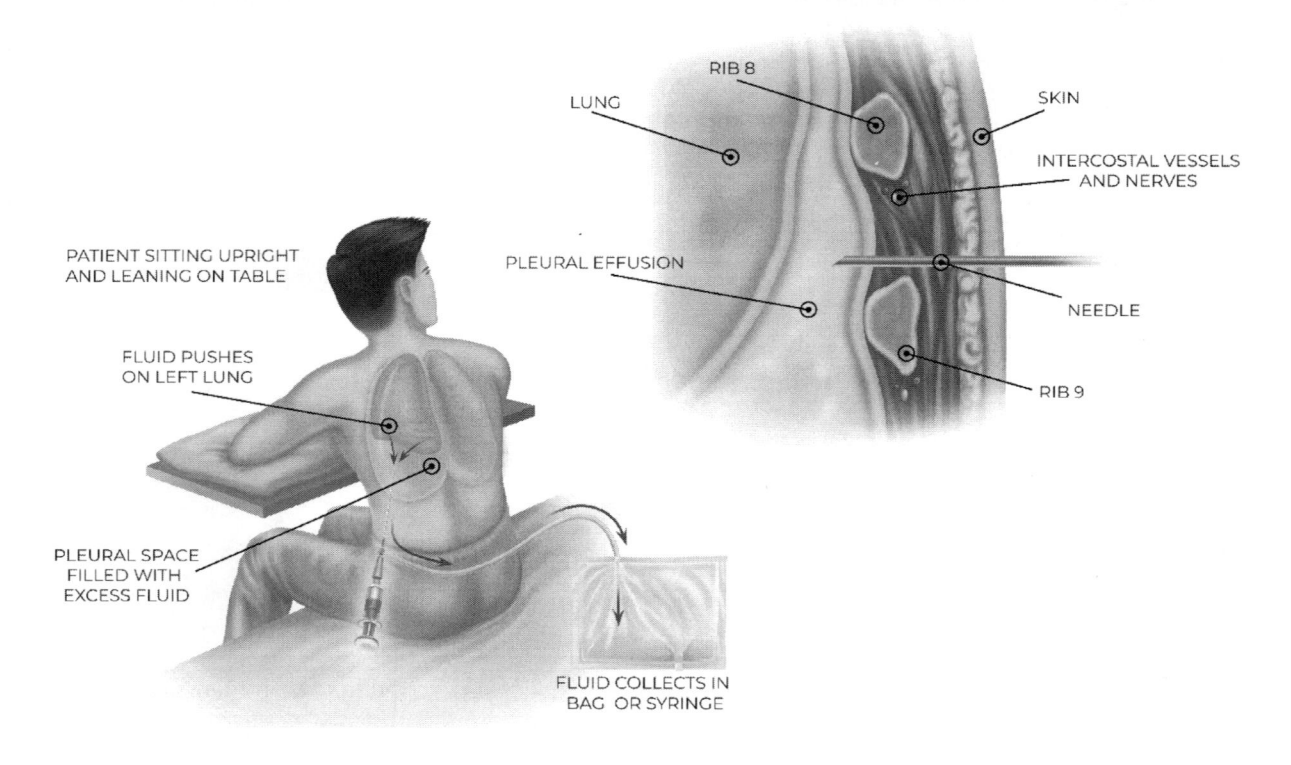

BRONCHOSCOPY

Bronchoscopy utilizes a thin, flexible fiberoptic bronchoscope to inspect the larynx, trachea, and bronchi for diagnostic purposes. It is also used to collect specimens, obtain biopsies, remove foreign bodies or secretions, treat atelectasis, and to excise lesions. The patient is in supine position during the procedure. The Mallampati classification may be used to determine difficulty of airway. The patient receives local anesthesia to the nares (lidocaine gel) and oropharynx (lidocaine gel, spray, or nebulizer), and usually receives a benzodiazepine (commonly midazolam or lorazepam), an opioid (fentanyl or meperidine), or propofol. Medications are usually given in small incremental doses throughout the procedure and may be combined. Over-sedation may cause physiologic depression, but undersedation may result in recall and agitation with sympathetic activation. The tube is advanced through the nares and down the trachea to the bronchi. Airway patency, respiratory rate, and oxygen saturation must be constantly monitored. Complications can include bleeding, arrhythmias, obstruction, laryngospasm, and respiratory failure.

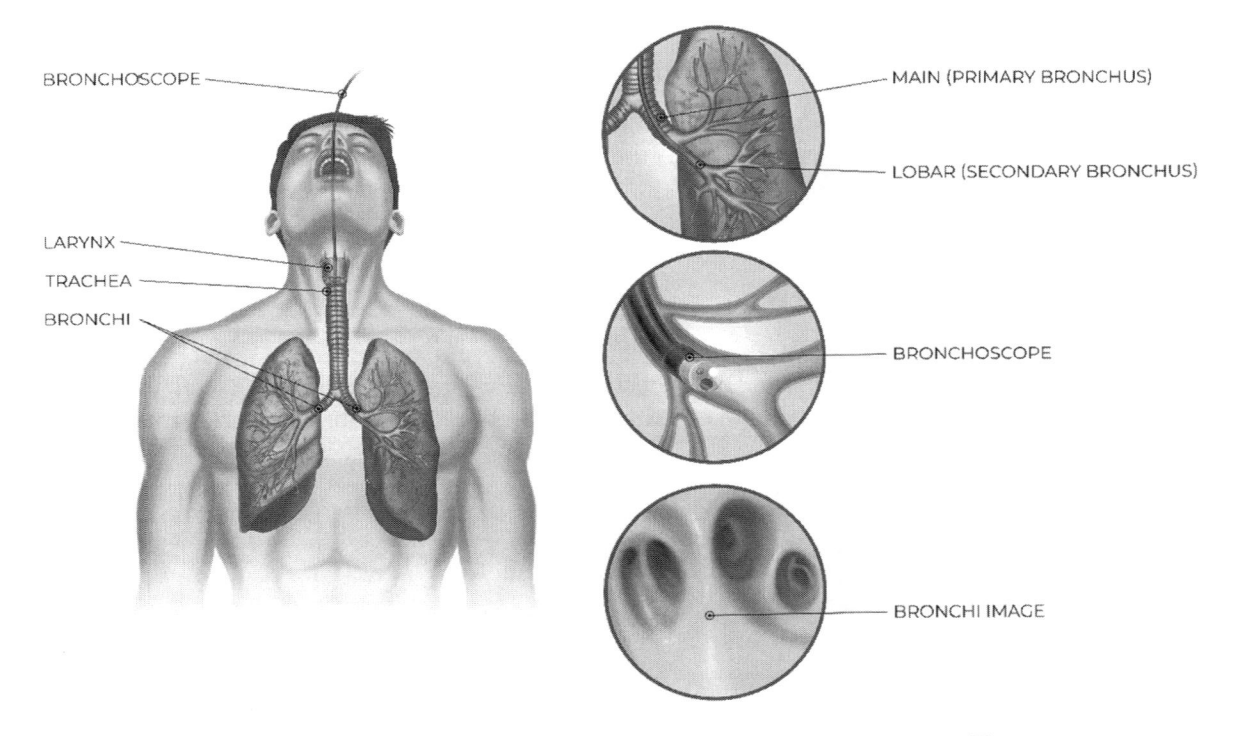

AHA PEDIATRIC ADVANCED LIFE SUPPORT GUIDELINES FOR RESPIRATORY EMERGENCIES

RESPIRATORY DISTRESS/ARREST

According to the PALS guidelines, if a child experiences respiratory distress and arrest, the **ABC protocol** is recommended:

- **Airway**: Open and support the airway. Begin CPR with 2 respirations. Insert OPA/NPA if necessary.
- **Breathing**: monitor oxygen saturation, provide oxygen as needed and endotracheal intubation, ventilation as needed.
- **Circulation**: Monitor heartrate, rhythm, and BP and place IV. Begin standard CPR with chest compressions if cardiac arrest occurs.

The type of respiratory problem must be identified and treatment instituted:

- **Upper airway obstruction** (croup, RSV, epiglottitis, anaphylaxis, foreign body): Treatment depends on the cause. For example, epinephrine and corticosteroids for croup and epinephrine, albuterol, antihistamines, and corticosteroids for anaphylaxis.
- **Lower airway obstruction**: For bronchiolitis, nasal suctioning and bronchodilator and for asthma, albuterol and ipratropium, corticosteroids, epinephrine, $MgSO_4$, and terbutaline.
- **Disordered work of breathing**: Manage ICP, provide ventilatory support, and provide antidote in the case of poison/overdose.
- **Lung-tissue disease**: For pulmonary edema provide ventilatory support, a diuretic, and vasoactive support. For pneumonia provide albuterol, antibiotics, and CPAP.

HEIMLICH MANEUVER FOR CHILDREN <1 YEAR

Indications of choking in infants of less than one year include lack of breathing, gasping, cyanosis, and inability to cry. Procedures for the **Heimlich chest thrusts** include:

- Position the infant in prone (face down) position along the forearm with the infant's head lower than the trunk, being sure to support the head so the airway is not blocked.
- Using the heel of the hand, deliver 5 forceful upward blows between the shoulder blades.
- Sandwich the child between the two arms and turn the infant into supine position and drape over thigh with head lower than trunk and head supported.
- Using two fingers (as for CPR compressions), give up to 5 thrusts (about 1.5 inches deep) to lower third of sternum.
- Only do finger sweep and remove foreign object if the object is visible. Repeat 5 back blows followed by 5 chest thrusts until the foreign body is ejected or emergency personnel take over.
- If the infant loses consciousness, begin CPR. If a pulse is noted but spontaneous respirations are absent, continue ventilation only.

HEIMLICH MANEUVER FOR CHILDREN ≥1 YEAR

The universal sign of choking is when a person clutches the throat and appears to be choking or gasping for breath. If the person can speak ("Can you speak?") or cough, a **Heimlich maneuver** is not usually necessary. The Heimlich maneuver can be done with the victim sitting, standing, or supine. The Heimlich procedure for children (≥1 year) and adults:

- Wrap arms around the victim's waist from the back if sitting or standing. Make a fist and place the thumb side against the victim's abdomen slightly above the umbilicus. Grasp this hand with the other and thrust sharply upward to force air out of the lungs.
- Repeat as needed and call 911 if no response.
- If the victim loses consciousness, ease into supine position on the floor, place hands similarly to CPR but over the abdomen while sitting astride the victim's legs. Repeat upward compressions 5 times. If no ventilation occurs, attempt to sweep the mouth and ventilate lungs, mouth to mouth. Repeat compressions and ventilations until recovery or until emergency personnel arrive.

Cardiovascular Pharmacology

ANTI-HYPERTENSIVE MEDICATIONS

The classes of anti-hypertensive medications are as follows: Diuretics, sympatholytics, vasodilators, calcium channel blockers, and angiotensin-converting enzyme inhibitors (ACE inhibitors).

- Diuretics include hydrochlorothiazide, chlorthalidone, chlorothiazide, indapamide, metolazone, amiloride, spironolactone, triamterene, furosemide, bumetanide, ethacrynic acid, and torsemide.
- Sympatholytics are clonidine, methyldopa, guanabenz, guanadrel, guanethidine, reserpine, labetalol, prazosin, and terazosin.
- Vasodilators include diazoxide, hydralazine, minoxidil, and nitroprusside sodium.
- Calcium channel blockers include amlodipine, nimodipine, isradipine, nicardipine, nifedipine, bepridil, diltiazem, and verapamil.
- ACE inhibitors include benazepril, captopril, enalapril, fosinopril, lisinopril, moexipril, quinapril, ramipril, and losartan.

> **Review Video: Side Effects of ACE Inhibitors and ARBs**
> Visit mometrix.com/academy and enter code: 525864

DIURETICS

Diuretics increase **renal perfusion and filtration**, thereby reducing preload and decreasing peripheral and pulmonary edema, hypertension, CHF, diabetes insipidus, and osteoporosis. There are different types of diuretics: loop, thiazide, and potassium sparing.

LOOP DIURETICS

Loop diuretics inhibit the reabsorption of sodium and chloride (primarily) in the ascending loop of Henle. They also cause increased secretion of other electrolytes, such as calcium, magnesium, and potassium, and this can result in imbalances that cause dysrhythmias. Other side effects include frequent urination, postural hypotension, and increased blood sugar and uric acid levels. They are short-acting so are less effective than other diuretics for control of hypertension.

- **Bumetanide** (Bumex) is given intravenously after surgery to reduce preload or orally to treat heart failure.
- **Ethacrynic acid** (Edecrin) is given intravenously after surgery to reduce preload.
- **Furosemide** (Lasix) is used for the control of congestive heart failure as well as renal insufficiency. It is used after surgery to decrease preload and to reduce the inflammatory response caused by cardiopulmonary bypass (post-perfusion syndrome).

> **Review Video: Diuretics**
> Visit mometrix.com/academy and enter code: 373276

THIAZIDE DIURETICS

Thiazide diuretics inhibit the **reabsorption of sodium and chloride** primarily in the early distal tubules, forcing more sodium and water to be excreted. Thiazide diuretics increase secretion of potassium and bicarbonate, so they are often given with supplementary potassium or in combination with potassium-sparing diuretics. Thiazide diuretics are the first line of drugs for treatment of **hypertension**. They have a long duration of action (12–72 hours, depending on the drug) so they are able to maintain control of hypertension better than short-acting drugs. They may be given daily or 3–5 days per week. There are numerous thiazide diuretics, including:

- Chlorothiazide
- Chlorthalidone
- Hydrochlorothiazide

Side effects include, dizziness, lightheadedness, postural hypotension, headache, blurred vision, and itching, especially during initial treatment. Thiazide diuretics cause sensitivity to sun exposure, so people should be counseled to use sunscreen.

POTASSIUM-SPARING DIURETICS

Potassium-sparing diuretics inhibit the **reabsorption of sodium** in the late distal tubule and collecting duct. They are weaker than thiazide or loop diuretics, but do not cause a reduction in potassium level; however, if used alone, they may cause an increase in potassium, which can cause weakness, irregular pulse, and cardiac arrest. Because potassium-sparing diuretics are less effective alone, they are often given in a combined form with a thiazide diuretic (usually chlorothiazide), which mitigates the potassium imbalance. Typical side effects include dehydration, blurred vision, nausea, insomnia, and nasal congestion, especially in the first few days of treatment.

- **Spironolactone** (Aldactone) is a synthetic steroid diuretic that increases the secretion of both water and sodium and is used to treat congestive heart failure. It may be given orally or intravenously.
- **Eplerenone** is an antimineralocorticoid similar to spironolactone but with fewer side effects.

ANTIDYSRHYTHMIC DRUGS

Antidysrhythmic drugs include a number of drugs that act on the conduction system, the ventricles and/or the atria to control dysrhythmias. There are four classes of drugs that are used as well as some that are unclassified:

- **Class I:** 3 subtypes of sodium channel blockers (quinidine, lidocaine, procainamide)
- **Class II:** β-receptor blockers (esmolol, propranolol)
- **Class III:** Slows repolarization (amiodarone, ibutilide)
- **Class IV:** Calcium channel blockers (diltiazem, verapamil)
- **Unclassified:** Miscellaneous drugs with proven efficacy in controlling arrhythmias (adenosine, electrolyte supplements)

Endocrine Pharmacology

ORAL HYPOGLYCEMIC AGENTS

Oral hypoglycemic agents are **anti-diabetic treatments** generally used in the treatment of Type II Diabetes. There are five classic categories of oral hypoglycemic agents: sulfonylureas, biguanides, meglitinides, competitive inhibitors of alpha-glucosidases (located in the intestinal brush border), and thiazolidinediones. More recently, two additional novel classes of oral hypoglycemics, DPP-4 inhibitors and SGLT2 inhibitors, were introduced with proven effectiveness when used in conjunction with changes in diet and exercise. Some examples of sulfonylurea oral hypoglycemic agents include the first-generation agents tolbutamide, tolazamide, chlorpropamide, and acetohexamide; and second-generation agents glyburide, glimepiride, and glipizide. The biguanide oral hypoglycemic agent is metformin. Metformin has the distinct advantage of not causing weight gain or hypoglycemic reactions. The meglitinide agent is repaglinide. Examples of alpha-glucosidase inhibitors are acarbose and miglitol. Alpha-glucosidase inhibitors bind tightly to intestinal alpha-glucosidases and decrease the postprandial rise in glucose levels. The only available thiazolidinedione oral hypoglycemic agent is currently pioglitazone; troglitazone was removed from US market in 2000, and rosiglitazone was removed from US market in 2011. Examples of DPP-4 inhibitors include linagliptin, vildagliptin, sitagliptin, and saxagliptin. Examples of SGLT2 inhibitors include canagliflozin, dapagliflozin, and empagliflozin.

INSULIN USED TO TREAT GLYCEMIC DISORDERS

There are a number of different types of **insulin** with varying action times. Insulin is used to metabolize **glucose** for those whose pancreas does not produce insulin. People may need to take a combination of insulins (short- and long-acting) to maintain glucose control. Duration of action may vary according to the individual's metabolism, intake, and level of activity:

- **Humalog** (Lispro H) is a fast-acting, short-acting insulin with onset in 5–15 minutes, peaking at 45–90 minutes and lasting 3–4 hours.
- **Regular** (R) is a relatively fast-acting insulin with onset in 30 minutes, peaks in 2–5 hours, and lasts 5–8 hours.
- **NPH** (N) insulin is intermediate-acting with onset in 1–3 hours, peaking at 6–12 hours, and lasting for 16–24 hours.
- **Insulin Glargine** (Lantus) is a long-acting insulin with onset in 3–6 hours, no peak, and lasting for 24 hours.
- **Combined NPH/Regular** (70/30 or 50/50) has an onset of 30 minutes, peaks at 7–12 hours, and lasts 16–24 hours.

Gastrointestinal Pharmacology

HISTAMINE RECEPTOR ANTAGONISTS

Histamine (H) receptor antagonists (actually reverse agonists) are used to treat conditions in which excessive stomach acid causes heartburn and GERD. They block histamine 2 (H_2) (parietal) cell receptors in the stomach, thereby decreasing acid production. These drugs are used less commonly now than proton-pump inhibitors. **Common H_2 antagonists** include:

- **Cimetidine**: The first H_2 antagonist, it is used less frequently than others because of inhibition of enzymes that results in drug interactions, especially with contraceptive agents and estrogen.
- **Famotidine (Pepcid)**: This may be combined with an antacid to increase the speed of effects as it has a slow onset. It may be used pre-surgically to reduce post-operative nausea.
- **Nizatidine**: The last H_2 antagonist developed, it is used to treat ulcers and GERD. It is about equal in potency and action to ranitidine, which was discontinued due to the presence of NDMA, a cancer-causing contaminant, when stored in high temperatures.

ANTACIDS

Antacids are medications used to reduce stomach acids by raising the pH and neutralizing the acids present. They are commonly used to treat heartburn or indigestion. Adverse reactions are relatively rare unless taken to excess or with renal impairment. Drugs include:

- **Aluminum hydroxide** may cause constipation and with renal impairment, hypophosphatemia and osteomalacia.
- **Magnesium hydroxide** (Milk of Magnesia) may cause diarrhea and with renal impairment can cause hypermagnesemia.
- **Aluminum hydroxide with magnesium hydroxide** may cause nausea, vomiting and diarrhea, yeast infection (thrush), or hypophosphatemia.
- **Calcium carbonate** (TUMS, Titralac) may cause gastric distention. Excess calcium intake may cause toxic reactions, including kidney stones and renal failure, so excess intake should be avoided.
- **Alka-Seltzer** combines sodium bicarbonate with aspirin and citric acid so this compound may cause gastric irritation, nausea and vomiting, and tarry stools.
- **Bismuth subsalicylate** (Pepto-Bismol). Pepto-Bismol may react with sulfur in the body to create a black tongue and black stools, but this is temporary. Pepto-Bismol has been associated with Reye's syndrome in children with influenza or chickenpox.

PROTON PUMP INHIBITORS

Proton pump inhibitors (PPIs) are now used more frequently than histamine receptor antagonists. PPIs interfere with an acid-producing enzyme in the stomach wall, reducing stomach acid. PPIs are used to treat GERD, stomach ulcers, and *H. pylori* (with antibiotics). PPIs are similar in action and include:

- Esomeprazole (Nexium)
- Lansoprazole (Prevacid)
- Omeprazole (Prilosec)
- Pantoprazole (Protonix)
- Rabeprazole (Aciphex)
- Omeprazole/sodium bicarbonate (Long-acting form of omeprazole)

Common side effects include gastrointestinal upset (nausea, diarrhea, and constipation), headache, and rash. In rare instances, PPIs may cause severe muscle pain; however, they are usually well-tolerated with few adverse effects. PPIs may interfere with the absorption of some drugs, such as those that are affected by stomach acid. Absorption of ketoconazole is impaired, and absorption of digoxin is increased, sometimes leading to toxicity. Omeprazole impacts the hepatic breakdown of drugs more than other PPIs and may cause increased levels of diazepam, phenytoin, and warfarin.

ANTI-LIPIDS

Anti-lipid medications are frequently used to **lower cholesterol levels** if dietary modifications are unsuccessful in order to decrease coronary artery disease. Four primary **types** of medications include the following:

- **Statins** (3-hydroxy-3-methylglutaryl coenzyme A reductase inhibitors), such as atorvastatin (Lipitor), rosuvastatin (Crestor), fluvastatin (Lescol), lovastatin (Altoprev), pravastatin, and simvastatin (Zocor), inhibit the liver enzyme that produces cholesterol, but different statins vary in the ability to reduce cholesterol and in drug/other interactions (protease inhibitors, erythromycin, grapefruit juice, niacin, and fibric acids). Adverse effects include rhabdomyolysis (which causes severe muscle pain and weakness), headache, rash, weakness, and gastrointestinal disorders.
- **Nicotinic acid** (Niacor) decreases synthesis of lipoprotein, lowers low-density lipoprotein (LDL) and triglycerides, and increases high-density lipoprotein (HDL). It is used for low elevations of cholesterol and may be combined with statins. Adverse effects include flushing, hyperglycemia, gout, upper gastrointestinal disorders, and hepatotoxicity. Liver function must be monitored.
- **Bile acid sequestrants,** such as cholestyramine (Questran, Prevalite), colesevelam (WelChol), and colestipol HCL (Colestid), decrease LDL, increase HDL, and do not affect triglyceride levels. They bind to bile acids in the intestines so that more are excreted in the stool rather than returned to the liver, so the liver has to produce bile acids by converting cholesterol. Adverse effects include gastrointestinal disorders and decrease in absorption of other drugs.

SEROTONIN ANTAGONISTS

Serotonin antagonists block $5\text{-}HT_2$ receptors of serotonin in the central and peripheral nervous systems and gastrointestinal system. An open channel can result in agitation, nausea, and vomiting, but antagonists close the channel and reduce these symptoms. Serotonin antagonists are frequently used to prevent and treat nausea associated with chemotherapy and anesthesia. Medications include:

- **Metoclopramide** (Reglan) is used to reduce nausea and vomiting from a wide range of causes. It is also a prokinetic drug that increases gastrointestinal contractions and promotes faster gastric emptying, so it is used for heartburn, GERD, and diabetic gastroparesis.
- **Ondansetron** (Zofran) reduces vagal stimulation of the medulla oblongata (vomiting center) and is used for nausea related to chemotherapy.
- **Granisetron** (Sancuso) is used to reduce nausea related to chemotherapy, surgery, and radiation.

Serotonin antagonists have fewer side effects than other antiemetics, but they may cause muscle cramping, agitation, diarrhea/constipation, dizziness, and headache.

LAXATIVES

The following are different types of laxatives:

- **Bulk formers** have high fiber content and both soften stool and create more formed stools. These include products such as Metamucil, Citrucel, and FiberCon, which are usually added to liquids because without adequate fluids, they can increase constipation.
- **Lubricants** include both oral mineral oil and glycerin suppositories. They coat the stool, preventing fluid absorption and keeping the stool soft. Mineral oil absorbs fat soluble vitamins and should be used only temporarily
- **Saline**, such as Milk of Magnesia and Epsom Salt, contain ions, such as magnesium phosphate, magnesium hydroxide, and citrate, which are not absorbed through the intestines and draw more fluid into the stool. The magnesium in the preparations also stimulates the bowel. People with impairment of kidney function should avoid magnesium products, and saline laxatives should be used infrequently to avoid dependence. Epsom Salt often has a purging effect and is rarely used.
- **Stool softeners** (emollients, such as Colace) use wetting agents, such as docusate sodium, to increase liquid in the stool, thereby softening it. They should not be used with mineral oil because of increased absorption of the oil through the intestines.
- **Hyperosmotics** (available by prescription) contain materials that are not digestible and serve to retain fluid in the stool. Products, such as Kristalose and MiraLAX soften the stool but may result in increased abdominal distension and flatus, especially initially. There are three types of hyperosmolar laxatives: lactulose, polymer, and saline. Lactulose types use a form of sugar and work similarly to saline laxatives, but more slowly, and may be used for long-term treatment. The salines empty the bowels quickly and are used short-term. The polymers contain polyethylene glycol, which retains fluid in the stool and is used short-term.
- **Combinations** use two or more types, such as stool softener with stimulant, and should be used only short-term.

STIMULANTS

Stimulants increase intestinal motility, moving the stool through the bowel faster and reducing the absorption of fluids so that the stool remains softer. Common ingredients include cascara in Castor oil and senna in Senokot. Stimulants work quickly and are effective but can result in electrolyte imbalance, Abdominal distension, and cramping. Chronic use may cause a cycle of constipation and diarrhea. Stimulant suppositories, such as Dulcolax, are also available.

> **Review Video: Gastrointestinal Drugs**
> Visit mometrix.com/academy and enter code: 455152

Integumentary Pharmacology

PHARMACOLOGIC TREATMENT OF WOUND PAIN

TOPICAL ANESTHETICS

There are numerous different types of pain medications that may be used to control pain from wounds, including **topical anesthetics**:

- **Lidocaine 2–4%** is frequently used during debridement or dressing changes. Lidocaine is useful only superficially and may take 15–30 minutes before it is effective.
- **Eutectic Mixture of Local Anesthetics (EMLA Cream)** provides good pain control. The wound is first cleansed and then the cream is applied thickly (1/4 inch) extending about 1/2 inch past the wound to the periwound tissue. The wound is then covered with plastic wrap, which is secured and left in place for about 20 minutes. The wrapped time may be extended to 45–60 minutes if necessary, to completely numb the tissue. The tissue should remain numb for about 1 hour after the plastic wrap is removed, allowing time for the wound to be cleansed, debrided, and/or redressed.

> **Review Video: Dermatology Drugs List**
> Visit mometrix.com/academy and enter code: 886820

REGIONAL ANESTHESIA

Regional anesthesia (injectable subcutaneous and perineural medications) is administered locally about the wound or as nerve blocks. Medications include lidocaine, bupivacaine, and tetracaine in solution. Epinephrine is sometimes added to increase vasoconstriction and reduce bleeding, although it is avoided in distal areas of the limbs (hands and feet) to prevent ischemia.

- **Field blockade** involves injecting the anesthetic into the periwound tissue or into the wound margins. The effect may be decreased by inflammation. The effects last for limited periods of time.
- **Regional nerve blocks** may involve single injections, the effects of which are limited in duration but can provide pain relief for treatments. Techniques that use continuous catheter infusions are longer lasting and can be controlled more precisely. Blocks may involve nerves proximal to affected areas, such as peripheral nerve blocks, or large nerve blocks near the spinal cord, such as percutaneous lumbar sympathetic blocks (LSB). Long-term blocks may use alcohol-based medications to permanently inactivate the nerves.

Respiratory Pharmacology

PHARMACOLOGICAL AGENTS USED FOR ASTHMA

Numerous pharmacological agents are used for control of asthma, some that are long-acting to prevent attacks and others that are short-acting to provide relief for acute episodes. Listed with each are the standard med and dosage used for urgent care:

- **β-Adrenergic agonists** include both long-acting and short-acting preparations used for relaxation of smooth muscles and bronchodilation, reducing edema, and aiding clearance of mucus. Medications include salmeterol, sustained-release albuterol and short-acting albuterol, and levalbuterol. Albuterol 2.5–5.0 mg every 20 minutes, 3 doses by nebulizer.
- **Anticholinergics** aid in preventing bronchial constriction and potentiate the bronchodilating action of β-Adrenergic agonists. The most commonly used medication is ipratropium bromide 500 mcg every 20 minutes, 3 doses by nebulizer.
- **Corticosteroids** provide anti-inflammatory action by inhibiting immune responses and decreasing edema, mucus, and hyper-responsiveness. Because of numerous side effects, glucocorticosteroids are usually administered orally or parenterally for ≤5 days (prednisone, prednisolone, methylprednisolone) and then switched to inhaled steroids. If a person receives glucocorticoids for more than 5 days, then dosages are tapered. Methylprednisolone 60–125 mg IV is the standard dose for respiratory failure. The Global Initiative for Asthma (GINA) recommends daily inhaled corticosteroids for all individuals with severe asthma to reduce the risk of exacerbations.
- **Methylxanthines** are used to improve pulmonary function and decrease the need for mechanical ventilation. Medications include aminophylline and theophylline.
- **Magnesium sulfate** is used to relax smooth muscles and decrease inflammation. If administered intravenously, it must be given slowly to prevent hypotension and bradycardia. When inhaled, it potentiates the action of albuterol. Standard dosage: 2 g (8 mmol), 1 dose by IV over 20 minutes.
- **Heliox** (helium-oxygen) is administered to decrease airway resistance with airway obstruction, thereby decreasing respiratory effort. Heliox improves oxygenation of those on mechanical ventilation.
- **Leukotriene inhibitors** are used to inhibit inflammation and bronchospasm for long-term management. Medications include montelukast.

ADDITIONAL PULMONARY PHARMACOLOGY

There is a wide range of agents used for pulmonary pharmacology, depending upon the type and degree of pulmonary disease. Agents include:

- **Opioid analgesics**: Used to provide both pain relief and sedation for those on mechanical ventilation to reduce sympathetic response. Medications may include fentanyl or morphine sulfate.
- **Neuromuscular blockers**: Used for induced paralysis of those who have not responded adequately to sedation, especially for intubation and mechanical ventilation. Medications may include pancuronium and vecuronium. However, there is controversy about the use of such blockers, as induced paralysis has been linked to increased mortality rates, sensory hearing loss (pancuronium), atelectasis, and ventilation-perfusion mismatch.
- **Human B-type natriuretic peptides**: Used to reduce pulmonary capillary wedge pressure. Medications include nesiritide.
- **Surfactants**: Reduces surface tension to prevent the collapse of alveoli. Beractant (Survanta) is derived from bovine lung tissue and calfactant from calf lung tissue. They are administered as inhalants.
- **Alkalinizers**: Used to treat metabolic acidosis and reduce pulmonary vascular resistance by achieving an alkaline pH. Medications include sodium bicarbonate and tromethamine (THAM).
- **Pulmonary vasodilator (inhaled nitric oxide)**: Used to relax the vascular muscles and produce pulmonary vasodilation. Some studies show it reduces the need for extracorporeal membrane oxygenation (ECMO).
- **Methylxanthines**: Used to stimulate muscle contractions of the chest and stimulate respirations. Medications include aminophylline, caffeine citrate, and doxapram.
- **Diuretics**: Used to reduce pulmonary edema. Medications include loop diuretics such as furosemide and metolazone.
- **Nitrates**: Used for vasodilation to reduce preload and afterload, which in turn reduces myocardial need for oxygen. Medications include nitroglycerin and nitroprusside sodium.
- **Antibiotics**: Used for treatment of respiratory infections, including pneumonia. Medications are used according to the pathogenic agent and may include macrolides such as azithromycin (Zithromax) and erythromycin.
- **Antimycobacterials**: Used for treatment of TB and other mycobacterial diseases. Medications include isoniazid, ethambutol, rifampin, streptomycin sulfate, and pyrazinamide.
- **Antivirals**: Used to inhibit replication of a virus early in a viral infection. Effectiveness decreases as time passes because the replication process has already begun. Medications include ribavirin and zanamivir.

NEBULIZERS

Nebulizers are used to provide respiratory treatments for conditions that can cause respiratory distress or wheezing, such as asthma. A nebulizer comes with several different parts, which often need to be assembled, depending on the model. The compressor works to power the machine to deliver the medication. Oxygen tubing is connected to the compressor, which travels from the machine to the patient. The other end of the oxygen tubing may be connected to either a mask that fits over the patient's mouth and nose or a mouthpiece that an older child may hold. Respiratory medication is available through vials or small, plastic bullets, which are emptied into a cup near the mouthpiece. Air flows from the compressor through the tubing to change the liquid into a mist that the patient can breathe during treatment.

INHALERS FOR CHILDREN

Inhalers used by children are typically one of two types: metered-dose inhalers or dry-powder inhalers.

- **Metered-dose inhalers** have a set amount of medication that is delivered with each use. The patient places the mouthpiece in his mouth and compresses the inhaler while breathing in the medication at the same time. For young children, a spacer may be added **(shown below)**, which holds the medication for the patient to inhale at his or her own pace. This may also be connected to a mask, which makes breathing the medication easier for young children.

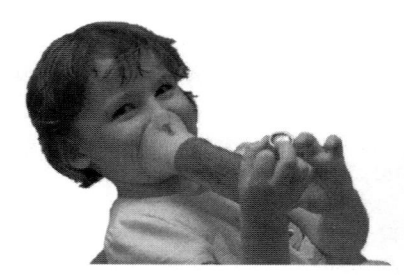

- With **dry-powder inhalers**, medication is inhaled in powdered form. The prescribed amount of medication is available in the inhaler, which is then inhaled at the patient's pace, without having to coordinate compressing the device and taking a breath.

Infectious Disease Pharmacology

ANTIBIOTICS

Antibiotics, produced from microorganisms (such as fungi), are used to combat bacterial infections. Bacteria are critical for human survival and most are benign, but some are pathogenic, leading to infection. Bacteria have simple prokaryote structures, with no membrane-encased nucleus or organelles. Instead, they have a tangle of looped DNA called a nucleoid. Bacteria also have plasmids, which are double strands of DNA outside of the nucleoid that allow for transmission from cell to cell or by attaching to viruses. Essentially, bacteria are able to trade genes, making them very adaptable. The cell membrane of most bacteria, except the Mollicutes (mycoplasmas), is surrounded by a cell wall, the composition of which varies. It is the composition of this cell wall that determines the Gram-staining, either negative or positive. Common side effects include nausea, vomiting, diarrhea, rash, and vaginal yeast infections. Severe reactions include anaphylaxis, super-infection with Clostridioides difficile, and bone marrow, liver, and renal impairment.

> **Review Video: Antibiotics: An Overview**
> Visit mometrix.com/academy and enter code: 165628

CLASSIFICATION

Antibiotics may be classified according to their chemical nature, origin, action, or range of effectiveness. There are hundreds of antibiotics. Broad-spectrum antibiotics are useful against both Gram-positive and Gram-negative bacteria. Medium spectrum antibiotics are usually effective against Gram-positive bacteria although some may be effective against Gram-negative as well. Narrow spectrum antibiotics are effective against a small range of bacteria. Depending on the type, antibiotics can kill bacteria by interfering with its biological functions (bactericidal) or by preventing reproduction (bacteriostatic). The **main classes of antibiotics** used in children include:

- **Macrolides**: Medium spectrum antibiotics. They prevent protein production by bacteria and are primarily bacteriostatic but may be bactericidal at high doses. They may be irritating to the gastric mucosa, but are less likely to cause allergic responses than penicillins or cephalosporins. Macrolides include erythromycin, clarithromycin, and azithromycin.
- **Sulfonamides**: Sulfonamides are medium spectrum with action against Gram-positive and many Gram-negative organisms as well as Plasmodium and Toxoplasma. Some people are sensitive and may develop an allergic response. Resistance to sulfa drugs is widespread. Sulfa drugs interfere with folate synthesis and prevent cell division, so they are bacteriostatic. Sulfonamides include co-trimoxazole (Bactrim) and trimethoprim.
- **Aminoglycosides**: Effective against Gram-negative bacteria. They interfere with protein production in the bacteria and are bactericidal. Aminoglycosides cannot be taken orally. They are often given in conjunction with other classes of antibiotics, such as penicillin. Aminoglycosides include gentamicin and tobramycin, neomycin, and streptomycin.
- **Penicillins**: Medium spectrum antibiotics may be combined with β-lactamase inhibitors. They are bactericidal and cause breakdown of the bacterial cell wall. They may cause severe allergic reactions in sensitive individuals. Penicillins include ampicillin and amoxicillin.
- **Cephalosporins**: Medium spectrum antibiotics are effective against Gram-negative organisms. They are bactericidal and inhibit cell wall synthesis. They are divided into different "generations" according to antimicrobial properties, with succeeding generations having a more powerful effect against resistant strains. First generation includes cephazolin, cephalexin (Keflex), and cefadroxil. Second generation includes cefaclor, cefuroxime, cefotetan (Cefotan), and cefprozil. Third generation includes cefotaxime, cefixime, cefpodoxime, ceftazidime, and cefdinir (Omnicef). Fourth generation includes cefepime.
- **Polymyxins**: Narrow spectrum antibiotics are effective against Gram-negative organisms. Interferes with cell membrane of bacteria and are bactericidal. Polymyxins have both neurotoxic and nephrotoxic properties and are not used unless other antibiotics are ineffective. They must be given intravenously.

ANTIFUNGAL AGENTS

Even though antifungal agents are available, systemic fungal infections are difficult to treat. Fungi were originally classified as plants, but they do not produce their own food through photosynthesis and must, like animals, get food from another source. Fungi vary widely, from one-celled microorganisms to multi-celled chains that are miles long. Fungi are used to make antibiotics, but they can also cause infection and disease. Two common classifications of fungi are **molds** (including mushrooms) and **yeast**. Fungi are not motile, but some produce spores, which can be inhaled. Some, such as the yeast Candida albicans, are part of the normal flora of the skin but can overgrow in an opportunistic infection. As microorganisms, fungal infections can invade the sinuses, the mouth, the respiratory system, and the vagina. Antibiotics may affect the balance between bacteria and yeast, causing infection. Fungal infections include histoplasmosis, blastomycosis, and coccidioidomycosis. Fungal infections, such as *Pneumocystis jiroveci* (formerly carinii), pose a serious problem for the immunocompromised.

Fungal infections are common on the skin and mucous membranes, but the use of vascular access devices and other invasive devices has increased the incidence of fungemia in patients. Additionally, powerful antibiotics contribute to fungal infections by altering the balance of organisms. Fungal cells are more difficult to eradicate than bacterial cells because they are more similar to human cells, so treating a fungus can damage other cells and result in serious side effects, such as nausea, diarrhea, anorexia, rash, and itching. Amphotericin B especially has serious side effects, which can cause fever and chills, headache, hypotension, dyspnea, multiple organ damage, and even death. There are a number of different classes of antifungal agents. Below are those most commonly used in the pediatric population:

- **Triazole antifungals** have similar action to imidazole but are newer and less toxic. Fluconazole (Diflucan) may be used for both superficial (skin, mucous membranes) and systemic fungal infections. It is used for both treatment and prophylaxis against candidiasis. It is effective for coccidioidomycosis, cryptococcosis, and histoplasmosis.
- **Polyene antifungals** attack the fungal cell membrane, leading to death of the organism. These antifungals are derived from *Streptomyces* sp. Amphotericin B may be used orally for treatment of thrush, but it is more commonly used intravenously for systemic fungal infections, including aspergillosis and candidiasis.
- **Echinocandin antifungals** also inhibit cell wall synthesis. Anidulafungin (Eraxis) is primarily used for the treatment of systemic candidiasis. It degrades chemically in the presence of normal body pH and is safe to use with liver or kidney impairment. Caspofungin (Cancidas) is used intravenously for treatment of aspergillosis and candidiasis and is often effective when patients have shown resistance to other drugs. Micafungin (Mycamine) is used intravenously to treat a wide variety of candidal infections, including candidiasis, candida peritonitis, and esophageal candidiasis. It is also used as a prophylaxis for those having hematopoietic stem cell transplantation.

ANTIPARASITIC AGENTS

Antiparasitic agents are used for protozoan diseases. **Protozoa** are one-celled organisms from a number of different phyla. Protozoa consume bacteria, so they have a critical role in the cycle of life, but about 10,000 species are parasites that can infect vertebrates. Protozoan infections, especially of the gastrointestinal tract, have become more prevalent in those who are immunocompromised:

- *Giardia intestinalis* has become the most common cause of water-borne disease and non-bacterial diarrhea in the United States. Antiparasitic agents include metronidazole (Flagyl), nitazoxanide, and tinidazole.
- *Dientamoeba fragilis* occurs worldwide, especially in children, and those who live or travel to areas with poor sanitation. Antiparasitics include iodoquinol, paromomycin, and metronidazole.
- *Entamoeba histolytica* is more prevalent in developing countries, but increasing rates of infection have been found in Hispanics (33%), Asian and Pacific Islanders (17%), recent immigrants, travelers, institutionalized populations, and men having sex with men. Antiparasitics for asymptomatic infections include iodoquinol, paromomycin, and diloxanide furoate. For mild to severe disease, metronidazole and tinidazole.

Antiparasitic agents include **anthelmintic agents** for treatment of parasitic worms:

- **Nematodes** are unsegmented roundworms, including pin worms, hookworms, whipworms, and roundworms. There are over 80,000 varieties. Those that infest humans range from as small as 0.3 mm to as long as 1 m in length. People usually become infected by ingestion of contaminated food or touching contaminated hands to the mouth. Antiparasitic drugs useful against nematodes include albendazole, mebendazole (Emverm), pyrantel pamoate (Pin-Away), and ivermectin.
- **Cestodes** are segmented flatworms, also called tapeworms, which live in the intestinal tracts of some animals and fish and infect humans who eat raw or undercooked meat/fish. Antiparasitic drugs include praziquantel (Biltricide), nitazoxanide, and niclosamide.
- **Trematodes** are a type of flatworm called flukes, which can cause diseases in the intestines, blood, liver, and lungs. Fluke infections are caused by ingestion of uncooked meat, plants, or fish from contaminated waters. Antiparasitic drugs include praziquantel and albendazole.
- *Balantidium coli* occur most commonly in the tropics among those in contact with pigs, but outbreaks have occurred in psychiatric hospitals in the United States. Antiparasitics include metronidazole and iodoquinol (topically only).
- *Cryptosporidium parvum* and *Cryptosporidium hominis* have caused a number of outbreaks since first identified in 1976, sometimes related to swimming in pools contaminated with feces or handling dirty diapers. The antiparasitic agent used for treatment is nitazoxanide, which is effective only in those without HIV. Antiretroviral treatment received for HIV infection is, however, effective against cryptosporidia.
- *Isospora belli* occurs worldwide, primarily in tropical areas, but can occur in travelers and those with HIV. The only effective antiparasitic agent is trimethoprim-sulfamethoxazole. There is no alternative for those allergic to sulfa.
- *Cyclospora cayetanensis* occurs worldwide and has been implicated in a number of food-borne outbreaks in the United States since 1996. The antiparasitic agent is trimethoprim-sulfamethoxazole. Those sensitive to sulfa may be treated with nitazoxanide.

Microsporidia are now commonly believed to be basic fungi, closer to fungi than other protozoa, and increasingly recognized worldwide as opportunistic infectious agents, especially in immuno-compromised individuals, such as those with HIV/AIDS, causing microsporidiosis. Fourteen species have been identified as **pathogenic** to humans, some affecting the eyes and muscles. Enterocytozoon bieneusi and Encephalitozoon intestinalis cause most cases of microsporidiosis with gastrointestinal manifestations and are common in HIV/AIDS patients, but there are increasing infections in non-HIV infected travelers and those living in tropical areas. Antiparasitic agents include thalidomide, which is used for chronic diarrhea unresponsive to other medications. Metronidazole is also useful for the treatment of diarrhea. On-going treatment may be needed to prevent recurrence of symptoms. Drugs of choice include:

- *E. Intestinalis*: Albendazole 400 mg daily for children ≥2 years old (200 mg for younger) for 14 days
- *E. Bieneusi*: Fumagillin 60 mg daily for 14 days

ANTIRETROVIRAL AGENTS FOR HIV AND AIDS

There are four primary classes of antiretroviral agents used for the treatment of HIV/AIDS:

- **Non-nucleoside reverse transcriptase inhibitors** (NNRTIs), such as efavirenz, and nevirapine, bind to reverse transcriptase and disable it. Reverse transcriptase is a protein required for HIV replication.
- **Nucleoside reverse transcriptase inhibitors** (NRTIs), such as abacavir (Ziagen), zidovudine (Retrovir), and lamivudine (Epivir), are defective versions of building blocks necessary for replication. When HIV binds to the defective version, it is unable to complete replication.
- **Fusion inhibitors**, such as enfuvirtide (Fuzeon), are entry blockers.

Pharmacologic Pain Management

WHO Pain Ladder

The WHO pain ladder was developed as an algorithm for treating pain through medications with progressively increasing potency. The approach can be used effectively with both adult and pediatric patients. Beginning with the least potent medication option, each step adds a stronger analgesic until optimum pain relief is reached.

The **WHO pain ladder** has three steps.

- **Step 1**: The patient is given a non-opioid medication which may be used alone or in conjunction with other adjuvant therapies.
- **Step 2**: If the patient reports no change in the pain level, mild- to moderate-level pain-relieving opioids are introduced along with adjuvants if they have not been previously introduced.
- **Step 3**: Uncontrolled pain is then treated with opioids for moderate to severe pain. Adjuvants may also be continued.

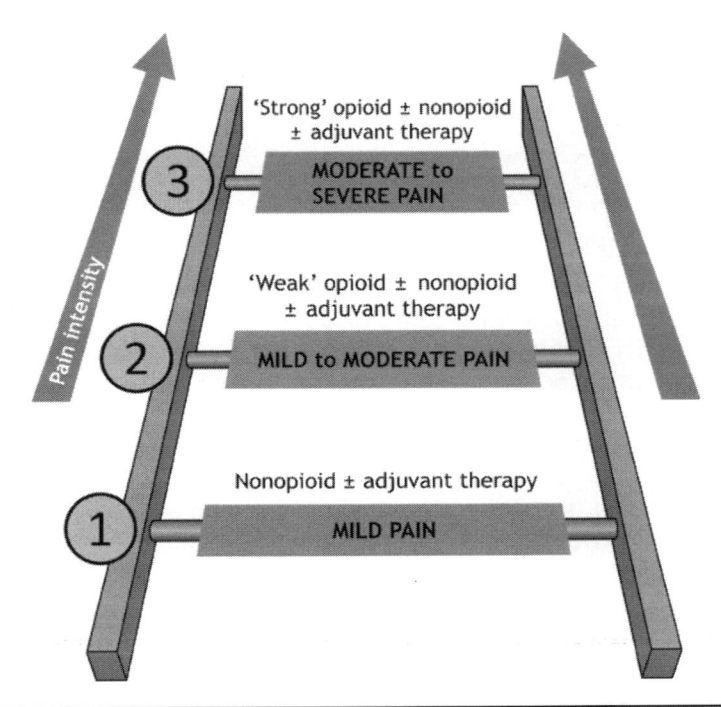

Review Video: Adjuvants
Visit mometrix.com/academy and enter code: 178200

Scheduling of Pain Medications

For mild to moderate pain, patients may take **acetaminophen** alternating with an **NSAID** such as ibuprofen on a regularly scheduled basis or as needed (PRN) at the onset of pain or when pain is anticipated (such as before a dressing change). However, for severe chronic pain, long-acting **opioid pain medications**, such as time-released morphine, fentanyl, and oxycodone, should be given regularly around the clock, because these medications help not only control but also prevent pain. The patient should not skip a dose when free of pain, because this makes control more difficult when the pain recurs. In addition to **time-scheduled medications**, the patient may need **short-acting supplementary medications**, such as Percocet, to take on a PRN basis. When taking short-acting medications, the patient should take the medication at the onset of pain, before anticipated pain, or at the onset of increased pain, rather than waiting until the pain is severe, because the goal should always be to keep the pain under control.

Acetaminophen

Acetaminophen remains one of the safest analgesics for **long-term use**. It can be used to treat mild pain or as an adjuvant with other analgesics for more severe pain. Nonspecific musculoskeletal pain and osteoarthritis are particularly responsive to acetaminophen therapy. Acetaminophen also has a limited **anti-inflammatory nature**.

Acetaminophen should, however, be used cautiously in persons with altered liver or kidney function, as well as those with a history of significant alcohol use, regardless of liver function compromise. It should be dosed separately from any opioid analgesic, which should be given separately as well. This allows for individual titration of each drug to assess the individual needs and side effects separately.

NSAIDs

NSAIDs act by inhibiting the cyclooxygenase (COX) enzyme, which controls prostaglandin formation. COX-1 affects platelet clumping, gastric blood flow, and mucosal integrity. COX-2 affects pain, inflammation, and fever. COX-1 and 2 inhibitors include aspirin and ibuprofen. Ibuprofen has a lower occurrence of side effects, such as gastric bleeding, than aspirin does. A COX-2 inhibitor, such as Celebrex, must be used with caution due to increased cardiovascular risks when used for over 18 months. NSAIDs are useful for both arthritis and bone cancer pain and work well with opioids for relief of postoperative and other severe pain. NSAIDs may increase the effects of antiseizure drugs and warfarin. Smaller doses are needed if kidney function is impaired.

> **Review Video: NSAID Side Effects**
> Visit mometrix.com/academy and enter code: 569064

Local Anesthetic Pain Relief

Local anesthetics block neural conduction of pain through the application of the anesthetic directly to the nerve endings in the area of pain. It can be injected prior to minor surgery or suturing. It can be injected intercostally for thoracic or high abdominal surgeries. The addition of a vasoconstrictor prolongs effectiveness of the anesthetic. A cream containing local anesthetics (EMLA) can be rubbed on the skin to decrease pain from IV starts or lumbar punctures. It should be applied 60–90 minutes prior to the procedure. A lidocaine 5% patch is approved to relieve pain from postherpetic neuralgia. The patient applies up to 3 patches for 12 hours at a time. Local anesthetics can be applied via the use of an epidural catheter to provide pain control for surgery, childbirth, or postoperative pain control. Opioids can be infused along with the anesthetic agent. Patients using an epidural catheter for postoperative pain tend to ambulate sooner, suffer fewer complications as a result, and go home more quickly.

Opioids

Guidelines for Opioid Use

Opioid analgesic therapy is a widely used method of chronic pain control. By adhering to clinical guidelines, pain control can be safely optimized. **Intramuscular administration** should be used as a last resort except in the presence of a "pain emergency" when no other treatment is readily available. Such cases are rare since subcutaneous delivery is almost always an alternative. Noninvasive routes such as **transdermal** and **transmucosal**, which bypass the enteral route, are optimal for continuous pain control and are often effective in eliminating breakthrough pain as well. Changing from one opioid to another, or altering the delivery method, may become necessary under the assumption that incomplete cross-tolerance among opioids occurs. Changing analgesics or method of delivery may result in a decreased drug requirement. When altering opioid delivery regimens, use **morphine equivalents** as the common factor for all dose conversions. This method will help reduce medication errors. Side effects such as sedation, constipation, nausea, and myoclonus should be anticipated in every care plan, and require both prevention and treatment methods.

Side Effects of Opioid Analgesics

Examples of **opioid analgesics** are numerous and include morphine, hydromorphone, oxymorphone, methadone, meperidine, fentanyl, sufentanil, levorphanol, codeine, oxycodone, hydrocodone, nalbuphine, and buprenorphine. Opioid analgesics have multiple effects on most of the organ systems of the body. Central nervous system (CNS) effects include respiratory depression, analgesia, euphoria, sedation, miosis, cough suppression, truncal rigidity, nausea, and vomiting. Cardiovascular effects are usually slight and include bradycardia, hypotension, reduced blood volume, and increased cerebral blood flow. Gastrointestinal effects can include constipation, decreased gastric motility, and decreased hydrochloric acid. Genitourinary effects are urinary retention and decreased renal function. Other effects are sweating, flushing, and histamine release with itching.

Opioid Use During Last Few Hours of Life

Assessment of pain continues in the **last hours of life**, and medication is adjusted according to assessment. Pain does not necessarily increase as death approaches. It can be assumed that if pain was present prior to loss of consciousness it will continue in the patient's unconscious state. It should be assessed for and treated accordingly. Research has confirmed that administering opioids at the end of life does not hasten nor prolong the dying process. The patient's **prior medication regimen** should be continued. However, adjustments may be made in consideration of reduced renal or hepatic clearance. The **route of administration** should also be assessed for appropriateness and adjusted as needed (e.g., loss of consciousness, inability to swallow).

Oral Transmucosal Fentanyl Citrate

Oral transmucosal fentanyl citrate consists of **fentanyl** on an oral applicator. The patient applies the dosage (starting at 200 mcg) to the **buccal mucosa** between the cheek and gum for rapid absorption and subsequent pain relief. This makes transmucosal fentanyl particularly useful for managing **breakthrough pain**. Pain relief generally begins within 5 minutes, but the patient should be instructed to wait 15 minutes after the previous dose has been completed before taking another dose. Swallowing even part of the dose rather than having it completely absorbed through the oral mucosa can affect the timing of pain relief onset. **Peak effect** occurs in 20–40 minutes with the total pain relief duration lasting 2–3 hours. Side effects can include somnolence, nausea, and dizziness. Consuming drinks such as coffee, tea, and juices that alter the oral secretion pH can also alter the absorption rate of transmucosal fentanyl.

Methadone

Methadone is useful for treating **severe or chronic pain** and may be particularly helpful in the presence of **neuropathic pain**. It has a long-acting pain relief factor for a lower cost than many comparable medications. However, the exact dosing ratios with morphine remain unclear within the available research. Metabolism of methadone can also be swayed (either increased or decreased) by many other medications normally taken by patients with chronic conditions. Methadone can also be used to treat opioid addiction. US law for the prescription of methadone for addiction in detoxification or maintenance programs requires a special license and patient enrollment. The words "for pain" need to be clearly stated in the prescription. Methadone can cause drowsiness, weakness, headache, nausea, vomiting, constipation, sweating, and flushing, as well as sedation, decreased respirations, or an irregular heart rate.

Oxycodone

Oxycodone, a synthetic formulation, is a long-acting opioid for **moderate to severe pain relief**. Side effects are similar to those of morphine. It has a similar pain relief ratio, with the possibility of less nausea and vomiting. Because of its extended-release nature, the medication cannot be cut or crushed for administration. Oxycodone does not carry any greater addiction risk than other types of opioids; however, public sensationalism related to this formulation may create hesitation for use among patients. Pharmacies may also limit the amount of this medication they will make available to an individual. Oxycodone should be used cautiously in patients with a history of hypothyroidism, Addison disease, urethral stricture, prostatic hypertrophy, or lung or liver disease.

Hydromorphone

Hydromorphone is available as tablets, liquid, suppository, and parenteral formulations. It offers the advantage of being synthetic, allowing for its use in the presence of a true **morphine allergy**. It is also helpful when significant side effects have occurred in the past or pain has been inadequately controlled with other medications. It may also be useful for controlling cough. However, neurotoxicity may occur, particularly myoclonus, hyperalgesia, and seizures. It should also be used cautiously in the presence of kidney, liver, heart, and thyroid disease, seizure disorders, respiratory disease, prostatic hypertrophy, or urinary problems. Common *side effects* include dizziness, lightheadedness, drowsiness, upset stomach if taken without food, vomiting, and constipation.

Titration of Morphine for Pain Control

Morphine titration protocols vary according to the type of morphine used, the severity of pain, and the patient's tolerance:

Type	Peak	Duration (hours)
Short-acting	60 minutes	4–5
Long-acting	3–4 hours	8–24
IM	30–60 minutes	4–5
SQ	50–90 minutes	4–5
IV	20 minutes	4–5
Rectal	20–60 minutes	3–7

For example, **optimal dosage** is usually calculated by starting with short-acting oral morphine at 30 mg every 3–4 hours with doses increased by 25–50% for moderate pain or 50–100% for severe pain each time until the patient has at least 50% reduction in pain on a scale of 1–10 or a behavior scale. The dose may need to be reduced if excessive sedation occurs. Once the patient's pain is controlled on short-acting morphine and 24-hour dosage needs are calculated, the patient could be switched to extended-release. **Breakthrough pain** is usually treated with dosages that are 10% of the 24-hour dose. Dosages may be repeated or increased if there is inadequate relief of pain at the peak time. Increasing the dose prior to peak time will result in increased drowsiness.

Morphine Use for Chronic Cancer Pain

One advantage of morphine for chronic cancer pain is that it has no **ceiling dose**. As tolerance to the medication increases or the disease progresses in severity, the dose can be gradually increased to an infinite level. It is also available in many different forms for administration, including intravenous, intramuscular, immediate release, sustained release, long-acting, liquid oral preparations, and suppositories. Morphine is often used as the **equivalency standard** for other opioid analgesics. Common *side effects* of morphine include sedation, respiratory depression, itching, nausea, chronic spasms or twitching of muscle groups, and constipation. Constipation is experienced by all patients receiving opioids. This inevitability should be planned for and treated aggressively. Hallucinations are common when morphine is initiated. After the first few days, most patients will overcome the respiratory depression, nausea, itching, and extreme sedation as tolerance for the medication is developed.

Dosages for Morphine, Codeine, Hydromorphone, and Levorphanol

The dosages for both the enteral and parenteral routes of morphine, codeine, hydromorphone, and levorphanol are as follows:

- **Morphine**: Enteral dosage is 30 mg (available as continuous and sustained-release formulations to last 12–24 hours); parenteral dosage is 10 mg.
- **Codeine**: Enteral dosage is 200 mg (not generally recommended); parenteral dosage is 130 mg.
- **Hydromorphone**: Enteral dosage is 7.5 mg (available as a continuous-release formula lasting 24 hours); parenteral dosage is 1.5 mg.
- **Levorphanol**: In acute pain episodes, enteral dosage is 4 mg; parenteral dosage is 2 mg. For chronic pain, dosage is equivalent for both enteral and parenteral at 1 mg. Levorphanol has a long half-life, increasing the chances of dosage accumulation over time.

Adhering to the statement "If the gut works, use it," as much as 90 percent of all patients will at least start out able to use oral medications instead of other routes.

Calculation for Converting Medication Regimen Between Two Opioids

Calculate the current 24-hour drug dose, or the total amount given in a 24-hour period. Multiply the current 24-hour dose times the ratio of the 24-hour equivalent dose for the new drug over the 24-hour equivalent of the old drug. This calculation provides the **equivalent 24-hour dose** for the new drug. Divide the new dose amount by the number of doses to be provided during the day. This amount equals the new **target dosage**.

$$\text{current 24 hr dose} \times \frac{\text{new drug 24 hr equiv dose}}{\text{current drug 24 hr equiv dose}} = \text{new 24 hr dose}$$

$$\frac{\text{new 24 hr dose}}{\text{doses per day}} = \text{new target dosage}$$

Ketamine

Ketamine is a dissociative anesthetic that can provide pain relief as an alternate or complement to an opioid. The dissociative quality is an effective way to help the patient separate from the sensation of pain. Ketamine treatment begins with an initial bolus of 0.1 mg/kg IV. If there is no improvement, a second bolus with double the dosage is provided in 5 minutes. This can be repeated as needed. Boluses should be followed by a decrease in the patient's current opioid dose by 50% and an infusion of ketamine. **Infusion dosing** for ketamine is 0.015 mg/kg/min, or about 1 mg/min for a 70 kg person. If IV access cannot be attained, subcutaneous infusion is a possibility with dosing of 0.3–0.5 mg/kg. Consider concurrent treatment with a **benzodiazepine** to prevent hallucinations or frightful dreams and observe for increased secretions, as these are all possible side effects of ketamine. The secretions may be treated with glycopyrrolate, scopolamine, or atropine as needed.

Treating Breakthrough Pain

The three basic types of breakthrough pain, and their treatment measures are as follows:

- **Incident pain**: Pain that can be specifically tied to an activity or event, such as a dressing change or physical therapy. These events can be anticipated and treated with a rapid-onset, short-acting analgesic just prior to the painful event.
- **Spontaneous pain**: This type of pain is unpredictable and cannot be pinpointed to a relationship with any certain time or event. There is no way to anticipate spontaneous pain. In the presence of neuropathic pain, adjuvant therapy may be useful. Otherwise, a rapid-onset, short-acting analgesic is used.
- **End-of-dose failure**: Pain that specifically occurs at the end of a routine analgesic dosing cycle when medication blood levels begin to taper off. Careful evaluation of end-of-dose failure can help prevent it sooner. It may indicate an increased dose tolerance and the need for medication dose alterations.

TREATING NEUROPATHIC PAIN

Treatment options for neuropathic pain are often different from the methods used to treat other types of pain. The three drug classes most commonly used and proven effective for treating neuropathic pain are **anticonvulsants**, **anesthetics**, and **antidepressants**. Some are given on an as-needed basis, but most require consistent dosing with **24-hour symptom control**. Examples of the most common medications include amitriptyline, nortriptyline, duloxetine, gabapentin, topical lidocaine, opioids, and pregabalin. Medication choice is dependent on factors such as the type and progression of the disorder and the associated physical and emotional problems, such as nerve injury, muscle weakness or spasms, anxiety, depression, or sleep disturbances.

> **Review Video: Neuropathic Pain**
> Visit mometrix.com/academy and enter code: 780523

TREATING BONE PAIN

Treatment options for bone pain may depend on the causative agent related to the pain, such as the primary cancer site, severely weakened bones, or fractures. **Systemic treatment choices** include chemotherapy, radiation, and hormone therapy. **Hormone therapy** is used in the presence of estrogen and androgen receptors within the cancer cells. **Bisphosphonates**, such as ibandronate, zoledronate, and alendronate, may help strengthen the bones, slow damage, and prevent fractures; they can also help reduce pain. However, side effects can include fatigue, fever, nausea, vomiting, and anemia. **Surgery** may also be considered to remove cancerous cells or reinforce weakened areas of bone. **Opioids** and **NSAIDs/COX-2 inhibitors** are most often used for pain relief and need to be provided on a consistent basis.

Morphine combined with ibuprofen provides the benefit of a centrally acting opioid with a peripherally acting NSAID. Ibuprofen also acts as an effective adjuvant analgesic agent to enhance the relief provided by the opioid without increasing opioid side effects.

MEASURES TAKEN DURING PAIN CRISIS

During a pain crisis, assess for a change in the mechanism or location of the pain and attempt to differentiate between **terminal anxiety** or agitation and the **physical causes** of pain. Begin with a rapid increase in **opioid treatment**. If the pain is unresponsive to opioid titration, switching to **benzodiazepines**, such as diazepam and lorazepam, may produce a more effective response. If terminal symptoms remain unresponsive, assess for **drug absorption**. While invasive routes of medication delivery are generally avoided unless necessary, the only guaranteed route of drug delivery is the IV route. If there is any question about absorption, it is appropriate to establish parenteral access. IM delivery should be considered as a last resort. When all accessible resources have been exhausted, seek a pain management consultation as quickly as possible. Alternative methods of terminal pain control include radiotherapy, anesthetic, or neuroablative procedures.

CONCERNS SURROUNDING USE OF PAIN MEDICATIONS WITH END-OF-LIFE PATIENTS

Common concerns surrounding the use of pain medications with end-of-life patients include:

- **Adequacy**: Patients are often concerned that medication may not be adequate to control pain and that chronic or breakthrough pain will occur. Patients may be concerned that if they take adequate pain medication, it will be less effective later when pain may be worse.
- **Sedation/addiction**: Some patients and family members are concerned about the risks of addiction, and others may be concerned about the effects of the medication on the patient's cognition, as some patients may become confused, disoriented, or sedated, depending on the medication or dosage.
- **Adverse effects**: Nausea and vomiting may be almost as debilitating to a patient as the pain it is intended to alleviate. Constipation, a common adverse effect, may be very uncomfortable for a patient. Some medications may result in itching and others may cause myoclonus, both of which are uncomfortable for the patient.

Prescribing Controlled Substances to Patients with Advanced Illness and Addiction Challenges

In the presence of **addiction challenges**, it becomes important to choose a **long-acting opioid** that can facilitate around-the-clock dosing and minimize the need for short-term medications used for breakthrough doses. **Short-term medication** use should be very limited or eliminated entirely if possible. Whenever possible, **nondrug adjuvants** such as relaxation techniques, distraction, biofeedback, TNS, and therapeutic communication should be used in place of short-term medications. When short-term medication therapy is needed, a **nonopioid** is best. Limit the amount of medication available to the patient at any given time and monitor for compliance with pill counts and urine toxicology screens as necessary. In some instances, a referral to an addictions specialist is recommended.

Equianalgesia

Equianalgesia is a comparison of doses of different analgesics that provide equivalent analgesia/sedation. Children may vary in their ability to metabolize drugs, so they must be monitored carefully with all analgesics. Intravenous analgesics usually take effect within 15 to 30 minutes while oral medications take twice as long. Dosage must be calculated according to age and weight:

Drug	Parenteral	Oral
Morphine sulfate	0.025–0.03 mg/kg/dose	0.08–0.1 mg/kg/dose (comes in 2 mg/mL or 4 mg/mL)
Dilaudid	0.015 mg/kg/dose	0.03–0.08 mg/kg/dose
Fentanyl	1-2 mcg/kg/dose	Varies (patches)
Codeine	Not recommended for children	0.5–1 mg/kg/dose (max dose 60 mg)
Vicodin	Not available parenterally	0.1–0.2 mg/kg/dose

Acetaminophen and NSAID Pediatric Dosing and Side Effects

Drug	Dosage	Side Effects
Acetaminophen	Dosages may be repeated every 4 hours to the maximum of 5 doses in 24 hours. Dosage is based on 10-15 mg/kg with adult dosing at 12 years: • 0-3 months: 40 mg • 4-11 months: 80 mg • 1-2 years: 120 mg • 2-3 years: 160 mg • 4-5 years: 240 mg • 6-8 years: 320 mg • 9-10 years: 325–400 mg • 11 years: 480 mg	Allergic response with itching, rash, and edema. Liver toxicity with overdose.
Choline Magnesium Trisalicylate	• <37 kg (81.5 lb): 50 mg/kg/day divided in 2 doses • >37 kg (81.5 lb): 2250 mg/day divided in 2 doses	Tinnitus. GI irritation with nausea, vomiting, diarrhea, constipation, and epigastric discomfort.
Ibuprofen	• <6 months to 12 years: 5-10 mg/kg every 6-8 hours to maximum of 40 mg/kg/day • 12-18 years: 200 to 400 mg every 4 to 6 hours to maximum of 2400 mg/day	Nausea, vomiting, and diarrhea. Gastrointestinal irritation with ulcerations and bleeding. Bleeding nephritis. Retention of fluid.

Drug	Dosage	Side Effects
Naproxen	• >2 years: 20 mg/kg/day divided in 2 doses	Same as ibuprofen
Tolmetin	• >2 years: 15–30 mg/kg/day divided in 3-4 doses	Same as ibuprofen

> **Review Video: NSAIDs and Their Side Effects**
> Visit mometrix.com/academy and enter code: 569064

COX INHIBITORS

Cyclooxygenase (COX) inhibitors are NSAIDs that block COX enzymes that develop with inflammation and with precancerous/cancerous tissues. COX enzymes form prostanoids:

- **Prostaglandins**: Cell growth, inflammatory reactions, sensitivity to pain, platelet aggregation/disaggregation, and hormone and calcium regulation
- **Prostacyclin**: Platelet aggregation and vasodilation
- **Thromboxane**: Platelet aggregation and vasoconstriction

COX inhibitors are used as anti-inflammatory analgesics and antiplatelet drugs. Some drugs, such as ibuprofen and aspirin, block both COX-1 and COX-2 enzymes (non-selective inhibitors). Non-selective NSAIDs are associated with irritation of gastric mucosa because of inhibition of COX-1, which has a protective effect on gastrointestinal mucosa. Other drugs, such as celecoxib, block only COX-2 enzymes (selective inhibitors) and these tend to have fewer gastrointestinal adverse effects, but they have been implicated in increased risk for cardiovascular disease and thrombus formation. COX-2 NSAIDs specifically target inflammation. A third COX enzyme, COX-3, has been identified, and some speculate acetaminophen (which has no anti-inflammatory properties) may target this enzyme, but research is inconclusive.

PATIENT-CONTROLLED ANALGESIA

Patient-controlled analgesia (PCA) allows the child to control administration of pain medication by pressing a button on an intravenous delivery system with a computerized pump. The device is filled with opioid (as prescribed) and must be programmed correctly and checked regularly to ensure that it is functioning properly and that controls are set. The most-commonly administered medications include morphine, meperidine, fentanyl, and sufentanil. Most devices can be set to deliver a continuous infusion of opioid as well as patient-controlled bolus. Each element must be set:

- **Bolus**: Determines the amount of medication received when the patient delivers a dose
- **Lockout interval**: Time required between administrations of boluses
- **Continuous infusion**: Rate at which opioid is delivered per hour for continuous analgesia
- **Limit** (usually set at 4 hours): Total amount of opioid that can be delivered in the preset time limit

With Authorized Agent Controlled Analgesia (AACA), people who are trained and authorized (such as a nurse, family member, and caregiver) may administer the medication as well as the child.

Psychosocial Pharmacology

ANTIPSYCHOTIC MEDICATIONS

FIRST-GENERATION

There are a variety of first-generation antipsychotics available, though their use is becoming less prominent now that atypical antipsychotic agents are available. Some **first-generation antipsychotics** include:

- Chlorpromazine
- Thioridazine hydrochloride
- Haloperidol
- Pimozide
- Fluphenazine hydrochloride
- Molindone hydrochloride
- Trifluoperazine hydrochloride

Possible side effects include photosensitivity, sexual dysfunction, dry mouth, dry eyes, nasal congestion, blurred vision, constipation, urinary retention, exacerbation of narrow-angle glaucoma, various cardiac effects, extrapyramidal effects, dyskinesia, sedation, cognitive dulling, amenorrhea, menstrual irregularities, hyperglycemia or hypoglycemia, increased appetite, and weight gain. The most common extrapyramidal symptom caused by antipsychotic agents is tardive dyskinesia, in which clients are unable to control their movements, such as tics, lip-smacking, and eye blinking. The extrapyramidal system is a group of neural connections outside of the medulla that control movement. **Extrapyramidal effects** are the result of drug influence on the extrapyramidal system and include:

- Akinesia (inability to start movement)
- Akathisia (inability to stop movement)
- Dystonia (extreme and uncontrolled muscle contraction, torticollis, flexing, and twisting)

SECOND-GENERATION

Second-generation antipsychotics (SGAs), also called atypical antipsychotics, are used for bipolar disorders, schizophrenia, and psychosis, and include aripiprazole (Abilify), clozapine (Clozaril), olanzapine (Zyprexa), quetiapine (Seroquel), risperidone (Risperdal), and ziprasidone (Geodon). Females report more side effects than males, but the recommended doses for males and females are identical. Women were underrepresented when SGAs were clinically tested, because researchers feared teratogenic effects on fetuses:

- Side effects include constipation, increased appetite, weight gain, urinary retention, various sexual side effects, increased prolactin, menstrual irregularities, increased risk of diabetes mellitus, decreased blood pressure, dizziness, agranulocytosis, and leucopenia.
- Atypical antipsychotics may interact with fluvoxamine, phenytoin, carbamazepine, barbiturates, nicotine, ketoconazole, phenytoin, rifampin, and glucocorticoids.
- The use of atypical antipsychotic agents correlates with significant weight gain. Overweight and obese clients are likely to develop insulin resistance and glucose intolerance, which may lead to diabetes mellitus. Data show clozapine and olanzapine as the greatest offenders. Ziprasidone seems to present the lowest risk.

> **Review Video: Antipsychotic Drugs**
> Visit mometrix.com/academy and enter code: 369601

ANTIDEPRESSANTS

INDICATIONS FOR TREATMENT WITH ANTIDEPRESSANT

The main **indicator** for use of an antidepressant is simply **depression**. This can be further expanded to include major depression, atypical depression, and anxiety disorders. Depression-type symptoms commonly include loss of interest in usual or pleasurable activities, decreased levels of energy, having a depressed mood, decreased ability to concentrate, loss of appetite, or suicidal thoughts. Antidepressants are also commonly used to treat **anxiety disorders** that include panic attacks, obsessive-compulsive disorder (OCD), social phobias, and post-traumatic stress disorder. They may also be beneficial in treating chronic pain syndromes, premenstrual syndrome, insomnia, attention deficit hyperactivity disorder, or bed-wetting.

SSRIs

Selective serotonin reuptake inhibitors (SSRIs) prevent the reuptake of serotonin at the presynaptic membrane. This increases the amount of serotonin in the synapse for neurotransmission. This class of antidepressants has been shown to reduce depression and anxiety symptoms. Common side effects are usually short in duration and include headache, GI upset, and sexual dysfunction. They do not cause significant anticholinergic, cardiovascular, or significant patient sedation side effects. Examples of SSRIs include citalopram (Celexa), escitalopram (Lexapro), fluoxetine (Prozac), fluvoxamine (Luvox), paroxetine (Paxil), and sertraline (Zoloft). These drugs are not highly lethal in overdose.

MONITORING

SSRI monitoring includes the following:

- Monitor for increased depression and suicidal ideation, especially in adolescents.
- Inform patients of the following:
  - Smoking decreases effectiveness.
  - Fatal reactions may occur with monoamine oxidase inhibitors.
  - Taking SSRIs with benzodiazepines or alcohol has an additive effect.
  - Some drugs, such as citalopram, may increase the effects of β-blockers and warfarin.
- Avoid cimetidine, which is prescribed for ulcers and gastroesophageal reflux disease, and St. John's wort.
- Inform patients of possible decreased libido and sexual functioning.
- Monitor for insomnia and gastrointestinal upset.

TRICYCLIC ANTIDEPRESSANTS

Tricyclic antidepressants not only block the reuptake of serotonin and norepinephrine, they also act to block muscarinic cholinergic receptors, histamine H1 receptors, and alpha1 noradrenergic receptors. These receptors do not affect depression symptoms, but their blockade is implicated in some of the side effects associated with tricyclics. The blockade of the muscarinic receptors produces anticholinergic side effects such as dry mouth, blurred vision, constipation, urinary retention, and tachycardia. The blockade of the histamine receptors is associated with drowsiness, low blood pressure, and weight gain. The alpha1 noradrenergic receptor blocking action produces the side effects associated with orthostatic hypotension, vertigo, and some memory disturbances.

MECHANISM OF ACTION AND NECESSARY EVALUATIONS

Most of the tricyclic antidepressants have very similar mechanisms of action and side effects. Although their exact **mechanism of action** is unknown, they are believed to act to inhibit the reuptake of both serotonin and norepinephrine. These drugs have a high **first-pass rate of metabolism** and are excreted by the kidneys. A complete **physical and history** should be obtained before starting a patient on tricyclic drugs. Because this class of antidepressants can cause death with an overdose, an initial **suicide risk assessment** must be obtained, and continued assessments for this risk are necessary. This class of drug can cause a prolongation in the electrical conduction of the heart. Therefore, a **baseline ECG** should be performed in children, young teenagers, anyone with cardiac electrical conduction problems, and adults over age 40.

MONITORING

Tricyclics monitoring includes the following:

- Observe for toxicity.
- Inform patients not to take with monoamine oxidase inhibitors.
- Observe for decreased therapeutic response to hypertensives (e.g., clonidine, guanethidine).
- Monitor other medications; the patient should avoid other central nervous system depressants, including alcohol. Some medications potentiate the effects of tricyclics, including bupropion, cimetidine, haloperidol, selective serotonin reuptake inhibitors, and valproic acid.
- Inform the patient to avoid prolonged exposure to sunlight or sunlamps.
- Administer major dosage of the drug at bedtime if the patient experiences drowsiness.
- Monitor for sedation, cardiac arrhythmias, insomnia, gastrointestinal upset, and weight gain.

MAOIs

The **mechanism of action** for monoamine oxidase inhibitors (MAOIs) is exactly what their name indicates. These drugs act to inhibit the enzyme **monoamine oxidase (MAO)**. There are actually two of these enzymes, **MAO-A** and **MAO-B**, and this class of medication inhibits both. These enzymes act to metabolize serotonin and norepinephrine. By inhibiting the production of these enzymes, there are increased levels of **serotonin** and **norepinephrine** available for neurotransmission. Medications that selectively inhibit MAO-B have no antidepressant effects and can be used to treat disease processes such as Parkinson's.

SIDE EFFECTS

Side effects associated with the use of monoamine oxidase inhibitors (MAOIs) are similar to antipsychotic medications. They can include symptoms such as GI upset, vertigo, headaches, sleep disturbances, sexual dysfunction, dry mouth, visual disturbances, constipation, peripheral edema, urinary hesitancy, weakness, increased weight, or orthostatic hypotension. The elderly population is at greatest risk for problems with **orthostatic hypotension** and should have lying, sitting, and standing blood pressure checks to monitor for this side effect. Orthostatic hypotension can lead to injuries related to falls, such as fractures. The most dangerous side effect can be an extreme **elevation in blood pressure** or **hypertensive crisis**. Hypertension can develop due to the presence of increased levels of **tyramine**. These levels increase because **monoamine oxidase**, which normally metabolizes tyramine, is inhibited. Increased levels of tyramine produce a vasoconstrictive response by the body that leads to increased blood pressure. Symptoms associated with hypertensive crisis can include severe occipital headache, palpitations, chest pain, diaphoresis, nausea and vomiting, flushed face, or dilated pupils. Complications associated with hypertensive crisis include hemorrhagic stroke, severe headache, or death. It is vital that patients receive in-depth education about the symptoms of hypertension, the need for close monitoring of blood pressure, and methods for sustaining a low-tyramine diet.

DIET RESTRICTIONS

Monoamine oxidase inhibitors can lead to increased levels of **tyramine** in the nerve cell. These increased levels can lead to a dangerous and possibly fatal increase in **blood pressure**. Certain **foods that contain tyramine** should be avoided to help prevent hypertensive episodes. Foods high in tyramine include strong or aged cheeses, cured meats, smoked or processed meats, pickled or fermented foods, sauces, such as soy or teriyaki sauce, soybeans, snow peas or broad beans, dried or overripe fruits, meat tenderizers, products containing monosodium glutamate, yeast-extract spreads, alcoholic beverages, and improperly stored foods or spoiled foods.

ANTI-ANXIETY MEDICATIONS
BENZODIAZEPINES

Benzodiazepines are the most commonly prescribed medications for **anxiety**. Some of the more commonly prescribed include chlordiazepoxide, lorazepam, diazepam, flurazepam, and triazolam. Benzodiazepines act to enhance the neurotransmitter **GABA**. This neurotransmitter inhibits the firing rate of neurons and therefore leads to a decline in anxiety symptoms. Indications for their use can include anxiety, insomnia disorders, alcohol withdrawal, seizure control, skeletal muscle spasticity, or agitation. They can also be utilized to reduce the anxiety symptoms preoperatively or before any other type of medical procedure such as cardiac catheterization or colonoscopy. This class of drug is also the treatment of choice for alcohol withdrawal.

SIDE EFFECTS

There are several common side effects associated with the use of benzodiazepines. One of the most common is the effect of **drowsiness**. Patients should be advised to use caution when operating motor vehicles or machinery. Activity will help decrease this effect. Other side effects include feelings of detachment, irritability, emotional lability, GI upset, dependency, or development of tolerance. The elderly population is at high risk for the development of **dizziness** or **cognitive impairment**, which places them at high risk for falls with associated injuries. When discontinuing a benzodiazepine after long-term use, the drug should be weaned off to prevent withdrawal side effects.

TREATMENT OF INSOMNIA

Benzodiazepines are used to treat **insomnia** because of their **sedative-hypnotic effects**. There are three different types of insomnia, which include the inability to fall asleep, inability to stay asleep, or the combination of both. Many times, insomnia can be helped by a change in habits or talking about worries or stress the patient may be experiencing. When using a sedative-hypnotic to treat sleep disturbances, the medication should have rapid onset and allow the patient to wake up feeling refreshed instead of tired and groggy. When administered at bedtime, most benzodiazepines will produce a sleep-inducing effect and should be used on a short-term basis.

> **Review Video: Sedatives, Hypnotics, and Insomnia Management**
> Visit mometrix.com/academy and enter code: 666132
>
> **Review Video: Chronic Insomnia**
> Visit mometrix.com/academy and enter code: 293232

USE OF BUSPIRONE FOR TREATMENT OF ANXIETY

Due to the addictive potential of benzodiazepines, the use of **nonbenzodiazepines** to treat anxiety has increased. One of the most commonly used nonbenzodiazepine medications is the drug **buspirone**. This medication is highly effective in treating anxiety and its associated symptoms such as insomnia, poor concentration, tension, restlessness, irritability, and fatigue. Buspirone has no addiction potential, is not useful in alcohol withdrawal and seizures, and is not known to interact with other CNS depressants. Because it may take several weeks of continual use for the effects of this drug to be realized by the patient, it cannot be used on an as-needed basis. Buspirone does not increase depression symptoms and therefore is useful in treating anxiety associated with depression. Side effects associated with medication can include GI upset, dizziness, sleepiness, excitement, or headache.

SSRIs FOR CHILDREN

Escitalopram (Lexapro) and fluoxetine (Prozac for children ages 8 and older) are the only two SSRIs approved by the FDA for children. They are the first-line pharmacologic treatment in pediatric depression. All SSRIs have similar action but may have different chemical properties that cause various side effects, so some people tolerate one better than others. Side effects include nausea, weight gain, sexual dysfunction, excitation and agitation, and insomnia, drowsiness, increased perspiration, headache, and diarrhea. In rare cases, **serotonin syndrome** may occur from high levels of serotonin from overdose or combination with monoamine oxidase (MAO) inhibitors, so SSRIs must not be taken within two weeks of each other. Symptoms include severe anxiety and agitation, hallucinations, confusion, blood pressure swings, fever, tachycardia, seizures, and coma. SSRIs are not addictive but abrupt cessation may trigger discontinuation syndrome (flu-like symptoms).

SECOND-GENERATION/ATYPICAL ANTIPSYCHOTICS FOR CHILDREN

Second-generation antipsychotics (SGAs), also called atypical antipsychotics, are used for bipolar disorders, schizophrenia, and psychosis in children. Children may also receive atypical antipsychotics for a wide range of non-psychotic disorders, such as mood disorders (most common), eating disorders, developmental disorders (autism spectrum), and tic disorders. Use is most common during adolescence. Children should receive the lowest effective dose of medication.

LITHIUM

Lithium carbonate (Lithobid) is used to control the manic episodes associated with bipolar disorder. While it is FDA-approved only for children over age 12, it is increasingly used for younger children. Children should be started on ≤30 mg/kg/day with blood levels monitored every other day initially. Lithium has a very narrow therapeutic window, and toxicity is a medical emergency that can lead to death. Target serum levels are 0.6-1.2 mEq/L. Increased blood levels can cause **toxicity**:

- 1.5-2.5 mEq/L: Severe vomiting and diarrhea, increased muscle tremors and twitching, lethargy, body aches, ataxia, ringing in the ears, blurry vision, vertigo, or hyperactive deep tendon reflexes.
- >2.5 mEq/L: Elevated temperature, low urine output, hypotension, ECG abnormalities, decreased level of consciousness, seizures, coma, or death.

Plasma levels will usually decrease to an acceptable level within 48 hours after discontinuation of the medication; however, in severe cases involving acute renal failure, dialysis may be necessary.

Immunizations

IMMUNIZATION VS. VACCINATION

Immunization refers to the body's buildup of defenses (antibodies) against specific diseases. It has an important role in preventing the spread of infection. Immunization prevents the individual from contracting a disease or lessens the severity of the disease, and can also prevent the complications (encephalitis, hearing loss, paralysis) associated with the infectious diseases. **Vaccination** is one method of creating immunity through the introduction of a small amount of the virus's or bacteria's antigen to the body, which then stimulates the body's creation of antibodies against that disease. Vaccination prevents the spread of infection to infants who are too young to have developed immunity and to those who are immunocompromised (cancer patients, transplantation recipients). Herd immunity results from a majority of the population being immune to a disease, therefore minimizing transmission. It is defined in terms of the percentage of the population that must be immunized in order to prevent outbreaks. This percentage may range from 80-85% for some disorders, but those that are highly contagious, such as measles, may require a herd immunity of 93-95%. Herd immunity can be obtained via widespread vaccination or widespread infection, though it is not recommended that individuals avoid immunization and rely on herd immunity for protection, as rates of immunization vary from one community to another.

TYPES OF VACCINES

There are a number of different types of vaccines:

- **Conjugated forms**: An organism is altered and then joined (conjugated) with another substance, such as a protein, to potentiate immune response (such as conjugated Hib).
- **Killed virus vaccines**: The virus has been killed but can still cause an immune response (such as inactivated poliovirus).
- **Live virus vaccines**: The virus is live but in a weakened (attenuated) form so that it doesn't cause the disease but confers immunity (such as measles vaccine).
- **Recombinant forms**: The organism is genetically altered and, for example, may use proteins rather than the whole cell to stimulate immunity (such as Hepatitis B and acellular pertussis vaccine).
- **Toxoid**: A toxin (antigen) that has been weakened by the use of heat or chemicals so it is too weak to cause disease but stimulates antibodies.

Some vaccines are given shortly after birth; others begin at 2 months, 12 months, or 2 years and some later in childhood.

DTAP AND TDAP VACCINES

Diphtheria and pertussis (whooping cough) are highly contagious bacterial diseases of the upper respiratory tract. Cases of diphtheria are now rare in the United States, although they still occur in some developing countries. There have, however, been recent outbreaks of pertussis in the United States. Tetanus is a bacterial infection contracted through cuts, wounds, and scratches. The **diphtheria, tetanus, and pertussis (DTaP) vaccine** is recommended for all children. DTaP is a newer and safer version of the older DTP vaccine, which is no longer used in the United States. **Tdap** is the DTaP booster shot meant to continue immunity to these diseases through adulthood, given every 10 years starting at age 11.

DTaP requires 5 doses:

- 2 months
- 4 months
- 6 months
- 5-18 months
- 4-6 years (or at 11-12 years if booster missed between 4-6)

According to recent ACIP recommendations, DTaP may now also be administered to children ages 7-9 as part of a catch-up series, but children will then require their routine Tdap dose at age 11-12. If DTaP is administered to children ages 10-18 it can be counted as their adolescent Tdap booster. Adverse reactions can occur, but they are usually mild soreness, fever, and/or nausea. About 1 in 100 children will have high fever (>105 °F) and may develop seizures. Severe allergic responses can occur.

HPV Vaccine

Human papillomavirus (HPV) comprises >100 viruses. About 40 are sexually transmitted and invade mucosal tissue, causing genital warts, which are low risk for cancer, or changes in the mucosa, which can lead to cervical cancer. Most HPVs cause little or no symptoms, but they are very common, especially in those 15-25. Over 99% of cervical cancers are caused by HPV and 70% are related to HPVs 16 and 18. The HPV vaccine, Gardasil, protects against HPVs 6 and 11 (which cause genital warts), along with 16 and 18, which can cause cancer. Protection is only conveyed if the female has not yet been infected with these strains. The vaccine is currently recommended for females under 26 but studies have determined that those not adequately covered over the age of 26 and up to 45 can benefit. A series of 3 injections is required over a 6-month period:

- Initial dose 11-12 years (but may be given as young as 9 or ≥18)
- 2 months after first dose
- 6 months after first dose

PPV

Pneumococcal polysaccharide-23 vaccine (PPV) (Pneumovax and Pnu-Immune) is a vaccine that has been available since 1977 to protect against 23 types of pneumococcal bacteria. It is given to adults ≥65 and children ≥2 years in high-risk groups that include:

- Children with chronic heart, lung, sickle cell disease, diabetes, cirrhosis, alcoholism, and leaks of cerebrospinal fluid
- Children with lowered immunity from Hodgkin's disease, lymphoma, leukemia, kidney failure, multiple myeloma, nephrotic syndrome, HIV/AIDS, damaged or missing spleen, and organ transplant

Children ≤2 may not respond to this vaccine and should take PCV-7. Administration is as follows:

- One dose is usually all that is required although a second dose may be advised for children with some conditions, such as cancer or organ/bone marrow transplantations.
- If needed, a second dose is given 3 years after the first for children ≤10 and 5 years after the first for those ≥10.

Hepatitis A Vaccine

Hepatitis A is a contagious virus that causes liver disease and can cause serious morbidity and death. It is spread through the feces of a person who is infected and often causes contamination of food and water. The **Hep A vaccine** is now recommended for all children at one year of age. It is not licensed for use in younger infants. Two doses are needed:

- 12 months (12-23 months)
- 18 months (or 6 months after previous dose)

Older children and teenagers may receive the two-injection series if they are considered at risk, depending upon lifestyle, such as young males having sex with other males or those using illegal drugs. It is also recommended if outbreaks occur. Adverse reactions are mild and include soreness, headache, anorexia, and malaise although severe allergic reactions can occur as with all vaccines.

Hepatitis B Vaccine

Hepatitis B is transmitted through blood and body fluids, including during birth; therefore, it is now recommended for all newborns as well as all those <18 and those in high-risk groups >18. Hepatitis B can cause serious liver disease leading to liver cancer. Three injections of **monovalent HepB** are required to confer immunity:

- Birth (within 12 hours)
- At 1-2 months
- ≥24 weeks

Note: If combination vaccines are given after the birth dose, then a dose at 4 months can be given.

If the mother is Hepatitis B positive, the child should be given both the monovalent HepB vaccination as well as HepB immune globulin within 12 hours of birth. Adolescents (11-15) who have not been vaccinated require 2 doses, 4-6 months apart. Adverse reactions include local irritation and fever. Severe allergic reactions can occur to those allergic to baker's yeast.

Rotavirus Vaccine

Rotavirus is a cause of significant morbidity and mortality in children, especially in developing countries. Most children, without vaccination, will suffer from severe diarrhea caused by rotavirus within the first 5 years of life. The new **rotavirus vaccine** is advised for all infants but should not be initiated after 12 weeks or administered after 32 weeks, so there is a narrow window of opportunity. Three doses are required:

- 2 months (between 6 and 12 weeks)
- 4 months
- 6 months

An earlier vaccine was withdrawn from the market because it was associated with an increase in intussusception, a disorder in which part of the intestine telescopes inside another. Rates of intussusception in those receiving the current (RotaTeq) vaccine have been investigated and incidence of intussusception was within the range of normal occurrences with no evidence linking the occurrences to the vaccine.

Inactivated Poliovirus Vaccine

Poliomyelitis is a serious viral infection that can cause paralysis and death. Prior to introduction of a vaccine in 1955, there were >20,000 cases of polio in the United States each year. There have been no cases of polio caused by the poliovirus for >20 years in the United States, but it still occurs in some third world countries, so continuing vaccinations is very important. Oral polio vaccine (OPV) is no longer recommended in the United States because it carries a very slight risk of causing the disease (1:2.4 million). Children require 4 doses of injectable polio vaccine (IPV):

- 2 months
- 4 months
- 6-18 months
- 4-6 years (booster dose)

IPV is contraindicated for those who have had a severe reaction to neomycin, streptomycin, or polymyxin B. Rare allergic reactions can occur, but there are almost no serious problems caused by this vaccine.

Varicella Vaccine

Varicella (chickenpox) is a common infectious childhood disease caused by the varicella zoster virus, resulting in fever, rash, and itching, and it can also cause skin infections, pneumonia, and neurological damage. After infection, the virus retreats to the nerves by the spinal cord and can reactivate years later, causing herpes zoster (shingles), a significant cause of morbidity in adults. Infection with varicella conveys immunity, but because of associated problems, it is recommended that all children receive varicella vaccine. Two doses are needed:

- 12-15 months
- 4-6 years (or at least 3 months after first dose)

Children ≥13 years and adults who have never had chickenpox or previously received the vaccine should receive 2 doses at least 28 days apart. Children should not receive the vaccine if they have had a serious allergic reaction to gelatin or neomycin. Most reactions are mild and include soreness, fever, and rash. About 1:1000 may experience febrile seizures. Pneumonia is a very rare reaction.

MMR Vaccine

Measles is a viral disease characterized by fever and rash but can cause pneumonia, seizures, severe neurological damage, and death. Mumps is a viral disease that causes fever and swollen glands but can cause deafness, meningitis, and swelling of the testicles. Rubella, also known as German measles) is also a viral disease that can cause rash, fever, and arthritis, but the biggest danger is that it can cause a woman who is pregnant to miscarry or deliver a child with serious birth defects. The **measles, mumps, and rubella (MMR) vaccine** is given in 2 doses:

- 12-15 months
- 4-6 years

Children can get the injections at any age if they have missed them, but there must be at least 28 days between injections. Children with severe allergic reactions to gelatin or neomycin should not get the injection. Severe adverse reactions are rare, but fever and mild rash are common. Teenagers may have pain and stiffness in joints. Occasional seizures (1:3000) and thrombocytopenia (1:30,000) occur.

PCV-7

Heptavalent pneumococcal conjugate vaccine (PCV-7) (Prevnar) was released for use in the United States in 2001 for treatment of children under 2 years old. It provides immunity to 7 serotypes of *Streptococcus pneumoniae* to protect against invasive pneumococcal disease, such as pneumonia, otitis media, bacteremia, and meningitis. Because children are most at risk ≤1, vaccinations begin early:

Administration is in 4 doses:

- 6-8 weeks
- 4 months
- 6 months
- 12-18 months

Although less effective for older children, PCV-7 has been approved for children between 2 and 5 years of age who are at high risk because of the following conditions:

- Chronic diseases: sickle cell disease, heart disease, lung disease, liver disease
- Damaged or missing spleen
- Immunosuppressive disorders: diabetes, cancer
- Drug therapy: chemotherapy, steroids

PCV-7 may also be considered for all children ≤ 5, especially those ≤3 and in group day care and in some ethnic groups (Native American, Alaska Natives, and African Americans).

MENINGOCOCCAL VACCINE

Meningitis is severe bacterial meningitis that can result in severe neurological compromise or death. A number of different serotypes of *meningococci* can cause meningitis and current vaccines protect against 4 types although not against subtype B, which causes about 65% of meningitis cases in children. However, the vaccines provide 85-100% protection against sub-types A, C, Y, and W-135. There are 2 types of vaccine:

- **Meningococcal polysaccharide vaccine (MPSV4)** is made from the outer capsule of the bacteria and is used for children 2-10.
    - One dose is given at 2 years, although those at high risk may receive 2 doses, 3 months apart.
    - Under special circumstances, children 3-24 months may receive 2 doses, 3 months apart.
- **Meningococcal conjugate vaccine (MCV4)** is used for children ≥11 (who have not received MPSV4). One dose is required:
    - Ages 11-12, all children should receive the vaccine.
    - If not previously vaccinated, high school and college freshmen should be vaccinated.
- Side effects are usually only local tenderness.

HIB VACCINE

***Haemophilus influenzae* type b (Hib) vaccine** (HibTITER and PedvaxHIB) protects against infection with *Haemophilus influenzae,* which can cause serious respiratory infections, pneumonia, meningitis, bacteremia, and pericarditis in children ≤5 years old. *Administration* is as follows:

- 2 months
- 4 months
- 6 months (may be required, depending upon the brand of vaccine)
- 12-15 months (this booster dose must be given at least 2 months after the earlier doses for those who start at a later age than 2 months)

Children over age 6 usually do not require Hib, but it is recommended for older children and adults. Here are some conditions that place them at risk:

- Sickle cell disease
- HIV/AIDS
- Bone marrow transplant
- Chemotherapy for cancer
- Damaged or missing spleen

Some chemotherapy drugs, corticosteroids, and other immunosuppressive drugs may interact with the vaccine.

INFANT IMMUNIZATION SCHEDULE SUMMARY

The recommended schedule for immunizations for the infant is summarized below:

- All newborns receive **ophthalmic drops or ointment**, to prevent blindness from possible gonorrhea infection, and an injection of vitamin K to prevent hemorrhagic disease.
- Before discharge, newborns are tested for **phenylketonuria** and **hypothyroidism**, and will possibly have their **hematocrit** and **hemoglobin** checked.
- **Hepatitis B vaccine** is given at birth, 1-2 months, and 6-18 months.
- **Diphtheria/tetanus/pertussis vaccine** is administered at 2 months, 4 months, 6 months, and 15-18 months.
- **Hib (Haemophilus influenza type b) vaccine** is given at 2 months, 4 months, and 12 months or later.
- **Poliovirus vaccine** is given at 2 months, 4 months, and 6-18 months.
- **MMR vaccine** is given at 12-18 months.
- **Varicella (chickenpox) vaccine** can be given at 12 months.

> **Review Video: Child Immunizations and Schedule**
> Visit mometrix.com/academy and enter code: 167190

REQUIRED IMMUNIZATION HISTORY FOR CHILDREN UP TO 6 YEARS OF AGE

According to the Centers for Disease Control and Prevention, by 6 years of age, children in the United States should receive a three-part series of hepatitis B, three doses of rotavirus prevention; four injections protecting against diphtheria, tetanus, and pertussis; four doses of *Haemophilus influenzae* type b; four doses of pneumococcal vaccine; four doses of polio vaccine; two injections that protect against measles, mumps, and rubella; two varicella vaccinations; one hepatitis A vaccination; and a yearly influenza prevention injection.

VACCINATION OF CHILDREN WITH UNCERTAIN IMMUNIZATION HISTORIES

Children who have uncertain immunization histories may need vaccinations to meet guidelines. The number of vaccinations needed depends on the child's history. For children who are not up-to-date on immunizations, the necessary injections must be determined. These vaccinations can then be given on a schedule so that the child can catch up. For children with no immunization history or uncertain status, such as refugees or internationally adopted children, restarting the immunization series may be necessary to ensure adequate coverage with all vaccines, particularly measles, mumps, and rubella; varicella; hepatitis B; *Haemophilus influenzae* type b; and polio.

POSSIBLE SIDE EFFECTS

Immunization reactions can be minimized and the child made more comfortable by giving acetaminophen prior to the immunizations. Common reactions to immunizations include irritability, decrease in appetite, fever less than 102 °F, and swelling, redness and tenderness at injection site. These may last for the first 1-2 days and can be treated with acetaminophen every 4-6 hours for the first day. If more severe reactions occur, such as fever greater than 102 °F, severe prolonged irritability, or high-pitched crying, or the symptoms last more than 2 days, the parents should call the healthcare provider immediately.

Important Considerations When Giving Immunizations

Every time a child comes into contact with the healthcare system, his **immunization status** should be assessed. Children are required, by all states, to be immunized before entering a licensed school or day care. Specific requirements will vary from state to state. Vaccines must be handled and stored according the manufacturers guidelines. Immunizations must be documented according to specific guidelines and parents must sign a consent form every time a vaccine is administered. Common illnesses such as colds, ear infections and diarrhea will not usually preclude giving vaccines. The MMR and varicella vaccines should not be given during pregnancy. There are two situations in which immunizations are contraindicated: a previous severe allergic reaction to a vaccine or one of its components and encephalopathy occurring within 7 days of giving a DTP or DTaP vaccine.

The Anti-Vaccination Movement

While **opposition to vaccination** is not a new concept, it is a movement that has gained momentum with the power of information sharing via social media. Opposers to vaccination, often referred to as "Anti-Vaxxers," believe that vaccinations can cause complications such as autism and SIDS, especially when administered in infancy and early childhood, and believe that these risks far outweigh the benefits. There are also those who oppose such medical interventions due to religious beliefs.

While the therapeutic effects of vaccinations have been supported by evidence for both individuals and communities, it is important that healthcare professionals be equipped to respectfully inform and care for those that oppose vaccinations. Individuals should be educated regarding the evidence supporting vaccinations and the vaccinations required by law. The CDC offers a wealth of resources for healthcare workers and for individuals regarding vaccinations. The most notable resource is the CDC's Vaccine Information Statement, a living document that outlines the benefits and risks of vaccines, that healthcare workers can use to inform individuals and parents. If, despite efforts to educate, the individual or caregiver still refuses vaccination, there are ICD codes that providers are required to use to document this refusal (for example, ICD-10-CM: Z28.82: Immunization not carried out because of caregiver refusal). The healthcare worker must also document that preventive medical counseling was provided.

Infection Control

NOSOCOMIAL INFECTIONS

Nosocomial infections are those that are healthcare-associated or hospital-acquired. The following is a list of common nosocomial infections.

- *Enterococci* infections include urinary infections, bacteremia, endocarditis as well as infections in wounds and the abdominal and pelvic areas.
- *Enterobacteriaceae* cause about half of the urinary tract infections and a quarter of the postoperative infections.
- *Escherichia coli* primarily causes urinary tract infections (especially related to catheters), diarrhea, and neonatal meningitis but it can also lead to pneumonia, and bacteremia (usually secondary to urinary infection).
- Group B β-hemolytic *Streptococci* (GBS) has increasingly been a cause of infections in neonatal units, causing pneumonia, meningitis, and sepsis. GBS infections may occur as wound infections after Cesarean sections, especially in those immunocompromised.
- *Staphylococcus aureus* is a major cause of nosocomial post-operative infections, both localized and systemic, and from indwelling tubes and devices.
- Methicillin-resistant *Staphylococcus aureus (MRSA)* is a common cause of surgical infections.
- *Clostridioides difficile* causes more nosocomial diarrhea cases than any other microorganism.
- *Candida*, a yeast fungal pathogen, can overgrow and lead to mucocutaneous or cutaneous lesions and sepsis.
- *Aspergillus* spp., filamentous fungi, produce spores that become airborne and can invade the respiratory tract, causing pneumonia.

CATHETER-RELATED INFECTIONS

Intravenous catheter-related infections are a significant cause of morbidity and mortality in the hospital setting. Usually, these infections are due to *Staphylococcus aureus, enterococcus*, or fungal infection such as *Candida*. These infections are important because they may progress and eventually lead to bacteremia, infective endocarditis, septic pulmonary emboli, septic shock, osteomyelitis, or superficial thrombophlebitis. Therefore, vigilance should be maintained to prevent these infections. The patient may exhibit fevers, chills, and discomfort around the catheter site. The site itself may show purulence or erythema. The subclavian vein is the preferred intravenous site and the femoral is the least-preferred site due to high infection rates. Infections are diagnosed with blood cultures and catheter tip cultures. Initial treatment includes removal of the catheter and antibiotic treatment. Antibiotics should be empiric at first, then directed toward culture results. Treatment duration should be 2 weeks at first, but 4–6 weeks if there is a complicated infection.

INFECTION CONTROL MEASURES

Standard infection control measures are designed to prevent transmission of microbial substances between patients and/or medical providers. These measures are indicated for everyone and include frequent handwashing, gloves whenever bodily fluids are involved, and face shields and gowns when splashes are anticipated. For more advanced control with tuberculosis, SARS, vesicular rash disorders (such as VZV), and COVID-19, **airborne precautions** should be instituted to prevent the spread of tiny droplets that can remain suspended in the air for days and travel throughout a hospital environment. Therefore, negative pressure rooms are essential, and providers and patients should wear high-efficiency N95 masks and be fitted in advance. For disorders such as influenza or other infections spread by droplets (spread by cough or sneeze) basic surgical masks should be worn (**droplet precautions**). For **contact precautions** in the setting of fecally-transmitted infection or vesicular rash diseases, gowns/gloves should be used and contact limited. White coats are not a substitute for proper gowning. In the case of a *Clostridioides difficile* infection, contact precautions should be used in addition to washing hands with soap and water (rather than alcohol-based hand sanitizer) after patient contact.

INFECTION CONTROL PLAN

The purpose of an infection control/surveillance plan should be clearly outlined and may be multifaceted, including the following elements:

- **Decreasing rates of infection**: The primary purpose of a surveillance plan is to identify a means to decrease nosocomial infections, including a notification system and laboratory surveillance.
- **Evaluating infection control measures**: Surveillance can evaluate effectiveness of infection control measures. (Surgical checklists, handwashing, housekeeping, ventilation).
- **Establishing endemic threshold rates**: Establishing threshold rates can help to enact control measures to reduce rates.
- **Identifying outbreaks**: About 5–10% of infections occur in outbreaks, and comparing data with established endemic threshold rates can help to identify these outbreaks if analysis is done in a regular and timely manner.
- **Achieving staff compliance**: Objective evidence may convince staff to cooperate with infection control measures.
- **Meeting accreditation standards**: Some accreditation agencies require reports of infection rates.
- **Providing defense for malpractice suits**: Providing evidence that a facility is proactive in combating infections can decrease liability.
- **Comparing infection rates with other facilities**: Comparing data helps focus attention and resources.

PROTOCOL FOR NEEDLESTICK INJURY AND POSTEXPOSURE PROPHYLAXIS

If the healthcare provider experiences a **needlestick injury**, the individual's initial response should be to irrigate the wound with soap and water. As soon as possible, the incident must be reported to a supervisor and steps taken according to established protocol. This may include testing and/or prophylaxis, depending on the patient's health history. In some cases, the patient may also be tested for communicable diseases, such as HIV, in order to determine the risk to the healthcare provider. PEP (post-exposure prophylaxis) is available for exposure to HIV (human immunodeficiency virus) and hepatitis B virus (hepatis B immune globulin). However, no PEP is available for HCV (hepatitis C virus) although the CDC does provide a plan for management. PEP should be initiated within 72 hours of exposure. All testing and treatments associated with the needlestick injury must be provided free of cost at a hospital or medical facility.

Alternative, Complementary, and Non-Pharmacologic Interventions

COMPLEMENTARY THERAPY

Complementary therapies are often used, either alone or in conjunction with conventional medical treatment. These methods should be included if this is what the patient/family chooses, empowering the family to take control of their plan of care. Complementary therapies vary widely and most can easily be incorporated. The **National Center for Complementary and Alternative Medicine** recognizes the following:

- **Whole medical systems**: Chinese medicine (acupressure, acupuncture), naturopathic and homeopathic medicines, and Ayurveda
- **Mind-body medicine**: Prayer, artistic creation, music and dance therapy, biofeedback, focused relaxation, and visualization
- **Biological medicine**: Aromatherapy, herbs, plants, trees, vitamins and minerals, and dietary supplements
- **Manipulation**: Massage and spinal manipulation
- **Energy medicines**: Magnets, electric current, pulsed fields, Reiki, qi gong, and laying-on of the hands

PRECAUTIONS

The use of alternative and complementary therapies should be thoroughly discussed by patients and their physician. Patients should be encouraged to use therapies that are shown to have a beneficial, complementary effect on conventional medical treatment. These therapies include the use of massage, superficial stimulation, relaxation, distraction, hypnosis, and guided imagery.

- Encourage patients to practice the techniques until they are proficient in their use to give them a chance to prove their value.
- Teach the patient how the therapies work to encourage the patient to believe in them to contribute to the placebo effect.
- Caution the patient against abandoning current medical treatment.
- Inform the patient of the high cost of alternate therapies that can divert needed funds and result in little or no benefit.
- Provide the patient with resources in the form of books, pamphlets, and informative websites that prove the results of scientific research so that they can evaluate alternative therapies for themselves.

WHOLE MEDICAL SYSTEMS

Whole medical systems are different philosophies and methods of explaining and treating health and illness. Some systems include:

- **Homeopathic medicine**: This European system uses small amounts of diluted herbs and supplements to help the body to recover from disease by stimulating an immune response.
- **Naturopathic medicine**: This is a European system that uses various natural means (herbs, massage, acupuncture) to support the natural healing forces of the body.
- **Chinese medicine**: Centers on restoring the proper flow of life forces within the body to cure disease by using herbs, acupressure and acupuncture, and meditation.
- **Ayurveda**: This is an Indian system that tries to bring the spirit into harmony with the mind and body to treat disease via yoga, herbs, and massage.

ESSENTIAL OILS

Essential oils (concentrated oils from plants) are either inhaled (aromatherapy) or diluted and applied to the skin. Essential oils are believed to reduce stress, aid sleep, improve dermatitis, and aid digestion. Commonly used essential oils include eucalyptus, lavender, lemon, peppermint, rosemary, rose, and tea tree. Oils may cause skin irritation when applied to the skin.

Cupping

Cupping is an ancient practice still used in Southeast Asia and the Middle East to reduce pain, promote healing, and improve circulation. With dry cupping, cups are heated by placing something flammable (such as paper or herbs) inside the cup and setting it on fire to heat the cup, which is then immediately placed on the back along the meridians (generally on both sides of the spine) to form a vacuum that draws blood to the skin and causes circular bruises believed to heal that part of the body. Wet cupping includes leaving the heated cup in place for three minutes, removing it, making small cuts in the skin, and then applying suction cups again to withdraw blood. Cupping should be avoided in children under 4 and limited to short periods in older children.

Acupuncture

Alternative systems of medical practice include acupuncture, homeopathy, and naturopathy. **Acupuncture**, an ancient Oriental practice, uses stainless steel or copper needles inserted into superficial skin layers at points where energy or life force called *qi* is believed to occur. The needles are supposed to restore balance and the flow of *qi*. The NIH has recognized the effectiveness of acupuncture for certain side effects of other cancer treatments, such as nausea, vomiting, and pain. However, there is no documented scientific evidence to support the principles expounded. Acupuncturists are certified through either formal coursework or apprenticeships, and there is also board certification in this area for physicians. The needles used are classified as class II, which means they have manufacturing and labeling requirements.

Herbal Remedies and Regulations

In the United States, most **herbal preparations** are classified as dietary supplements. That means that they are not subject to the same rigorous manufacturing, safety, efficacy, and control practices as pharmaceutical drugs. Herbal supplements are only governed by the Dietary Supplement and Health Education Act (DSHEA). As long as no specific disease treatment or curative claims are made, the supplement can be marketed without limitation and safety concerns must be pursued by the FDA after the fact. Nevertheless, some herbal remedies have been undergoing clinical trials in the U.S. to substantiate their health-enhancing or traditional/historical or international use claims. However, the focal point of these studies is still only on the effectiveness of the specific supplement. In Europe, there has been some movement toward greater regulation and licensing of herbal products, but not to the extent of formal drug regulations.

Toxicities Associated with Herbal Remedies

Use of herbal preparations has been associated with a variety of **toxicities**, primarily in categories such as cardiovascular problems, hypersensitivity reactions, disorientation, gastrointestinal problems, and liver malfunction. Because quality control measures are relatively lax for these remedies, contamination from infectious agents and toxic metals can potentially cause other side effects. Many of these herbal medicines **interact with conventional drugs**, thus altering their pharmacodynamics. For example, St. John's wort, which is primarily used for depressive disorders or as a sedative, interacts with a wide range of traditional pharmacologic agents and suppresses their levels in the bloodstream. Kava kava, made from dried roots of a type of pepper bush, is used as a sedative, but it also has been associated with hepatic failure and via interactions with several other drugs can actually induce a comatose state. Ginseng is an Asian remedy touted for its curative properties in a number of diseases. However, it can react with steroidal drugs and induce shaking and manic episodes. These are just a few examples of potential dangers.

Non-Pharmaceutical Pain Relief

Non-pharmaceutical methods to relieve pain that can be used exclusively or combined with medications include massage, heat, cold, electrical stimulation, distraction, relaxation, imagery, visualization, and music. Other **alternatives or adjuncts to pain medication** include hypnosis, magnets, acupuncture, acupressure, and therapeutic touch. Herbs, aromatherapy, reflexology, homeopathic medicine, and prayer may also be accepted by the patient. Any method that the patient feels may help that isn't harmful should be used to help get relief.

MIND-BODY MEDICINE FOR PAIN AND DISEASE

Mind-body medicine (prayer, artistic creation, music and dance, biofeedback, relaxation, and visualization) can help distract people from pain or other symptoms if they are able to concentrate on the method. This can result in the transfer of less painful stimuli to the brain by stimulating the **descending control system**. These methods work if the patient can use them to create alternate sensations in the brain, but will not work if the patient is unable to concentrate due to intense pain.

Relaxation that occurs as a result of using these methods helps to reduce muscular tension that can make pain worse and reduces fatigue caused by chronic pain. Relaxation has been proven to be the most helpful after surgery. Postoperative patients report a greater feeling of control over their pain and tend to request fewer opioids to control pain. Biofeedback can help patients to recognize the feelings of both tension and relaxation and provide a way to indicate their success in managing muscle tension.

USE OF VISUALIZATION

There are a number of methods used for **visualization** to reduce anxiety and promote healing. Some include audiotapes with guided imagery, such as self-hypnosis tapes, but the patient can be taught basic **techniques** that include:

- Sit or lie comfortably in a **quiet place** away from distractions.
- Concentrate on **breathing** while taking long slow breaths.
- **Close the eyes** to shut out distractions and create an image in the mind of the place or situation desired.
- Concentrate on that **image**, engaging as many senses as possible and imaging details.
- If the mind wanders, breathe deeply and **bring consciousness back** to the image or concentrate on breathing for a few moments and then return to the imagery.
- End with positive imagery.

Sometimes, patients are resistive at first or have a hard time maintaining focus, so **guiding** them through visualization for the first few times can be helpful.

STIMULATION OF THE SKIN TO REDUCE PAIN

Skin, muscles, fascia, tendons, and the cornea contain **nociceptors** that are nerve endings that respond to painful stimuli. Massage, transcutaneous electrical nerve stimulation (TENS), heat and cold provide stimulation to other nerves that transfer only sensation, not pain. These signals block some of the transfer of the nociceptor impulses:

- **Massage** not only sends alternate sensation to the brain, but also results in relaxation that decreases the muscular tension that contributes to pain.
- **TENS** works well on incisional and neuromuscular pain by providing a gentle electrical stimulation that overrides the painful impulses from the area and may stimulate endorphins.
- **Heat therapy** increases blood flow and oxygen to promote healing and stimulates neural receptors, decreasing pain. Heat also helps loosen tense muscles that may be contributing to pain.
- **Cold therapy** decreases circulation and reduces production of chemicals related to inflammation, thereby reducing pain.

Temperature-Controlled Therapies
Methods of Heating and Cooling

There are a number of different ways to **heat** (thermotherapy) or **cool** (cryotherapy) for **healing**:

- **Conduction**: Conveyance of heat, cold, or electricity through direct contact with the skin, such as with hot baths, ice packs, and electrical stimulation.
- **Convection**: Indirect transmission of heat in a liquid or gas by circulation of heated particles, such as with whirlpools and paraffin soaks.
- **Conversion**: Heating that results from converting a form of energy into heat, such as with diathermy and ultrasound.
- **Evaporation**: Cooling caused by liquids that evaporate into gases on the skin with a resultant cooling effect, such as with perspiration or vapo-coolant sprays.
- **Radiation**: Heating that results from transfer of heat through light waves or rays, such as with infrared or ultraviolet light.

Superficial Heat

Superficial heat with externally applied heat sources penetrates only the superficial layers of the skin (1–2 cm after about 30 minutes), but it is believed to relax deeper muscles by reflex, decrease pain, and increase metabolisms (2–3 times for every 10 °C increase in skin temperature). Therapeutic temperature range is 40–45 °C. **Superficial heat modalities** include:

- **Moist heat packs** placed on the skin and secured by several layers of towels to provide insulation, applied for 15–30 minutes.
- **Paraffin baths** (52–54 °C) with the hand, foot, or elbow dipped 7 times, cooling between dippings, and then wrapping with plastic and towels for 20 minutes.
- **Fluidotherapy** uses hot-air warmed (38.8–47.8 °C) cellulose particles into which a hand or foot is submerged for 20–30 minutes.

Passive and active range of motion exercises are done after superficial heat treatment. Contraindications include cardiac disease, peripheral vascular disease, malignant tumor, bleeding, and acute inflammation.

Deep heat differs from superficial heat in that the heat is generated internally using ultrasound, short wave, and microwave diathermy rather than applied to the surface of the skin. Deep heating has penetrance to 3–5 cm.

Rehabilitation
SAID Principle of Rehabilitation and Reconditioning

The Specific Adaptation to Imposed Demands (SAID) principle suggests that when a person is injured or stressed, that person attempts to overcome the problem by **adapting** to the demands of the situation. This is based on **Wolff's law** (systems adapt to demands). For example, if one hand is not usable, the person adapts and uses the other hand. Unfortunately, this adaptation can lead to increasing disability, so when the SAID principle is applied to rehabilitation, it means that the person must do exercises that specifically aim to correct the problem. Thus, the functional needs of the person should always be considered when designing a specific exercise program for that individual (such as treadmill running for soccer players). The exercise activities should as closely mirror the functional activities as possible. For example, if the goal is increased strength rather than endurance, then the exercise program should rely more heavily on strengthening exercises.

Massage for Rehabilitation and Reconditioning

Massage therapy is commonly used in sports and may be employed before activities, at breaks during activities, and after the activity is completed. Many types of massage are used in sports, and some massage therapists specialize in sports massage, but all nurses who work with athletes of any age should know the basic techniques of **sports massage** as it is used to both treat and prevent injuries. Sports massage is based primarily on Swedish massage although the massage may be deeper and targeted toward a particular injury, and other types of massage may be incorporated into a sports massage program. Massage of an injured area is delayed for the first **48–72 hours** to prevent further injury to tissues. Different techniques include:

- **Compression**: Deep rhythmical compressions of the muscles are done to increase circulation and temperature and make muscles more pliable. It may be used prior to deeper massage techniques.
- **Effleurage**: This is usually the beginning massage and begins softly and increases in intensity with the hands gliding over the tissue, so it is done with some type of oil or emollient. Massage is done in rhythmical broad strokes with the palms of the hands. This massage helps to relax the athlete and identify areas of tightness or pain that may require additional attention.
- **Friction**: These are massages either in line with muscle fibers or across the muscle fibers to create stretching and to reduce adhesions and scarring during healing. The tissue is pressed firmly against the underlying tissue and then pressure moves the underlying tissue until resistance is felt. Friction massage may be done deeply, and this can be uncomfortable. Usually, the thumb or fingers are used for this type of massage.
- **Petrissage**: This is kneading massage and is usually used on large muscle areas, such as the calf or thigh. It increases circulation, so it is useful to relax and to improve circulation and drainage as well as to stretch muscles. The full hand is used for this massage with the heel and thumb stabilizing the tissue while the fingers squeeze the tissue.
- **Tapotement**: This type of massage uses quick rhythmic tapping, usually with the edge of the palm and little finger or the heel of the hand with the fingers elevated. It is done to increase circulation or relieve cramped muscles.
- **Vibration**: Vibratory massage is used for deep muscle relaxation and reduction of pain. Usually, the entire hand is placed against the skin, compressing the muscle and then vibrating the hand to cause movement.
- **Trigger point**: Pressure is applied with a finger or thumb to areas of point tenderness to reduce spasticity and pain.

Progression in Strengthening Exercises

Strengthening exercise progression includes the following exercises:

- **Isometric exercises** are done with the muscle and limb in static position with no movement of the joint or lengthening of the muscle. The muscle is contracted against resistance.
- **Isotonic exercises** include movement of the joint during exercise (such as running, weight lifting) and both shortening and lengthening of the muscles through eccentric or concentric contractions. Isotonic refers to tension, so the tension is constant during shortening and lengthening of the muscle.
- **Isokinetic exercises** utilize machines (such as stationary bicycles that can be set with various parameters) to control the rate and extent of contraction as well as the range of motion. Both speed and resistance can be set so the athlete is limited by the settings of the machine.
- **Plyometrics** is a particular type of exercise program that uses activities to allow a muscle to achieve maximal force as quickly as possible, and the sequence is a fast, eccentric movement (to stretch) followed quickly by a strong concentric movement (to contract).

APRN Scope and Standards

ADVANCED PRACTICE REGISTERED NURSING

Advanced practice registered nursing (APRN), according to the National Council of State Boards of Nursing (NCSBN), is acting as a nurse with a foundation on **information and proficiency** that was obtained in basic nursing school. This nurse has a license to be an RN and has completed and received a diploma from graduate school in an APRN program that has been accredited from a nationwide accrediting body. This nurse has up-to-date **certification** from a nationwide certification board to work in the proper APRN specialty.

STANDARDS OF PRACTICE

Standards of practice for the APRN are defined by the ANA (from 1998) and meant to act as professional guidelines regarding the excellence of performance, service, and learning. They outline the level of work deemed satisfactory to meet the requirements of the role. These standards also provide patients with a reference to determine the quality of the treatment that was given to them. There are both **broad and particular standards** to each area of expertise. Some particular areas of expertise have their own standards as well, such as National Association of Pediatric Nursing Practitioners (NAPNP) and Association for Women's Health, Obstetric, and Neonatal Nurses (AWHONN). PNP also has separate standards. All standards may be used in legal proceedings, but they are not originally meant for this purpose.

SCOPE OF PRACTICE

The scope of practice for the APRN is dependent on each state and what the APRN in this position can do according to the Nurse Practice Act for that state. The **scope** provides **guidelines** instead of particular directives, which may be wide in range, depending on the state. Many times, the scope is founded on what is allowed legally both in the state and in the nation. The initial Scope of Practice for PNPs was created in 1983 by the National Association of Pediatric Nurse Practitioners, and has been updated multiple times since. The APRN's scope of practice is always changing and improving to meet the needs of the community, state, and country at large.

CREDENTIALS

Advanced practice registered nurses (APRN) are comprised of nurse anesthetists, nurse midwives, nurse practitioners, and clinical nurse specialists. These specialties must have proper **credentials** and take responsibility for the patient's care. Some other nurses who hold leadership responsibilities are not included under the term APRN. These nurses who are not included may have professional responsibilities but not in a clinical setting, such as teachers, administrators, or researchers, even though these nurses may have the same knowledge as an APRN. Someone that is not working in direct patient care with patients or in a family medical clinic cannot be considered an APRN.

PURPOSES OF CREDENTIALS

Purposes of credentials for the APRN are to:

- Ensure there is accountability for proficient work.
- Authenticate that the practitioner has received the correct education, has a license, and is certified.
- Ensure that the local and national laws are followed.
- Recognize the growing scope for the APRN.
- Allow an avenue for patients to make a grievance.
- Ensure a responsibility to the community by making sure standards of practice are met.

Responsibilities

Advanced practice registered nurse (APRN) **responsibilities** include but are not limited to the following:

- Evaluate the patient, produce and assess information; comprehend complex nursing practice and practice critical thinking.
- Assess many kinds of information; compile the differential diagnosis; determine proper medical care.
- Without supervision, determine how to handle difficult patient issues.
- Create a way to identify the condition, create objectives for the patient's medical management, and stipulate the medical routine or plan.
- Plan, modify and implement the medical plan. This includes prescribing and administering drugs that fall within the APRN's scope and specialty.
- Treat the patient's physical and mental condition.
- Maintain the privacy of the patient.
- Conduct care within a therapeutic environment.

Consultation, Referral, and Coordination

As part of the scope of practice, the advanced practice nurse is able to provide and augment primary care to patients through a number of different services:

- **Consultation** services may include a variety of services, such as assessment of growth and development and risk factors, providing interventions, such as diet and exercise programs, and educating patients.
- **Referral services** include referring patients to physicians, such as orthopedic specialists, and to organizations or agencies, such as drug rehabilitation programs.
- **Coordination services,** with the nurse maintaining contact and receiving reports from referrals in order to provide an integrated plan of care, serves as a valuable service to patients, who often must deal with many different healthcare providers who have little or no contact with each other. This type of service can prevent unnecessary duplications of service but also ensure that findings are not overlooked.

Prescription and Diagnostics

Both prescribing medications and treatment and ordering diagnostic tests are within the scope of practice of nurse practitioners, but as with other aspects of practice, each state establishes how that will be carried out. Additionally, insurance reimbursement varies from one area to another and must be considered:

- **Prescription:** Terminology varies from state to state with nurse practitioners allowed to "furnish" or "prescribe" some types of medications. In some states they may do so independently; in others, they must be "supervised" by a physician under whose auspices they provide care to patients. The nurse practitioner should maintain a list of medications and consider cost-effectiveness when ordering medications.
- **Diagnostics:** Nurse practitioners can order laboratory, EKG, and radiographic tests for routine screening and health assessment as well as diagnosis based on assessment. There are limitations, depending upon the individual state nursing practice act.

Medicare

Medicare, a federally directed program, was introduced by the Title XIX Social Security Act in 1965. It provides health insurance to elderly patients and to patients with disabilities. The patient who is covered will receive hospital, doctor, and further medical care as needed. The patient's income is not a factor for eligibility. **Original Medicare** consists of **Part A** and **Part B**, and covers the majority of medical care when the patient seeks care at a facility that accepts Medicare. If the patient requires prescription drug assistance, they may opt into **Part D**, which is the Medicare drug plan, or they may opt into the **Medicare Advantage Plan (Part C)**, which bundles Parts A, B and D.

Medicare Part A

Medicare Part A covers hospital care (inpatient), care at a skilled nursing facility or nursing home, hospice care, and home health care. Anyone 65 years of age or older that is eligible to receive **Social Security** is automatically enrolled even if still working. Patients are also able to receive Social Security if they or their spouse put money into the system by way of working for at least 40 quarters. If the patient has less than 40 quarters of work, Medicare Part A requires a payment each month. If the patient is not yet 65 but has a complete disability that will remain for the rest of their life, Medicare Part A can be used after receiving Social Security benefits for 2 years. A patient with ongoing renal disease who needs either dialysis or transplant can become eligible for Part A without waiting for 2 years.

Medicare Part B

Medicare Part B covers both medically necessary services and preventive services such as doctor visits, physical therapy, occupational therapy, speech therapy, medical equipment, assessments, clinical research, mental health support and wellness visits. The patient has to **pay a monthly premium for Medicare Part B,** which is either directly billed to the patient or deducted from their Social Security or other benefit payment. The program covers 80% of the authorized expense for any medical attention that is required (following a yearly deductible).

Medicaid

1965 Title XIX Social Security Act introduced **Medicaid** as a federal/state matching plan for low-income individuals supervised by the federal government. Funding comes from federal and state taxes, with no less than 50%, but no more than 83% being funded federally. Each state is able to add optional eligibility criteria on the list, and they may also put restrictions (to a point) on federally directed aid. Patients who receive Medicaid cannot get a bill for the aid, but states are able to require small copayments or deductibles for particular types of help.

Federal regulations require that states support certain individuals or groups of individuals through Medicaid, although not everyone who falls below the federal poverty rate is eligible. **Mandatory eligibility groups** include the following:

- Patients deemed categorically needy by their state, and receive financial support from various federal assistance programs.
- Individuals receiving Federal Supplemental Security income (SSI).
- Patients that are older than 65 that are blind or have complete disability.
- Pregnant women and children younger than 6 years of age who live in families that are up to 133% of the federal poverty level (some states allow for a higher income to meet eligibility in this class).
- Adults under the age of 65 that make less than or equal to 133% of the federal poverty level and are not receiving Medicare.

> **Review Video: Medicare & Medicaid**
> Visit mometrix.com/academy and enter code: 507454

Third Parties That Give Compensation

Other than Medicare and Medicaid, the following are some **third parties** that give compensation for medical care:

- **Private insurance**: Will reimburse according to contract; particular for each state insurance commission.
- **TRICARE**: Used by patients in the armed forces, their dependents that may be living beyond a time when they have died, their families, or retirees.
- **Federal Employees Health Benefit Program** (FEHBP): Provided to non-military federal employees and their family.

Billing and Coding for Reimbursement in the Pediatric Office Setting

International Classification of Diseases

International Classification of Diseases, 10th revision, Clinical Modifications (ICD-10-CM) is a coding system used to code diagnoses. While the World Health Organization (WHO) has released the 11th revision of the ICD (ICD-11), the United States has not begun implementation of this version. ICD-10-CM codes are used for billing purposes to ensure that procedure codes match appropriate diagnoses. The codes all have at least 3 characters but may have up to 4 additional sub-categories. The first character must be alpha, the second and third, numeric, and the remaining alpha or numeric. A decimal point is placed after the first 3 characters. Diagnoses are classified by type of disease or system involved. For example, main categories include neoplasms and diseases of the respiratory systems. With ICD-10-CM, injuries are grouped by body part rather than category of injury. Thus, all injuries to the thorax (S20-S29) are grouped together. The chapter dealing with injuries, poisoning and other consequences of external causes are divided by two letters, S and T. The S-coded injuries are grouped by single body regions; however, some injuries are not localized, such as poisonings, and these are T-coded injuries.

CPT Codes

Current procedural terminology (CPT) codes were developed by the American Medical Association (AMA) and used to define those licensed to provide services and to describe medical and surgical treatments, diagnostics, and procedures. CPT 2012 codes specific procedures as well as typical times required for treatment. CPT codes are usually updated each October with revisions (additions, deletions) to coding. The use of CPT codes is mandated by both CMS and HIPAA to provide a uniform language and to aid research. These codes are used primarily for billing purposes for insurances (public and private). Under HIPAA, HHS has designed CPT codes as part of the national standard for electronic healthcare transactions:

- Category I codes are used to identify a procedure or service.
- Category II codes are used to identify performance measures, including diagnostic procedures.
- Category III codes identify temporary codes for technology and data collection.

HCPCS Level II Codes

Healthcare Common Procedure Coding Systems (HCPCS Level II) codes are used when filing claims for equipment, supplies and services that are not covered by CPT codes (Level I codes), including non-physician products such as durable medical equipment, ambulance services, laboratory service, orthotics, and prosthetics. HCPCS codes are also used for outpatient hospital care, chemotherapeutic drugs, and Medicaid:

- D codes are used for dental procedures.
- E codes are used for durable medical equipment, such as bedside commodes.
- L codes are used for orthotic and prosthetic procedures and devices, such as orthopedic shoes.
- P codes are used for pathology and laboratory services.

HCPCS Level II codes are comprised of 5 alphanumeric characters, beginning with a letter that indicates the grouping. For example, metal underarm crutches would be coded as E0114. The letter E indicates the item is durable medical equipment. The codes are updated on a quarterly basis.

Diagnostic-Related Groups

Diagnostic-related groups (**DRGs**) were instituted in 1982 as a way to classify patients who shared similar diseases and treatments for billing purposes, under the assumption that patients who shared symptoms and/or diseases use the same amount of resources and should be **billed the same amount**. There are approximately 500 different DRGs, and patients are placed into specific DRGs using **International Classification of Disease (ICD) codes**, along with specific patient information such as sex, age, and the presence of comorbidities. By placing patients into DRGs, Medicare is able to determine how much the hospital should be reimbursed for patient care. The institution of DRGs has changed the health care system from one that was provider-driven (meaning the individual clinician determined the billable amount) into one that is payer-driven (meaning that Medicare determines reimbursement).

Patient Education

BANDURA'S THEORY OF SOCIAL LEARNING

In the 1970s, Bandura proposed the theory of social learning, in which he posited that learning develops from observing, organizing, and rehearsing behavior that has been modeled. Bandura believed that people are more likely to adopt the behavior if they value the outcomes, if the outcomes have functional value, and if the person modeling the behavior is similar to the learner and is admired because of status. Behavior is the result of observation of behavioral, environmental, and cognitive interactions. There are **four conditions** required for modeling:

- **Attention**: The degree of attention paid to modeling can depend on many variables (physical, social, and environmental).
- **Retention**: People's ability to retain models depends on symbolic coding, creating mental images, organizing thoughts, and rehearsing (mentally or physically).
- **Reproduction**: The ability to reproduce a model depends on physical and mental capabilities.
- **Motivation**: Motivation may derive from past performances, rewards, or vicarious modeling.

TRANSTHEORETICAL MODEL OF CHANGE

The transtheoretical model of change puts forth concepts applicable to the process of educating patients and their family members. The **stages** of the transtheoretical model of change include the following:

- The first stage is **precontemplation**. At this point, the patient is not aware of any need for a change in the health behavior.
- In the next stage, **contemplation**, the patient begins to realize why the change may be necessary after recognizing that the health behavior in question is unhealthy and weighing the consequences of continuing this behavior.
- During the stage of **preparation**, the patient imagines making the change at a future time and starts to formulate a plan to do so.
- The **action** stage occurs when the patient makes specific modifications in health behavior and begins to note the resulting positive changes.
- During the **maintenance** stage, the patient is able to implement the change over time by utilizing strategies to prevent a return to previously unhealthy behaviors.
- **Termination** is the stage at which a patient has incorporated the changed behavior into daily functioning, and the patient will not resume the previous unhealthy behavior.

KURT LEWIN

FORCE FIELD ANALYSIS

Force field analysis was designed by Kurt Lewin, a social psychologist, to analyze both the driving forces and the restraining forces for change:

- **Driving forces** instigate and promote change, such as leaders, incentives, and competition.
- **Restraining forces** resist change, such as poor attitudes, hostility, inadequate equipment, or insufficient funds.

The educator can use this force field analysis diagram to discuss variables related to a proposed change in process:

- Write the proposed change in the center column.
- Brainstorm and list driving forces and opposed restraining forces. Score the forces. (When driving and restraining forces are in balance, this is a state of equilibrium or the status quo.)
- Discuss the value of the proposed change.
- Develop a plan to diminish or eliminate restraining forces.

Lewin's Model of Change Theory

Lewin's model of change theory may be used to help some patients make decisions for change. Patients can be educated about the need for change and can be assisted with making alterations in behavior or thoughts in order to better facilitate change; however, only the patient can truly implement the change permanently. Lewin's concept of change theory involves a three-part process:

- **Unfreezing** is the part of the model in which the patient becomes open to change, sees a need for it, and removes the boundaries inhibiting change.
- The patient then makes the **actual change** according to expected outcomes and goals.
- Finally, **refreezing** is the process of maintaining the change so that it becomes a habit, and one that the patient is likely to uphold for a long period of time.

Lewin's theory also involves either driving forces or restraining forces. Driving forces are those outside measures that support the change, while restraining forces inhibit success in implementing the change.

Principles of Adult Learning

Adults have a wealth of life and/or employment experiences. Their attitudes toward education may vary considerably. There are, however, some **principles of adult learning** and typical characteristics of adult learners that an instructor should consider when planning strategies for teaching parents, families, or staff.

- Practical and goal-oriented:
  - Provide overviews or summaries and examples.
  - Use collaborative discussions with problem-solving exercises.
  - Remain organized with the goal in mind.
- Self-directed:
  - Provide active involvement, asking for input.
  - Allow different options toward achieving the goal.
  - Give them responsibilities.
- Knowledgeable:
  - Show respect for their life experiences/education.
  - Validate their knowledge and ask for feedback.
  - Relate new material to information with which they are familiar.
- Relevancy-oriented:
  - Explain how information will be applied.
  - Clearly identify objectives.
- Motivated:
  - Provide certificates of professional advancement and/or continuing education credit for staff when possible.

> **Review Video: Adult Learning Processes and Theories**
> Visit mometrix.com/academy and enter code: 638453

Learning Styles

Not all people are aware of their preferred **learning style**. A range of teaching materials and methods that relate to all three major learning preferences (visual, auditory, and kinesthetic) and that are appropriate for different ages should be available. Part of assessment for teaching involves choosing the right approach based on observation and feedback. Often, presenting learners with different options gives a clue to their preferred learning style. Some people have a combined learning style.

Visual learners learn best by seeing and reading:

- Provide written directions or picture guides, or demonstrate procedures. Use charts and diagrams.
- Provide photos or videos.

Auditory learners learn best by listening and talking:

- Explain procedures while demonstrating and have the learner repeat.
- Plan extra time to discuss and answer questions.
- Provide audio recordings.

Kinesthetic learners learn best by handling, doing, and practicing:

- Provide hands-on experience throughout teaching.
- Encourage handling of supplies and equipment.
- Allow the learner to demonstrate.
- Minimize instructions and allow the person to explore equipment and procedures.

APPROACHES TO TEACHING

There are many approaches to teaching, and the educator must prepare, present, and coordinate a wide range of educational workshops, lectures, discussions, and one-on-one instructions on any chosen topic. All types of classes will be needed, depending upon the purpose and material:

- **Educational workshops** are usually conducted with small groups, allowing for maximal participation. They are especially good for demonstrations and practice sessions.
- **Lectures** are often used for more academic or detailed information that may include questions and answers but limits discussion. An effective lecture should include some audiovisual support.
- **Discussions** are best with small groups so that people can actively participate. This is a good method for problem solving.
- **One-on-one instruction** is especially helpful for targeted instruction in procedures for individuals.
- **Online learning modules** are good for independent learners.

Participants should be asked to evaluate the presentations in the forms of surveys or suggestions, but ultimately the program is evaluated in terms of patient outcomes.

READINESS TO LEARN

The patient/family's readiness to learn should be assessed because if they are not ready, instruction is of little value. Often, readiness is indicated when the patient/family asks questions or shows an interest in procedures. There are a number of factors related to readiness to learn:

- **Physical factors:** There are a number of physical factors that can affect ability. Manual dexterity may be required to complete a task, and this varies by age and condition. Hearing or vision deficits may impact a person's ability to learn. Complex tasks may be too difficult for some because of weakness or cognitive impairment, and modifications of the environment may be needed. Health status, age, and gender may all impact the ability to learn.
- **Experience:** People's experience with learning can vary widely and is affected by their ability to cope with changes, their personal goals, motivation to learn, and cultural background. People may have widely divergent ideas about what constitutes illness and/or treatment. Lack of English skills may make learning difficult and prevent people from asking questions.
- **Mental/emotional status:** The external support system and internal motivation may impact readiness. Anxiety, fear, or depression about one's condition can make learning very difficult because the patient/family cannot focus on learning, so the nurse must spend time to reassure the patient/family and wait until they are emotionally more receptive.

- **Knowledge/education:** The knowledge base of the patient/family, their cognitive ability, and their learning styles all affect their readiness to learn. The nurse should always begin by assessing what knowledge the patient/family already has about their disease, condition, or treatment and then build from that base. People with little medical experience may lack knowledge of basic medical terminology, interfering with their ability and readiness to learn.

METHODS TO ASSIST CAREGIVERS

Caregivers for children are most often the parents, with the greatest burden of care often falling on the mother. Caregiving can be extremely stressful, especially if the child suffers from a chronic or serious disease. Part of caring practices is to recognize that the caregivers need care as well.

- **Conflict resolution** brings people with conflict together with a neutral person or group in order to attempt to negotiate or reach agreement. Nurses are in a unique position to assist with conflict resolution because they see people at their most vulnerable, when they are dealing with stress.
- **Debriefing** allows the caregiver to talk about experiences that have caused trauma or stress.
- **Crisis intervention** takes place when an individual is overwhelmed by a situation and is not able to function adequately. It involves intervening during the crisis in order to help the person stabilize and to help him or her to function and to facilitate problem solving.

EFFECTS OF DEVELOPMENTAL STAGE OF THE LEARNER ON TEACHING

Many children have chronic conditions, such as those receiving insulin or managing colostomies, and the nurse must **guide the child** and family in helping the child become independent in care based on the **development stage** of the child and the learner:

- **Infant/toddler:** Caregivers provide care; instruction encourages bonding and acceptance.
- **Early childhood:** Children learn by participation, such as role-playing, simple explanation, and teaching dolls. Children should be independent in emptying colostomy pouch by kindergarten.
- **Childhood:** By age 6, children should be independent in care at school. They should have supplies at school, and the school nurse should know about care so the nurse can provide assistance. Child should be completely independent in care by 6th grade. Parents and child should be taught together.
- **Adolescence/young adulthood:** The adolescent may be angry and resistive. Extra time and guidance, including visits with other young patients facing the same or similar challenges may help. Parents should allow adolescents to be independent in care.

INCREASING KNOWLEDGE BASE OF HEALTHCARE COMMUNITY

There are numerous ways to contribute to and advance the **knowledge base** of the healthcare community:

- **Research** may be a review of literature and compilation of findings on a given subject or may be clinical research in which different treatment approaches are used and evaluated.
- **Presentations** may include any variety of informal or formal presentations in meetings, workshops, or classes.
- **Publications** may include research results or nurse-related educational courses, such as continuing education courses related to a field of expertise. Publications may be in journals, online, or intended for in-house use only.
- **Involvement in professional organizations** is especially important in the field of nursing because changes occur rapidly, not only in medical treatments but also in regulations. Professional organizations provide up-to-date information and provide a means to lobby legislators about issues related to nursing practice, such as nurse-patient ratios.

Telehealth

TELEHEALTH NURSING

Telehealth nursing is a process that provides nursing care for patients over the telephone or other medium of non-physical interaction. Through telehealth services, patients are able to call in and speak with nurses about their symptoms or current condition, and in turn, telehealth nurses can provide health information and guidance to patients without seeing them in person. In addition to phone calls, these visits may also be conducted through videoconferencing, the internet, or other types of media. Some nurses who perform case management services for clients may also utilize telehealth to contact patients and review their current states of health. This type of technology allows these nurses to make assessments with the information provided from the patient, and to then compare these data with former conversations or visits to determine if the patient is moving toward expected outcomes in management of illness.

NECESSARY SKILLS

The nurse must master certain skills in order to be able to provide quality care via telehealth:

- The nurse must have excellent **verbal skills** and be able to effectively communicate over the phone to meet patient needs.
- The nurse must have a knowledge of **cultural differences** and be competent in communicating by telephone with patients of different cultures.
- The nurse must be able to **prioritize** the needs of the patient, using the standards of care provided by the *Telehealth Nursing Standards of Practice*, most recently revised in 2017.
- The nurse must be able to **perform** telehealth nursing in a variety of environments, including, but not limited to, clinics, physician's offices, emergency departments, and call centers.
- The nurse must be able to **ask specific questions** that will lead to the optimum treatment plan for the patient and assist in triaging for both nonemergent and emergent states of health.

TELEPHONE TRIAGE

Telephone triage is the process in which the receiving nurse uses protocols and guidelines to assess and prioritize the needs of a patient as they describe their condition over the phone. Telehealth does not allow the nurse to physically see the patient, so the nurse must be skilled at asking the appropriate questions and prioritizing needs based on the patients responses. The nurse must develop a plan of care that may include education, wellness promotion, and preventative education. The telehealth nurse is an extension of the clinic; therefore, he or she must also advocate for the patient and provide additional emotional support. Telehealth nursing increases patient satisfaction by providing the patient with a reliable source of information, direction, and emotional support.

ALGORITHMS

In the telehealth process, patients are guided through triage questions to help the nurse reach a decision for care. **Algorithms** may be used as part of protocol for this triage process. Algorithms are a set of rules designed to solve a certain problem. They are different than a guideline because algorithms direct the nurse toward the best line of treatment. Algorithms also provide a systematic way to evaluate a broad problem or issue. They cover six areas of evaluation, which include the following:

- Assessment and data collection.
- Classification of acuity.
- Degree of advice or intervention.
- Education of caller.
- Validation of the caller.
- Evaluation/Follow-up.

The process follows a chain of logic and relies on the nurse's ability to assess, analyze, and interpret the patient's responses to questions posed by the nurse. The nurse may use algorithms as a direct line of questioning with "yes or no" answers. Each answer directs the nurse to the next type of question, ultimately guiding the nurse to the appropriate way to manage the situation by ruling out other conditions. The use of algorithms in telehealth nursing helps nurses to effectively triage patients over the phone, thereby potentially reducing the frequency of unnecessary emergency department visits and elevated costs.

Efficient Use of Protocols or Guidelines

Protocols and guidelines in telehealth provide structure to the assessment process tailored to the patient's symptoms. They help to promote quality care when followed universally by telehealth nurses. Universal guidelines ensure that no matter where a patient lives, he or she is getting information based on the universal nursing standards of care. Some guidelines may be used to educate the patient on upcoming procedures such as ocular exams or hearing tests. Preoperative instructions can also be given through telehealth using standardized guidelines, as are post-hospitalization follow-up instructions. Guidelines are symptom-based and do not require a confirmed medical diagnosis. For example, if a patient calls in with a suspected sprain or break to the leg, the telehealth nurse would refer to the guideline for care that applies to an injury to an extremity (more generally). The nurse must listen carefully to what a patient is saying, but also to what is not being said in order to carefully prioritize the symptoms the patient is describing.

Necessary Professional Competencies and Professional Development

As with nurses in any other specialty, telehealth nurses must demonstrate professional nursing competencies and an ongoing knowledge of health care practices. They must show clinical expertise with the populations they serve. **Professional competencies** for the telehealth nurse include the following:

- A knowledge of health and illness across all age groups.
- Assessment skills specific for telephone triage.
- Communication skills, both verbal and written.
- Assertiveness and excellent listening skills.
- Critical thinking skills and effectiveness at educating patients over the phone.
- Customer service skills, including the knowledge of how to refer patients to internal and external resources, and the use of guidelines and protocols.
- Skills in written documentation.
- Skills in electronic documentation (including computers, telephones, fax machines, and other electronic forms of communication).

Forms of Documentation

The telehealth nurse must understand and use proficiently the nursing process. The process should be **documented** in the patient record regardless of whether the patient was seen in person or attended to by telephone. Included in the patient record is the assessment of complaint(s), allergies, a history of the present illness/injury, and a medical history. The nurse's categorization of the call as urgent, nonurgent, etc. should also be documented. The plan provided by the nurse should be documented, including a referral if one is made. An evaluation of the patient's understanding and acceptance of the plan of care should also be conducted and documented. It must be remembered that the telehealth nurse may not meet every need of the patient in a single call. Rather, the telehealth nurse's focus should be to prioritize what needs to meet first. Documentation is important to evaluate and ensure that follow-up is conducted.

Application of HIPAA Standards to Telemedicine

The Health Insurance Portability and Accountability Act (HIPAA) was passed in 1996 as a measure to protect private health information of patients. Health care centers have enacted protocols to protect this information by limiting those with access to protected health information and maintaining confidentiality standards set forth by the act. The same standards apply in telemedicine, although there is an additional component of needed safety measures because the information is passing through media or telecommunications. These systems may require increased security to prevent hacking or the transmission of data into the wrong hands. Additional security systems should be in place, such as antiviral software, encryption systems, and password-protected files. Patients should be educated about the security measures being used in order to instill confidence that their personal information is protected.

Therapeutic Relationships

THERAPEUTIC COMMUNICATION
FACILITATING COMMUNICATION

Therapeutic communication begins with respect for the patient/family and the assumption that all communication, verbal and nonverbal, has meaning. Listening must be done empathetically. The following are some techniques that facilitate communication.

Introduction:

- Make a personal introduction and use the patient's name: "Mrs. Brown, I am Susan Williams, your nurse."

Encouragement:

- Use an open-ended opening statement: "Is there anything you'd like to discuss?"
- Acknowledge comments: "Yes," and "I understand."
- Allow silence and observe nonverbal behavior rather than trying to force conversation. Ask for clarification if statements are unclear.
- Reflect statements back (use sparingly): Patient: "I hate this hospital." Nurse: "You hate this hospital?"

Empathy:

- Make observations: "You are shaking," and "You seem worried."
- Recognize feelings:
    o Patient: "I want to go home."
    o Nurse: "It must be hard to be away from your home and family."
- Provide information as honestly and completely as possible about condition, treatment, and procedures and respond to the patient's questions and concerns.

Exploration:

- Verbally express implied messages:
    o Patient: "This treatment is too much trouble."
    o Nurse: "You think the treatment isn't helping you?"
- Explore a topic but allow the patient to terminate the discussion without further probing: "I'd like to hear how you feel about that."

Orientation:

- Indicate reality:
    o Patient: "Someone is screaming."
    o Nurse: "That sound was an ambulance siren."
- Comment on distortions without directly agreeing or disagreeing:
    o Patient: "That nurse promised I didn't have to walk again."
    o Nurse: "Really? That's surprising because the doctor ordered physical therapy twice a day."

Collaboration:

- Work together to achieve better results: "Maybe if we talk about this, we can figure out a way to make the treatment easier for you."

Validation:

- Seek validation: "Do you feel better now?" or "Did the medication help you breathe better?"

AVOIDING NON-THERAPEUTIC COMMUNICATION

While using therapeutic communication is important, it is equally important to avoid interjecting **non-therapeutic communication**, which can block effective communication. *Avoid the following:*

- Meaningless clichés: "Don't worry. Everything will be fine." "Isn't it a nice day?"
- Providing advice: "You should…" or "The best thing to do is…." It's better when patients ask for advice to provide facts and encourage the patient to reach a decision.
- Inappropriate approval that prevents the patient from expressing true feeling or concerns:
  - Patient: "I shouldn't cry about this."
  - Nurse: "That's right! You're an adult!"
- Asking for an explanation of behavior that is not directly related to patient care and requires analysis and explanation of feelings: "Why are you so upset?"
- Agreeing with rather than accepting and responding to patient's statements can make it difficult for the patient to change his or her statement or opinion later: "I agree with you," or "You are right."
- Making negative judgments: "You should stop arguing with the nurses."
- Devaluing the patient's feelings: "Everyone gets upset at times."
- Disagreeing directly: "That can't be true," or "I think you are wrong."
- Defending against criticism: "The doctor is not being rude; he's just very busy today."
- Changing the subject to avoid dealing with uncomfortable topics;
  - Patient: "I'm never going to get well."
  - Nurse: "Your family will be here in just a few minutes."
- Making inappropriate literal responses, even as a joke, especially if the patient is at all confused or having difficulty expressing ideas:
  - Patient: "There are bugs crawling under my skin."
  - Nurse: "I'll get some bug spray,"
- Challenging the patient to establish reality often just increases confusion and frustration:
  - "If you were dying, you wouldn't be able to yell and kick!"

COMMUNICATING WITH PATIENTS WITH DISABILITIES

Guidelines for communicating with individuals with disabilities:

- Do not assume that the person with disabilities also has impaired cognition.
- Always treat the person with respect and dignity.
- Use first names with the patient if asked to do so, but start out formally as with any patient.
- Offer to shake hands even when a prosthesis is present.
- Be patient if communication is impaired.
- Offer assistance, but allow the patient to tell you what is helpful; otherwise don't assist.
- When a wheelchair is used, sit down so the patient does not have to strain their neck to speak with you.
- If providing directions, consider the obstacles that may be in the way and assist the person to find an appropriate way around them.

Communication with Patients with Cognitive Disabilities

The person with cognitive disabilities may be easily distracted, so verbal communication should be attempted in a quiet area:

- Address people with dignity and respect.
- Do not try to discuss abstract ideas but stick with concrete topics.
- Keep words and sentences very simple and try rephrasing when necessary. People may have difficulty in distinguishing your spoken words and deriving the meaning from them.
- Be very patient with people's attempts to speak to you since they may have difficulty in processing thoughts and changing them into spoken words.
- Use objects around you and gestures to illustrate your words since the patient may also use pointing and gesturing when unable to find the words to communicate with you. The person may prefer written communication, although some may be unable to read.
- Use touch to convey your regard during communication, as this is recognized by the patient as reassurance of your care and concern for them.
- Give a few instructions at a time as to not overwhelm them.

Communicating with Deaf or Hearing-Impaired Patients

Communicating with a person with deafness or hearing impairment:

- Try to communicate in a quiet environment if possible.
- Wave or touch the person to let him or her know you are trying to communicate.
- Determine the method the person uses to communicate: sign language, lip reading, hearing devices, or writing.
- Fingerspell or use some signs if able to do so.
- Address the person directly when you speak even though the person may be looking at an interpreter or your lips.
- Look at the person as the interpreter tells you what was said.
- Speak slowly so the interpreter can keep up with you.
- If the person reads lips, face the person and speak clearly and normally, using normal volume.
- If writing a communication, do not speak while writing.
- Do not be afraid to check that the person understands you, and ask questions if you do not understand the person.

Communication with People with Low Vision or Blindness

Communicating with a person with low vision or blindness:

- Greet the person with low vision or blindness, identifying yourself and others present.
- Always say goodbye when you are leaving.
- Alert the person to written communications, such as warning signs or printed notices.
- Face the person and touch briefly on the arm to let the person know you are speaking to him or her if you are in a group.
- Speak at normal loudness.
- Make any directions given specific in terms of the length of walk and obstacles, such as stairs.
- Use the position of hands on a clock face to give directions (potatoes at 3 o'clock) as well as using *right* or *left*.
- Mention sounds that the person may hear in transit or on arrival at a destination.

COMMUNICATING WITH A PATIENT ON A VENTILATOR

When a patient on a ventilator is conscious, he or she may still be able to communicate by blinking, nodding, shaking the head, or pointing to a picture or word board:

- If the person is able to write, try to reposition the IV line to leave the dominant hand free to communicate.
- Discuss the need for communication with the physician and ask if a valve or an electric larynx can be used to permit speech.
- Help the patient practice lip reading of single words.
- Remember the patient's glasses or hearing aids when attempting to communicate.
- Enlist the aid of a speech therapist if there is frustration on the part of the patient and family due to communication difficulty.

COMMUNICATING WITH PERSONS WITH SPEECH PROBLEMS DUE TO A STROKE

Methods to communicate with stroke patients with speech problems:

- **Dysarthria**: Patients have problems forming the words to speak them aloud. Give them time to communicate, offer them a picture board or other means of communicating, and give encouragement to family members who are frustrated with the difficulty of trying to communicate.
- **Expressive aphasia**: The patients' efforts at speech come out garbled when they try to say sentences, but single words may be clear. Encourage the patients to try to write and to practice the sounds of the alphabet. Resist the urge to finish sentences for the patients.
- **Receptive aphasia**: The patients have a problem comprehending the speech they hear. Communicate in simple terms and speak slowly. Test comprehension of the written word as an alternative method of communication.
- **Global aphasia**: The patient has both receptive and expressive aphasia. Use simple, clear, slow speech augmented by pictures and gestures.

COMMUNICATION PROBLEMS OF PATIENTS WITH PARKINSON'S DISEASE

Parkinson's disease causes problems with speaking in the majority (75–90%) of patients. The reason for this is not clear but may relate to increasing rigidity and changes in movement. Speech is often very low-pitched or hoarse, given in a monotone and with a soft voice. Speech production may decrease because of the effort required to speak. **Speech therapy** can develop exercises for the patient that can assist them in remembering to speak slowly and carefully, as patients are not always aware that their **communication** is impaired:

- Allow time for the patient to communicate, asking for repetition if you do not understand the message.
- Help family by teaching ways to facilitate communication with the patient and encouraging them to assist the patient to do the exercises provided by the therapist.
- If speech volume is very low, suggest amplification devices that can be obtained through speech therapy.

Communication with Patients with Psychiatric Problems

Persons with psychiatric disorders appreciate being addressed with respect, dignity, and honesty:

- Speak simply and clearly, repeating as necessary.
- Encourage patients to discuss their concerns regarding treatment and medications to improve compliance.
- Use good eye contact and be attentive to your body language messages.
- Be alert, but unless the person is known to be violent, try to relax and listen to them.
- Don't try to avoid words or phrases pertaining to psychiatric problems, but if you do say something inappropriate, apologize honestly to the patient.
- Offer patients outlets for their thoughts and feelings.
- Learn more about their disorder and ways to use therapeutic communication to help them with their problem, such as re-orienting them as needed.

Cultural Competence

Different cultures view health and illness from very different perspectives, and patients often come from a mix of many cultures, so the nurse must be not only accepting of cultural differences but must be sensitive and aware. There are a number of characteristics that are important for a nurse to have **cultural competence**:

- **Appreciating diversity**: This must be grounded in information about other cultures and understanding of their value systems.
- **Assessing own cultural perspectives**: Self-awareness is essential to understanding potential biases.
- **Understanding intercultural dynamics**: This must include understanding ways in which cultures cooperate, differ, communicate, and reach understanding.
- **Recognizing institutional culture**: Each institutional unit (hospital, clinic, office) has an inherent set of values that may be unwritten but is accepted by the staff.
- **Adapting patient service to diversity**: This is the culmination of cultural competence as it is the point of contact between cultures.

Evaluation

Ethical Behavior

BIOETHICS

Bioethics is a branch of ethics that involves making sure that the medical treatment given is the most morally correct choice given the different options that might be available and the differences inherent in the varied levels of treatment. In the health care unit, if the patients, family members, and the staff are in agreement when it comes to values and decision-making, then no ethical dilemma exists; however, when there is a difference in value beliefs between the patients/family members and the staff, there is a bioethical dilemma that must be resolved. Sometimes, discussion and explanation can resolve differences, but at times the institution's ethics committee must be brought in to resolve the conflict. The primary goal of bioethics is to determine the most morally correct action using the set of circumstances given.

ETHICAL DECISION-MAKING MODEL

There are many ethical decision-making models. Some general guidelines to apply in using ethical decision-making models could be the following:

- Gather information about the identified problem
- State reasonable alternatives and solutions to the problem
- Utilize ethical resources (for example, clergy or ethics committees) to help determine the ethically important elements of each solution or alternative
- Suggest and attempt possible solutions
- Choose a solution to the problem

It is important to always consider the **ethical principles** of autonomy, beneficence, nonmaleficence, justice, and fidelity when attempting to facilitate ethical decision-making with family members, caregivers, and the healthcare team.

ETHICAL ASSESSMENT

While the terms *ethics* and *morals* are sometimes used interchangeably, ethics is a study of morals and encompasses concepts of right and wrong. When making **ethical assessments,** one must consider not only what people should do but also what they actually do, as these two things are sometimes at odds. Ethical issues can be difficult to assess because of personal bias, which is one of the reasons that sharing concerns with other internal sources and reaching consensus is so valuable. Issues of concern might include options for care, refusal of care, rights to privacy, adequate relief of suffering, and the right to self-determination. Internal sources might include the ethics committee, whose role is to make decisions regarding ethical issues. Risk management can provide guidance related to personal and institutional liability. External agencies might include government agencies, such as the public health department.

ETHICAL ANALYSIS OF A SITUATION

Assessment of the situation is done to reveal the ethical, legal, and professional **conflicts** that are present. Those who are involved are identified, including the patient, family, and healthcare personnel. The decision maker is determined if it is not the patient. Information about the situation is collected to determine medical facts about the disease and condition of the patient, options for treatment, and nursing diagnoses. Any pertinent legal information is included. The patient and family's cultural, religious, and moral values are determined. Possible courses of action are listed and compared in terms of outcomes for the patient using the utilitarian or deontological theory of ethics. Professional codes of ethics are also applied. A decision is made and evaluated as to whether it is the most morally correct action. Ethical arguments for and against the decision are given and responded to by the decision maker.

Professional Boundaries

Gifts

Over time, patients may develop a bond with nurses they trust and may feel grateful to the nurse for the care provided and want to express thanks, but the nurse must make sure to maintain professional boundaries. Patients often offer **gifts** to nurses to show their appreciation, but some adults, especially those who are weak and ill or have cognitive impairment, may be taken advantage of easily. Patients may offer valuables and may sometimes be easily manipulated into giving large sums of money. Small tokens of appreciation that can be shared with other staff, such as a box of chocolates, are usually acceptable (depending upon the policy of the institution), but almost any other gifts (jewelry, money, clothes) should be declined: "I'm sorry, that's so kind of you, but nurses are not allowed to accept gifts from patients." Declining may relieve the patient of the feeling of obligation.

Sexual Relations

When the boundary between the role of the professional nurse and the vulnerability of the patient is breached, a boundary violation occurs. Because the nurse is in the position of authority, the responsibility to maintain the boundary rests with the nurse; however, the line separating them is a continuum and sometimes not easily defined. It is inappropriate for nurses to engage in **sexual relations** with patients, and if the sexual behavior is coerced or the patient is cognitively impaired, it is **illegal**. However, more common violations with adults, particularly elderly patients, include exposing a patient unnecessarily, using sexually demeaning gestures or language (including off-color jokes), harassment, or inappropriate touching. Touching should be used with care, such as touching a hand or shoulder. Hugging may be misconstrued.

Attention

Nursing is a giving profession, but the nurse must temper giving with recognition of professional boundaries. Patients have many needs. As acts of kindness, nurses (especially those involved in home care) often give certain patients extra attention and may offer to do **favors**, such as cooking or shopping. They may become overly invested in the patients' lives. While this may benefit a patient in the short term, it can establish a relationship of increasing **dependency** and **obligation** that does not resolve the long-term needs of the patient. Making referrals to the appropriate agencies or collaborating with family to find ways to provide services is more effective. Becoming overly invested may be evident by the nurse showing favoritism or spending too much time with the patient while neglecting other duties. On the other end of the spectrum are nurses who are disinterested and fail to provide adequate attention to the patient's detriment. Lack of adequate attention may lead to outright neglect.

Coercion

Power issues are inherent in matters associated with professional boundaries. Physical abuse is both unprofessional and illegal, but behavior can easily border on abusive without the patient being physically injured. Nurses can easily **intimidate** older adults and sick patients into having procedures or treatments they do not want. Regardless of age, patients have the right to choose and the right to refuse treatment. Difficulties arise with cognitive impairment, and in that case, another responsible adult (often the patient's child or spouse) is designated to make decisions, but every effort should be made to gain patient cooperation. Forcing the patient to do something against his or her will borders on abuse and can sometimes degenerate into actual abuse if physical coercion is involved.

Personal Information

When pre-existing personal or business relationships exist, other nurses should be assigned care of the patient whenever possible, but this may be difficult in small communities. However, the nurse should strive to maintain a professional role separate from the personal role and respect professional boundaries. The nurse must respect and maintain the confidentiality of the patient and family members, but the nurse must also be very careful about **disclosing personal information** about him or herself because this establishes a social relationship that interferes with the professional role of the nurse and the boundary between the patient and the nurse. The nurse and patient should never share secrets. When the nurse divulges personal information, he or she may become vulnerable to the patient, a reversal of roles.

Evidence-Based Practice

CLASSES OF EVIDENCE-BASED PRACTICE

Evidence-based practice is treatment based on the best possible evidence, including a study of current research. Literature is searched to find evidence of the most effective treatments for specific diseases or injuries, and those treatments are then utilized to create clinical pathways that outline specific multi-departmental treatment protocols, including medications, treatments, and timelines. Evidence-based guidelines are often produced by specialty organizations that undertake the task of searching and analyzing literature to produce policies, procedures, and guidelines that become the standard of care for the disease. These guidelines are then used when a patient fits the disease criteria for that guideline.

Evidence-based nursing aims to improve the quality of nursing care by examining the reasons for all nursing practices and determining those that have the most positive outcomes. Evidence-based nursing focuses on the individual nurse utilizing evidence-based observations to influence decision-making.

EVIDENCE-BASED PRACTICE GUIDELINES

The creation of evidence-based practice guidelines includes the following components:

- **Focus on the topic/methodology:** This includes outlining possible interventions and treatments for review, choosing patient populations and settings, and determining significant outcomes. Search boundaries (such as types of journals, types of studies, dates of studies) should be determined.
- **Evidence review:** This includes review of literature, critical analysis of studies, and summarizing of results, including pooled meta-analysis.
- **Expert judgment:** Recommendations based on personal experience from a number of experts may be utilized, especially if there is inadequate evidence based on review, but this subjective evidence should be explicitly acknowledged.
- **Policy considerations:** This includes cost-effectiveness, access to care, insurance coverage, availability of qualified staff, and legal implications.
- **Policy:** A written policy must be completed with recommendations. Common practice is to utilize letter guidelines, with "A" being the most highly recommended, usually based on the quality of supporting evidence.
- **Review:** The completed policy should be submitted to peers for review and comments before instituting the policy.

CRITICAL PATHWAYS

Clinical/critical pathway development is done by those involved in direct patient care. The pathway should require no additional staffing and cover the entire scope of an illness. Steps include:

1. Selection of patient group and diagnosis, procedures, or conditions, based on analysis of data and observations of wide variance in approach to treatment and prioritizing organization and patient needs
2. Creation of interdisciplinary team of those involved in the process of care, including physicians to develop pathway
3. Analysis of data including literature review and study of best practices to identify opportunities for quality improvement
4. Identification of all categories of care, such as nutrition, medications, and nursing
5. Discussion and reaching consensus
6. Identifying the levels of care and number of days to be covered by the pathway
7. Pilot testing and redesigning steps as indicated
8. Educating staff about standards
9. Monitoring and tracking variances in order to improve pathways

LEVELS OF EVIDENCE IN EVIDENCE-BASED PRACTICE

Levels of evidence are categorized according to the scientific evidence available to support the recommendations, as well as existing state and federal laws. While recommendations are voluntary, they are often used as a basis for state and federal regulations.

- **Category IA** is well supported by evidence from experimental, clinical, or epidemiologic studies and is strongly recommended for implementation.
- **Category IB** has supporting evidence from some studies, has a good theoretical basis, and is strongly recommended for implementation.
- **Category IC** is required by state or federal regulations or is an industry standard.
- **Category II** is supported by suggestive clinical or epidemiologic studies, has a theoretical basis, and is suggested for implementation.
- **Category III** is supported by descriptive studies, such as comparisons, correlations, and case studies, and may be useful.
- **Category IV** is obtained from expert opinion or authorities only.
- **Unresolved** means there is no recommendation because of a lack of consensus or evidence.

OUTCOME EVALUATION

Outcome evaluation is an important component of evidence-based practice, which involves both internal and external research. All treatments are subjected to review to determine if they produce positive outcomes, and policies and protocols for outcome evaluation should be in place. **Outcome evaluation** includes the following:

- **Monitoring** over the course of treatment involves careful observation and record-keeping that notes progress, with supporting laboratory and radiographic evidence as indicated by condition and treatment.
- **Evaluating** results includes reviewing records as well as current research to determine if outcomes are within acceptable parameters.
- **Sustaining** involves discontinuing treatment but continuing to monitor and evaluate.
- **Improving** means to continue the treatment but with additions or modifications in order to improve outcomes.
- **Replacing** the treatment with a different treatment must be done if outcome evaluation indicates that current treatment is ineffective.

EVIDENCE-BASED NURSING INTERVENTIONS

Evidence-based nursing interventions enable nurses to provide high-quality patient care that is based upon research and knowledge, as opposed to giving care that is based upon tradition or information that is out of date. An evidence-based nursing approach is based on the integration of practical clinical experience with medical and clinical research; it utilizes proven clinical guidelines and assessment practices. Evidence-based nursing interventions allow nurses to make patient care decisions based on cutting-edge research that has been scientifically validated. Studies show that evidence-based nursing practice yields improved patient outcomes, enables nurses to practice up-to-date methods, improves nurse confidence and decision-making skills, and enhances Joint Commission standards.

Resources

There are numerous information resources for evidence-based nursing interventions. These resources include evidence-based textbooks; databases such as CINAHL Plus, COCHRANE library, Mosby's Nursing Index, NursingConsult, and Nursing@Ovid; evidence-based nursing metasites such as the Academic Center for EBN, Joanna Briggs Institute, McGill University, ONS-EBN section, and EBN-University of Minnesota; online evidence-based nursing journals such as Clinical Nurse Specialist, Clinical Nursing Research, Evidence-Based Nursing, Journal of Nursing Care Quality, Journal of Advanced Nursing, Journal of Nursing Scholarship, Nurse Researcher, Nursing Research, Western Journal of Nursing Research, and Worldviews on Evidence-Based Nursing; and various online tutorials.

Obtaining Results of Research to Use in Evidence-Based Practice

When searching for **current evidence** in print and online literature, the nurse should look for **systematic reviews, analyses, and reports**. PUBMED lists all literature and can be searched for all published articles on a particular subject. These articles can be analyzed to determine treatments that have the best evidence of efficacy. Subject and methodological terms and clinical filters can be used to find necessary information, including a specific medical subject heading (MH), subheading (SH), publication type (PT), and text word (TW). The nurse should also search the National Guideline Clearinghouse, Cochrane Databases, Agency for Healthcare Research and Quality, and US Preventive Services Task Force Recommendations for evidence and guidelines. When trials of a treatment provide evidence of effectiveness, the evidence is weighed for strength and confidence. Those that provide the strongest evidence of efficacy become recommendations and guidelines for use in the field. Research is also done on a smaller scale by specialists who publish in peer-reviewed journals their research results related to the use of a particular intervention.

FNP Practice Test #1

1. An adult patient needs treatment for *Chlamydia trachomatis* urethritis. Which one of the following drugs is useful as a single-dose regimen?
   a. Ceftriaxone intramuscularly.
   b. Levofloxacin.
   c. Azithromycin.
   d. Doxycycline.

2. A patient who gave birth to an infant two months previously seems disengaged and withdrawn. The family nurse practitioner is concerned that the patient may have postpartum depression. Which three of the following symptoms are characteristic of postpartum depression?
   a. Insomnia or hypersomnia.
   b. Disorientation and confusion.
   c. Feeling of worthlessness or inadequacy.
   d. Poor concentration and inability to make decisions.
   e. Delusions associated with the infant.

3. A child with fetal alcohol syndrome (FAS) is likely to exhibit which one of the following findings?
   a. Growth deficiency.
   b. Normal IQ.
   c. Thickened upper lip.
   d. Macrocephaly.

4. To evaluate a child for esotropia, which one of the following is a rapid and convenient diagnostic screening test?
   a. Slit lamp examination.
   b. Corneal light reflex test.
   c. Snellen test.
   d. Fluorescein test.

5. According to Dr. Elisabeth Kübler-Ross, dying patients experience several emotional stages during terminal illness. Which one of these emotions persists throughout all the stages of terminal illness?
   a. Anger.
   b. Hope.
   c. Denial.
   d. Bargaining.

6. A family nurse practitioner is assessing an 11-month-old African-American child who was brought in by his mother for concerns about swelling in both hands and both feet. On examination, the nurse practitioner finds tenderness and obvious swelling of the hands and feet. Vital signs, including temperature and blood pressure, are normal. The most likely diagnosis is:
   a. osteomyelitis.
   b. hand-foot-mouth disease.
   c. glomerulonephritis.
   d. sickle cell disease.

7. A 65-year-old woman complains of urinary incontinence. She is experiencing leakage of urine when she coughs, sneezes, or laughs. This form of urinary incontinence is called:
   a. stress incontinence.
   b. urge incontinence.
   c. overflow incontinence.
   d. functional incontinence.

8. A full-term newborn weighed 7 pounds, 9 ounces at birth. Three days after hospital discharge, the family nurse practitioner is seeing the baby for his first checkup. He now weighs 7 pounds, 4 ounces. This level of weight loss is:
   a. worrisome because it is below birth weight.
   b. Indicative of inadequate nutrition.
   c. A sign of dehydration.
   d. Normal at this age.

9. Which of the following drugs is NOT associated with human teratogenicity?
   a. Valproic acid.
   b. Warfarin.
   c. Phenytoin.
   d. Amoxicillin.

10. The family nurse practitioner is assessing an infant for indications of developmental hip dysplasia utilizing the Ortolani-Barlow maneuver. The maneuver begins by placing the infant on the back and includes the following steps:
    1. Grasp the infant's knees with the thumbs over the inner thighs.
    2. Slowly abduct the infant's hips and observe for equal movement, resistance, or an abnormal "clunk" sound.
    3. Flex the infant's knees and hips to 90 degrees.
    4. Touch the infant's knees together, and then press down on the one femur at a time, observing for dislocation.

Place the steps to this maneuver in sequential order, from first to last:
   a.
   b.
   c.
   d.

11. An adolescent patient presents with severe sore throat, fever, cervical lymphadenopathy, and difficulty opening the mouth. On examination, the family nurse practitioner sees that the uvula is deviated from the midline and there is some bulging of the soft palate near the tonsillar area. What is the most likely diagnosis?
    a. Epiglottitis.
    b. Viral pharyngitis.
    c. Peritonsillar abscess.
    d. Retropharyngeal abscess.

12. Most cases of infectious pharyngitis are caused by:
    a. viruses.
    b. group A streptococcus.
    c. streptococcus pneumoniae.
    d. haemophilus influenzae.

13. A pediatric patient has a tender, boggy lesion on the scalp. There are numerous pustules overlying the lesion. Occipital lymphadenopathy is also present, and there are also three to four small scaly areas of hair loss scattered over the scalp. A Wood's lamp examination shows no fluorescence. What is the most likely diagnosis?
    a. Scalp abscess.
    b. Tinea capitis.
    c. Impetigo.
    d. MRSA infection.

14. Which one of the following is a typical characteristic of *Mycoplasma pneumoniae* infection?
    a. Consolidated infiltrate on chest x-ray.
    b. Headaches.
    c. Hypoxia.
    d. Myositis.

15. Thelarche begins in girls during which Tanner stage?
    a. Stage I.
    b. Stage II.
    c. Stage III.
    d. Stage IV.

16. A nurse practitioner is examining a 55-year-old diabetic man who reports a bilateral pretibial rash. The physical exam reveals a thin epidermis with brown–yellow ulcerated plaques that are oozing blood. What is the most likely diagnosis?
    a. Erythema nodosum.
    b. Myxedema.
    c. Cutaneous Candida albicans infection.
    d. Necrobiosis lipoidica diabeticorum (NLD).

17. Red blood cell (RBC) casts in the urine indicate:
    a. interstitial nephritis.
    b. myoglobinuria.
    c. renal tubular damage.
    d. glomerular disease.

18. Which of the following is a criterion for diagnosis of diabetes mellitus?
    a. Single fasting blood glucose > 126 mg/dL.
    b. HgA1c of 6.5%.
    c. Polydipsia and polyuria.
    d. Single nonfasting blood glucose > 200 mg/dL.

19. According to federal law, a family nurse practitioner can care for nursing home patients under which of the following conditions?
    a. A physician must be available for emergencies.
    b. Patients must be younger than 80 years of age.
    c. The caseload must not exceed five patients.
    d. All of the above.

20. The public health department has noted a recent increase in cases of West Nile fever, and the family nurse practitioner has begun to see patients with the infection. Which three of the following signs or symptoms does the family nurse practitioner recognize as being typical of West Nile fever?
    a. Alterations of consciousness.
    b. Weakness of facial muscles.
    c. Transient maculopapular rash on the chest, stomach, and back.
    d. Fever, headache, and body aches.
    e. Nausea and vomiting.
    f. Seizures.

21. An African-American woman asks a nurse practitioner about sickle cell disease. She informs the practitioner that she is homozygous for hemoglobin A (AA) and her husband has sickle cell trait (AS). What is the probability that they would have a child with sickle cell disease?
    a. 0%.
    b. 25%.
    c. 50%.
    d. 100%.

22. The percentage of persons with dementia cared for in the home by family members is closest to:
    a. 33%.
    b. 52%.
    c. 65%.
    d. 80%.

23. A family nurse practitioner observes the interaction between a parent and a seven-year-old child. Which three of the following parental behaviors indicate that the parent has an authoritarian parenting style?
    a. Parent issues commands and expects obedience.
    b. Parent communicates little with the child.
    c. Parent shows unconditional love to the child.
    d. Parent sets reasonable limits on behavior.
    e. Parent has rules that are inflexible.
    f. Parent provides little guidance to the child.

24. Which of the following is a HIPAA violation?
    a. Discussing patient treatment information with another provider via e-mail.
    b. Leaving patient charts outside patient exam rooms while they wait to see the provider.
    c. Revealing protected health information with a pharmaceutical representative who needs feedback on his new product.
    d. Releasing health information to the police to aid in an investigation.

25. Which of the following is NOT a cause of secondary hypertension?
    a. Sepsis.
    b. Cocaine use.
    c. Kidney disease.
    d. Oral contraceptive use.

26. An otherwise healthy patient was diagnosed with influenza B within 48 hours of onset of symptoms and was treated with oseltamivir (Tamiflu). Within 24 hours, he reports intermittent heart palpitations. The most likely cause of the palpitations is:
   a. a routine symptom of the flu virus.
   b. high fever.
   c. viral myocarditis.
   d. a side effect of Tamiflu.

27. The family nurse practitioner has noted that a nursing team member has engaged in professional boundary violations. Which three of the following actions may indicate boundary violations?
   a. The nurse accepts a $20 tip from a patient.
   b. The nurse is upset about a family situation and confides in a patient.
   c. The nurse touches a patient's arm when comforting the patient.
   d. The nurse exchanges patients with another nurse in order to care for a favorite patient.
   e. The nurse calls a priest for a patient who wants spiritual support.

28. A three-year-old-boy has had fever of 104 to 105 degrees for six days. While examining the patient, a nurse practitioner notes a strawberry tongue, a maculopapular rash on the trunk, unilateral cervical lymphadenopathy, and nonexudative conjunctivitis. He also has cracked lips and edema of the hands and feet. A physician treated the patient three days prior with antibiotics for a presumed strep infection. What is the most likely diagnosis?
   a. Toxic epidermal necrolysis.
   b. Resistant strep infection.
   c. Kawasaki disease.
   d. Juvenile rheumatoid arthritis.

29. An American elderly person is most likely to be abused by which one of the following?
   a. A sibling.
   b. A spouse.
   c. An adult child.
   d. An unrelated caregiver.

30. Which one of these conditions is associated with the highest suicide rate?
   a. COPD.
   b. Diabetes.
   c. AIDS.
   d. Osteoporosis.

31. An eight-year-old child has had severe nausea and vomiting from enteritis and is at risk for hypokalemia. Which three of the following signs or symptoms are characteristic of hypokalemia?
   a. Bradycardia.
   b. Muscle weakness, cramps, and hyporeflexia.
   c. Renal calculi.
   d. Confusion.
   e. Hypotension.
   f. Lethargy and fatigue.

32. The most common cause of viral pneumonia in adults is:
   a. adenovirus.
   b. RSV.
   c. Haemophilus influenzae.
   d. influenza virus.

33. A family nurse practitioner is evaluating a 21-year-old patient with bilateral eye irritation. He has had several similar episodes in the past, but this one is more severe. The palpebral conjunctivae are edematous and velvety red and the bulbar conjunctivae are injected. No eye discharge is visible. Which one of these other clinical findings would the nurse practitioner expect to see in this case?

   a. Increased intraocular pressure.
   b. Fever.
   c. Myopia.
   d. Pruritus.

34. A 35-year-old male has been an insulin-dependent diabetic for five years and now is unable to urinate. Which of the following would the nurse practitioner most likely suspect?

   a. Atherosclerosis.
   b. Diabetic nephropathy.
   c. Autonomic neuropathy.
   d. Somatic neuropathy.

35. The most common cause of cancer-related deaths in the 25- to 44-year-olds group is:

   a. lung cancer.
   b. Hodgkin's lymphoma.
   c. breast cancer.
   d. colon cancer.

36. An adult patient with iron deficiency anemia asks his family nurse practitioner about foods that are rich in iron. Which one of the following is highest in iron?

   a. Oranges.
   b. Whole milk.
   c. Beans.
   d. Egg whites.

37. A 21-month old child has a fever of 103 degrees, fussiness, drooling, and lack of appetite. On exam, the family nurse practitioner notes a red throat with several ulcerations over the tonsillar pillars. What is the most likely diagnosis?

   a. Herpangina.
   b. Strep pharyngitis.
   c. Gingivostomatitis.
   d. Epiglottitis.

38. Which of the following is not an etiologic agent of bronchiolitis?

   a. RSV.
   b. Coronavirus.
   c. Norovirus.
   d. Rhinovirus.

39. According to Erikson's psychosocial theory, children go through four stages:

   1. Autonomy versus shame and doubt.
   2. Trust versus mistrust.
   3. Industry versus inferiority.
   4. Initiative versus guilt.

Place the stages (in numbers) in sequential order, from infancy to school age.
- a. Infancy:
- b. Early childhood:
- c. Late childhood:
- d. School age:

40. A family nurse practitioner has a patient who is habitually at least 30 minutes late for her appointments. She is a 42-year-old Hispanic woman with several health issues. Which of the following statements demonstrates cultural competence on the part of the healthcare provider?
- a. The provider should not take cultural differences into account in healthcare situations.
- b. Refusing to see the patient unless she arrives on time will teach her a lesson.
- c. Consider that the patient belongs to a culture where being on time is flexible or approximate rather than exact.
- d. Making a reminder call to the patient the day before will solve the problem.

41. Pneumococcal polysaccharide vaccine (PPSV 23, Pneumovax) is:
- a. recommended for all adults age 65 or over.
- b. administered intradermally.
- c. recommended yearly for asplenic patients.
- d. not given concurrently with other vaccines.

42. The family nurse practitioner is actively engaged in preventive health maintenance activities. Which two of the following nursing actions are examples of primary prevention?
- a. Administering immunizations.
- b. Conducting vision screening.
- c. Instructing parents about car safety seats.
- d. Screening adolescents for scoliosis.
- e. Developing rehabilitation activities for a child.

43. The number-one cause of blindness in the elderly is:
- a. cataracts.
- b. age-related macular degeneration.
- c. glaucoma.
- d. diabetic retinopathy.

44. A family nurse practitioner is evaluating a three-year-old child with suspected Henoch–Schönlein purpura (HSP). Which one of the following is NOT true about HSP?
- a. Patients may complain of joint pain.
- b. The purpura is due thrombocytopenia.
- c. HSP may be associated with abdominal pain.
- d. Microscopic hematuria may be present.

45. Which one of the following is good advice for a patient with gastroesophageal reflux disease (GERD)?
- a. Take anticholinergics to speed gastric emptying.
- b. Increase fat intake.
- c. Raise the head of the bed on two-inch blocks.
- d. Eat a high-fiber diet.

46. A family nurse practitioner is instructing a 65-year-old patient on taking psyllium (Metamucil). Which of the following is appropriate advice?
    a. Sprinkle psyllium into a half cup of applesauce, and eat the entire serving.
    b. Take the psyllium dose mixed in one cup of fluid followed by a second glass of fluid.
    c. Psyllium is most effective when taken with a calcium supplement.
    d. The onset of action of psyllium is usually within 30 to 45 minutes.

47. What is the treatment of choice for a routine tooth abscess?
    a. Extraction of the tooth.
    b. Erythromycin.
    c. Penicillin VK.
    d. Levaquin.

48. A nurse practitioner is seeing an adult patient with a 72-hour history of fever, cough, and runny nose. Her in-clinic flu test is positive for flu type B. She wants a prescription for antibiotics. Which one of the following would be the best thing to tell her?
    a. "The virus will just have to run its course. Be patient."
    b. "There's just nothing I can do to cure a virus."
    c. "Everybody knows antibiotics are not effective for treating the flu."
    d. "You must feel miserable and I sympathize with you. Let's discuss some things that will relieve your symptoms."

49. Which of the following statements is true about an infantile umbilical hernia?
    a. It will most likely require surgical repair.
    b. It will get worse if the baby cries excessively.
    c. The baby should wear a band around the abdomen to keep the hernia "in."
    d. It will heal on its own because it is less than 2 cm in diameter.

50. The family members of a patient with Alzheimer's disease are having difficulty coping with the patient's repetition of questions and phrases. This phenomenon is known as:
    a. perseveration.
    b. denial.
    c. confabulation.
    d. contrivance.

51. A nurse practitioner is instructing a newly diagnosed diabetic on the symptoms of hypoglycemia. Which one of the following is NOT a symptom of hypoglycemia?
    a. diaphoresis.
    b. tremors.
    c. hunger.
    d. diplopia.

52. Which of these choices best describes the classic presentation of viral croup in a toddler?
    a. Drooling and sitting in a tripod position.
    b. Seal-like cough and rhinorrhea.
    c. Fever of 104.5 and cough.
    d. Oxygen saturation of 92% and severe retractions.

53. A nurse practitioner is performing a breast exam on a 44-year-old woman and detects a painless irregular-shaped mass on the right breast. Which one of these findings is most likely to be associated with breast cancer?
   a. Breast lump fixed to muscle or skin.
   b. A tender nodule.
   c. Nodule that feels rubbery.
   d. Lumps in both breasts.

54. A 20-year-old marathon runner is running a race in 100-degree weather, and partway through the race, the runner is unable to continue and complains of severe muscle cramps. His family immediately takes him to see the family nurse practitioner, who finds that the patient is alert, pale, diaphoretic, and slightly dizzy with skin that is cold and clammy. The patient's temperature is 102° F/39° C. Which three of the following initial treatments does the family nurse practitioner employ?
   a. Evaporative cooling.
   b. Alcohol baths.
   c. Benzodiazepines and barbiturates.
   d. Oral rehydration with 0.1% isotonic NaCl solution.
   e. Intravenous (IV) fluids.
   f. Monitor vital signs (VS), temperature, and urinary output.

55. The mechanism of injury in a nursemaid's elbow is usually:
   a. pulling.
   b. twisting.
   c. bending.
   d. compression.

56. A family nurse practitioner is conducting a follow-up visit with a 60-year-old woman who is on Coumadin for a history of deep vein thrombosis originally treated in the hospital. She is in the clinic today for an exam and to have her INR checked. The goal for her INR is:
   a. 1.5 to 2.0.
   b. 2.0 to 3.0.
   c. 3.0 to 4.0.
   d. 4.0 to 4.5.

57. A 42-year-old man wants to quit smoking. He wants to know the symptoms of nicotine withdrawal. All of the following are symptoms EXCEPT:
   a. difficulty sleeping.
   b. tachycardia.
   c. anxiety.
   d. impotence.

58. A 68-year-old patient with osteoarthritis of both knees has been treating his chronic pain with acetaminophen 650 mg four times daily and drinks approximately six to eight alcoholic beverages daily. The patient's diet is poor, leading to a weight loss of 10 pounds in the past three months. The patient's mobility is impaired, causing a decreased activity level. The family nurse practitioner compiles a problem list:
   1. Chronic pain.
   2. Risk of hepatotoxicity.
   3. Impaired physical mobility and activity.
   4. Risk for imbalanced nutrition.

In which order of priority should the nurse address the patient's problems, from most critical to least critical?

a.
b.
c.
d.

59. A mother brings her nine-month-old son to see the nurse practitioner for a tight foreskin. What is the best management approach?

    a. Force the foreskin back under direct physician supervision.
    b. Refer the baby to a urologist.
    c. Advise the mother to retract the foreskin little by little at each diaper change until it loosens.
    d. Explain to the mother that a tight foreskin is normal at this age.

60. Which one of the following is a conjugated vaccine?

    a. Inactivated polio vaccine.
    b. Hepatitis B vaccine.
    c. Hib vaccine.
    d. Acellular pertussis vaccine.

61. The rotavirus vaccine is given to children to protect against a potentially severe diarrheal infection. An early version of the vaccine was removed from the market because of its association with:

    a. a high risk of developing the rotavirus infection after vaccination.
    b. a contaminant in the vaccine.
    c. an increased risk of intussusception.
    d. poor development of immunity after vaccination.

62. A family nurse practitioner has given an influenza vaccine to an adult patient. The patient wants to know how long it will take for his body to form antibodies to the virus. The nurse practitioner's answer is:

    a. 4 to 6 weeks.
    b. 72 hours.
    c. 48 hours.
    d. 2 weeks.

63. Due to visual impairment and problems with mobility, an elderly patient is unable to care for himself. In reference to barriers against self-care, these two specific impairments are classified as:

    a. cognitive barriers.
    b. physical barriers.
    c. psychological barriers.
    d. psychosocial barriers.

64. Which of these is NOT associated with infant tooth decay?

    a. Exclusive breastfeeding.
    b. Sleeping with a bottle of formula in the mouth.
    c. Frequent pacifier use.
    d. Presence of only one to four erupted teeth.

65. At what age(s) can one begin to obtain reliable hearing screening results?
   a. Newborn.
   b. Age six months.
   c. Age nine months.
   d. Ages two to three years.

66. Which of the following is true about eye contact in the clinical setting?
   a. Eye contact occurs in generally the same way from one culture to another.
   b. In some cultures, direct eye contact is considered to be rude.
   c. In American culture, avoiding eye contact is usually a signal of respect for the other person.
   d. Avoiding direct eye contact is always a sign of disapproval.

67. A 24-year-old female comes to the clinic with confusion. This patient has a history of a myeloma diagnosis, constipation, intense abdominal pain, and polyuria. Which of the following would the family nurse practitioner most likely suspect?
   a. Diverticulosis.
   b. Hypercalcemia.
   c. Hypocalcemia.
   d. Irritable bowel syndrome.

68. Which of the following is an example of medical negligence?
   a. Delegating a routine task to a trained assistant.
   b. Failure to monitor a patient.
   c. Providing medical advice over the phone.
   d. Referring a patient to a specialist.

69. The family nurse practitioner is examining a five-year-old child. Which three of the following physical skills should the child be able to carry out?
   a. Uses scissors.
   b. Draws shapes such as circles and squares.
   c. Jumps rope.
   d. Roller skates or ice skates.
   e. Rides tricycle or bicycle with training wheels.

70. Which of these statements is true about the nurse practitioner scope of practice?
   a. Nurse practitioners may not prescribe narcotics in most states.
   b. Nurse practitioner scopes of practice vary widely from state to state.
   c. Most states allow nurse practitioners to practice independently.
   d. A nurse practitioner cannot evaluate the psychosocial status of a patient.

71. Scabies is an infestation caused by:
   a. mites.
   b. insects.
   c. ticks.
   d. protozoans.

72. Which of these is NOT a potential complication of rosacea?
   a. Folliculitis.
   b. Oral lesions.
   c. Facial pyoderma.
   d. Dry eyes.

73. Which three of the following are age-associated changes of the cardiovascular system expected in the older adult?
   a. Heart increases in size.
   b. Adipose tissue accumulates around the heart.
   c. Cardiac output decreases.
   d. Veins become increasingly more elastic.
   e. The heart's sympathetic nervous response to exertion decreases.

74. A possible complication of gallstones is:
   a. hepatitis.
   b. gastritis.
   c. acute cholecystitis.
   d. cancer of the gallbladder.

75. Which of the following is the most appropriate treatment for a single tinea corporis lesion that is less than 2 cm in diameter?
   a. Topical betamethasone.
   b. Oral griseofulvin.
   c. Topical diphenhydramine.
   d. Topical clotrimazole.

76. The percentage of patients with Bell's palsy that experience full and spontaneous resolution is closest to:
   a. 25%.
   b. 50%.
   c. 70%.
   d. 90%.

77. A key component in the initial overall management of osteoarthritis is:
   a. nonpharmacologic treatment.
   b. etanercept (Enbrel).
   c. joint replacement surgery.
   d. arthroscopy.

78. Management of a 34-year-old man with Type 2 diabetes routinely includes all of these EXCEPT:
   a. referral to an ophthalmologist for periodic retinal exams.
   b. measuring lipid levels periodically.
   c. screen for proteinuria periodically.
   d. measuring HbA1c once yearly.

79. A nurse practitioner is assessing a "suspicious" mole on a 78-year-old man's face. He is concerned about skin cancer. The most common type of skin cancer is:
   a. squamous cell carcinoma.
   b. melanoma.
   c. basal cell carcinoma.
   d. mycosis fungoides.

80. A nurse practitioner is performing a Denver II Developmental Screening Test on a toddler. Which of the following is NOT a developmental category screened by the test?
   a. Fine motor development.
   b. Language development.
   c. Gross motor development.
   d. Emotional development.

81. A nurse practitioner is counseling a pregnant woman about the risks of smoking during pregnancy. Which one of the following is associated with smoking during pregnancy?
   a. Gestational diabetes.
   b. Preeclampsia.
   c. Low birth weight.
   d. Molar pregnancy.

82. Which of the following has a protective effect against the development of neural tube defects during pregnancy?
   a. Vitamin B12.
   b. Iron sulfate.
   c. Folic acid.
   d. Vitamin C.

83. A patient has been diagnosed with Alzheimer's disease and is at stage 5: moderate cognitive decline, early dementia. Which four of the following signs or symptoms are typical of stage 5?
   a. Patient needs some assistance with personal hygiene.
   b. Patient is oriented to self but may be disoriented to place and time.
   c. Patient may sometimes forget names of friends and family members.
   d. Patient may experience urinary and/or fecal incontinence.
   e. Patient may begin to exhibit wandering and sundowning.
   f. Patient may forget addresses and telephone numbers.

84. The mother of a nine-year-old girl is concerned that the child is already showing signs of breast development. What would the family nurse practitioner do next?
   a. Reassure the mother that breast development at this age is within normal limits.
   b. Make a diagnosis of premature breast development.
   c. Refer the child to an endocrinologist.
   d. Obtain bone age radiographs.

85. During a routine physical exam, a family nurse practitioner notices peripheral edema of both legs in a 48-year-old diabetic woman who also suffers from high blood pressure and depression. Of the following medications, which of the following is most likely causing the edema?
   a. Hydrochlorothiazide.
   b. Fluoxetine (Prozac).
   c. Rosiglitazone (Avandia).
   d. Metformin.

86. The family nurse practitioner is completing a neurologic exam for a patient who is complaining of unexplained weakness and ataxia. The neurologic exam includes:
   1. reflexes.
   2. motor system.
   3. mental status.
   4. cranial nerves.
   5. sensory system.

Place the elements of the neurologic exam (in numbers) in the correct sequence, starting from the first element to the last.

a.
b.
c.
d.
e.

87. In general, all of the following should have a preoperative electrocardiogram EXCEPT
    a. men over age 45
    b. patients with known heart disease
    c. patients with a history of costochondritis
    d. patients with hypertension

88. At what age would it be appropriate to stop performing Pap smears on a 53-year-old woman whose previous Pap smears have all been normal? Both she and her husband have been monogamous for 30 years.
    a. 60 years.
    b. 65 years.
    c. 70 years.
    d. She should continue Pap screenings indefinitely.

89. A 66-year-old woman with asthma states she has not received any immunizations since age 14. Aside from her asthma, she is healthy. She asks her nurse practitioner if she currently needs any vaccines. Which one of the following would the nurse practitioner recommend?
    a. FluMist.
    b. Pneumovax.
    c. MMR.
    d. Hib.

90. A family nurse practitioner has diagnosed a 32-year-old woman with influenza A. She wants prophylaxis with oseltamivir (Tamiflu) for her two children, ages 2 months and 2 years. Which of these choices represents the current influenza prophylaxis recommendations?
    a. Only the 2-month-old may receive prophylaxis.
    b. Only the 2-year-old may receive prophylaxis.
    c. Both may receive prophylaxis.
    d. Neither may receive prophylaxis.

91. In reference to patient education, which one of these statements is true?
    a. Patients usually recall and understand most information given by their provider.
    b. Most patients feel their providers overload them with information.
    c. When behavioral changes are medically necessary, patients like to be given options for change and then select from the list.
    d. Leaning toward the patient while giving instructions does not increase recall.

92. A family nurse practitioner is working in a clinic that sees many Native-American patients. Which of these health conditions has a higher prevalence among Native Americans when compared to other American population groups?
    a. Tuberculosis.
    b. Hypertension.
    c. Coronary artery disease.
    d. Obesity.

93. Which one of the following is NOT one of the three fundamental principles of professionalism?
   a. Principle of professional appearance.
   b. Primacy of patient welfare.
   c. Principle of patient autonomy.
   d. Principle of social justice.

94. A 42-year-old man has terminal cancer. He will most likely die within one year. He asks his nurse practitioner not to disclose this prognosis to his wife. The nurse practitioner sees his wife as he is walking out of the hospital and she asks him to "tell her the truth" about her husband's condition. The nurse practitioner feels she has a right to know, and he tells her about the grim prognosis. This is a violation of:
   a. Patient autonomy.
   b. Patient welfare.
   c. Patient confidentiality.
   d. Professional competence.

95. The family nurse practitioner is conducting a physical examination of a two-year-old child. Which three of the following signs may indicate hearing impairment?
   a. The tympanic membranes are slightly red.
   b. The child has no speech.
   c. The child cannot follow simple age-appropriate commands.
   d. The child turns away when addressed by the nurse.
   e. The child does not make distinct age-appropriate speech sounds.

96. Which of the following is NOT an area of concern when giving parents anticipatory guidance for a two-year-old?
   a. Physical development.
   b. Emotional development.
   c. Sexual development.
   d. Safety issues.

97. A 46-year-old man presents for evaluation of a red rash on both cheeks. This is his third flare-up of the same problem. Some red papules and pustules are visible in the involved areas. On closer inspection, the nurse notices some telangiectasias on his nose and cheeks. There are no comedones present. What is the most likely diagnosis?
   a. Lupus erythematosus.
   b. Acne.
   c. Rosacea.
   d. Seborrheic dermatitis.

98. A patient was diagnosed with right temporomandibular joint dysfunction several months ago. She now presents for evaluation of right ear pain. The most likely etiology of her ear pain is:
   a. eustachian tube dysfunction.
   b. otitis media.
   c. otitis externa.
   d. referred pain.

99. Which of these conditions most commonly predisposes a patient to recurrent bacterial sinusitis?
   a. Immune system deficiency.
   b. Allergic rhinitis.
   c. GERD.
   d. Cigarette smoking.

100. A family nurse practitioner is discussing a treatment plan with an adult patient. The patient is sitting with arms folded across his chest, his legs crossed at the knees, and he is leaning backward. Which type of nonverbal communication is he exhibiting?
   a. Body language.
   b. Gestures.
   c. Facial expressions.
   d. Empathy.

101. A family nurse practitioner is caring for a patient who speaks only Vietnamese. A Vietnamese interpreter is present to help. Which of these statements best describes appropriate behavior when using an interpreter?
   a. Express two to three ideas at a time before pausing for the interpreter to speak to the patient.
   b. Speak clearly and loudly.
   c. Face the interpreter when speaking.
   d. If the patient gives an unusual response to a question, ask the question in a different way.

102. The assistant at the clinic reports the following vital signs to the nurse practitioner. Which of the following vital signs is abnormal?
   a. 11-year-old male – 90 bpm, 22 resp/min, 100/70 mm Hg.
   b. 13-year-old female – 105 bpm, 22 resp/min, 100/70 mm Hg.
   c. 5-year-old male- 102 bpm, 24 resp/min, 90/65 mm Hg.
   d. 6-year-old female- 100 bpm, 26 resp/min, 90/70mm Hg.

103. According to Peplau's framework for psychodynamic nursing, the nurse carries out a number of different nursing roles. Which nursing roles do the following statements exemplify?
   1. "I heard you yelling at other patients and staff members. Let's talk about what you are feeling and explore other ways to express those feelings."
   2. "BiPAP delivers two different levels of pressure while you sleep. This is where we set those pressures. One pressure is for when you breathe in, and the other pressure is for when you breathe out."
   3. "It's important to take your pulse each morning before you take your digoxin. You must not take the medication if your pulse is lower than 60 because the medicine can slow your heart too much."
   4. "The home health agency can monitor your care when you go home, and the Meals on Wheels program can bring in daily meals until you are able to prepare meals yourself."

Match the statements (in numbers) to the appropriate nursing role.
   a. Teacher:
   b. Counselor:
   c. Technical expert:
   d. Resource person:

104. Which of the following is a "red flag" for patient drug-seeking behavior?
   a. The patient claims allergies to multiple classes of non-narcotic pain medications
   b. The patient is using relaxation techniques under medical supervision for relief of pain
   c. The patient has tried acupuncture
   d. The patient becomes upset when not treated with antibiotics for a virus

105. An adult female with a vaginal discharge presents for evaluation. The nurse practitioner orders a KOH prep on the discharge. The laboratory reports the presence of clue cells. The best treatment for this patient is:
    a. doxycycline.
    b. ceftriaxone.
    c. terconazole.
    d. metronidazole.

106. Fifth disease is caused by:
    a. a parvovirus.
    b. an enterovirus.
    c. a paramyxovirus.
    d. an adenovirus.

107. Which one of the following medications is clearly contraindicated during pregnancy?
    a. Amoxicillin.
    b. Ondansetron (Zofran).
    c. Permethrin 5% cream (Elimite).
    d. Isotretinoin (Accutane).

108. The problem-solving process has various components. When identifying a problem, a family nurse practitioner employs the nursing process of:
    a. planning.
    b. assessment.
    c. implementation.
    d. evaluation.

109. If two nurse practitioners have incompatible differences in values and patient care beliefs, which type of conflict exists between them?
    a. Organizational.
    b. Intrapersonal.
    c. Interpersonal.
    d. Psychological.

110. A nurse practitioner is treating a patient with conjunctivitis. Which of the following microorganisms is related to this condition?
    a. *Yersinia pestis.*
    b. *Helicobacter pylori.*
    c. *Vibrio cholera.*
    d. *Haemophilus influenzae* biogroup *aegyptius.*

111. When two or more states recognize licensure by other state boards that have equivalent licensing requirements, this is known as:
    a. temporary license.
    b. licensing by waiver.
    c. licensure by examination.
    d. reciprocity.

112. A nurse practitioner is reviewing a new patient's medication list. The drug pentoxifylline is present on the list. Which of the following conditions given in the patient's history listed below is being treated with this medication?
   a. COPD.
   b. CAD.
   c. PVD.
   d. MS.

113. All of the following are categories of medication errors EXCEPT:
   a. wrong patient.
   b. incorrect dosage.
   c. failure to note patient allergies.
   d. surgical removal of wrong body part.

114. A twenty old male has a tender lump area in his left groin. His abdomen is distended and he has been vomiting for the past 24 hours. Which of the following would the nurse practitioner most likely suspect?
   a. Ulcerative colitis.
   b. Biliary colic.
   c. Acute gastroenteritis.
   d. Strangulated hernia.

115. A process that analyzes, identifies, and treats potential hazards in a specific setting is known as:
   a. risk management.
   b. quality assurance.
   c. standards of care.
   d. patient rights.

116. Which of the following blood therapeutic concentrations is abnormal?
   a. Phenobarbital   10-40 mcg/ml.
   b. Lithium   0.6-1.2 mEq/L.
   c. Digoxin   0.5-1.6 ng/ml.
   d. Valproic acid   40-100 mcg/ml.

117. Which of the following blood therapeutic concentrations is abnormal?
   a. Digitoxin   9-25 mcg/ml.
   b. Vancomycin   5-15 mcg/ml.
   c. Primidone   2-14 mcg/ml.
   d. Theophylline   10-20 mcg/ml.

118. Which of the following blood therapeutic concentrations is abnormal?
   a. Phenytoin   10-20 mcg/ml.
   b. Quinidine   2-6 mcg/ml.
   c. Haloperidol   5-20 ng/ml.
   d. Carbamazepine 5-25 mcg/ml.

119. Five days after a patient hiked through the nearby woods, the patient consulted the family nurse practitioner about a bull's-eye rash (erythema migrans) on the leg. The nurse suspects Lyme disease. Which three additional symptoms are commonly associated with early-stage Lyme disease?
   a. Headache.
   b. Facial palsy.
   c. Myalgia.
   d. Enlarged lymph glands near the rash.
   e. High fever.
   f. Disorientation and confusion.

120. All of the following are true about incident reports EXCEPT:
   a. Incident reports can be useful in improving patient care and in identifying risks.
   b. Incident reports should be completed accurately.
   c. The report form should be copied and placed in the patient record.
   d. The report should be filled out following specific documentation guidelines.

121. A 25-year-old patient is having trouble with recurrent conjunctivitis, having had four episodes in the past year. She wears contact lenses. What type of organisms should be strongly suspected as a cause of eye infections in contact lens wearers?
   a. Gram-negative organisms.
   b. Fungi.
   c. Adenoviruses.
   d. Mixed organisms.

122. The family nurse practitioner is evaluating an eight-month-old child whose mother reports a history of frequent vomiting over the past two months. She has mentioned it to other providers, but she has been told the baby would "outgrow it." In looking over his medical record, the nurse notices the patient has also been seen for recurrent episodes of wheezing. However, he is currently not wheezing, is afebrile, and appears healthy. Which of the following is the most likely cause of the vomiting?
   a. Pyloric stenosis.
   b. Gastroesophageal reflux (GER).
   c. Gastroenteritis.
   d. Reactive airway disease.

123. A 30-year-old woman has a body mass index (BMI) of 28. According to her BMI, the patient is:
   a. normal weight.
   b. overweight.
   c. obese.
   d. extremely obese.

124. The percentage of Americans that are overweight (based on BMI) is closest to:
   a. 20%.
   b. 35%.
   c. 50%.
   d. 65%.

125. A four-year-old child presents with a complaint of rust-colored urine. She has no dysuria and no history of urinary tract infections in the past. She has been healthy except for a recent case of impetigo, which has since resolved. Her mother states that the child's eyes looked "a little puffy" this morning, but look fine now. Which of the following is the most likely diagnosis?

   a. UTI.
   b. Kidney stone.
   c. Poststreptococcal glomerulonephritis.
   d. Nephrotic syndrome.

126. An adult patient with persistent sinusitis has failed treatment with amoxicillin, trimethoprim/sulfa, and amoxicillin clavulanate. Which of the following is the best choice for the next round of treatment?

   a. A first-generation cephalosporin.
   b. Clarithromycin.
   c. A fluoroquinolone.
   d. Erythromycin ethylsuccinate.

127. A 38-year-old man developed lower back pain that started two days after lifting up his four-year-old son. He has limited spinal range of motion, but his neurological exam is normal. The nurse practitioner suspects nerve root irritation from a herniated disk. Which of the following would help corroborate the diagnosis?

   a. An MRI.
   b. Plain lumbosacral radiographs.
   c. Testing range of spinal motion.
   d. Bend-over test.

128. The parent of a 15-year-old girl is concerned that the girl may be involved in substance abuse. Which four of the following signs or symptoms may be indicative of substance abuse?

   a. Abnormal physical changes.
   b. Falling grades and school attendance.
   c. Periods of moodiness.
   d. Repeated unexplained falls and accidents.
   e. Constant use of social media.
   f. Labile mood and behavior.

129. The family nurse practitioner is discussing avoidance of asthma triggers with an adult patient. Which of these offers the best advice?

   a. Vacuum carpets daily to remove allergens.
   b. Use ceiling fans throughout the home instead of air conditioning.
   c. Maintain home humidity levels over 50%.
   d. Encase his mattress and pillows in allergen-blocking covers.

130. Which of these antidepressants is least likely to cause sexual side effects?

   a. Bupropion (Wellbutrin).
   b. Escitalopram (Lexapro).
   c. Amitriptyline (Elavil).
   d. Fluoxetine (Prozac).

131. The family nurse practitioner is assessing the development of a five-month-old child. Which four of the following fine and gross motor abilities does the family nurse practitioner expect to observe?
   a. Exhibits no head lag when pulled to a sitting position.
   b. Uses pincer grasp.
   c. Crawls or creeps.
   d. Turns from abdomen to back.
   e. Uses palmar grasp.
   f. Grasps and manipulates objects such as rattles.

132. A 55-year-old woman has swelling of the proximal interphalangeal joints of the first and second digits of both hands. She also complains of prolonged morning stiffness and often experiences excessive fatigue. What is the most likely diagnosis?
   a. Gout.
   b. Osteoarthritis.
   c. Rheumatoid arthritis.
   d. Psoriatic arthritis.

133. A 64-year-old man presents with acute onset of redness and severe pain in his right eye. He also complains of blurred vision, headache, nausea, and seeing halos around lights. After examining the patient and taking a history, what is the next course of action?
   a. Reassure the patient and prescribe antibiotic eye drops for conjunctivitis.
   b. Apply tetracaine drops to relieve pain.
   c. Perform a fluorescein test to check for a corneal abrasion.
   d. Arrange for immediate referral to an ophthalmologist.

134. A 6-month-old infant has been diagnosed and hospitalized with pertussis. The infant is not in daycare. The only known sick contact is a 12-year-old sibling who has had a cough for 3 weeks. Which of the following represents the best option for chemoprophylaxis in this case?
   a. Treat all household contacts and other close contacts with erythromycin.
   b. Treat only the sibling who has the cough and the sick infant.
   c. Treat all household and other close contacts with either azithromycin or clarithromycin.
   d. If all other close contacts are current on their immunizations, there is no need for prophylaxis.

135. A nine-month-old Caucasian child has been seen in the clinic for frequent respiratory infections and frequent bouts with loose stools. Stool cultures and ova and parasites have been negative. During her routine physical examination, the nurse practitioner discovers that in the past four months her growth parameters have dropped from the 60th percentile to the 10th percentile for weight and from the 75th percentile to the 25th percentile for height. What is the best thing to do next?
   a. Order thyroid function tests.
   b. Order a sweat chloride test.
   c. Admit the child to the hospital to see if she gains weight when fed appropriately.
   d. Evaluate for tuberculosis.

136. A family nurse practitioner is evaluating a newborn infant for a Moro reflex. Of the following, which is the best way to elicit the reflex?
   a. Gently stroke the perioral area with a finger.
   b. Turn the newborn's head to one side, and observe his arm movements.
   c. Apply firm pressure to the palm of the baby's hand.
   d. Clap hands loudly and suddenly.

137. The family nurse practitioner is providing guidance to nurses caring for preschoolers after a bus accident resulted in the hospitalization of six children. Which four of the following nursing management techniques should the family nurse practitioner recommend?

    a. Encourage parents to stay with their children.
    b. Allow the child to make choices when possible.
    c. Explain all procedures to the child.
    d. Encourage the child to discuss fears.
    e. Encourage peer interaction.
    f. Provide a night light.

138. Which of the following is useful as a rescue medication in the treatment of asthma?

    a. Corticosteroid inhaler.
    b. Leukotriene inhibitor.
    c. Anti-allergic medications.
    d. Short-acting beta-2 agonist.

139. Which of the following is most likely to be the first symptom of tuberculosis?

    a. Chest pain.
    b. Cough productive of bloody sputum.
    c. Mild cough with nonbloody mucoid sputum.
    d. Shortness of breath.

140. An 11-month-old baby recently completed a course of oral antibiotics for otitis media. She now presents with a beefy red rash in the diaper area. The rash is surrounded by small satellite lesions and has not responded to diaper rash ointments. What is the best way to manage this rash?

    a. Prescribe topical nystatin cream.
    b. Advise the parents to apply talcum powder at each diaper change.
    c. Prescribe mupirocin ointment.
    d. Prescribe oral fluconazole.

141. The family nurse practitioner is examining a 16-year-old male patient who is active in sports. Which three of the following teaching topics are important as part of injury prevention education?

    a. Protective gear.
    b. Bicycle, skateboard, and automobile safety.
    c. Sexuality.
    d. Drinking and driving.
    e. Social media safeguards.
    f. Study habits.

142. A 10-year-old girl has a two-week history of a mucocele inside her lower lip. There is no pain or bleeding. What is the next course of action?

    a. Manually rupture the lesion and let the contents flow out.
    b. Cauterize the lesion with silver nitrate.
    c. Advise the parents that spontaneous rupture will occur.
    d. Refer immediately to an oral surgeon.

143. Which one of the following is true about primary enuresis in children?

    a. A physical etiology, such as a UTI, is found in about 20% of children.
    b. Bed wetting is more common in boys than girls.
    c. The patient should take imipramine.
    d. It is crucial to perform a renal ultrasound as soon as possible.

144. A four-year-old child presents with a four-day history of cough and nasal congestion. He had a temperature of 100.8 for the initial 24 hours only. Today, his nasal mucus is thicker and yellow. What is the most likely diagnosis?
   a. Allergic rhinitis.
   b. Sinusitis.
   c. Viral upper respiratory infection (URI).
   d. Foreign body in the nose.

145. A 21-year-old asymptomatic woman has a positive purified protein derivative (*PPD*) test result of 13 mm. What is the next step in managing this patient?
   a. Chest x-ray.
   b. Chest x-ray and six to nine months of treatment with isoniazid (INH).
   c. Sputum culture.
   d. Repeat the PPD in three months.

146. Which of the following patients is at increased risk for recurrent otitis media?
   a. A teenager on the school swimming team.
   b. A child with narrow ear canals.
   c. A child with cleft palate.
   d. An infant with blocked tear ducts.

147. All of the following are associated with childhood exposure to cigarette smoke EXCEPT:
   a. colic.
   b. bacterial conjunctivitis.
   c. SIDS.
   d. wheezing.

148. The family nurse practitioner is carrying out an assessment of a two-week-old newborn and observes indications of developmental delay. Which two of the following signs indicate the need for a complete medical and developmental evaluation?
   a. Infant sucks poorly and feeds very slowly.
   b. Respiratory rate at rest is 45 beats per minute.
   c. Limbs are loose and floppy.
   d. Infant exhibits occasional jitteriness.
   e. Infant frequently moves arms and legs.

149. Which of these illnesses is most frequently reported by patients who have recently traveled overseas?
   a. Hepatitis A.
   b. Traveler's diarrhea.
   c. Malaria.
   d. Amoebiasis.

150. Which of the following types of patients is most likely to be interested in using alternative medical therapies?
   a. Patients older than age 65.
   b. Men.
   c. Women.
   d. High school and college students.

151. The parents of a 17-year-old child who was involved in an auto accident have been told that their child died. The parents repeatedly say, "This can't be true!" and appear unable to believe that their child is dead, refusing to allow the child's body to be removed. Which two of the following responses are most therapeutic?

    a. "I'm so sorry for your loss."
    b. "I'm afraid that nothing can bring your child back."
    c. "It is almost unbelievable."
    d. "You must accept that your child has died."
    e. "Take the time you need to be with your child."

152. A two-year old child has viral diarrhea. Several other children in his daycare have the same illness. He is not vomiting and is eating well. His mother asks for treatment recommendations. What should be done next?

    a. Advise his mother to keep the child well hydrated.
    b. Recommend Imodium AD.
    c. Prescribe Levsin.
    d. Tell the mother to stop solid foods for now.

153. A 72-year-old man complains of cramping pain in both calves after walking. The pain disappears after resting. His condition is most likely:

    a. restless legs syndrome.
    b. multiple sclerosis.
    c. intermittent claudication.
    d. normal for his age.

154. Which one of the following about the erythrocyte sedimentation rate (ESR) is true?

    a. It measures the rate red blood cells fall in an upright tube of anticoagulated blood in a 30-minute period.
    b. It is a specific test for inflammation.
    c. It is an acute phase reactant.
    d. The faster the red blood cells fall, the higher the sedimentation rate.

155. A young and inexperienced mother brings in her 6-month-old infant for evaluation of vomiting and diarrhea. Because he has been vomiting his formula, the baby's mother has been giving him nothing but plain water for the past 24 hours. The infant suddenly has a seizure in the clinic. Of the following choices, he is most likely suffering from:

    a. hyponatremia.
    b. sepsis.
    c. idiopathic epilepsy.
    d. carotenemia.

156. A 65-year-old client states that he has received no immunizations since childhood. The client had chickenpox when he was eight years old. Which four immunizations should the family nurse practitioner recommend?

    a. Tetanus, diphtheria, and pertussis (Tdap).
    b. Varicella (chickenpox).
    c. Influenza.
    d. Herpes zoster (shingles).
    e. Pneumococcal vaccine (PCV13 and PPSV23).
    f. Measles, mumps, and rubella (MMR).

157. The Adams forward bend test is used to:
   a. screen for scoliosis.
   b. test for a herniated disk.
   c. assess cerebellar function.
   d. assess for spinal arthritis.

158. Contributory negligence occurs when:
   a. the healthcare provider willfully disregards the safety of the patient.
   b. the healthcare provider fails to provide appropriate standard of care.
   c. the patient contributes to his own negative outcome.
   d. a percentage of negligence is assigned to each party involved.

159. A patient weighs 64 kilograms and is 1.6 meters tall. What is her body mass index (BMI)?
   a. 22.
   b. 25.
   c. 28.
   d. 30.

160. A mother tells her family nurse practitioner that her two-year-old child refuses almost all solid foods. She states, "All he'll take is whole milk." This child is most at risk for:
   a. hemolytic anemia.
   b. developing milk allergy.
   c. gastroesophageal reflux.
   d. iron deficiency anemia.

161. A 79-year-old multiparous woman complains of a pulling sensation in her vagina and bloody spotting on her underwear. She has also started to have some mild urinary incontinence. As the nurse practitioner prepares to examine the area, she notices a rather large ulcerated soft tissue mass at the vaginal introitus. What is the most likely diagnosis?
   a. Urethral prolapse.
   b. Uterine prolapse.
   c. Vaginal neoplasm.
   d. Pelvic hernia.

162. Which of the following is NOT a symptom of retinal detachment?
   a. Eye pain.
   b. Flashes of light.
   c. Floaters.
   d. Loss of central vision.

163. Which of the following hernias is most likely to be acquired?
   a. Indirect inguinal hernia.
   b. Direct inguinal hernia.
   c. Infant umbilical hernia.
   d. Hiatal hernia in a child.

164. An elderly, immobile patient in a nursing home has an area of dark purple, boggy skin that is intact in the sacral area. The skin is still intact. What is the most likely explanation for this condition?
   a. Stage I Pressure Injury.
   b. Stage II Pressure Injury.
   c. Suspected Deep Tissue Injury.
   d. Unstageable Pressure Injury.

165. All of the following are grounds for nursing malpractice EXCEPT:
   a. failure to report a change in a patient's condition.
   b. neglecting to monitor a patient properly.
   c. administering a medication not ordered by the physician.
   d. failure to maintain continuing education requirements.

166. An adolescent complains of acute left ear pain. The ear hurts with manipulation of the external ear. On examination, the ear canal is red, swollen, and very tender. The nurse practitioner also notices flaky debris in the ear canal. Which of the following is the most appropriate treatment?
   a. Antipyrine/benzocaine ear drops (Auralgan).
   b. Combination antibiotic and corticosteroid ear drops.
   c. Ibuprofen and warm compresses to the ear.
   d. Oral antibiotics.

167. A patient is receiving citalopram (Celexa) for depression. Which three of the following adverse effects are commonly associated with citalopram?
   a. Sedation and lethargy.
   b. Orthostatic hypotension.
   c. Agitation, anxiety, and insomnia.
   d. Heart block.
   e. GI distress.
   f. Increased sex drive.

168. The family nurse practitioner is performing a developmental exam on a child. He is able to use a pincer grasp, pull up to stand, and he understands the word "no." His age is closest to:
   a. 4 months.
   b. 5 months.
   c. 6 months.
   d. 9 months.

169. An obviously distressed 14-year-old boy has recently noticed that one of his breasts has grown larger than the other and is also somewhat tender. His mother seems equally concerned. What is the best management course to follow?
   a. Treat for mastitis.
   b. Offer reassurance that this is temporary and benign.
   c. Check testosterone levels.
   d. Refer him to an endocrinologist.

170. Which of the following is the best way to stop a nosebleed?
   a. Apply an ice pack to the forehead.
   b. Apply pressure on the bridge of the nose.
   c. Pinch nostrils shut and apply pressure for 10 continuous minutes.
   d. Have the patient relax and tilt his head back.

171. An 81-year-old woman complains of darkening of the skin right above her ankles, itching, thinning of the skin, and progressive irritation. Her ankles swell intermittently. What is the most likely diagnosis?
   a. Venous stasis dermatitis.
   b. Zinc deficiency.
   c. Atopic dermatitis.
   d. Id reaction.

172. A known asthmatic has a peak flow meter reading that is 78% of his personal best. This measurement is in the:
   a. normal zone.
   b. green zone.
   c. yellow zone.
   d. red zone.

173. In reference to adult CPR, the currently recommended ratio of chest compressions to breaths is:
   a. 15:2.
   b. 10:2.
   c. dependent on the age of the patient.
   d. 30:2.

174. Which of the following is the best prophylactic treatment for traveler's diarrhea in an adult?
   a. Amoxicillin.
   b. Ciprofloxacin.
   c. Trimethoprim/sulfa.
   d. Doxycycline.

175. Which of the following is the treatment of choice for an adult female with gonococcal cervicitis?
   a. Intramuscular penicillin.
   b. Intramuscularly ceftriaxone.
   c. Oral doxycycline.
   d. Oral cefixime.

176. A nurse practitioner is examining a 12-year-old female patient and notes in the chart that her Tanner stage is B-2, Ph-2. This means she has:
   a. breast buds and a light growth of long pubic hair, mainly on the labia.
   b. breast and areola enlargement without a differentiation of the contours and dark, coarse pubic hair connecting over the mons pubis.
   c. no breast enlargement and no pubic hair.
   d. breast enlargement with protrusion of the areola from the breast and thick, coarse pubic hair completely covering the mons pubis.

177. A new mother expresses concern over the tiny white bumps on her newborn's nose and chin. The best explanation for her is:
   a. she can usually remove these by applying some pressure and pinching the bumps.
   b. she will need a referral to Dermatology for further evaluation of this.
   c. there is a special cream the nurse practitioner can prescribe to help resolve this.
   d. this is due to plugged pores in the skin and it will go away on its own.

178. A 52-year-old female was having irregular periods for approximately one year followed by a full year of no bleeding. Which of the following lab results could confirm that she has reached menopause?
   a. High normal levels of estradiol of 350 pg/mL or higher.
   b. FSH levels consistently elevated to 30 mIU/mL or higher.
   c. Elevated progesterone level of 90 ng/mL or higher.
   d. Elevated testosterone level of 80 ng/dL or higher.

179. A 44-year-old male is being seen by the nurse practitioner as a new patient to establish care. His blood pressure reading is 142/92. He is not aware of his blood pressure ever being elevated in the past and he has not had any subjective symptoms of hypertension. The most appropriate action is to:
   a. start him on a low dose of an ACE inhibitor or diuretic and advise him to monitor and record his blood pressure daily.
   b. start him on a low dose of a beta blocker and advise him to monitor and record his blood pressure daily.
   c. provide him with information on how to lower his blood pressure through diet and exercise and advise him to monitor and record his blood pressure daily.
   d. refer him to the ED for treatment of malignant hypertension.

180. Which of the following is NOT a reliable test to check for dehydration in an elderly patient?
   a. Hypotension.
   b. Tenting of skin.
   c. Elevated heart rate.
   d. Dizziness or confusion.

181. A 67-year-old male presents to the clinic with complaints of vision changes causing some yellowish discoloration in his visual field. He has a past medical history of hypertension, coronary artery disease, and congestive heart failure. He is currently taking lisinopril, metoprolol, digoxin, and Plavix. Which of these medications is most likely causing his symptoms?
   a. Plavix.
   b. Metoprolol.
   c. Digoxin.
   d. Lisinopril.

182. Which of the following drugs would be least likely to help with bradykinesia associated with Parkinson's disease?
   a. Amantadine.
   b. Anticholinergics.
   c. Levodopa.
   d. MAOIs.

183. A 3-year-old male is brought to the pediatrician's office for evaluation of sore throat. The nurse practitioner enters the exam room and sees the patient sitting on the exam table leaning forward and drooling. His vital signs are as follows: temperature 102.2, pulse 146, respiratory rate 34, and O2 saturation 91%. The next appropriate step would be to:
   a. let the parents know he most likely has a viral illness and to treat symptomatically.
   b. perform a throat swab to check for strep throat.
   c. give the child some cool water or a popsicle.
   d. have a staff member contact emergency services to arrange transport to the closest ED and gather supplies to assist in maintaining the patient's airway.

184. A nurse practitioner is riding in the elevator with a co-worker at the end of shift, along with a few hospital visitors. The co-worker is complaining about the very demanding family members of one of the patients she cared for today. The most appropriate response is to:
   a. quietly let her know she should not be discussing patient care in a public place.
   b. try to lighten the mood and make her feel better after a hard shift.
   c. tell her about some difficult patients she had during her shift, also.
   d. say nothing, but report the conversation to the Risk Management Department at the hospital.

185. Using the patient-centered medical home model of healthcare delivery, the main person coordinating the patient's care is:
   a. the primary care provider.
   b. the lead nurse within the primary care office.
   c. an assigned social worker.
   d. the patient coordinates their own care.

186. The purpose of quality improvement is to:
   a. improve employee satisfaction.
   b. monitor the leadership skills of the administration of a healthcare facility.
   c. implement specific changes in healthcare which have a measurable improvement for a specific group of patients.
   d. provide specific training and education opportunities to employees to ensure the quality of the care provided is reaching high standards.

187. A nurse practitioner works in the ER at a local children's hospital. At her child's soccer game, another mother asks how the daughter of a mutual friend is doing who was brought into the ER the day before with a broken arm. The most appropriate response is:
   a. the daughter is doing well and will be seeing Orthopedics.
   b. deny having seen the child.
   c. tell her the child was seen, but that her care cannot be discussed with anyone else.
   d. explain to her that you are not able to discuss the care or prognosis of any patients.

188. What is the difference between palliative care and hospice care?
   a. Palliative care can be started at the time of diagnosis during treatment, and hospice care is started when the patient is not going to survive the illness and the end of life is nearing.
   b. Palliative care is for inpatient end of life care, and hospice care is performed in the home.
   c. Palliative care can be provided by a patient's primary care provider, and hospice care is provided by a certified hospice care agency.
   d. Palliative care specializes in only the different forms of therapy that a patient needs, and hospice care specializes in end-of-life comfort care.

189. The fastest growing emerging cultural population in the United States is:
   a. Hispanic.
   b. Asian.
   c. Middle Eastern.
   d. Eastern European.

190. A dressing change is being performed on a patient and his family is present bedside. They are devout, practicing Muslims. Knowing this, it is important to:
   a. keep as much of the patient's skin covered at all times during the dressing change.
   b. try not to talk while touching the patient.
   c. ask everyone to leave the room except for the male head of the family.
   d. explain what is being done to the female head of the family only.

191. A teenage Vietnamese girl is interested in starting oral contraceptive pills, but is concerned that her parents will find out and be disappointed because of their cultural beliefs. This is because:
   a. the Vietnamese culture does not believe in birth control of any kind.
   b. the Vietnamese culture believes that men should be responsible for birth control.
   c. the Vietnamese culture is firmly against premarital sex, and they may ostracize her for this.
   d. the Vietnamese culture believes that OCPs can cause handicapped babies.

192. When communicating with a non-English speaking patient and her family, it is best to:
   a. have another family member interpret if possible.
   b. improvise with using pictures and video to teach.
   c. hold most of the conversation through an online translating program.
   d. arrange to have an interpreter familiar with medical terminology present.

193. When teaching a patient who has a hearing impairment, it is important to:
   a. face them directly so the face and lips are clearly visible to them.
   b. give them educational materials in print to take home and read on their own.
   c. have the patient be the only person receiving educational material so they can feel more involved in their treatment plan.
   d. discuss the treatment plan with the parents so that they can communicate with the patient in the way that best suits her needs.

194. A 10-year-old child with muscular dystrophy has been treated as an inpatient for pneumonia. The discharge plan is being prepared and the nurse practitioner is reviewing the treatments he will need at home. While doing the teaching for the patient and his family, it is important that:
   a. they know that home health and respiratory therapy will be coming in daily for evaluations and nebulizer treatments, so they will not need to worry about how to do these.
   b. the primary focus be on the parents because it is not as important that the child understand his treatment.
   c. give all of the educational material in writing rather than reviewing it in person to save time.
   d. the patient be included to help him maintain some independence in his treatment.

195. A 52-year-old female presents to the clinic with a bad sore throat and low-grade fever. She tests positive for strep pharyngitis. Her past medical history includes hyperlipidemia and a past history of SVT with her last episode being 1 year ago. She is currently taking atorvastatin and atenolol. Which of the following antibiotics would be contraindicated for this patient?
   a. Amoxicillin.
   b. Cefdinir.
   c. Azithromycin.
   d. Penicillin.

196. Which of the following medications is most likely to cause pupil dilation, photophobia, and blurred vision?
   a. Warfarin (Coumadin).
   b. Diphenhydramine (Benadryl).
   c. Oseltamivir (Tamiflu).
   d. Ketorolac (Toradol).

197. A 39-year-old female is started on levothyroxine for hypothyroidism. When should she return for lab work to check the effectiveness of the dosage of her medication?
   a. 6 to 8 weeks.
   b. 4 weeks.
   c. 2 weeks.
   d. 1 week.

198. A 50-year-old female presents to the clinic with complaints of epigastric abdominal pain, right shoulder pain, nausea, vomiting, and decreased appetite. Of the following differential diagnoses, which would be the most like diagnosis?
   a. Peptic ulcer disease.
   b. Pancreatitis.
   c. Acute cholecystitis.
   d. Urinary tract infection.

199. When interpreting pulmonary function test results, the expected FEV1 value for a patient with severe COPD (stage 3) would be:
   a. 0-10% below normal.
   b. 10-15% below normal.
   c. 15-30% below normal.
   d. 30-50% below normal.

200. A 55-year-old male is being seen as a new patient to establish in a family practice. He has no known chronic medical problems and does not take any medications. He tells the nurse practitioner that he was told several years before that he had "borderline diabetes." He has baseline labs checked while in the office and his hemoglobin A1C is 6.2%. This is interpreted as:
   a. a normal blood sugar level.
   b. prediabetes that can be initially treated through lifestyle changes, diet, and exercise.
   c. diabetes that will require oral medication to control.
   d. severe diabetes that will require insulin to control.

Answer Key and Explanations for Test #1

1. C: Only azithromycin has shown effectiveness when taken as a single dose for treatment of chlamydial urethritis. Levofloxacin and doxycycline are also effective treatment choices, but would have to be taken for seven days. Ceftriaxone (Rocephin) is not effective in this case.

2. A, C, and **D**: A patient who has given birth within the previous two to three months and seems disengaged and withdrawn may be exhibiting signs of postpartum depression. Characteristic symptoms include:

- Insomnia or hypersomnia.
- Feeling of worthlessness or inadequacy.
- Poor concentration and ability to make decisions.
- Lack of interest and pleasure.
- Recurrent thoughts of death.
- Lack of energy and constant fatigue.
- Marked change in appetite.
- Consistently sad or depressed mood.

Postpartum psychosis often begins early and is more acute and dangerous and can include disorientation, confusion, hallucinations, and delusions associated with the infant.

3. A: FAS is caused by alcohol consumption during pregnancy. Pregnant women should be counseled against drinking any amount of alcohol because there is no known "safe" amount to drink. Pregnant women should abstain from alcohol during all trimesters. Alcohol has a wide range of permanent effects on children, particularly on the nervous system. Some common characteristics include abnormal facial features (thin upper lip and smooth philtrum), microcephaly, growth deficiency, hyperactivity, learning disabilities, and low IQ.

4. B: Corneal reflex tests are useful to diagnose strabismus (e.g., esotropia). To perform the test, shine a light directly onto both corneas at the same time with the patient looking straight at the light source. In patients with strabismus, the light reflected on the cornea appears off-center in the affected eye. Note that corneal light reflex tests may not detect an intermittent strabismus.

5. B: The five emotional stages of dying are hope, denial, isolation, anger, and bargaining. The hope of a cure (even if slim) persists throughout all the other stages of terminal illness. Isolation and denial help handle the shock of approaching death. After this, the patient experiences anger followed by bargaining.

6. D: Dactylitis (hand-foot syndrome) is often the first manifestation of sickle cell disease in an infant or toddler. Swelling and pain are usually symmetric and result from ischemia of small bones. Bone marrow is expanding and compromising circulation to the bones of the hands and feet. X rays are not helpful in the acute phase, but they eventually show bone destruction and repair. Management includes hydration and pain control. Patients who present with dactylitis before 24 months of age often go on to have a severe course of sickle cell disease.

7. A: Stress incontinence refers to leakage of urine by performance of an activity that puts pressure on the bladder. These activities include laughing, sneezing, lifting something heavy, or coughing. Urge incontinence is present when a patient develops a sudden, strong urge to urinate and begins passing urine before making it to the bathroom. Patients who have functional incontinence have a physical or mental disability that prevents normal urination even though the urinary tract is normal. Examples are Parkinson's disease, dementia, and severe depression.

8. D: Most babies lose several ounces during the first week of life. They usually get back to birth weight and start gaining weight by two weeks of age. Breastfed babies may take a little longer to get back to birth weight. A weight loss of between 5% and 10% in the first week is within normal range.

9. D: Valproic acid (Depakene, Depakote) is an anticonvulsant associated with an elevated risk of neural tube defects, such as spina bifida and meningocele, among others. Phenytoin (Dilantin) affects the developing fetus and may cause such defects as cleft lip, cleft palate, mental deficiency, and hypoplastic fingers and nails. Warfarin (Coumadin), a common anticoagulant, is known to cause nasal deformities, brain abnormalities, and stillbirth. Of the answer choices given for this question, only amoxicillin is not known as a teratogen.

10. The infant is placed on the back for the Ortolani-Barlow maneuver. Steps to the maneuver include:

- a. 1. Grasp the infant's knees with the thumbs over the inner thighs.
- b. 3. Flex the infant's knees and hips to 90 degrees.
- c. 4. Touch the infant's knees together, and then press down on the one femur at a time, observing for dislocation.
- d. 2. Slowly abduct the infant's hips and observe for unequal movement, resistance, or an abnormal "clunk" sound.

11. C: Peritonsillar abscesses are typical in teens. Symptoms include sore throat, fever, and difficulty swallowing and opening the mouth (trismus). In fact, the exam may be difficult due to trismus. The abscess causes bulging of the soft palate in the tonsillar area. Cultures usually grow group A strep and mixed anaerobes. Retropharyngeal abscesses occur most frequently in children under five years of age and are less common in older patients whose retropharyngeal nodes have involuted. Epiglottitis also causes sore throat and fever, but it is accompanied by respiratory distress and typically occurs in younger children.

12. A: Viruses cause over 62% of infectious pharyngitis. The remaining answer choices are bacterial agents. Contrary to what patients often believe, group A strep pharyngitis is significantly less common than viral pharyngitis.

13. B: This patient has tinea capitis. The boggy lesion on the scalp is a kerion, which is often mistaken for an abscess. Itchy, scaly areas on the scalp and scattered areas of hair loss are common, as are swollen occipital lymph nodes. Most cases of tinea capitis in the United States are caused by *Trichophyton tonsurans,* which does not fluoresce on Wood's lamp examination. While impetigo can occur on the scalp, it is not associated with hair loss. All clinical information provided in this clinical scenario points to tinea capitis, making all other choices incorrect.

14. B: Constitutional symptoms such as malaise and headaches are typical with *Mycoplasma* infection. The expected norm for chest x-ray findings is diffuse infiltrates as opposed to a consolidated infiltrate. Myalgias and myositis are more common with viral pneumonia. Hypoxia is also atypical for pneumonia due to *Mycoplasma*.

15. B: Breast bud development (thelarche) starts during Tanner stage II. Stage I represents preadolescent girls who have not yet developed secondary sex characteristics. Stages III and IV are more advanced stages of sexual development. Stage V is the highest level of sexual development and is equivalent to an adult in sexual characteristics.

16. D: NLD is characterized by collagen degeneration, granulomatous reaction, fat deposits, and thickened blood vessel walls. The specific cause is unknown, but several theories hint at peripheral blood vessel disease, vasculitis, or trauma. Erythema nodosum usually also occurs on the pretibial areas, but consists of tender red subcutaneous nodules. Myxedema is a nonpitting edema associated with hypothyroidism. Candida infections most commonly occur in warm, moist skin folds.

17. D: Urinary casts may be composed of red blood cells, white blood cells, or renal cells. To perform a test for casts, the patient provides a midstream clean-catch urine specimen. RBC casts indicate bleeding into the renal tubule, commonly seen in glomerular diseases such as lupus nephritis, IgA nephropathy, and Wegener's granulomatosis. With renal tubular damage, renal tubular epithelial cell casts are present in the urine. Neither UTIs nor interstitial nephritis is associated with RBC casts.

18. B: Diabetes mellitus is diagnosed with an HgA1c of greater than or equal to 6.5%. A single high fasting or nonfasting blood glucose level is not diagnostic of diabetes mellitus, as these elevations must be present on separate occasions. Polydipsia and polyuria are generally present in the context of excessively high blood sugar, but are not diagnostic criteria alone.

19. A: A nurse practitioner can care for nursing home patients as long as a physician is available in case of emergency. There are no age restrictions for a FNP's patient population, nor is there a caseload limit.

20. C, D, and **E**: West Nile infections are classified as viremia, West Nile fever, or West Nile encephalitis/meningitis, depending on the severity of symptoms. West Nile fever is characterized by fever, headache and body aches, nausea and vomiting, eye pain (occasional), swollen lymph glands (occasional), and maculopapular skin rash on the chest, stomach, and back (occasional). West Nile fever affects about 20% of those who become infected, with symptoms lasting from a few days to several weeks.

21. A: None of their children will have sickle cell disease. For this couple, with each pregnancy, there is a 50% probability of having a child with sickle cell trait and a 50% probability of having a child who is homozygous (AA), but a 0% chance that the child will have sickle cell disease.

22. D: The percentage of patients with dementia that are cared for in the home by family members is about 80%.

23. A, B, and **E**: An authoritarian parent is highly controlling and tends to show little warmth. Authoritarian behavior includes:

- Issuing commands and expecting obedience without question.
- Communicating little with the child outside of giving orders.
- Maintaining inflexible rules.
- Permitting little independence on the child's part.

This parenting style results in a child with poor negotiation skills and an inability to initiate independent activities or achieve autonomy. Additionally, the child may become unassertive and withdrawn. During adolescence, girls often become passive and dependent and boys may become rebellious and aggressive.

24. C: It is not a HIPAA violation to communicate with another provider via email. It is permissible by law to release health information to the police, but the practitioner should verify the identity of the police officer. It is acceptable to leave charts outside patient rooms, but care should be done that PHI is not in open view.

25. A: Most people with high blood pressure have primary hypertension, meaning that there is no known cause. Secondary hypertension refers to high blood pressure with a known cause. Cocaine use, renal disease, and oral contraceptive use are all causes of secondary hypertension. Sepsis is associated with hypotension rather than hypertension.

26. D: Tamiflu (oseltamivir) is indicated for the treatment of uncomplicated illness due to influenza. To be effective, it must be started within 48 hours of onset of symptoms. Nausea, vomiting, and diarrhea are all common side effects of Tamiflu. Heart palpitations are not a symptom routinely associated with influenza.

27. A, B, and **D**: The following actions may indicate boundary violations:

- Accepting a $20 tip from a patient. The nurse should not accept personal gifts for professional services.
- Confiding to a patient about a family situation. Personal situations should only be shared very judiciously for therapeutic purposes, such as telling a patient who struggles with quitting cigarettes about a similar successful struggle.
- Exchanging patients in order to care for a favorite patient. It's always a warning sign if a nurse begins to show favoritism or wants to avoid a patient.

28. C: High fever for more than five days, cervical lymphadenopathy, nonexudative pharyngitis, red strawberry tongue, and maculopapular rash are hallmarks of Kawasaki disease. The fact that the illness did not respond to antibiotics and duration of fever makes the diagnosis of strep infection unlikely. This group of symptoms is not characteristic of either toxic epidermal necrolysis or juvenile rheumatoid arthritis.

29. B: A spouse is most likely to perpetrate abuse. The abuse may be either active or passive. Spouses feel most trapped in their situations of being caregivers and feel no hope of escape. A day-shift unrelated caregiver, by contrast, can leave and "decompress" after her shift.

30. C: The risk of suicide is over 60 times greater than normal in people with AIDS. In patients with chronic lung disease, the risk is 10 times greater. Comparatively speaking, diabetes and osteoporosis do not have high suicide rates.

31. B, E, and **F**: Hypokalemia is a risk factor for those with severe nausea and vomiting as well as those on nasogastric suctioning. Symptoms of hypokalemia include muscle weakness, cramps, and hyporeflexia as well as hypotension, lethargy, and fatigue. Although this child has diarrhea, hypokalemia can lead to abdominal distention and constipation. Hypokalemia can eventually impair kidney function and result in polyuria and polydipsia. Electrocardiogram (ECG) changes characteristic of hypokalemia include premature ventricular contractions (PVCs), a prolonged QT interval, depressed ST segment, and flat or inverted T-waves.

32. D: Influenza virus is the most common cause of viral pneumonia in adults. Respiratory syncytial virus may be associated with pneumonia in children. *Haemophilus influenzae* is a bacterium, not a virus.

33. D: This patient has allergic conjunctivitis, which is associated with pruritus. Causes are allergens or environmental agents. Allergic conjunctivitis is not associated with increased intracranial pressure, fever, or myopia.

34. C: Autonomic neuropathy can cause inability to urinate. The autonomic system innervates many organs including the bladder and urinary tract. As the nerves become damaged, in this case due to diabetes, the nerves of the bladder can't respond to pressure normally when the bladder fills.

35. C: Breast cancer causes the most cancer-related deaths in the 25- to 44-year age range. Lung cancer is the overall leading cause in patients of all ages. Hodgkin's disease occurs commonly in the 15- to 34-year age group and over age 60. The incidence of colon cancer peaks between 60 to 75 years of age. It is the second leading cause of cancer death in Western countries.

36. C: Iron-rich foods include leafy green vegetables, beans, egg yolks, fish, and poultry. Oranges are rich in vitamin C. Milk is rich in calcium and is typically not fortified with iron.

37. A: Herpangina is a viral illness caused by Coxsackie virus. Symptoms include fever, fussiness, throat pain, and drooling. In the early stages, vesicles appear on the tonsillar pillars. The vesicles subsequently ulcerate. Strep pharyngitis is uncommon at this age and is not associated with ulcerations. Gingivostomatitis, also viral, is associated with inflamed, bleeding gums, and mucosal ulcers over the anterior oral cavity. Epiglottitis is a severe, life-threatening bacterial infection associated with respiratory distress.

38. C: Norovirus (also called Norwalk-like virus) causes gastroenteritis. RSV, coronavirus, and rhinovirus have all been shown to cause bronchiolitis. Rhinovirus has recently been implicated in severe bronchiolitis illness. Human metapneumovirus is also an etiologic agent. In fact, the list of pathogens is growing.

39. According to Erikson's psychosocial theory, children go through four stages, followed by four additional stages leading through adolescence to old age. Childhood development impacts later adult development. Stages of childhood include the following:

a. Infancy (birth to 1 year): 2. Trust versus mistrust.
b. Early childhood (1 to 3 years): 1. Autonomy versus shame and doubt.
c. Late childhood (3 to 6 years): 4. Initiative versus guilt.
d. School age (6 to 12 years): 3. Industry versus inferiority.

40. C: People can have different concepts of time based on their cultures. Americans have more exacting standards for being on time. Hispanics (and others as well), often have a flexible interpretation of time and are more likely to be more approximate with their timelines. Providers should take cultural differences into account in healthcare settings.

41. A: Pneumovax is recommended for all patients 65 years and over. It can be administered with other vaccines but must be injected using a separate syringe at a different injection site. It should never be injected intradermally.

42. A and C: Preventive health maintenance activities may focus on primary prevention, secondary prevention, and tertiary prevention. Primary prevention occurs before illness or injury and attempts to prevent it. Primary prevention includes administering immunizations and instructing parents about car safety seats. Secondary prevention aims to lessen the severity of an illness through early diagnosis and treatment. Examples of secondary prevention include conducting vision screening and screening adolescents for scoliosis. Tertiary prevention aims to prevent deterioration and maintain optimum function. Tertiary prevention measures would include developing rehabilitation activities for a child.

43. B: About one in three people over age 65 has some form of visual impairment. The number-one cause of loss of vision in this age group is age-related macular degeneration.

44. B: HSP is a type of vasculitis seen mostly in children. Patients with HSP often complain of abdominal pain. GI bleeding may also be present as well as joint pains. Patients should also be monitored for renal involvement by checking for hematuria. Purpura typically occurs on the buttocks and lower legs. Patients with HSP do not have thrombocytopenia, but may in fact have thrombocytosis.

45. D: A high-fiber diet is good advice for patients with GERD. Anticholinergic drugs are to be avoided, as they delay gastric emptying and thus would be counterproductive to the management of GERD. Excessive fat intake also delays gastric emptying, and it increases acid secretion in the stomach. Elevating the head of the bed helps prevent the flow of acid into the lower esophagus during sleep; however, the recommendation for elevation is 6 to 8 inches.

46. B: Bulk-forming laxatives such as psyllium (Metamucil) should be taken with a glass of water or other suitable liquid, immediately followed by a second glass. If not taken with enough fluid, it may cause choking or impaction of psyllium in the gastrointestinal tract. It is not necessary to take it with a calcium supplement.

47. C: The treatment of choice for an uncomplicated tooth abscess is penicillin VK. Erythromycin may also be used if the patient is allergic to penicillin. Extraction of the tooth is not necessary.

48. D: It is important maintain therapeutic communication with patients. Answers A, B, and C are nontherapeutic statements because of their defensive nature. Answer A has a punitive tone, implying a punishment of waiting an extra hour for attention. Answer B implies that the patient's problem is not worth the doctor's time. The correct answer, D, is therapeutic because it does not have a negative tone and it reinforces validation of the patient's feelings.

49. D: Umbilical hernias that are less than 2 cm in diameter will heal on their own. It is normal for an umbilical hernia to pouch out when intra-abdominal pressure increases, such as when the baby crying. This does not cause harm and will not cause enlargement of the abdominal wall defect that is present. Wrapping a band around the abdomen will not heal the hernia.

50. A: Perseveration is a repetitive, involuntary pathologic verbal or motor response to stimuli. It occurs in patients with organic mental disorders such as Alzheimer's disease and other forms of dementia. Repeating the same questions over and over is an example of perseveration. Contrivance refers to development of a clever scheme. By confabulating, a person makes up a plausible story or experience to compensate for memory lapses.

51. D: Symptoms of hypoglycemia include hunger, diaphoresis, light-headedness, tremors, nervousness, irritability, sleepiness, and confusion. Diplopia is not a symptom of low blood sugar.

52. B: Croup, also known as viral laryngotracheobronchitis, is associated with subglottic swelling, URI symptoms, and mild to moderate fever. The parainfluenza virus is a common cause. Routine croup is characterized by normal oxygen saturation and mild, if any, retractions. The hallmark is a barking or seal-like cough. On the other hand, fever of 104.5, tripod position, and drooling are signs of a life-threatening acute airway obstructive bacterial infection known as epiglottitis.

53. A: Breast cancer masses tend to be unilateral, firm, painless and irregular in shape. As the disease progresses, there may be redness and retraction of the nipple or the skin overlying the mass. A rubbery, smooth consistency is characteristic of a fibroadenoma, which is most common in women in their twenties and thirties.

54. A, D, and F: The patient's symptoms are consistent with heat exhaustion. The initial treatment for heat exhaustion is evaporative cooling. Alcohol baths are no longer recommended, and ice immersion is reserved for severe cases of heat stroke. Oral rehydration with 0.1% isotonic NaCl solution is given, usually at the rate of four ounces every 15 to 20 minutes, although IV fluids may be given in severe cases or if oral rehydration does not bring about a positive response. The patient's VS, temperature, and urinary output must be carefully monitored.

55. A: Nursemaid's elbow (radial head subluxation) is common in toddlers, usually 1 to 4 years of age. When taking a history of the mechanism, it usually reveals that a parent suddenly pulled the child up by the arm as he started to fall. When the nursemaid's elbow is successfully reduced, the radial head relocates into its ligament. The clinician can usually feel a "pop" as it goes back into place.

56. B: Most anticoagulant treatment is directed toward a goal international normalized ratio (INR) of 2 to 3. An INR over 3 increases risk of bleeding. Specifically, for DVT, a goal of 2.0 to 3.0 drastically reduces the chances of bleeding when compared to having a higher INR without a reduction in effectiveness.

57. B: Nicotine withdrawal is associated with bradycardia rather than tachycardia. Answers A, C, and D are all symptoms of nicotine withdrawal. Additional symptoms include poor concentration, irritability, depression, restlessness, and weight gain.

58. The order of priority in which the nurse should address the patient's problems, from most critical to least critical, is as follows:

a. 2. Risk of hepatotoxicity: Risks markedly increase when drinking more than three alcoholic beverages daily combined with acetaminophen.
b. 1. Chronic pain: Better methods of pain control should be explored.
c. 4. Risk for imbalanced nutrition: Excessive drinking often interferes with nutrition. This patient may benefit from nutritional counseling.
d. 3. Impaired physical mobility and activity: Physical therapy and better pain control may help to improve mobility.

59. D: The penile foreskin serves a protective function for the glans penis. During the first 12 months of age, nearly all uncircumcised boys will have foreskin that tightly adheres to the glans. By 3 years of age, 90% will retract spontaneously. For some boys, it is normal to achieve retraction by age 5 or 6 years of age. Never forcibly retract the foreskin, as it is painful and may cause infection, phimosis, or paraphimosis.

60. C: Of all the choices given, only Hib (*Haemophilus influenzae*) vaccine is a conjugated vaccine. A conjugated vaccine is made from an altered organism that has been combined with a protein. Conjugation heightens the immune response to the vaccine.

61. C: Rotavirus has long been recognized as a cause of substantial morbidity in pediatric patients from infancy to age five years. An earlier version of the vaccine was taken off the market because of an associated incidence of intussusception, an obstructive condition in which one section of intestine "telescopes" into an adjacent section. Since the introduction of the current vaccine, intussusception rates have not increased beyond the expected range for this age group.

62. D: Antibodies to the killed influenza viruses used to prepare the vaccine form in approximately 2 weeks. The other answer choices are obviously incorrect.

63. B: Physical barriers are impediments that result from inadequate functioning of one or more systems of the body. These include vision, hearing, and mobility. In the case of this patient, his eyesight is impaired and he has limited mobility. Other barriers are psychological (such as emotional instability) and cognitive (such as dementia).

64. C: Frequent pacifier use is not associated with an increased risk of infant tooth decay. Decay may occur when an infant sleeps with a bottle of formula in his mouth and occurs regardless of the number of teeth present. Even babies who are exclusively breastfed can develop dental caries.

65. A: Reliable hearing screening results can be obtained as early as the newborn period.

66. B: Eye contact utilization varies from one culture to another. In some cultures, direct eye contact is considered rude, while in others, it is the desired norm. Observation of eye contact behaviors through experience working with different cultures can help the nurse practitioner appreciate differences in eye contact customs.

67. B: Hypercalcemia can cause polyuria, severe abdominal pain, and confusion. The acronym CRAB is part of the criteria to help diagnose myeloma (calcium elevation, renal insufficiency, anemia, and bone disease). More than 25% of patients with a diagnosis of multiple myeloma will experience hypercalcemia.

68. B: Failure to monitor a patient is an example of medical negligence. Delegating routine tasks to a trained assistant, giving sound medical advice over the telephone, and referring a patient to a specialist are all appropriate actions.

69. A, B, and **E**: During the preschool years (ages three to six), the child should be able to carry out a number of physical skills:

- Uses scissors to cut.
- Draws shapes such as circles and squares.
- Rides tricycle or bicycle with training wheels.
- Ties own shoes.
- Buttons clothes.
- Brushes teeth and washes hands.
- Climbs well with good coordination of arms and legs.
- Learns letters and numbers and may recognize some words and have rudimentary reading skills.

70. B: Nurse practitioner scopes of practice do vary widely from state to state. Contrary to the statements in the answer choices, nurse practitioners may prescribe narcotics in most states and can also perform evaluations of psychosocial status.

71. A: Scabies is caused by the mite *Sarcoptes scabiei.* Mites are in the arachnid family and have eight legs. Insects have six. Ticks and protozoans are not etiologic factors in scabies infestation.

72. B: Rosacea is a chronic dermatosis. Characteristic features include facial redness, papules, and rhinophyma (hyperplasia of nasal tissue). It is commonly found on the cheeks, chin, forehead, and nose. Complications are dry eyes, deep painful facial nodules (pyoderma faciale), folliculitis, and blepharitis.

73. B, C, and **E**: Age-associated changes of the cardiovascular system expected in the older adult include

- Adipose tissue accumulates about the heart.
- Cardiac output decreases.
- The veins become decreasingly elastic.
- The heart's sympathetic nervous response to exertion decreases.
- Mitochondrial DNA in the cardiac muscle is damaged.
- Specialized conduction cells decrease in number.

In a healthy individual, the heart does not increase in size but does so in response to hypertension and heart failure.

74. C: Approximately 30% of patients who have gallstones experience biliary colic, and about 10% will develop acute cholecystitis. Less common (< 1%) complications are gallbladder hydrops, small bowel obstruction, pancreatitis, and gallbladder perforation.

75. D: Because the lesion is localized, topical antifungal treatment is sufficient. In cases where lesions are generalized, oral antifungal therapy is appropriate and more practical. Topical corticosteroids, such as betamethasone, only suppress itching and inflammation. Topical diphenhydramine is not an antifungal medication, but rather an anti-itch product.

76. C: Over two-thirds of Bell's palsy patients recover completely and spontaneously. Approximately 15% have only mild sequelae.

77. A: Key components of overall management of osteoarthritis are nonpharmacological including exercise, physical therapy, thermal therapy, and weight loss if indicated. Joint replacement surgery and arthroscopy may eventually be needed, but not initially. Etanercept (Enbrel) is indicated for treatment of rheumatoid arthritis.

78. D: Hemoglobin A1c is typically measured every three to six months, depending on the desired tightness of glycemic control. Diabetics should also receive retinal exams at least once yearly to screen for retinopathy. In addition, urine should be tested for protein. If protein is negative, a screen for microalbuminuria would also be appropriate. Lipid measurement and control are routine in the management of Type 2 diabetes.

79. C: Basal cell carcinoma accounts for approximately 60% of primary skin cancers, while squamous cell carcinoma comprises 20%. Although most skin cancer deaths are from malignant melanoma, it is relatively rare and accounts for only 1% of skin cancers. Mycosis fungoides is a cutaneous T-cell lymphoma that initially appears in the skin but involves the whole reticuloendothelial system.

80. D: Developmental categories of Denver II are gross motor, fine motor, language, and personal/social. The test evaluates development in children from ages one month to six years.

81. C: Tobacco use in pregnancy is associated with numerous adverse outcomes. Maternal smoking accounts for over 20% of low-birth-weight infants. Other associated problems are placenta previa, preterm birth, placental abruption, and an increased risk of miscarriage.

82. C: Neural tube defects (NTDs) are congenital malformations caused by failure of neural tube closure during embryologic development. The neural tube forms the brain, spinal cord, and other central nervous system tissues. Folic acid protects against development of NTD. According to the Centers for Disease Control, all women who may potentially become pregnant should take folic acid daily.

83. A, B, C, and **F**: Alzheimer's disease is characterized by stages ranging from 1 to 7, with no apparent symptoms at stage 1 and severe cognitive decline and dementia at stage 7. Stage 5, moderate cognitive decline, early dementia, is characterized by

- Needing some assistance with personal hygiene and other activities of daily living.
- Being oriented to self but sometimes being disoriented to place and time.
- Sometimes forgetting names of friends or family.
- Being frustrated at lapses in memory and withdrawing and becoming increasingly self-absorbed.

84. A: Normal breast development may start as early as 8 years of age or as late as age 13 years. The girl in this clinical scenario is not, therefore, developing breasts prematurely and does not need medical evaluation.

85. C: Numerous medications are known to cause the side effect of peripheral edema. Rosiglitazone, an insulin sensitizer, can cause peripheral edema as in this patient. Neither SSRIs (Paxil and others) metformin, nor thiazide diuretics (hydrochlorothiazide) are associated with this side effect.

86. The neurologic exam is conducted following a logical sequence that proceeds from the top down:

a. 3. Mental status: Various instruments may be used, depending on the patient's age and condition.
b. 4. Cranial nerves: Cranial nerves I through XII.
c. 2. Motor system: Includes evaluation of muscles and cerebellar function.
d. 5. Sensory system: Includes assessment of the spinothalamic tract and posterior column tract.
e. 1. Reflexes: Includes assessment of the stretch or deep tendon reflexes and the superficial cutaneous reflexes.

87. C: The majority of experts agree that routine preoperative electrocardiograms should be conducted on all men over age 45, patients with a history of heart disease, and patients with hypertension. Costochondritis is an inflammation of the anterior chest wall and is not associated with an abnormal ECG.

88. C: The patient in this clinical scenario is low risk. The incidence of an abnormal Pap test is low in women who have been screened at 65 years of age. According to the American Cancer Society, the recommendation for stopping is 70 years.

89. B: Of the choices given, only Pneumovax is appropriate. It is recommended for all persons over 65. FluMist is given to healthy patients under age 50. People born before 1957 are considered immune and do not need MMR. Hib vaccine is given to children under 6 years of age.

90. B: Only the 2-year-old may receive prophylaxis with Tamiflu. Oseltamivir (Tamiflu) is generally not recommended in children under 12 months of age.

91. C: Patients appreciate the opportunity to make choices from a list of viable options when they are available. Contrary to what many believe, patients often feel they have not received enough information rather than too much. Leaning toward patients has been shown to improve recall. Patients often do not understand or recall information, making it important to use techniques that help improve patient recall such as moving closer to the patient and increasing eye contact.

92. D: Of the choices given, obesity has a higher prevalence among Native Americans. Other conditions that are more prevalent in Native Americans when compared to other populations are diabetes, alcoholism, and suicide.

93. A: The principle of professional appearance is not one of the fundamental principles of professionalism. The true principles are as follows: primacy of patient welfare (serving the interest of the patient and not doing harm), patient autonomy (empowering patients to make informed treatment decisions), and social justice (eliminating discrimination in healthcare).

94. C: Disclosing this information would be a violation of patient confidentiality. The desire not to disclose protected information is the patient's prerogative, even if his wife asks for disclosure.

95. B, C, and **E**: Indications of possible hearing impairment in a two-year-old child include the following:

- The child has no speech. Although language acquisition varies, at two years old, a child should say some words, such as "No."
- The child cannot follow simple age-appropriate commands, such as "Show me your toy." Children's comprehension usually precedes language production.
- The child does not make distinct age-appropriate speech sounds. Children should make a wide range of sounds even before they begin speaking in words.

96. C: Family nurse practitioners often give anticipatory guidance to children and parents. Because children move from one developmental phase to another, parents need guidance on what to expect in certain areas of concern. Common areas for discussion for two-year-olds are growth and development, nutrition, emotional development, and safety. As children grow older, sports, exercise, sexual development, and warnings about drug abuse become important.

97. C: Rosacea is a chronic skin problem that is common in middle age. Most people with rosacea develop a cyclic pattern of disease. It may be confused with acne, but unlike acne, patients with rosacea do not develop comedones. Telangiectasia is common on the cheeks and nose with rosacea. The classic lupus malar rash is butterfly shaped and involves the cheeks and bridge of the nose. Seborrheic dermatitis appears on the face, upper chest, and any other areas of oily skin. There are often flaky, greasy white, or yellow scales present.

98. D: Temporomandibular dysfunction is a common cause of referred ear pain, making the other choices unlikely.

99. B: All of the choices given predispose patients to recurrent sinus infections. However, allergic rhinitis is the most common one of those listed. Allergic rhinitis is seen in approximately 60% of patients with recurrent sinusitis.

100. A: This patient is exhibiting body language that poses a barrier to communication with the provider by him appearing disinterested. Gestures are performed with hands or with the head as in nodding in agreement or waving hands to mimic an activity. Facial expressions show emotions such as happiness or fear. Empathy is not a type of nonverbal communication.

101. D: It is sometimes necessary to use an interpreter in a clinical setting. The interpreter should be medically trained. The provider should address the patient directly, as if the interpreter was not there. Use a normal voice volume and try to employ simple language, expressing one concept at a time. Place chairs in a triangular configuration and face the patient while speaking.

102. B: HR and Respirations are slightly increased. BP is decreased from normal for this age range. Normal pedi heart rate: 1-3 yrs: 70-110; 3-6 yrs: 65-110; 6-12 yrs: 60-95; >12 yrs: 55-85. Normal pedi respiratory rate: 1-3 yrs: 20-30; 3-6 yrs: 20-25; 6-12 yrs:14-22; >12 yrs: 12-18.

103. According to Peplau's framework for psychodynamic nursing, the nurse carries out a number of different nursing roles:

a. Teacher: 3. "It's important to take your pulse each morning before you take your digoxin. You must not take the medication if your pulse is lower than 60 because the medicine can slow your heart too much."
b. Counselor: 1. "I heard you yelling at other patients and staff members. Let's talk about what you are feeling and explore other ways to express those feelings."
c. Technical expert: 2. "BiPAP delivers two different levels of pressure while you sleep. This is where we set those pressures. One pressure is for when you breathe in, and the other pressure is for when you breathe out."
d. Resource person: 4. "The home health agency can monitor your care when you go home, and the Meals on Wheels program can bring in daily meals until you are able to prepare meals yourself."

104. A: Drug-seeking patients often claim "allergies" to various pain medications and claim that only one specific narcotic works for their pain. In addition, drug seekers usually hop from one doctor to another to get the drugs they want. The term "drug seeker" applies to a person who is trying to obtain narcotics. The term is not usually used to refer to patients who want antibiotics.

105. D: This patient has bacterial vaginosis. A KOH prep characteristically reveals a fishy odor and clue cells. The treatment is metronidazole. Doxycycline is used to treat Chlamydia. Terconazole is used to treat vaginal candidiasis and ceftriaxone is used to treat gonococcal infections.

106. A: Fifth disease is primarily a disease of children. It produces the so-called slapped cheek rash and is caused by parvovirus B19. The other answer choices are incorrect.

107. D: Accutane (an acne drug) is a known teratogen that belongs to pregnancy category X. In fact, it is best not taken by women of childbearing age unless acne is extremely severe and unresponsive to other therapies. It is associated with a high potential for fetal injury. Healthcare providers perform a pregnancy test on the patient before starting Accutane and will likely continue doing pregnancy tests monthly prior to prescription renewal.

108. B: By identifying a problem, the nurse practitioner is employing the process of assessment. Planning involves the process of determining an action plan. Implementation carries out the plan, and evaluation involves examining and appraising the plan of action.

109. C: Interpersonal conflict exists between one person and another, whereas intrapersonal conflict is an internal conflict involving only one person.

110. D: *Haemophilus influenzae* biogroup *aegyptius* is related to conjunctivitis. *Yersinia pestis* is linked to Plague, *Helicobacter pylori* is linked to peptic ulcers, and *Vibrio cholera* is linked to Cholera.

111. D: Licensure by examination is required when a state does not grant licensure by reciprocity and a candidate must pass an examination in that state. A temporary license allows a nurse to practice while the license is pending. Licensure by waiver occurs if the candidate meets or exceeds some licensure requirements. These requirements can be waived, but the nurse must be able to demonstrate other requirements.

112. C: Pentoxifylline is a hemorheological agent that helps blood viscosity. This drug is used for symptomatic PVD. It is contraindicated in patients with a sensitivity to caffeine or theophylline.

113. D: While surgically removing the wrong body part is an egregious error, it does not involve a medication-related error.

114. D: A hernia is the most likely indicated in this case. The tender lump in the groin cannot be explained by any of the other diagnoses listed. Moderate or more pain in a hernia is not normal and should make the case to consider strangulation in conjunction with the other symptoms. The patient may be febrile, have nausea/vomiting, and systemic symptoms of sepsis.

115. A: This process is known as risk management. Quality assurance is an evaluation of medical services, their results, and how they compare to the accepted standards. Patient rights are a form of nursing intervention involving healthcare rights.

116. C: The normal range for Digoxin is 0.7-1.4 ng/ml.

117. C: The normal range for Primidone is 4-12 mcg/ml.

118. D: The normal range for Carbamazepine is 10-20 mcg/ml.

119. A, C, and D: Other symptoms that are typical of early-stage Lyme disease include headache, myalgia, and enlarged lymph glands near the rash. Typically, the first erythema migrans is at the site of the tick bite. As the disease progresses, multiple rash sites may appear as well as more pronounced signs of infection, such as fever and facial palsy. Arthritic and neurological symptoms may occur as the disease disseminates.

120. C: Answer choices A, B, and D are all correct. The incident report form should not be copied nor placed in the patient's record.

121. A: The nurse practitioner should strongly suspect gram-negative organisms as the cause of conjunctivitis in contact lens wearers. Topical gentamicin or tobramycin would therefore be a good choice for treatment. In people who do not wear contact lenses, bacterial conjunctivitis is most commonly caused by either *Staphylococcus aureus* or *Streptococcus pneumoniae*.

122. B: GER is a common cause of vomiting in infants. It may also be associated with episodes of recurrent wheezing. This patient is too old to be presenting with pyloric stenosis, which typically manifests itself with recurrent vomiting within three to five weeks after birth and is rare in babies over three months of age. Viral gastroenteritis is self-limited and does not last two months. Reactive airway disease is associated with wheezing but not with vomiting.

123. B: To determine BMI, divide the patient's weight in kilograms by their height in meters squared. A BMI greater than 25 is overweight. If the BMI is more than 30, the patient is considered obese. Morbidly obese patients have BMIs over 35.

124. D: An estimated 65% of Americans are overweight and about 35% are obese.

125. C: The patient in this clinical scenario has post-streptococcal glomerulonephritis (PSGN). The source of the strep infection was the impetigo. Children often present with periorbital edema because of a loss of protein in the urine. A diagnosis of UTI is not likely, given the symptoms of painless hematuria and edema. Painless hematuria requires investigation. Kidney stones are associated with intermittent severe colicky pain.

126. C: A fluoroquinolone such as levofloxacin is a good choice of antibiotic considering there was treatment failure with first-line drugs. First-generation cephalosporins and erythromycin are not recommended because they do not provide adequate coverage of major pathogens. In addition, clarithromycin may not provide coverage for resistant *Streptococcus pneumoniae*.

127. A: Of the choices given, an MRI is the best choice. A herniated disk will not show up on a plain radiograph. Bend-over tests screen for scoliosis. Loss of range of motion is nonspecific.

128. A, B, D, and **F:** Periods of moodiness and constant use of social media are fairly typical behavior associated with adolescents. However, signs or symptoms that may be indicative of substance abuse include abnormal physical changes (dental problems, skin color, rash, hair loss, and nasal discharge), falling grades and school attendance because of lack of motivation and inability to concentrate, repeated unexplained falls and accidents (including burns), and labile mood and behavior. The adolescent may have difficulty setting goals, act irresponsibly, and may feel hopeless and depressed. Appetite and sleep habits may change.

129. D: Placing allergen-blocking covers on the mattress and pillows are a good way to decrease asthma triggers. Frequent vacuuming and use of ceiling fans actually help spread allergen particles into the air. Home humidity levels should ideally be less than 50%.

130. A: Tricyclic antidepressants such as amitriptyline and SSRIs such as citalopram are often associated with sexual dysfunction. Of the choices given, bupropion is least likely to cause sexual side effects.

131. A, D, E, and **F:** Fine and gross motor abilities that are typical of a five-month-old child include

- Exhibits no head lag when pulled to a sitting position.
- Turns from abdomen to back and then from back to abdomen by six months.
- Uses a palmar rather than a pincer grasp. Able to pick up items.
- Grasps and manipulates objects such as rattles.
- Mouths objects, including pulling feet to mouth.
- Supports much of own weight if held in a standing position.

132. C: This patient is showing signs and symptoms of rheumatoid arthritis: proximal interphalangeal joint involvement of the hands, symmetrical swelling, fatigue, and prolonged morning stiffness. Symptoms of osteoarthritis usually develop gradually. Joints of the hips, back, base of the thumb and neck are often affected in osteoarthritis. Psoriatic arthritis occurs in patients who have psoriasis. In this type of arthritis, joints are less symmetrically involved. Gout most often involves the joints of the feet.

133. D: The patient in this scenario has symptoms of acute glaucoma. This is a medical emergency. The only correct answer is to refer the patient immediately to an ophthalmologist.

134. C: All household and close contacts should be treated with azithromycin or clarithromycin, which each have fewer side effects and are associated with better patient compliance with once-daily dosing. The medication is taken by close contacts and household members regardless of immunization status. This helps limit the transmission of infection to others.

135. B: This clinical scenario raises strong suspicion for cystic fibrosis. CF is more common in Caucasians and is associated with frequent respiratory infections and digestive problems such as diarrhea and greasy stools (high fat content). These finding are not characteristic of either thyroid disorders or tuberculosis. Performing a sweat chloride test will aid in the diagnosis of CF.

136. D: A newborn infant exhibits the Moro reflex in response to a loud noise such as a hand clap. This reflex is also known as the startle reflex. Stimulation of the perioral area elicits the rooting reflex. The tonic neck reflex occurs when the newborn's head is turned to one side and he assumes a "fencing posture."

137. A, B, C, and F: The family nurse practitioner should recommend the following nursing management techniques for nurses caring for preschoolers:

- Encourage parents to stay with children: Children often have separation anxiety and fear of abandonment.
- Allow the child to make choices when possible: Children may feel totally out of control and fearful.
- Explain all procedures to the child in age-appropriate terms: Children often have a poor understanding of medical procedures and may fear that tubes are permanent or that they will lose body parts.
- Provide a night light: Children often fear the dark or monsters, especially in a strange environment.

138. D: A short-acting beta-2 agonist, such as albuterol or levalbuterol, is appropriate for use as a rescue medication. Corticosteroid inhalers, leukotriene inhibitors, and anti-allergic medications are useful for long-term control.

139. C: An initial symptom of tuberculosis is a mild cough productive of nonbloody mucoid sputum. Bloody sputum production, chest pain, and breathing difficulty are all late symptoms.

140. A: The infant has a candida diaper rash, which is usually treated with nystatin cream. The use of talcum powder is no longer recommended due to the risk of aspiration of particles by the infant and because it was not shown to be effective in decreasing moisture in the diaper area. Oral fluconazole is not first-line treatment for cutaneous candidiasis. Mupirocin is useful in the treatment of localized bacterial skin infections.

141. A, B, and D: Although all of these topics are important, those that are specific to injury prevention education for a 16-year-old patient include:

- Protective gear.
- Bicycle, skateboard, and automobile safety.
- Drinking and driving.

Some injury prevention topics may be specific to the adolescent's environment. For example, farm safety measures should be covered for an adolescent living in a rural area but are not generally necessary for adolescents in urban areas. Other topics that should be covered for adolescents include sleep, school performance, peer interactions, discipline, and future planning.

142. C: Mucoceles are usually caused by trauma to the inner lining of the lip. They rupture easily and spontaneously. Most patients with mucoceles are under the age of 20. Unroofing or aspirating the lesion is associated with recurrences. If the patient has frequent recurrences, refer them to an oral surgeon.

143. B: Enuresis is more common in boys than girls. UTI is not a common cause of nocturnal enuresis. A renal ultrasound is usually not necessary. Imipramine has a success rate of less than 50%.

144. C: This child most likely has a viral URI. Allergic rhinitis and nasal foreign bodies are not associated with fever. In addition, nasal foreign bodies cause unilateral nasal discharge. The yellow color of the mucus is not significant. Symptoms of four days' duration are highly unlikely to be caused by sinusitis, which is uncommon at this age anyway.

145. B: A chest x-ray is recommended for asymptomatic patients with a positive PPD to rule out the slight possibility of an active TB infection. Treatment with INH decreases the progression of latent TB to active TB infection. Nine months is the optimal duration of treatment. A sputum culture is done if there are findings of old TB on chest x-ray.

146. C: Children with a cleft palate are at increased risk for recurrent otitis media. Children with clefts are more likely to develop fluid behind the tympanic membrane. Usually the fluid drains through the Eustachian tube, but the tube is often distorted by the cleft and interferes with proper drainage. During surgical repair of the cleft, surgeons usually insert ventilator tubes in the eardrum to allow fluid to drain.

147. B: Colic, sudden infant death syndrome (SIDS), and wheezing are all associated with cigarette smoke exposure. Bacterial conjunctivitis is not associated with exposure to smoking.

148. A and C: Indications of developmental delay should trigger a complete medical and developmental evaluation to determine the cause. Indications include

- Infant sucks poorly and feeds very slowly.
- Limbs are loose and floppy.
- Eyes don't blink in response to bright light and do not follow a nearby object moving from one side to the other.
- Movement of arms and legs is restricted or stiff.
- Lower jaw constantly trembles.
- Child does not respond to loud sounds.

149. B: About 50% of people who travel abroad become ill while traveling. The most common illness is traveler's diarrhea. The other illnesses listed as answer choices are less frequent.

150. C: Of all the choices given, women are most likely to be interested in using alternative medicine therapies.

151. A and E: Denial is not uncommon, especially with the unexpected death of a child. The most therapeutic responses are "I'm so sorry for your loss" and "Take the time you need to be with your child." Although the family nurse practitioner should not reinforce the denial, the nurse should also avoid arguing or forcing the parents to acknowledge the death until they are ready. Parents may need some quiet time with the deceased to come to terms with their feelings and to accept that their child has died.

152. A: The mainstay of treatment for viral diarrhea in children is to maintain adequate hydration. If the child with diarrhea is not vomiting, there is no need to stop feeding solid foods. Antidiarrheal and antispasmodic medications are not recommended for children.

153. C: Intermittent claudication is an aching, cramping, or burning in the legs due to poor circulation in the arteries. It often occurs with walking and disappears with rest. It is not normal and can be due to atherosclerosis or vasospasm. Restless legs syndrome is a neurologic disorder associated with an unpleasant sensation in the legs and with a compulsion to move the legs. Multiple sclerosis is also a neurologic disorder.

154. C: The ESR is an acute phase reactant. An elevated ESR is indicative of inflammation, but it is not specific for any disorder. In performing the test, red blood cells are allowed to settle in a tube of unclotted blood. At the end of one hour, the distance the cells have fallen is measured. Inflammation produces a change in blood proteins, causing red blood cells to aggregate and become heavier than normal and therefore take longer to form sediment at the bottom of the tube.

155. A: As in this case, an infant given free water is at risk for developing hyponatremia. Low levels of sodium are associated with seizures. Infants who need hydration should be given an oral electrolyte solution or intravenous fluids rather than plain water.

156. A, C, D, and E: A 65-year-old client who states that he has received no immunizations since childhood and had chickenpox as a child should receive the following immunizations:

- Tdap: The Tdap immunization one time and then Td boosters every 10 years.
- Influenza: The flu immunization every year before flu season.

- Herpes zoster: The shingles immunization one time.
- Pneumococcal: A series of two different injections.

Depending on risk factors, some adults may receive recommendations to receive the hepatitis A and B immunizations as well.

157. A: The Adams forward bend test is used to screen for scoliosis. The test is performed by asking the patient to bend forward 90 degrees at the waist, as if to touch his toes. The examiner looks for asymmetry of the trunk (an asymmetric thoracic prominence on one side). The test has its limitations in that it cannot detect the exact severity of scoliosis, nor can it detect lower spine curvatures.

158. C: Contributory negligence occurs when the patient contributes to his own negative outcome.

159. B: To calculate BMI, divide the weight in kilograms by the height in meters squared. In this example, BMI = 64 divided by (1.6 x 1.6) = 64/2.54 = 25.

160. D: A child subsisting on a diet of mostly whole milk is at risk for developing iron deficiency anemia. Whole milk is not iron fortified. Because he is not eating any solid foods, there are no other sources of iron in his diet.

161. B: The patient in this clinical scenario has a prolapsed uterus. The uterus is the only organ that can fall into the vagina. Depending on duration and severity, the uterus can become ulcerated and result in bleeding. This is often the result of child bearing and weakening of the pelvic tissues as a woman ages. It is common for urinary incontinence to exist in these cases.

162. A: Retinal detachment is typically not associated with eye pain. The patient complains of seeing floaters, flashes of light, and loss of the central portion of vision.

163. B: Direct inguinal hernias are generally acquired due to heavy lifting, straining, or coughing. Indirect inguinal hernias, hiatal hernias in children, and umbilical hernias in infants are congenital.

164. C: The National Pressure Injury Advisory Panel developed a staging system to ensure that definitions for pressure injuries were standardized. Stage I: Nonblanchable erythema: Intact, reddened area that does not blanch. Area remains intact but the physical appearance is altered. Stage II: Partial thickness: Destruction of the epidermis and/or dermis. This type of injury may be an intact blister, ruptured blister, or an open ulcer if it has a pinkish or a reddish wound bed. Stage III: Full thickness skin loss. Muscle, tendons, and bones have not been injured. Stage IV: Full thickness tissue loss: Damage has progressed to bone, muscle, or tendons. Unstageable/Unclassified Injury is present and involves full thickness, but cannot be staged until slough is removed. Suspected Deep Tissue Injury Discolored skin that is still intact but has been damaged. Area may feel boggy and appear deeper than stage I.

165. D: A nurse can be sued for malpractice for various reasons including failure to report a change in a patient's condition, failure to answer calls from a patient, neglecting to monitor a patient, administering the wrong medication, and administering a treatment not ordered by the physician. All nurses should maintain continuing education requirements, but failing to do so is not grounds for a malpractice suit.

166. B: This patient has otitis externa. Topical treatment with combination antibiotic and corticosteroid drops has been shown to be very effective. Because the inflammation is localized, systemic antibiotics are rarely indicated. Antipyrine/benzocaine drops are ineffective. Ibuprofen may help with pain, but by itself, it is not the best answer.

167. A, C, and E: Citalopram (Celexa) is a selective serotonin reuptake inhibitor (SSRI) that is used to treat depression. Common adverse effects include:

- Sedation and lethargy.
- Agitation, anxiety, and insomnia.
- GI distress: nausea, dry mouth, diarrhea, constipation, and anorexia.
- Vision disturbances: blurring, tunnel vision, dry eyes, and pain.
- Decreased sex drive, impotence, and erectile dysfunction.

Citalopram may cause suicidal ideation, especially in those younger than 18, and its use may result in a life-threatening interaction if taken with a monoamine oxidase (MAO) inhibitor. Citalopram is in Food and Drug Administration (FDA) pregnancy category C and can pass into breast milk.

168. D: The developmental milestones are closest to those of a 9-month-old. Infants that are 8 to 10 months old are able to use a pincer grasp, pull up to stand, and walk holding onto furniture, and recognize the word "no."

169. B: Breast development in adolescent boys can be very distressing. These patients are often teased at school. However, it is a temporary and benign condition due to hormonal imbalances of estrogen and testosterone during puberty. It affects 40 to 60% of male teens. No treatment, workups, or referrals are needed.

170. C: Routine nosebleeds often originate from Kiesselbach's plexus over the anterior nasal septum. To stop a nosebleed, pinch the nostrils shut and apply continuous pressure for 10 minutes. Applying pressure to the nasal bridge, tilting the head back, and applying ice packs to the forehead are common mistakes people make when treating nosebleeds.

171. A: Venous stasis dermatitis is an inflammatory skin disease that occurs in the lower extremities of middle-aged and elderly patients. It is caused by venous insufficiency that occurs when venous valves become incompetent.

172. C: Peak flow is a useful measure of asthma control. Peak flow meters measure the air flow out of the lungs as a patient blows forcefully into the device. Measurements between 80 to 100% of personal best are in the green zone, indicating good control. Measurements at 50 to 79% are in the yellow zone, a caution indicating some loss of asthma control. Adjustments may need to be made with medications. The red zone is a reading less than 50% of personal best and indicates a need for immediate medical attention.

173. D: The recommended ratio of chest compressions to breaths in adult CPR is 30:2. The same ratio applies to children.

174. B: Ciprofloxacin may be used safely and effectively for prophylaxis of traveler's diarrhea. Increased resistance has limited the effectiveness of trimethoprim-sulfa and doxycycline.

175. B: The treatment of choice for gonococcal cervicitis is intramuscular ceftriaxone in combination with oral azithromycin. Oral cefixime may be substituted if ceftriaxone is not available.

176. A: The Tanner stages are used to classify the physical symptoms of male and female adolescents as they progress through puberty. In females, the breasts and distribution of pubic hair are assessed, while in males the distribution of pubic hair and genital development are assessed. In females, the classifications range from B-1 when there is no breast development up to B-5 when the breasts have completed full development. Pubic hair is assessed on a scale of Ph-1 when there is none present up to Ph-5 when there is an inverse triangle of hair present that extends to the medial thighs.

177. D: Milia are very common and occur when flakes of skin become trapped within pores. It is most common in newborns and occurs most often on the nose and chin. It is important to not pick or pinch these lesions because this could damage the tissue or lead to a skin infection. The lesions usually resolve on their own within a few weeks.

178. B: When a woman has gone a full year without any menstrual bleeding and her FSH levels are consistently elevated at 30 mIU/mL or higher, she is considered to have reached menopause. Estrogen and progesterone levels will be low in a woman who has reached menopause. A normal testosterone level for a woman is 15-70 ng/dL. A thorough history should also be taken to identify other symptoms of menopause, such as hot flashes, sleep disturbances, vaginal dryness, and mood changes.

179. C: Hypertension is diagnosed after 3 readings of a blood pressure higher than 140/90. The most appropriate action in this case is to provide the patient with information about his blood pressure and the conservative measures he can take at home to help lower it without the use of medications. This includes watching his diet to decrease sodium intake, increase his activity level to include a regular exercise program, and monitor and record his blood pressure daily. This blood pressure log should be brought to his next appointment to review the readings and then determine whether he needs to start on an anti-hypertensive medication.

180. B: Skin will tent when pinched due to dehydration, but in the elderly patient this can also occur because of decreased elasticity of the skin. As the skin ages, the elastic connective tissue underneath loses its ability return to normal after it is pinched. It can take up to 30 seconds for elderly skin to return to its normal appearance even in a well-hydrated patient. The other choices listed are more reliable at identifying dehydration in the elderly patient than assessing skin turgor.

181. C: One of the earliest signs of digoxin toxicity is a yellowish discoloration in vision, especially while looking at light. This is called xanthopsia. A digoxin level should be checked regularly in patients who are taking this medication. The normal range is 0.5-2 ng/mL.

182. B: Anticholinergic drugs can help with some of the rigidity seen with Parkinson's, but they do little to help with the bradykinesia. The side effects seen with this class of drugs can be more severe in elderly populations. The other medications listed are helpful with all of the symptoms of Parkinson's disease.

183. D: The symptoms described are consistent with epiglottitis, a medical emergency. Airway compromise is the biggest risk with this illness. Epiglottitis is treated in the hospital and usually requires intubation to maintain the airway.

184. A: It is important to be aware of the conversations co-workers are having, especially in a public place. HIPAA regulations prohibit conversations in a public space regarding a patient. It would be appropriate to subtly remind co-workers of this if it occurs.

185. A: The patient-centered medical home model utilizes the primary care provider as the main person coordinating all care for the patient. This way, specific specialties or other medical care that is needed can be delegated by one person.

186. C: Quality improvement is instrumental in improving the way healthcare services are provided, while continually measuring the effect those changes have on the health status of the patients served. This is often measured through patient satisfaction information.

187. D: HIPAA regulations state that the care of a patient cannot be discussed to anyone without appropriate permission. This includes confirming or denying that the patient was seen at a specific healthcare facility. Most people understand this once it is explained to them.

188. A: Palliative care is often utilized to offer a patient the extra care of therapy they need when faced with a chronic illness. Some palliative care patients will "graduate" from this and others may need to transition to hospice care as their chronic disease progresses.

189. B: The Asian population has been the fastest growing in the United States since 2000. There are approximately 21 million people of Asian descent living in the U.S. today.

190. B: It is respectful to not speak while touching a person who practices the Muslim faith. Any explanations of what is being done, such as a dressing change, should be communicated before the procedure is performed and this should be explained to the patient and family.

191. D: In the Vietnamese culture, there are specific feelings regarding birth control. Oral contraceptive pills are thought of as a "hot" medication that may cause a newborn baby to be handicapped. They also believe the IUD can cause cancer and personality changes. Termination of a pregnancy is considered very dangerous because the spirit of the fetus may stay with the family to cause them problems.

192. D: Whenever possible, have an interpreter present in these types of situations who has undergone some training in medical terminology. Using a family member is not ensuring that any medical training or terms will be correctly translated. Online software may not be accurate and there is no way to verify that the terms and concepts are being interpreted appropriately.

193. A: Having a patient with a hearing impairment offers the opportunity to utilize different forms of teaching. Some of these patients may have some degree of hearing acuity left, but most have learned to adapt and read lips. It is important to be aware of any distracting background noises and to face the patient directly so that the face and mouth are clearly visible. Remember not to turn away when talking or cover the mouth with the hand as that will make it difficult for the patient.

194. D: Education should be done with the patient and the family. The patient should try to maintain as much independence as possible and be informed as to what treatments will need to be continued at home. Including the patient in the teaching process can also increase compliance to the treatment plan.

195. C: Azithromycin is very effective at treating Group A strep pharyngitis; however, it has been linked to an increased risk of cardiac dysrhythmias. This would make azithromycin contraindicated for this particular patient with a history of SVT. Azithromycin, and other macrolide antibiotics, increase the risk of developing QT prolongation. There have also been reported cases of torsades de pointes and ventricular dysrhythmias while taking azithromycin.

196. B: Benadryl can cause anticholinergic side effects, such as pupil dilation, photophobia, and blurred vision. This is most likely due to relaxation of the ciliary muscle and the decrease in accommodation of the eyes. Other medications that commonly cause anticholinergic side effects include antipsychotics, medications used to treat the symptoms of Parkinson's disease, and antispasmodics.

197. A: It usually takes approximately 6 to 8 weeks for the TSH to show changes in levels following when medication is started or after adjusting the dosage of medication. The TSH still remains the most reliable lab test for diagnosing or monitoring thyroid disease. If labs need to be performed before 6 to 8 weeks, the free T_4 and total T_3 levels can be checked. This should still be followed up with a check of the TSH at the appropriate time, though.

198. C: Abdominal pain with nausea and vomiting can occur with any of these choices. Only acute cholecystitis, however, also presents with right shoulder pain. This is called referred pain. Right shoulder pain occurs with gallbladder disease because of its proximity to the phrenic nerve. The phrenic nerve runs down each side of the next to the diaphragm in the upper abdomen. The gallbladder is close to this and can cause nerve impulses, such as pain, to pass through the phrenic nerve and refer pain to the right shoulder, or between the shoulders.

199. D: The FEV1 value that is associated with severe, or stage 3, COPD is 30-50% below normal. The FEV1 is the forced expiratory volume which measures the amount of air a person can forcibly exhale in 1 second. The worse the degree of COPD, the lower the FEV1 will be. This is also helpful to monitor in order to track the progression of COPD and the rate at which the disease has worsened.

200. B: Prediabetes is diagnosed when the hemoglobin A1C is between 5.7% and 6.4%. It is usually managed with lifestyle changes to include diet and exercise. A hemoglobin A1C less than 5.7% is normal, but patients with a strong family history of type 2 diabetes should be made aware of some of the steps they can take to help decrease their risk of diabetes. Diabetes is diagnosed when the hemoglobin A1C is greater than 6.4%.

FNP Practice Tests #2 and #3

To take these additional FNP practice tests, visit our bonus page:
mometrix.com/resources719/npfamily-28640

Online Resources

Due to our efforts to try to keep this book to a manageable length, we've created a link that will give you access to all of your online resources:

mometrix.com/resources719/npfamily-28640

It's Your Moment, Let's Celebrate It!

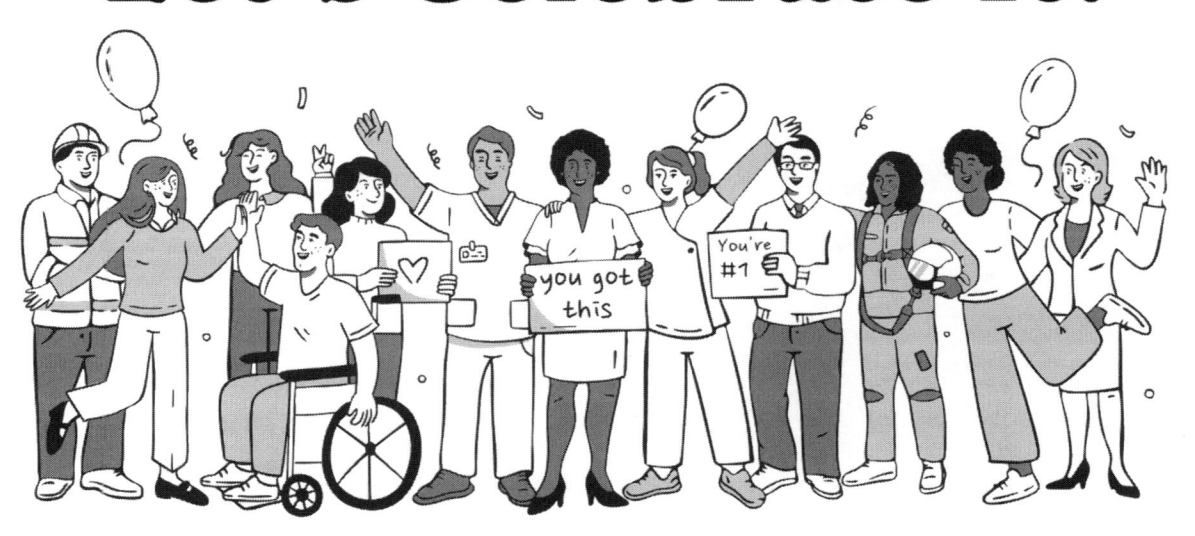

Share your story @mometrixtestpreparation